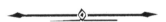

ISBN 978-0-428-95263-1
PIBN 10783312

TRANSACTIONS

—OF THE—

Medical & Chirurgical Faculty

—OF THE—

STATE OF MARYLAND,

—AT ITS—

Semi-Annual Session, Held at Hagerstown, Md., Nov., '89.

Ninety-Second Annual Session

—HELD AT—

BALTIMORE, MARYLAND, APRIL, 1890.

BALTIMORE:
GRIFFIN, CURLEY & Co., PRINTERS,
202 Baltimore St., East,
1890.

Officers, Committees, Sections and Delegates.

FOR THE YEAR 1890-91.

President.
T. A. ASHBY.

Vice-Presidents.
GEORGE H. ROHE,   J. McPHERSON SCOTT.

Recording Secretary.
G. LANE TANEYHILL.

Assistant Secretary,
ROBERT T. WILSON.

Corresponding Secretary.
J. T. SMITH.

Reporting Secretary.
WM. B. CANFIELD.

Treasurer.
W. F. A. KEMP.

Executive Committee.
P. C. WILLIAMS,   S. T. EARLE,   A. FRIEDENWALD,
J. W. CHAMBERS,   R. WINSLOW.

Examining Board of Western Shore.
C. H. JONES,   B. B. BROWNE,   WILMER BRINTON.
J. E. MICHAEL,   L. E. NEALE,   J. D. BLAKE,
J. H. BRANHAM.

Examining Board of Eastern Shore.
B. W. GOLDSBOROUGH,   G. T ATKINSON,   A. H. BAYLEY,
J. K. H. JACOBS,   W. F. HINES.

Library Committee.
I. E. ATKINSON,   T. BARTON BRUNE,   B. B. BROWNE.
WM. H. WELCH,   G. LANE TANEYHILL.

Publication Committee.
G. LANE TANEYHILL,   W. F. A. KEMP,   JOHN G. JAY,
GEO. J. PRESTON,   RANDOLPH WINSLOW.

Memoir Committee.
E. F. CORDELL,   D. W CATHELL,   W. STUMP FORWOOD,
T. B. EVANS,   JOHN R. QUINAN.

Committee on Ethics.
CHAS. H. JONES,   THOMAS S. LATIMER,   JOS. T. SMITH.
CHRISTOPHER JOHNSTON, Sr.,   H. M. WILSON.

Membership Committee.
T. A. ASHBY,   S. T. EARLE,   G. LANE TANEYHILL.
WM. LEE,   G. W. HUMRICKHOUSE,   W. F. HINES,
J. H. BRANHAM.   GEO. H. ROHE,   J. W. CHAMBERS.

Curator.
L. F. ANKRIM.

Section on Surgery.

L. McLANE TIFFANY,   J. W. CHAMBERS,   RANDOLPH WINSLOW,
JOHN McP. SCOTT,   JOHN D. BLAKE.

Section on Practice.

WM. OSLER,   JOS. T. SMITH,   SAMUEL C. CHEW,
DAVID STREETT.   W. F. HINES.

Section on Obstetrics and Gynæcology.

J. E. MICHAEL,   THOMAS OPIE,   W. E. MOSELY,
WM. S. GARDNER,   ROBT. T. WILSON.

Section on Materia Medica and Chemistry.

I. E. ATKINSON,   R. H. P. ELLIS,   J. L. INGLE,
CHAS. G. W. McGILL,   H. M. SALZER.

Section on Sanitary Science.

GEO. H. ROHE,   E. M. HARTWELL,   JACKSON PIPER,
E. G. WATERS,   JOHN NEFF.

Section on Anatomy, Physiology and Pathology.

H. NEWALL MARTIN,   J. H. BRANHAM,   HERBERT HARLAN,
GEO. J. PRESTON,   JOHN C. HEMMETER.

Section on Psychology and Medical Jurisprudence.

RICHARD GUNDRY,   JOHN MORRIS,   WM. LEE,
CHAS. G. HILL,   JOHN S. CONRAD.

Section on Microscopy, Micro-Chemistry, and Spectral Analysis,

WM. T. COUNCILMAN,   C. HAMPSON JONES,   N. G. KEIRLE,
A. K. BOND,   WM. B CANFIELD.

Section on Ophthalmology, Otology and Laryngology.

RUSSELL MURDOCK,   HIRAM WOODS,   J. H. HARTMAN,
J. W. HUMRICKHOUSE,   WM. T. CATHELL.

Delegates to American Medical Association.

I. E. ATKINSON,	B B. BROWNE,	T BARTON BRUNE,
JOHN D. BLAKE,	WILMER BRINTON,	SAMUEL C. CHEW,
E. F. CORDELL,	J. J. CHISOLM,	T. B. EVANS,
SAMUEL T. EARLE,	L. M. EASTMAN,	A FRIEDENWALD,
R. H. GOLDSMITH,	JOHN C. HEMMETER,	CHAS. H. JONES,
C. C. JACOBS,	J. A. KEENE,	W. F. A. KEMP,
T. S. LATIMER,	LEE J. McCOMAS,	R. L. RANDOLPH,
DAVID STREETT,	G. LANE TANEYHILL,	R. H. THOMAS,
E. G. WATERS,	E. R. WALKER,	ARTHUR WILLIAMS
P. C. WILLIAMS,	RANDOLPH WINSLOW,	WHITFIELD WINSEY.
JOHN C. HARRIS.		

Delegates to West Virginia State Medical Society.

L. McLANE TIFFANY,   GEO. H. ROHE,   CHAS. H. OHR,
H. H. BEIDLER,   J H. BRANHAM.

Delegates to Virginia State Medical Society,

I. E. ATKINSON,   THOMAS OPIE,   JAMES G. WILTSHIRE,
JOSEPH E. CLAGGETT,   H. P. C WILSON.

Delegates to North Carolina Medical Society.

GEO. J. PRESTON,   J. E. MICHAEL,   WM. H. NORRIS,
W. C. VAN BIBBER,   JNO. R. WINSLOW.

Delegates to the Tenth International Congress at Berlin.

G. LANE TANEYHILL,   JNO. WHITRIDGE WILLIAMS.

Delegates to the Pharmacopœial Convention of 1891.

E. F. CORDELL,   I. E. ATKINSON,   T. B. BRUNE.

DISCLAIMER. The Medical and Chirurgical Faculty of the State of Maryland, while formally accepting and publishing the reports of the various Sections and Volunteer Papers read at its sessions, *does not hold itself responsible* for the opinions, theories or criticisms therein contained.

To AUTHORS. Contributors to any volume of the TRANSACTIONS are requested to observe the following: 1st, Write on one side of the paper only. 2nd, Write without breaks, *i. e.*, do not begin a new sentence on a new line; when you want to begin a new paragraph, begin in the middle of the line. 3rd, Draw a line along the margin of such paragraphs as should be printed in smaller type—for instance, all that is clinical history in reports of cases, or that which is quoted, &c. 4th, Words to be printed in *italics* should be underscored once; in SMALL CAPITALS twice; in LARGE CAPITALS three times. 5th, Proofs sent for revision should be returned without delay: authors who contemplate a temporary absence from their regular residence any time during the summer, should notify the Recording Secretary, thus avoiding vexatious delays in the delivery of proof. 6th, Authors whose papers have been "accepted" by the Faculty and referred to the Publication Committee—such papers thus becoming the property of the Faculty—are expected to place the original or a verbatim printable copy on desk of the Recording Secretary immediately after the reading of the same. 7th, The Publication Committee is instructed by the Faculty to publish no paper that has been read before a local medical society prior to the publication of the TRANSACTIONS of the Faculty. 8th, Alterations in manuscript should be limited to what is of essential importance, they are equivalent to resetting, and cause additional expense, such changes, if they exceed half a page of printed matter, as also, all wood cuts, photographs and electrotypes are invariably to be paid for by authors.

MEMBERSHIP. Applications for membership in the Medical and Chirurgical Faculty should be addressed to the Recording Secretary, Corresponding Secretary, Treasurer, or Chairman of the Examining Board, and should state name in full, post office address, where graduated in medicine, date of graduation, and by whom recommended. They must be accompanied by the *initiation fee* of five dollars: no membership dues are required for the first current year: a copy of the annual TRANSACTIONS is mailed gratuitously to each member. *Blank applications* for membership will be mailed to any address on application to the Recording Secretary or Treasurer.

CONTENTS.

Semi-Annual Meeting.

The Semi-Annual Session of the Medical and Chirurgical Faculty of Maryland was called to order at Court Hall, Hagerstown, Md., November 12th, at 1.30 P. M., the President, Dr. A. Friedenwald, in the chair, Dr. Wm. B. Canfield, acting Recording Secretary.

Dr. A. S. Mason, Hagerstown, delivered the following—

ADDRESS OF WELCOME.

Mr. President: I am honored by my professional brothers of Hagerstown in being assigned to the agreeable office of expressing to you and your associates a few words of welcome, and to thank you for selecting our town for this meeting.

We have read with interest the announcement made by your committee of arrangements, and we desire to assure you of our full sympathy with its purposes.

You, the president, are the representative of an association, ripe in years and in usefulness, upon whose roster are inscribed the names of gentlemen eminent and honored, running down through a long line, now quite near a century, but Sir, it has remained for its present members to inaugurate this new departure, to widen and extend its usefulness, to come out into the counties of Maryland and offer to your country brothers its influence and its benefits, for this Sir, let me thank you, and in behalf of my brothers of Washington County I extend to you and each of you a most cordial welcome, trusting that this meeting which began here to-day, may end so auspiciously, that you may take courage to go on with your good work.

Dr. A. Friedenwald, in delivering the

PRESIDENT'S ADDRESS

responded very happily to the address of welcome, and in his remarks said: Before all else I desire to give some expression in behalf of the Faculty to the deep appreciation of the warm welcome we have received and the kind words that have been spoken to us in this goodly town. I regret I cannot do this as fittingly as the occasion deserves. I am sure that the cordiality with which we have been met here, will long be remembered by us, and that we all unite in the wish to have the opportunity at our next annual meeting in Baltimore to reciprocate the friendly greeting that has awaited us here.

I shall ask your permission, gentlemen, to refer to a bit of history in the life of this Faculty. Born over 90 years ago in the dawn of our National History it was a credit to the devoted men who stood around its cradle and shaped its future career and destiny. They labored earnestly, and consequently did that good work which makes their memories dear to us to-day. Those were men who did not wait for opportunities but who made them. They stood together to advance medical science and maintain the honor and dignity of their profession. Well as they did their work, and despite the prerogatives they had secured from the State which promised to endow this Faculty with a vigorous life during all time, there came a period when it almost seemed that its usefulness would end shorn of the legal rights with which it has been invested, and which enabled quackery to flourish. This was a great disappointment, and inaugurated a period of discouragement which culminated about the year 1840. This is the time to which I specially desire to call your attention, for some years previous to this time the Faculty had lapsed into a state of lethargy which threatened to become a deep and lasting sleep. This unfortunate condition was due largely to an indifference which took possession of many of its members, many had grown old, and there seemed to be nothing left in the Faculty that was calculated to attract new members. Meetings, it is true, were annually called, and officers were elected and this was about the only manifestation of life that remained. Gradually the membership had diminished, and the library was threatened with decay. About this time a new generation of physicians had entered the ranks of the profession in Baltimore.

They demonstrated by the local Medical Societies which they had organized and the successful career upon which these had entered, that the profession had been strengthened by a goodly number of new recruits of whom good work could be expected in the future. The veterans of the Medical and Chirurgical Faculty of that time, did not fail to recognize this. When they looked upon this band of active, earnest, able and enthusiastic young physicians, who had already done themselves so much credit, new hope revived in them as to the future of their time honored State Society. They met their young brethren in all frankness, and confessed that they were no longer able to bear the burdens of the Faculty alone, and appealed to them for their fellowship. This appeal met with a prompt and warm response, and from that time up to this hour, a period of over nineteen years, the history of the Faculty has been one of uninterrupted prosperity. The transactions which have been regularly published fully testify to the valuable work that has been done at the annual meetings. The library has been made a chief feature in the attractions of the Faculty, embracing not only a very large number of standard medical books, but also a large number of foreign and American journals. The membership has increased from year to year, and so has the number of those who are willing to do work, so that four or five days of the annual meetings hardly suffice for the presentation of the papers that are offered. There is one wish however, that has long been entertained by every one who has felt an interest in the welfare of the Faculty, which has not been sufficiently gratified. The counties of Maryland have not been adequately represented in the membership of this State Society.

There is need for more intimate relations, for a closer bond of fellowship between the medical practitioners residing in the various districts of this State than does now exist. This semi-annual meeting of the Faculty has for its purpose the inauguration of a new era in its history looking to the consummation of this important object. Now is the time, and the Medical and Chirurgical Faculty offers the best opportunity for the realization of this hope. The young men who responded to the call which brought about the renaissance of this Society, nineteen years ago have now in time become its veterans, and they with those who have since joined with them send the profession in all parts of this State their fraternal greetings, and request that every reputable physician whether he resides in hamlet, in town, or in city to enroll himself as a member of this organization.

Dr. Robert W. Johnson, Baltimore, then read a paper entitled

Some Practical Points on Hernia.

Simplicity marks the termini of science—complication the middle ground, but the simplicity of the beginning differs from the simplicity of the end ; the one is the result of ignorance, the latter the product of elimination. The complication of the intervening period is not fortuitous nor unnecessary, but the dictum of the law of development,—the compulsory trying in balances to see what is found wanting.

Surgery as a branch of science has run and is still running this course, but each year brings us nearer the goal, and each knot in advance cancels miles of tacking we had to make. The simplicity of early surgical dressing was akin to that of animals left to their own resources. The use of the saliva, the application of water, the use of earth and grass was, to say the least, better surgery than the application of the manifold, and in most instances, pernicious substances that were vaunted as panaceas as soon as a little knowledge had rendered men dangerous to themselves. The idea of punishing the part at fault by the use of disgusting ointments or pain-giving liniments took possession of men; they attempted to drive out devils and evict entities under the names of diseases.

No chapter in surgery is more replete with complexities than the subject of hernia. From the time it got its false and misguiding name of "rupture," to the near present, it has been the *bete noir* of the medical student and *pons asinorum* of the green room. The descent of the testicle has been studied by teachers and awaited by scholars with anxiety and acrostics as "some Surgeons, in cutting, tremble painfully," have been designed to recall the coverings of this mysterious lesson. Practically, when we come to operate on hernia by taxis or truss, we do not have to recall *all* of Gray; but we substitute the grooved director for our acrostics, and cut as many coverings as come up, without regard to Sharpey and Quain.

I have shown in a former paper, read before this Society, some of the absurd methods and disastrous line of treatment followed out by the tramp herniotomists of the middle ages. Most of you are familiar with the impression left by attempts to learn the radical cure of hernia of a decade ago—well have they been dubbed "Indian Puzzle" operations, for more complicated passages of needles and thread, and in most cases. impotent attempts to block up the inguinal rings, could hardly be devised, and in spite of all the detail enrolled many failures. But antiseptic surgery has lit up this corner of abdominal wall as well as the linea alba, and subcutaneous possibilities are now visible accomplished facts.

The anatomy of hernia is the anatomy of the part on the one hand, a projection of peritoneum enclosing omentum or gut, or both, on the other, and a variable element sometimes accompanying the sac in its escape, whose presence or absence, while satisfactory for diagnosis, has little effect on the practical question of treatment, now that we stand in so little awe of peritonitis. I do not mean by this to undervalue anatomical knowledge, which is always an acquisition and a positive necessity in intelligent treatment of hernia, but to emphasize the fact that a patient should not die of strangulated hernia because his attendant may feel that he is not able to point out the coverings as he goes, provided he can recog· nize the sac when he reaches it.

In regard to diagnosis, the books lay down practical rules, which I shall not rehearse, and some by placing hernial symptoms side by side with conditions which simulate it, bring out the contrast very sharply. There is one condition that occasions perplexity, and that is hydrocele in the negro, when the light test is defeated by the dark pigment of the scrotum. The aspirator or hyperdermic needle throws light on the question and can be used without detriment in either case. Indeed, the withdrawal of the fluid from the sac sometimes lessens it so that it can be reduced without herniotomy and is better outside than in at any rate.

At one time I was in hope that from the sac fluid I might be able to demonstrate a positive indication of its contents whether containing gut or omentum, by simple chemical means only, but unless there has been extravasation of feces, we can not make the distinction with certainty. Bacteriological studies of the transuded fluid conducted by Garre disprove the claims of Nepveau that bacteria were constantly found, without fecal extravasation. (*Fortschritte der Medicin*, B. 10, pp. 486-490.)

There are numerous and confusing divisions of hernia, based on the character of the sac; practically we can consider two the most important ; The acquired, when the peritoneal sac is pushed forward by the errant gut, and the congenital, when the gut enters a preformed sac made by the non-closure of the tubular vaginal process of the peritoneum after the descent of the testicle. The nomenclature based on location is simple, and should be used in the description of a hernia, which, for instance, is only begun to be described by stating that it is inguinal or femoral ; thus it may be clearly brought to the mind of the reader by stating it, for example, as an acquired irreducible indirect scrotal entero-epiplocele. Moreover, it is well to remember in suspicious cases that every aperture of the abdomen can have a hernial protrusion, and each abdominal organ has been found in it. It may

exist when the customary sites are entirely free, or, as in
Littre's hernia, only a portion of the circumference of the
gut be nipped by constriction.   It is generally stated that the
smaller the hernia the more dangerous,—this is not strictly
true, for we may have a large hernia gradually passing
through a small opening, but the smaller the aperture through
which a hernia passes, the more danger of strangulation, is
axiomatic.

The sac may be absent when the hernia forms at the seat
of a wound, and the same holds true when the cæcum or
colon protudes through the inguinal canal (Bryant's *Surgery*,
p. 527.)

It is not my purpose to go into the descriptions and methods
that are so well stated in text-books or to bore you with a
repetition in worse language of the ground that is so thoroughly gone over there.   I want to call your attention to
facts that I have not usually found mentioned, not claiming
them, however, as original with myself, so if you miss the
cardinal points of treatment in the paper do not lay these
omissions to my ignorance but rather to my certainty that
you know them as well, if not better, than I do.

After diagnosing hernia the first thing we do is to try to
reduce it.   One practical point here.   You will often find
that a patient who has been in the habit of reducing his rupture will know more of its peculiarities than the surgeon who
applies taxis on well marked anatomical grounds.   It is safe
to let the owner have a first chance at his own hernia when
there is not much danger of strangulation or weakening of
the walls of the intestine.   A case was reported not long ago
where a patient was about to be operated on, and while on
the table asked for this privilege, which was granted.   He
got his hernia between his thighs, and by crossing them exerted pressure sufficient and in the proper direction to reduce
it.   This is an extreme case, but one may get a hint of value
from observing the patient's methods.   Taxis is usually
thought so innocent that it is indulged in by the ordinary
practitioner immoderately.   It is, in fact, a two edged sword;
the moment it ceases to be beneficial it becomes malignant.
Hard and fast rules cannot be set for its use.   Five, ten, or

fifteen minutes have been allotted as the proper time. Each case is a law unto itself, and you might as well set out to pour medicine down a patient's throat five, ten or fifteen minutes as to regulate your taxis by the hands of the clock. I have seen cases of hernia where taxis was not to be thought of. I have had others where protracted taxis has been beneficial. One thing is certain, however, and that is medical men employ taxis too long in the main. It furthermore wastes valuable time to run the gamut of remedies suggested by text-books until you reach kelotomy. Ice, tobacco injection, etc., are all inferior to an anæsthetic, so that if your simple taxis fails without adjuncts give ether or chloroform and use taxis again ; do not go through a long list of remedies seriatim, following each by taxis. It is not necessary, because you have given a patient ether or chloroform to proceed with kelotomy immediately should taxis fail. If for any reason you think his hernia is irreducible and not strangulated, the anæsthetic is like any other innocent remedy and can be repeated if you want to operate later. In other words, use it early, as it is the most satisfactory and do not feel a moral obligation to cut unless there is a further indication than the readiness of the patient on the table.

Chloroform has the advantage of producing less vomiting after its use. Strangulated hernia *per se* at the outset is not a very dangerous condition. It is made one of the most fatal by the temporizing effect at reduction by men who are not surgeons, and treat on the expectant plan. Conservatism is a great merit, but delay is not conservative in these cases. If I had to place a bound beyond which delay may be said to be criminal, I would say that the appearance of stercoraceous vomiting is the latest signal for kelotomy, but many cases should not be compelled to wait that long for relief, because aseptic surgery has offered salvation without a fraction of the risk run by waiting. Are not exploratory incisions made every day into the peritoneum for chronic slow growing tumors ? Why then need we hesitate to make them in these cases when the patient's life is at the mercy of an hour's temporizing ? In the application of trusses as much care should be taken as in fitting a shoe to a deformity. A misfitting truss is almost worse than none from its false security. Their application should not be left to any ignorant, or perhaps avaricious instrument maker, who has a stock on hand he has found difficulty in disposing of. If you send your patient to the shop see that he returns and lets you examine his purchase and its qualities if you have not time to go with him to be fitted. In some of the great charities for the ruptured they make casts of the patient's body in difficult cases and apply a truss to fit it.

In restraining inguinal hernia of children, especially of babies, when there is difficulty in keeping the stiff instruments in position, I have found great convenience in applying a skein of worsted about the groin in the following manner : Tie a knot in one end of the skein. Apply the knotted end over the hernial opening ; bring the other end round the back over the opposite flank ; draw it through the loop made by the knot ; pass it over the perineum and attach it to the skein above the sacrum. The worsted is not expensive ; it is easily washed ; elastic, soft, adapts itself well to the parts and produces no abrasion, as is likely in the thin skins of· babies. The herniæ of children have a natural tendency to recover, which I do not believe is affected in any markéd degree by the pressure of the pad, except as far as it restrains the protrusion. At least you will find the worsted convenient until a truss can be fitted. A late publication (*Philadelphia Medical News*, October 5, 1889, p. 375,) recommends for umbilical hernia in children the use of "a hard rubber, slightly oval, plano-convex lens, with a greater diameter of 3 cm. and thickness of 6 or 7 mm. On the plain surface are two small wire loops·facing each other at a distance of 2 cm. This is attached to the centre of an adhesive plaster strap 2 cm. wide and long enough to embrace three fourths of the child's body by thrusting the wire loop through the plaster and a small safety pin through the loop. No plaster other than a reliable emplastrum resin, of the pharmacopœia should be used. This may remain three weeks at a time." Picture nail-heads are serviceable and handy. The prophylactics against hernia in the infant are the well adapted compress over the umbilicus, the avoidance of constipation with its consequent straining and an earnest endeavor on the part of the nurse to appease those terrific fits of crying, which for no better reason are put down to the child being mad. In fact, the above rules apply, with modification, to adults, for though most cases of hernia begin on some sudden exertion, a man or woman who feels that there is a weak point in the inguinal or umbilical region should fortify it by a truss before the actual escape of the gut. Some authors speak of the truss as an intolerable encumbrance. Such has not been my experience when they are well fitted. Patients become used to them and find they gird up the loins like a belt.

Therefore it seems to me highly practical and conservative to say to all patients who do not find a truss irksome and whose herniæ are retained comfortably enough by it to let well enough alone, and not to run even the slight risk of operation, which they can postpone until their hernia gives them trouble, unless, like sailors, they may be out of the reach of surgeons and instrument makers for weeks at a time.

There are cases where no truss will retain the gut comfortably and these are cases suitable for the operation for permanent cure.

I heard Mr. Durham, of Guy's Hospital, once say: "When you hear a man say that he treats all his cases of stricture in such a way, all his cases of pustatic diseases in such a way, and all his cases of stone in the bladder in such a way, then you may be sure, that, that man has either had a very small experience, or else that he is a great fool." He might have added the single way operator on hernia to the same list. There is now, however, so marked an agreement among herniotomists that the subcutaneous methods, except, perhaps, Heaton's are unworthy to be compared with the open operations, that I do not think we can go far wrong when we relegate these complicated proceedings to the ancient history of hernia, together with castration and the suture royale, the more so as they were seldom practically useful, post-mortems showing that the invaginated tissue pulled from the outside and pushed from within does not restrain the gut.

On account of the tendency of hernia, if restrained, in children to get well without operation there should be some very positive indication before we do the radical cure on them; an equally imperative demand exists to complete all operations for strangulated hernia with the one for permanent cure, provided the condition of the patient admits of the further proceeding.

I have spoken of the comparative freedom from danger in these operations, but I must amend that statement by adding, under the aseptic plan. Without aseptic precautions the dangers are as great as ever; with half aseptic methods the dangers are probably greater than before, but with a conscientious carrying out of every detail of cleanliness—not apparent nor chemical cleanliness, but surgical cleanliness—the danger is reduced to a minimum, as shown by the result of operations like McBirney's or Macewen's. Under these conditions we have the further advantage of opening the sac and seeing the contents and the state of preservation the strangulated parts are in. Formerly it was the wise operator who, unless certain that the gut and omentum were gangrenous, returned the sac unopened. If in doubt, even the slightest, now, we open the sac and see for ourselves the state of its contents. This advance removes another source of danger; the reduction of the sac with contents constricted by its neck, or as it is called, *en bloc;* that is impossible in an open sac, as in it we reduce the contents before the sac leaves our view.

Should we find the gut and omentum gangrenous and unfit to return after ligating with catgut, in several places, bearing in mind the tendency of bleeding arteries in the abdomen to continue to bleed no matter how small, unless ligated, we cut off the distl end; the gangrenous gut should be opened and after bringing down enough healthy intestine suture it to the sides of the wound. In ordinary cases suturing the intestines at the time of the operation protracts the patient's shock at a time when he can least bear it. That had better be reserved as a subsequent operation, unless his condition is good. In operating we should follow the injunction laid down in trephining the skull and equally applicable here;

consider that the parts to be cut are the thinnest possible, and on no account plunge your knife at random in tissues that may barely conceal bowel. The clinching precaution after operation for permanent cure is to keep the patient in bed for some time after operating, in order that the transposed tissues may become part and parcel of the region to which they are attached before any strain shall be put upon them, and follow this up with the application of a truss if there is the least indication of bulging at the old opening. For minute details I refer you to text-books excusing the old story element in the paper, on the ground that hernia has been a target for all surgeons, and it is difficult to find novelty in a subject so thoroughly discussed.

DISCUSSION.

Dr. J. W. Chambers, Baltimore, said he thought that an important fact had been brought out. Each case should be treated on its own merits. The question of time in taxis was very important. A hernia should be strangulated as short a time as possible. Consent of the patient should be obtained to an operation if taxis fail. The danger is not in the operation but in the condition of the gut found when the doctor is called. Temporizing cannot improve the gut, therefore waiting is uncalled for. Strangulated cases needed the radical operation unless they can be kept up by a truss. It is not easy to know what to do when the gut is gangrenous.

Dr. A. Friedenwald, Baltimore, related the case of an infant with inguinal hernia, in which the application of truss was enjoined. The child did not get the truss, however, and the rupture disappeared spontaneously.

He also reported a case of strangulated inguinal hernia which he reduced, but the symptoms continuing he feared that there was trouble in the returned gut. He called in two surgeons who differed from him, and who thought that these symptoms would subside. The patient died on the eighth day, and upon the post-mortem a small bit of the intestine was found engaged in the internal ring. Dr. Friedenwald made the point that when the symptoms produced by a hernia do not disappear completely after it has been reduced, the parts should be thoroughly explored.

Dr. T. W. Simmons, Hagerstown, said he would like to ask in connection with Dr. Johnson's very interesting and instructive paper which of the different methods for the radical cure of hernia did he advocate, and how far the operation should be regarded as a necessary part of every operation for strangulated hernia. That it did seem after a patient was so far subjected to the opening of the hernial tumor, and its accompanying dangers, the right to close it again without giving him the benefit of some of the approved methods looking to a radical cure, should at least be regarded as an important question, that he thought the tendency was to make the two operations more a unit.

Dr. J. E. Michael, of Baltimore, said that the importance of the subject of Dr. Johnson's paper, and especially the role which was being played in modern surgery by the radical operation, justified a full discussion. He wished especially to commend certain points in the paper. Dr. Johnson's conservative views on the treatment of hernia in children were most excellent. Doubtless there was a marked tendency to recovery and the proper use of conservative means during growth would often result in radical cure. This is especially true with regard to umbilical hernia. He had had experience in two cases among his own children, both of which had resulted in cure. He thought the picture nail-head suggested by Dr. Johnson presented too positive a convexity. The object was to close and not to fill the ring. He had used, with great comfort and success an ordinary large wooden button mould covered with chamois leather. This is fastened to a broad strip of mole-skin plaster and applied to the ring. Another position taken by the reader is especially worthy of support. He says that with regard to taxis and the length of time we should continue to use it each case should be a law unto itself. The circumstances are so different. What would be good surgery with a vigorous patient and recent hernia, would be very bad surgery with a feeble patient where hernia had been strangulated for a long time. He thinks much nonsense had been written and talked about caution and gentleness in taxis. Of course we must be gentle and cautious when circumstances demand it, but some cases demand vigor and persistence and he had reduced by active taxis many cases which under the fifteen or even twenty minute rule would have been doomed to operation. The radical operation had occupied much attention of late. Surgeons everywhere, he thought, were agreed that every kelotomy for strangulation should be followed by such measures for prevention of a return of the rupture as the condition of the parts justified. So thoroughly was he convinced of the safety and benefit of the radical operation, done under proper antiseptic precautions, that he was rather inclined to look upon success in reduction by taxis as a disaster for the patient. He could hardly subscribe to the very conservative views of the reader in regard to the radical operation. He would do it and recommend it in any active adult whose hernia was at all troublesome. For himself he would, if afflicted with hernia, accept radical operation in preference to the annoyance of a truss and the danger of strangulation. He believed it was true conservatism so to do. The doctor then described Bank's, Macewen's and McBirney's operation. His own procedure is like McBirney's, with the exception that he sews up all the tissues from sub-serous connective tissue to subcutaneous in one line of continuous catgut suture and the skin in another line. He is not yet convinced of the utility of allowing the canal to be closed by granulation. The treatment of the sac is the great bone of contention. It is used in many and various ingenious ways to close the canal, but he believes it best treated by removal. It should be opened in order that the surgeon may be sure of what he is doing, dissected clear of the canal throughout its whole extent and ligated off well within the abdominal cavity.

Dr. E. Tracy Bishop, Smithsburg, Md., asked for information as to the prevention of hernia. He believed it possible to prevent it by proper physical training. The tissues involved being modified forms of muscular tissues could be kept in proper condition of resistance by suitable gymnastic or other exercise. He related the history of a case in point where a young man found that he could relieve an inguinal hernia by taking exercise and who recovered entirely by keeping up his exercise throughout the year. The doctor considered congenital hernia to be due to defective muscular condition inherited from the parents. The doctor made the further observation that hernia would rarely be found among the American Indians.

Dr. J. McP. Scott, Hagerstown, expressed the pleasure he had in listening to the very practical address of Dr. Johnson upon one of the most important subjects which could claim the attention of the active practitioner. He must, however, except to the application of any inflexible rule as to the management of the incarcerated gut showing marked evidence of impaired vitality. He had recently had an experience which would hereafter be a lamp and guide. A few months since he was called to a remote portion of the county, late Saturday night, to operate upon a case of hernia, said to have been strangulated since Thursday. It was impossible to make the visit until the next morning, Sunday, and the patient was found with a left inguinal hernia which had come down on the Thursday previous. The history of the case indicated an old hernia and also made it questionable whether, although a truss had been worn, it was completely reducible. Taxis failed to reduce the tumor. Constipation and some vomiting were present. The symptoms, however, calling for operative interference were most urgent. This procedure, however, having been determined upon the operation was done. The sac having been exposed it was necessary to open it to sever the strangulation. Upon opening the sac the gut was found to be very dark and bordering upon gangrene. The bowel was adherent to the sac, and the vitality had been so far affected by the strangulation that the adhesion between the lower portion of the knuckle of bowel and sac had given way; the remainder of the sac and bowel were adherent. They were carefully separated by the handle of the scalpel and the constriction caused by the sac severed up to the peritoneal cavity. This was the condition of the bowel, threatening the patient with the most serious result, and placing upon the attendant the responsibility of adopting a treatment which had not been considered, as the mildness of the symptoms had not suggested damage to the bowel. You gentlemen of the city, surgeons of skill whose word is law with your patients, can hardly appreciate the feeling experienced by the country practitioner under such circumstances. The gut was thoroughly freed from its adhesions, washed with hot boiled water, and allowed to remain. The edges of the wound were brought together, a soft wad of cotton applied and retained by a spica bandage, and the case left to whatever result nature might effect. Subsequent visits showed the tumor had disappeared, which could only be accounted for by the restoration of vitality to the bowel, which free from its adhesions, had slipped by its peristaltic action back into the peritoneal cavity. The incision rapidly healed and the patient made an excellent recovery. As has been stated, every case is a law unto itself, and this case was specially instructive in two particulars: 1st, The gut in a hernial protrusion can be almost gangrenous without urgent indications for an operation by the absence of urgent general symptoms. 2nd, The bowel possesses remarkable recuperative power when free from the strangulation, and stimulated by hot applications, and hence an artificial anus should not be formed so long as the bowel is intact.

Dr. R. W. Johnson, Baltimore, in closing the discussion, could not agree with Dr. Chambers as to the propriety of leaving gangrenous gut in a newly made wound, especially when there was close connection with the peritoneum nor could he go as far as Dr. Michael, who stated that if he had a hernia himself he would have the radical permanent cure attempted, even if it was causing no trouble with a truss. In regard to the cure of hernia by exercise, the writer believed that a well developed muscular abdominal wall would do much to prevent the first appearance of hernia, but after it had once come, he found that abdominal gymnastics would do more harm than good. He heartily seconded the wise course pursued by Dr. Scott in an interesting case he narrated, and would like to emphasize the fact that because all operations are finished in text-books, there are cases where surgeons find it the usual course to ask time to solve questions, even after the early incisions have been made.

Dr. J. Edwin Michael, Baltimore, then read a

REPORT OF A CASE OF DOUBLE POPLITEAL ANEURISM CURED BY LIGATURE.

S. M. Swede, stevedore, æt. 37, entered the Maryland University Hospital Feb. 5, 1889, with the following history : His general health had always been good, and no syphilis or other constitutional disease could be diagnosticated. Two years ago a small swelling had appeared in the right ham. This swelling had gradually increased in size and he had suffered with much pain in the leg. The pain was of a jerking character, worse at night, and interferred very materially with locomotion ; so much so that he had to give up his occupation as stevedore. Four months ago a similar enlargement had appeared on the left ham and had been followed by similar symptoms. Upon examination, the diagnosis of double popliteal aneurism was arrived at without difficulty. Both swellings pulsated, gave a characteristic "bruit" on ausculation and decreased on pressure. Pressure on the femoral artery also caused the cessation of both pulsation and "bruit" in the tumors.

It having been found that flexion of the knee did not control the pulsation, it was determined to treat the case by the use of the antiseptic animal ligature. It was also thought wise not to operate on both arteries at the same time, on account of possible disturbance of the circulation.

On Feb. 10, the part having been prepared by scouring with soap, and the application for some hours of cloths wet with solution of bichloride of mercury (1-1000,) the patient was etherized, and the left superficial femoral artery ligated in the apex of Scarpa's triangle. The operation was easy, simple and almost bloodless. Carbolized cat-gut ligature was used, the ends being cut short.

Upon application of the ligature, pulsation ceased in the aneurism. The wound was dressed with sublimate gauze. No reaction followed the operation, and when the first dressing of the wound on Feb. 25th, was removed, healing was found to be complete, the size of the tumor having notably decreased in the meantime.

On March 14th, the same operation was done on the right side, the procedure being in all respects the same except that a small superficial vein was cut, and required clamping. Dressing as before. Wound healed under a single dressing, as before. With decrease of the aneurismal tumors, the patient improved in locomotion, and in a few weeks walked out of the hospital well and happy.

On April 11th, not quite a month after the last operation, the patient walked into the hospital to show himself. The tumors were very much reduced in size, he could walk without difficulty, felt well and looked well.

The report of the case is short and simple, but I think sufficiently interesting to justify presentation. It illustrates the well-known tendency of aneurisms to occur in persons who follow an especially laborious vocation, as well as the tendency to be multiple, and is interesting as bearing on the safety of operations which were formerly considered grave, when they are done under the protection of antisepsis.

Dr. William Lee, Baltimore, then read a paper entitled

Rachitis Considered in Regard to some of its Symptoms.

At the meeting of the American Medical Association, at Richmond, in 1882, I read a short paper on rickets, and made the assertion that there was a greater prevalence of this disease in the United States than the meagre literature on the subject would have us to suppose. With the exception of the late John S. Parry, of Philadelphia, and Dr. Jacobi, of New York, all who had treated on the subject had done so very unsatisfactorily.

I am glad to say much has been done since to infuse further interest, and of the many valuable articles on rickets that of Drs. Barlow and Bury (to be found in the *Cyclopædia of Diseases of Children*, compiled by Dr. John S. Keating,) shows the most careful study and research. One of the most important of the many reasons why this disease should be carefully considered is that after infantile paralysis, no disease contributes more frequently to the production of spinal curvatures and other orthopædic troubles.

Rickets is peculiarly a disease of infancy and childhood, affecting the entire body, and most often seen in those children having hereditary tendency to other diseases. Its early manifestations are, as a rule, overlooked, being usually attributed to more trivial constitutional derangements. It has as characteristic a general impairment of nutrition, which is followed by a special form of debility and peculiar bone lesions.

Etiology.—Rickets is caused by improper alimentation, by which is meant other food than mother's milk or properly prepared cow's milk, during the first months of infancy; irregular or too frequent nursing, or when the child is nursed naturally, the mother is debilitated, improperly nourished, or overworked, thus rendering her milk unfit for the off-spring. Again forcing upon the child at too early an age food which it cannot digest, such as meat, bread-pap or other farinaceous preparations ; or erring on the other side, by unduly prolonged lactation. All of these assist in setting up gastro-intestinal derangements and subsequent malnutrition, which is the ground-work of the disease under discussion. Then too, early marriages, intermarriages, or any excesses of the parents, may further rickets in the child. This disease is found most frequently among the poor, living in crowded tenement houses, or narrow, dirty courts, where the ventilation is bad and the air impure.

After carefully reviewing the various theories as to how rickets is produced, we find strong evidence pointing to that of acid fermentation, its excessive formation in the stomach being assigned as the mode by which the phenomena of the disease is produced. It has been supposed that a superabundance of acid thus finding its way into the blood, facilitates the removal of the earthy salts from the bones, and it is fully proven that in rickets as in most other constitutional diseases an over amount of free acid is constantly generated in the primæ viæ. The particular acid is the subject of various statements. Oxalic acid (Beneke, Inre, Schmidt, phosphoric acid (Weatherhead,) and lactic acid, by Heitzmann, have each in their turn been decided the special agent in bringing about the characteristic lesions of rickets. Of these, I think

that offered by Heitzmann most plausible. He asserts that
lactic acid exercises an irritating influence upon the osteo-
plastic tissue, and that it is this influence, combined with a deficiency of lime salts, which produces the disease.

There is little doubt that lactic acid is abundantly generated in the deranged digestive organs of rickety children, for
this acid has been detected in the urine, and it dissolves and
helps to eliminate the calcareous matter deposited in the
bone.

Much has been said to show that rickets is the outcome of
scrofula and syphilis ; but as yet we have no positive data
upon the subject, other than that the disease is intensified
where there is evidence of such hereditary diathesis.

Syphilis may of itself, however, produce symptoms which
simulate those of rickets, but the two diseases are separate
and distinct. Syphilis runs a more definite course and is
most often seen in the first offspring of syphilitic parents, notwithstanding the influence of anti-syphilitic remedies. It is
never initiated during convalescence from acute attacks ;
such as of the exanthemata or broncho-pneumonia. On the
other hand, rickets is constantly met with where most vigi-
lant inquiries and examinations fail to discover any history
of a veneral taint. Its symptoms are more general, and
there is a peculiar tendency to nervous disorders of functional
character ; it more frequently shows itself in the later children than in the first-born, and it is frequently ushered in after
an attack of broncho-pneumonia or one of the exanthemata.

Symptoms.—Indigestion, chronic dyspepsia, pasty looking
stools, diarrhœa, alternated with constipation, sleeplessness,
general tendency to sweating, day and night, especially of
the head; fretfulness upon the least exertion, progressive
emaciation, catching cold upon the lightest exposure, tendency to pulmonary catarrh, delayed detention, such teeth as
have appeared decay easily, quickly blacken and easily break
off. Lymphatic glands and spleen altered and swollen, general uneasiness, great irritability of temper, with disposition
to be left unmolested, crying and fretting from pain when
moved or carried in the arms of the nurse. The anterior
fontanelle, which is generally completely ossified by the

twelfth month, remains open, in rachitic cases, until about third year ; the sutures are also somewhat open, with their edge soft and yielding ; also in many instances both posterior fontanelles are quite membranous. From sleeping constantly on the back and rubbing its head against the pillow, the hair becomes decidedly thin at the back of the child's head. Across the forehead a well marked glazed line may be noticed, caused by the child sitting, during the day, with its hands supporting its head or resting it against the side of a chair when left alone. It assumes this position to relieve the chest of the weight of the head and at the same time assist chest expansion.

Alterations of the Bones, etc.—Unless the case be a mild one, when the only evidence is slight enlargement of the ankles and wrists, the most frequent alteration is that which is known as cranio-tabes. This unique symptom, the earliest and most constant feature in rachitis requires some care and diligent search to be found ; but by pursuing the plan adopted by Elsasser and Jacobi the difficulty will be overcome. Place yourself immediately before the child, put the heel of your hand upon either temple, carefully examine the upper portion of the occiput and posterior portion of the parietal bones with the fingers perpendicular to their surface. As this process is accomplished we find the occiput and parietes will feel soft on pressure of the fingers and spots of thinning detected over the bones. They are supposed to be caused by absorption of the imperfect ossified bone from its pressure between the pillow and brain as the child lies upon his cot. They are detectable as early as the fourth month and as late as the twelfth, and about the size of a grain of corn. When the head is decidedly affected it becomes elongated and flattened, the occiput projects and the frontal bosse is prominent ; the face is small looking and by contrast the head appears very large. We have further as an early symptom thickening of the clavicle with its ends enlarged.

Enlargement of the Joints.—If the general ill health is protracted we find very important changes noticeable in the bones of the upper and lower limbs. The epiphyses of the radius and ulna, especially the former, present a more or less striking thickening and broadening, so that in severe cases, especially in emaciated children, the hand appears as if separated from the arm by a groove, so with the tibia, the epiphysis of which, like that of the fibula, will be very much thickened. Following next in order is the characteristic bowing, bending and twisting of the bones of the upper and lower extremities, the former being very much increased if the child is allowed to crawl, the weight of the body then is thrown upon the wrists, and the latter by being permitted to stand up too frequently.

Chest Deformities.—This is never well marked in children before sixteen months, and even then by no means common.

Curvature of the Spine.—As stated before, apart from infantile paralysis, this is frequently produced by rickets.

Bending of the Ribs—(Rickety Rosary.)—Detected most often along the fifth, sixth and seventh ribs, and they also are the first to become unnaturally bowed or curved. The enlarged surfaces on the ribs are usually at their junction with the sternum which, projecting forward, gives rise to pectus carinatum—(chicken-breasted.)

The bones of the pelvis are early affected. When so there is usually a projecting of the sacrum and a depression of the acetabula from the weight of the trunk.

During the progress of the bone lesions there is a great tendency in this disease to involutions and we find as it commences in one region it subsides in another. This is especially observable in the cranial lesions where the bony changes, as a rule, run their full course before any other portion of the skeleton is involved.

With regard to the nervous element of rickets, laryngismus stridulus and convulsions stand out most prominently, but they do not appear as early symptoms, rarely before eight months, are of reflex origin and last but a short time.

Prognosis.—If the disease is recognized and treated early its prognosis should be favorable, except when complicated with some other disease, as laryngismus stridulus, bronchitis or broncho-pneumonia (the elasticity of the thoracic wall being lost, the lungs can neither receive nor expel a normal amount of air.)

Treatment.—We are unable to furnish a scientific basis for the treatment of rickets. The best plan, however, to pursue is to treat it as a general disease. Our aim, therefore should first be directed to the digestive organs, assist healthy action of the skin, and enjoin the strictest nursery hygiene.

If the mother is unable to nourish her child or provide a wet nurse, artificial food must then be resorted to, cow's milk being the best. In its preparation I always advise the use of saccharated liquor calcis instead of lime water, the latter containing but a limited quantity of lime and otherwise inferior for neutralizing the acid cow's milk and assisting its assimilation.

The manner of preparing and giving artificial food to infants is very important, particularly in the treatment of rickets, but neither time or place permits its further discussion. So far no specifics have been discovered for the disease, but great benefit is derived from the judicious use of cod liver oil, phosphorus and some of the preparations of iron, as citrate of iron and ammonia (or simple steel wine.) One agreeable way of giving cod liver oil is in combination with some of the maltine preparations which not only destroy the oily taste but very materially assist its proper digestion.

A good plan, and one which saves the child's stomach for its regular food, is to give the oil by inunction about twice a day. As soon as bone lesions are detected care should be taken to maintain the child in a horizontal position in order to support the back and limbs.

For obviating as much as possible the characteristic deformities, especially of the lower extremities, mild forms of support are not inappropriate, such as plaster of paris splints, which should be applied loosely and made to extend the entire length of the limb so as to furnish complete support and immovability.

DISCUSSION.

Dr. William B. Canfield, Baltimore, said that while Dr. Lee had only mentioned phosphorus as a mode of treatment, he had dwelt considerably on cod liver oil inunction, also he had mentioned other remedies. He thought it was strange that, while phosphorus had been so highly recommended by Cassowitz of Vienna,and others and the statistics had been so favorable to its use there, so little notice had been taken of it in this country.

Dr. V. M. Reichard, Fair Play, said he was very much interested in the reading of Dr. Lee's paper, as he had been so unfortunate as to have met with quite a considerable number of cases of *rachitis* in the last eight years. He would like to ask Dr. Lee, if, in his study of the disease, he had found it more frequent, proportionately in the negro than in the white race. The speaker had been struck, in his own practice, by the frequency with which the disease was encountered in negroes. A family would have the first of three or four children perfectly healthy and then every succeeding child would be rachitic. He would like to know if his experience was unique in this direction of if the observations of Dr. Lee were similar. Special stress should be laid on the part played by wasting diseases in the causation of the rickets. Any severe wasting malady, especially in young children, was liable to bring on this complication. His attention was painfully drawn to the truth of this in the last few months in observing the case of his own baby. At the age of five months the child was exceptionally hardy and robust. Suture lines apparently solid and anterior fontanelle almost shut. The posterior had been almost completely ossified at the birth of the child. At the age above mentioned the child fell into a severe ileo-colitis, which in six weeks reduced him to the most extreme degree of emaciation, and at this time, to his (the doctor's) horror he found the anterior fontanelle widely gaping, the sutures opened so as to permit full motion of the cranial bones and the posterior fontanelle much larger than it had been at any time in the child's extra-uterine life.

Arrest of the bowel trouble, with subsequent rapid fattening of the child, removed all anxiety.

The two most striking symptoms, and ones which roughly are diagnostic when present, he thought, are delayed dentition and a widely open fontanelle. He would make it a rule to regard all those cases as dangerous in which at the age of one year the child is not regularly cutting teeth and the anterior fontanelle is not either closed or rapidly closing.

There are of course, two indications in treatment : stop the disease and remove the effects. He knows of nothing more satisfactory than a good compound syrup of hypophosphites. He has given lacto-phosphate of lime, and cod liver oil ad nauseam—the latter by mouth and by inunction—and they always left the patient in worse condition than he was when their administration was begun. He now gives only the syrup hypophos. comp. This relieves the gastro-intestinal disorder which, as Dr. Lee has correctly pointed out, lies at the root of the disease, and at the same time supplies to the softened bones the earthy matter which they so much need.

The disease having been checked, there remains the resulting deformity to be relieved. The speaker could not at all say what he would do if he were in a city where deformed rachitics were in the most unsanitary surroundings. There he might perhaps find it necessary to have some operation performed for the correction of the deformity ; but here in Washington county, surrounded as they are by fine healthful air, he has never seen a case of deformity following rickets which nature could not cure more pleasantly than the surgeon, even if not so rapidly. When first observing these cases, he did not see how they could possibly become straight; but as year after year has passed, he now knows that with proper sanitary surroundings a child will grow out of the most exaggerated deformity. He had in his mind at that time the case of a negro boy, whose deformity was such as very seriously to interfere with his locomotion. His knees rubbed together to such extent as to form bursæ. He was completely wing-footed, so that he walked on his internal malleoli. He was, in short, the most crooked specimen of humanity that could well be imagined. Now, at the age of seven years, he is becoming really straight. And the speaker thought that in course of a few years yet, there might perhaps be left no trace of his disease, except, perhaps, a lump on the back.

Hard and fast rules could not be laid down, but he would not, as a rule, advise operation under five years from the cessation of the disease, and not at all if the deformity were gradually improving.

Dr. William B. Canfield, Baltimore, then read a paper entitled

THE EARLY DETECTION OF PULMONARY CONSUMPTION, WITH MICROSCOPICAL DEMONSTRATION OF THE BACILLUS, AS STAINED BY THE QUICK METHOD.

The relation of rare cases, the presentation of unusual specimens, and the reading of deep papers, make up the usual programme of our medical societies. Still we should not forget that in the absence of anything new under our present luminary, old subjects may often with advantage be renewed, typical cases and specimens may be exhibited, and indeed facts must be repeated and repeated until their importance becomes impressed upon each one of us. It is this reason that has induced me to take up the old theme of the early detection of pulmonary consumption. There can be no doubt in any one's mind but that prevention is better than cure. Unfortunately, in pulmonary consumption the physician is generally called in too late even to hope to effect a cure. Up to within a few years ago, consumption when detected was considered absolutely hopeless, and the physician's only duty was to try to alleviate the accompanying suffering and produce a painless euthanasia. This plan of treatment was followed because the disease was recognized at too late a stage. Although the judicious use of auscultation and percussion, and in fact, of what is called physical diagnosis in general, had done much toward mapping out with comparative accuracy, the locality and extent of the lung lesion, still even before this method was used, the keen observer by other signs and symptoms often suspected the fatal disease at a time when the most skilful diagnostician could have found no physical signs of it.

Now that the newer department of medicine, bacteriology, which too many consider unpractical and as belonging to the pathological laboratory, has given us a more certain evidence of the early approach of consumption, we need rarely be in doubt. Ever since the discovery of the bacillus tuberculosis by Koch, few or probably now no important observers will deny its causative relation to tuberculosis in general and pulmonary consumption in particular. The discovery by Koch has given us one solid fact. If we find the tubercle bacillus in the sputa, consumption is present, and if after a sufficient number of examinations the bacillus is not found, then there is, generally speaking, no consumption. I was in Vienna at the time that Koch's discovery was announced, and noticed there how at first it was received with incredulity by Nothnagel, Bamberger and others, and how they all gradually came over to Koch's opinion; and again and again have I seen the statement, no bacillus, no consumption, and where there is a bacillus there is consumption, proved in the wards of the General Hospital at Vienna, and in the Charite at Berlin. This ocular demonstration and positive proof was much more convincing to me than if I had simply read these statements in the various journals and in text books. In every case examined in the wards in the foreign hospitals, clinical and microscopical examinations are made of the secretion and excretion of each patient in the little laboratory attached to each ward, just as it is done at the Johns Hopkins Hospital. Thus it was that in a great many cases where little history and absolutely no physical signs could be found that the microscope showed the presence or absence of bacilli, and thus rendered the diagnosis certain.

In the large number of cases under my care in the Chest Department of the University Dispensary, Baltimore, and of some in private practice, I have had frequently cases presenting a history of obstinate continued tickling cough, hoarseness, fever, emaciation, but with no marked physical signs. In such cases I always examine a specimen of the morning sputa and I have often had the satisfaction of early detecting the bacilli. Although such an observer as von Ziemssen may say that tuberculosis of the larynx is always secondary to that disease of the lungs, still we know that the larynx often gives the first cause of complaint, and through this the disease has been detected when there were absolutely no physical signs in the lungs.* In most of my cases, even after the early diagnosis, the fatal result could not be averted, but in some, quick action has succeeded in staying the progress of the wasting, and a cessation of the symptoms. Of the poorer class at the dispensary, I sent a selected number to a small private hospital which I attend, and several times I have been rewarded by seeing great improvement, and in more than one case stopping the disease. In several cases detected very early by the presence of bacilli, the climatic cure was insisted upon at once, and, as you all know, this is the cure giving the most hope of success. 'The great trouble was that in young people, and especially men, as I noticed in one case, the desire to go on with their work has cut short the climatic treatment and started up the disease afresh. One case which I had last year was almost well, but a return to business renewed all the old symptoms, and before he could sufficiently rally he died. In another case, which went so far as to have breaking down of the right lung with a cavity, this cavity is now so small that it can only be found with great care.

In-examining sputa the two most important abnormal ingredients are elastic tissue and tubercle bacilli. The latter alone are pathognomonic of pulmonary consumption ; the former may be present in any breaking down of the lung whether tubercular or not. There has been an attempt made to measure the severity of the case by the number of bacilli found. This is not always practical, as many bad cases show few bacilli and light cases expectorate sputa laden with bacilli. What I claim then, from my own experience only, and it is nothing original, is that the microscopical examination of the sputa for tubercle bacilli is so easy, and in doubtful cases so important, that no physician should fail to undertake it or have it done for him for the sake of the patient. The early detection of such cases as apparently

---

*Since writing the above, a case which had been examined by several physicians and pronounced nervous cough, came into my hands. Auscultation and percussion yielded negative results, but the first examination of the sputa revealed bacilli in abundance.

begin in the larynx, or have sufficient cough, emaciation and fever to cast suspicion on the lungs, will enable the patient to be sent to a proper climate before it is too late, and from this treatment there is much to be expected as we all know by experience.

A few words about the technique will close this subject. The method of looking for these bacilli is soon learned after a little practice by one already familiar with the use of the microscope. Others may not find it so easy, and there may be danger of drawing too hasty conclusions by those not versed in these matters. To examine the sputa for tubercle bacilli, the patient is requested to bring a specimen coughed up in the morning when it is free from food on waking up. I generally have it expectorated into a wide-mouth bottle, and then tightly corked. This is labeled at once and may be examined at once which is best, or may be delayed several days without much harm. The bottle is tipped up on the side and a bit of those yellowish or opaque masses is spread out on a clean cover glass with a sterilized platinum needle, or is taken up with sterilized forceps and put in the centre of a clean cover glass upon which a second cover glass is pressed, and then the two are drawn apart and allowed to dry. They are then passed through the alcohol or Bunsen flame to coagulate the albuminous substance and fix the layer on the glass. Good microscopists, with the aid of strong lenses and strong light may have detected the bacilli unstained, but such a procedure is uncertain and time wasting. The principle of rendering the bacilli visible by staining them has been clearly enunciated by Koch and modified, *but not improved*, by a host of followers. This principle of all is about the same, namely, to overstain the specimen and then decolorize, experience having shown that the bacilli retain their color better than the cells and other matter. The stains most commonly used are fuchsine or magenta, properly called hydrochlorate of rosaniline, and methyl-violet or gentian-violet. The coloring fluid which I find most convenient and durable is made up of

Fuchsine (by weight) . . . . . 1 part.
Absolute alcohol . . . . 10 parts.
Solution carbolic acid (5 per cent.) . . . 100 "

This keeps better and longer than the ordinary aniline solutions, which should be prepared fresh for every examina - tion. The cover glass, with sputa side downwards, may be floated on the staining solution in a watch glass which is held on a wire gauze over the flame to hasten the coloring, or a few drops of the stain may be dropped on the cover glass, which is then cautiously held over the flame high above it until bubbles break on the surface ; the glass is then dipped into diluted nitric acid (one to three or four,) until slightly decolorized, then directly into water, to stop the de- colorizing process, or some prefer to pass it from the acid into alcohol. For immediate examination it is laid on a slide, the excess of liquid taken up by blotting paper and examined. An immersion lens is generally used to find these bacilli, but good dry lenses are made of sufficient strength and definition, such as the one I here show you, made by Queen, of Philadelphia. Indeed, the bacilli may be recognized with 350 diameters, although it is not desirable to use less than 500. The method of staining and double staining other than these I shall not mention, and will only add, in conclusion, that I shall be pleased after the session, to demonstrate to any of the members the method de- scribed here.

Dr. Joseph T. Smith, Baltimore, then read a paper on

Typhoid Fever. Its Prevention and Treatment.

"Typhoid fever is essentially a disease of continued type * * * it is in all respects a disease of a very formidable nature, producing lesions which profoundly impair vital or- gans, inducing organic changes of a permanent kind and implicating life, either immediately or remotely in a large number of cases. It may kill in the acute stage by the force of the fever exhausting the system, by perforation of the peritoneum and its consequences, by sphacelus of the intes- tine itself, by hæmorrhage, wasting and protracted diarrhœa, or, finally, by its extraordinary power of calling into play certain dyscrasiæ previously dormant in the system."

This is the disease we have thought advisable to bring to your attention this afternoon; we have endeavored to condense the subject as much as possible, to keep within the required limits, as to time.

Surely such a diseased condition should be continually kept before us; like phthisis and pneumonia, it has always received a large share of attention, and should continue to do so until its ravages are much less destructive to human life, than is the case at present.

In the city of Baltimore, during the past ten years (1879-1888, inclusive,) the deaths from typhoid fever numbered 1,623, an average of over 160 year; a small death rate, it is true, for a city of 400,000, but one which can be still further reduced. Our efficient Health Commissioner, Dr. Steuart, in his last report to the Mayor and City Council, says, "The reduction of the annual mortality from zymotic or preventable diseases in this city, since the enforcement of the 'Plumbing Ordinance,' Jan. 1, 1884, has been very remarkable—the percentage of deaths from zymotic diseases to the total mortality from all causes, during a period of 48 years (1836-1883, inclusive,) was 28.08, diminished during the past 5 years (1884-1888, inclusive,) to 22 per cent. * * * During a period of 24 years (1860-1883, inclusive,) the deaths (from typhoid fever,) averaging 190 annually, were reduced during the past five years to an average of 165." Such a condition of things in this city shows the gain that has accrued to us from the constant agitation and discussion of diseased conditions and their causes, in that way has the public conscience been aroused and their desire for better things stimulated. We have our reward in seeing such palpable fruits of the labor bestowed; as the report above quoted says, "This may well be claimed as a triumph in sanitation, demonstrating the value of good laws, diligently and strictly enforced."

Typhoid fever comes to us as a unique disease in many of its aspects, and we had intended to pass it in review, but the task would be too great for your time and patience; we have therefore noted but two points: its prevention and treatment.

We have fallen upon an era of preventive medicine; we are called upon not so much to put out the fire already kindled, but to take care that no sparks shall get near the combustible material. We point with just pride to the almost total extinction of small-pox by means of the preventive treatment; as with small-pox, so with typhoid fever—it should not exist. We heartily endorse what a recent writer has said; "Nothing is more disgraceful to the civilization of the 19th century than the existence of typhoid fever." "Obsta principiis" is the motto with which we should go forth to meet this disease. We do not need to go heavily armed; a few simple weapons well handled will give us the victory.

We find in typhoid fever a disease well suited to the attacks of preventive medicine. We are taught to believe that the disease is due to the presence of an infecting micro-organism, the typhoid bacillus, that it finds a lodgment in the intestinal canal, thus contaminating the stools, and that we have ample means at our command for its complete destruction; still further we know full well in what way it gains access to the intestinal tract. While the germs may be taken up from the atmosphere, while they may be ingested with milk and meat, water is the chief source from which the human family obtain their supply of typhoid fever germs. Instances innumerable are to be found in proof of this, but in this assembly to narrate them would be a waste of time; but I cannot refrain from noting one, as it comes so near home; the report noted above speaks of it thus : "In one instance, in the village of Woodberry, there were 15 cases of typhoid fever surrounding the locality of one pump, from which these people all derived water for cooking and drinking. The city water department was fortunately able to supply them with hydrant water, and not another case occurred after this supply was procured."

The prevalence of typhoid fever, then, can be largely prevented by keeping the water supply pure, and few diseases show the healthful influence of sanitary measures wisely carried out, as does this. The result speedily shows itself, and were no germs allowed to gain access to the water used for domestic purposes, or that used by the cattle of the fields, it takes no prophet to say that in a very short time typhoid fever would be as rare as small-pox.

The question of the hour, then, is how shall the typhoid bacillus be kept from our water supply? In the city of Baltimore much success, as we have seen, has attended the answer to the question as given in the "Plumbing Ordinance," enforced and carried out by the health commissioner. A plumber of large business in the city told me, a few days ago, that the health department held them very rigidly to the ordinance. Where new plumbing is done or the old to any extent repaired, the pipes can be so secured that no possible point of communication can exist between the cess-pool and the drinking water, thus in the cities we can measurably well be protected, as the water is brought to us from a distance in pipes, whereas elsewhere the cess-pool drains more or less directly into the main water supply. If the plumbing in every house in the city could be each year thoroughly examined, doubtless our death rate from typhoid fever would soon be a very insignificant factor in the year's mortality, but as this is impossible, leaks will sooner or later show themselves and contamination result.

While, then, a vast amount of good has been accomplished by a strict supervision of the plumbing, still, from the vast extent of the work required, it is hardly possible that it alone can lead us to a total extinction of the disease.

Outside of the cities, for reasons obvious to all of you, the problem is still more difficult of solution, and to keep the contents of the cess-pool from draining into the water-well is a matter very difficult to accomplish.

We have thus far gone upon the supposition that the cess-pool must of necessity contain the bacillus, but why need the micro-organism get into the cess-pool? Is it not easier to kill him than to let him live, and to try and control his movements? Instead, therefore, of undertaking the difficult task of controlling the movements of the germ, let us kill him as soon as he leaves the body of our patients. The evidence we have all goes to show that heat, carbolic acid, corrosive sublimate, etc., will readily destroy the bacillus; it is a germ easily destroyed, and by means which can be used in safety by any one; again, the germ is accessible.

If we have learned anything in regard to phthisis it is that a complete destruction of the bacillus after it leaves the body of our patients, would soon markedly reduce the mortality from that disease, but this seems a task impossible to accomplish, as the phthisical go freely about and their saliva is disposed of to suit their convenience, so that we get but a limited control in order to disinfect it. With typhoid fever all is different; we have our patients, as a rule, under control; the germ is thrown off in the stools; these can easily be watched and the contents of the intestines can at once be discharged into a disinfecting fluid. With the light at present thrown upon the subject, it seems as if this were a method capable of eradicating the disease. The dejecta should at once be discharged into a disinfecting fluid, the hands of the nurse immediately upon leaving the patient be disinfected, and anything in contact with the stools should also be at once disinfected. No one should be allowed to come in contact with the patient except the doctor and nurse. We, as physicians, may be trusted to do our duty in this matter, but it is needful that the public should be still further enlightened, and by the constant agitation of the subject made to feel its vital importance.

The evidence, we think, all goes to show that were a thorough system of disinfection carried out in each case of typhoid fever, it would no longer be able to spread its baneful influence. This is especially needful in towns and the rural districts. In our cities a combined system of thorough disinfection and careful sanitary inspection would soon we believe, made the disease rank very low, if not altogether banish it from the mortality list. We have purposely refrained from illustrating our subject or quoting from sanitary authorities, but have endeavored to present you with a few practical conclusions drawn from them.

Bartlett, in his *Fevers of the United States*, edition 1852, says of the treatment of typhoid fever, "There are few diseases of equal frequency and importance, the treatment of which is more unsettled, than that of typhoid fever, and there is certainly no disease the therapeutics of which has within the last few years, attracted more attention than this;" and this is true, in great part, of to-day, except that our methods are more uniform, a decided sign of progress. We have mostly come to endorse the opinion of Dr. Nathan Smith, as noted by Bartlett, in the book referred to, under the various methods of treatment then in vogue. He (Dr. Smith,) says "That he has never seen a single case in which he was satisfied that he had been able to cut short and arrest its progress; and that in all cases where the disease is going on regularly in its course, without any symptoms denoting danger and without any local distress, active interference will likely do more harm than good. Under such circumstances no medicine should be given." We need no better picture of the present method of treatment. The disease resists all our attempts at curative medication, and drugs hold but a poor place in our armory. Opium for rest and alcohol for its power of rousing the heart to increased activity being most frequently called upon.

The one prominent symptom which at this day is exciting much attention, as it always has, is the fever. What shall we do about the elevation of temperature? In regard to its danger, Prof. Welch seems to have answered it for us in his Cartwright Lectures, 1888, where he says: "We found that animals may be kept at high febrile temperature for at least three weeks without manifesting any serious symptoms * * * the conclusion seems justified that failure of the heart's power in fever is less an effect of high temperature than of other concomitant causes;" and again, "What is the significance of fever? Is a question which thrusts itself upon us no less than it has upon physicians of all ages. Unfortunately, we cannot to-day, any more than could our predecessors, give other than a speculative answer to this question.

There have been, in all ages, enlightened physicians who have held the opinion that fever is a process which aids in the elimination or destruction of injurious substances which gain access to the body. Under the influence of ideas which

sought in increased temperature, the origin of the grave symptoms of fever, we have in recent times in great part, lost
sight of the doctrine, once prevalent, that there may be in
fever, a conservative element. * * * The real enemy in
most fevers is the noxious substance which invades the body,
and there is nothing to prevent us from believing that fever
is a weapon employed by nature to combat the assaults of
the enemy. * * * It is impossible, with our present
knowledge, to say exactly in what way fever accomplishes a
useful purpose. * * * The supposition seems to me more
probable that the increased oxidation of fever aids in the destruction of injurious substances. According to this view, the
fever producing agents light the fire which consumes them. It
is not incompatible with this conception of fever to suppose
that the fire may prove injurious also to the patient."

We must, then, ever bear in mind these two points, when
at the bed-side of our fever-sick patients : that even high
febrile temperatures can be borne without giving rise to serious symptoms, and that in so far as we can know, the febrile
condition may be one of protection, and it is, to say the least,
remarkable how strenuously all our attempts to keep the
temperature within normal limits have been resisted. Let
the fire burn, but keep a hand on the draught, call upon
quinine, antipyrine, etc., if need be, to regulate, not extinguish the flame. The treatment by *cold baths* in the systematic and strict method brought to our attention by Brand,
Liebermeister and others, from all the evidence, is worthy
of the most careful consideration ; the good it does is not by
a simple reduction of the temperature—we are to use this as
a guide only. The remedial agent acts most beneficially by
its power of rousing to increased activity the dormant energies of the toxically depressed nervous system ; in this way,
all the bodily functions are energized, and go to work with
more vigor to throw off the toxic agent or resist the poisoning influence. The fact that many are timid in the use of the
bath, the necessity of keeping strictly to the rules laid down,
the number of baths required daily, in many cases, the force
of strong men to lift the sick one to and from the water, the
need of an intelligent director as to when and how long the

bath is to be employed, and the popular prejudice will doubt-less keep it from being much resorted to in private practice ; in hospital practice, where these conditions do not prevail, its record for good entitled the cold bath to be looked upon with favor as a means for overcoming the evil influences at work to destroy our patients.

Nourishment in as large an amount as the patient can digest, and fresh air in abundance are points noted by us all. That the air may not be contaminated, and have free egress and ingress, and as a prevention against infection, the sick room should be without carpet, the floor frequently cleaned, all hangings kept from the doors and windows, plain furni-ture, and but little of it, nothing allowed in the room except what is absolutely necessary, and disinfection thoroughly carried out.

We thus hope that preventive medicine, in the future, will be able to control more effectually than she does to-day the spread of typhoid fever, and that a successful method of treatment will be as little sought for, as in the cases of small-pox. We do not think this is too much to hope for, as we study the disease by the light we can at present throw upon it. All this can be accomplished only by the exertions of each physician, with this end in view, upon the community in which he labors.

DISCUSSION.

Dr. William B. Canfield, Baltimore, in speaking of what scientific study, combined with well enforced sanitary regula-tions, can accomplish in a practical way, referred to the im-proved condition of the city of Munich, which formerly had such a notoriously large mortality from typhoid fever that travellers frequently avoided that city, or remained there as short a time as possible, whereas now, since Pettenkofer and Voit had used such stringent measures to stamp out that dis-ease, it was with great difficulty that the medical school could find a case of typhoid fever for demonstration to the stu-dents.

Dr. George J. Preston, Baltimore, spoke of the effect of high temperature acting mainly on the nervous system   He had had the best effects from antifebrin as an antipyretic.

Dr. W. F. A. Kemp, Baltimore, spoke of a case of his with persistent high temperature, on which antipyretics had no effect.

Dr. E. Tracy Bishop, Smithsburg, Md., gave an account of an epidemic of typhoid fever, that occurred in his practice more than thirty years ago. The disease appeared scattered over an area of country fifteen miles in diameter; cases occurred out on the lime stone soils and in the mountains, in the deep valleys and on the high hills. Some of the sick used water from wells and some from springs. The epidemic began during a severe drought, and when the weather was excessively hot. Day after day the sky had a copper color. Dr. Bishop's father was guided in his treatment of the disease by the views of his preceptor, Dr. Nathan Smith, the father of Dr. N. R. Smith. Dr. Nathan Smith, in his book, is believed to have been first in the profession to distinguish and describe the disease. Dr. Bishop gave very little medicine, kept the patient cool and clean, used thorough ventilation, gave ice and milk, and when the patient craved it, as they sometimes did, he gave small beer. He employed small doses of nitrate of potash and calomel and Dovers' powder. A neighboring doctor gave large and continuous doses of calomel. When unusual symptoms occurred they had special treatment.

Dr. Bishop gave the history of a case in which acute general peritonitis seemed to develop. He covered the whole abdominal surface with a cantharides plaster, and directed the nurse to lift one corner of the cuticle, after the blister had formed, and smear in a small quantity of mercurial ointment. Next morning, when he went to see his patient, a woman, and she had evidently been told of his approach, he heard her crying out every half-minute, like the tolling of a bell, "Skinned alive! skinned alive! When he had reached the sick-room and asked what was the matter, the nurse told him that the blister hurt her after she (the nurse,) had taken the loose skin off and put on the salve. To his horror, he found that the whole abdomen had been first peeled off and then frescoed in blue. Upon examination, however, he found that her condition was good and that she was salivated. By way of comforting her, he said, "My good woman, you need not mind this; you are going to get well now. You are doing well and you are salivated.'

Then she yelled out, "Pizened! skinned alive and pizened!" The doctor rushed out of the house, mounted his horse and galloped off, followed by the haunting refrain. The patient recovered, is still alive and well, not having had a day's sickness since, and although pretty old now, has very good natural teeth yet. He thought the percentage of recoveries was about the same then as now.

Dr. T. A. Ashby, Baltimore, thought that drinking water has always, directly or indirectly, been the cause of typhoid fever.

Dr. J. W. Humrichouse, Hagerstown, remarked that since the introduction of mountain water there had been few cases of typhoid fever in Hagerstown. That the fever when observed could be traced to the drinking of well water. That in one house where all the members of the family had the fever the water used came from a cistern, the cemented sides of which were cracked, permitting the flowing into it of water from a sink. That recently, under the observation of Dr. A. S. Mason, there had occurred a number of cases in a public institution near that town where the water used came from a well about fifty feet distant. This institution was supplied with mountain water, but the well water was preferred on account of its coolness. An analysis of the well water by Dr. Onderdunk showed organic matter, chloride of sodium and ammonia. Dr. Mason had the pump locked and since then there have not been any new cases. Dr. Humrichouse also said that when cases were seen in the country it was found that the barnyard and the well or cistern were very near each other, thus allowing contamination of the drinking water.

Dr. John Montgomery, Chambersburg, Pa., advocated the use of frequent sponging, with cold or tepid water, or the use of the wet sheet as a means of paramount importance in the reduction of the high temperature of typhoid fever. The country practitioner was not so well prepared to give his patient the benefit of the bath, but the method suggested was always available and at hand and answers the purpose well.

He warmly endorsed the use of alcohol in high temperatures, as not only of great benefit in its reduction, but believed with Flint and others that it prevents the loss of tissue. He uses quinia, but not in the excessive dose, believing more benefit is derived from the tonic dose and without the toxic effect, which he thinks is to be feared.

Dr. Wm. Lee, Baltimore, was surprised that antypyrin and antifebrin had not reduced the temperature. He had used them both in large doses on children, in many cases with excellent results.

Dr. A. Friedenwald, Baltimore, does not regard antipyrin and antifebrin innocent medicines. He has repeatedly seen symptoms of a collapse following their administration. Noticing the colliquative sweats that were produced by five grain doses of antifebrin in some cases, he has reduced the dose to two and a-half grains, and subsequently to one and a-half grains. At first these small doses were well borne, but after a little time considerable depression followed and the remedy had to be abandoned.

Dr. W. H. Perkins, Hancock, Md., referred to a very remarkable case in his practice of typhoid fever which was interrupted by scarlet fever, and after the scarlet fever the typhoid went on. He had heard of scarlet fever interrupted by typhoid fever but never the reverse.

Dr Joseph T. Smith, Baltimore, said in conclusion : "We would say that the point desired to be made was that we can feel much more at our ease in regard to the fever than was formerly the case, inasmuch as we know that even quite high temperatures can be borne with impunity. True, we may treat the fever for the comfort of our patients, as it may become a necessary factor in the diseased condition, still it does not hold that high place in our regard it once did. It is often extremely difficult to trace the source from which the water supply becomes contaminated, but it is not often that a careful and painstaking search will not reveal it."

Second Day.

Dr. Randolph Winslow, Baltimore, read a paper on

SOME RECENT CASES OF ABDOMINAL SURGERY.

Abdominal surgery is an interesting subject to medical and surgical practitioners alike, as it illustrates perhaps better than anything else in the domain of medicine, what can be accomplished by a bold and yet conservative procedure. To one who has not paid attention to this branch of surgery it may seem contradictory to speak of abdominal section as being conservative, but such is nevertheless the case. It is certainly more conservative to remove an ovarian tumor and thereby save a life than to allow a patient to die for lack of such an operation. For many years the medical profession has recognized the propriety of removing ovarian growths, so that at this time there are but few physicians who would not recommend their patients to submit to ovariotomy in the case of a large ovarian cystoma. Some, however, might demur to subject their patients to the dangers of abdominal section in the case of small tumors, and still it is the part of conservatism to remove these as early as possible whilst they are small and free from adhesions to surrounding parts. The wonderful success of the ovariotomist has caused attention to be directed to other abdominal and pelvic affections, so that at the present time it is probable that more laparotomies are performed for other diseases than for the removal of ovarian tumors, whilst in many cases the abdomen is opened for the purpose of exploring the peritoneal cavities and thereby establishing a diagnosis. That which takes medicine from the realm of doubt to that of assurance is entitled to be considered conservative, and this is effected by laparotomy in very many instances. During the past summer I have had occasion to perform laparotomy five times for various affections of female pelvic organs, to the details of which I now invite your attention.

CASE I.—*Double Pyosalpinx and Pelvic Abscess. Laparotomy. Recovery.*—Miss M., age 29, has suffered more or less for ten years with pelvic distress. About a year ago had an acute attack of so-called "pelvic cellulitis," from which she slowly recovered. In March, 1889, was again taken with severe pelvic pain, difficulty in urination, requiring the use of the catheter, tenderness, etc. She was attended by my brother, Dr. John Winslow, for some weeks, by whose invitation I was called in consultation in April of this year. I found her a well formed, quite stout woman ; bed-ridden ; the least jar causing pain. She is single and has had no children, and there is no history of abortion or gonorrhœa, , though these exciting causes cannot be eliminated positively.

A bimanual examination under chloroform revealed a hard mass on the left side, pressing on the bladder, whilst on the right side a sausage-shaped mass was discovered which felt like small intestine. Diagnosis, pyosalpinx. Operation on May 5th, 1889, at a private hospital Ether narcosis. The belly had been shaved and disinfected over night, as follows : After a good scrubbing with soap and water it was washed off with ether and then well washed with bichloride 1-1000. The instruments, sutures and ligatures had been boiled and the sponges carefully rendered aseptic with sublimate solution. Simple boiled water was used for irrigation of the cavity. No difficulty was experienced in opening the abdomen. The pelvis was blocked up with an inflammatory mass on the left side, whilst a large pus tube, which proved to be the left Fallopian tube, was found upon the right side. After some difficulty the inflammatory mass was separated from the pelvic walls, during which an abscess which was situated between the mass and the bladder was opened, allowing a large quantity of foul pus to flood the pelvis and peritoneal cavity. The pelvis was immediately flushed with hot boiled water, under which the free hæmorrhage promptly ceased. The mass, consisting of a large ovarian abscess and the left tube, was freed from adhesions and ligated through the left angle of the uterus on account of the extreme friability of the tissues at the junction of the tube and uterus. The right tube and ovary were also removed, the tube containing pus, though in no large quantity. This tube was also adherent to the pelvis by its fimbriated extremity. The patient became quite collapsed and the operation had to be finished rather rapidly. After flushing the cavity again with hot boiled water, a glass drainage tube was introduced at the lower angle of the wound, the peritoneum sutured separately with catgut and the soft parts with silk. A rope of absorbent cotton was placed in the glass drainage tube to act as a capil· lary drain. Iodoform and bichloride gauze dressings to the wound. The patient being in considerable shock, hot bottles and blankets were placed about her and whiskey administered hypodermically. There was but little subsequent vomiting, and the pain was not excessive. She was allowed nothing to eat except a little cracked ice until flatus passed. I will not narrate in detail the variations which presented themselves ; suffice to say that the highest temperature occurred on the evening of the next day, when the thermometer indicated 101°, rapidly falling below 100°, the pulse also diminished in frequency. On the day succeeding that of the operation the urine became bloody and was the precursor of a violent cystitis. A half-ounce of bloody serum was removed from the tube on the second day, rapidly decreasing in quantity until the fifth day, when, as all discharge had ceased, the drainage tube was removed. On the sixth day the urine came through the abdominal wound, showing a perforation of the bladder. This perforation was due to sloughing of the bladder walls and not to direct injury during the operation. It is probable that the abscess which was opened into the peritoneal cavity would have broken into the bladder. Owing to the cystitis which was present an attempt was made to drain the bladder, but this caused so much irritation that the catheter had to be removed. Fluid extract of pichi was given in half teaspoonful doses three times daily, and the bladder was washed out daily, first with a weak sublimate solution, later with a solution of boracic acid. Under this treatment the cystitis subsided and in a week the urine ceased to flow through the abdominal wound and the opening soon closed. She sat up in two weeks and was discharged in three weeks with her wounds healed, cystitis cured and pain gone. This case, which was complicated with such a serious accident as a urinary fistula, terminated happily, and I hope it may serve to encourage some other operator who may be unfortunate enough to have a like mishap. The woman has never menstruated since and is now free from pelvic pain, but is suffering from the flushes and other nervous phenomena incident to the menopause.

CASE II.—*Salpingitis with Hydrosalpinx. Laparotomy. Recovery.*—M. R., white, aged 34 years, one child 2½ years old. She is a well developed woman who has had pelvic distress since the birth of her baby. The pain is especially severe on the left side. She is essentially bed-ridden and has been obliged to seek admission to a hospital on account of her inability to work. The previous diagnosis had been "pelvic cellulitis." Examination was painful, hence an anæsthetic was given. Not much pelvic deposit could be felt, but the left tube seemed to be enlarged.

Diagnosis, Salpingitis. An operation was proposed and accepted. As this was the first laparotomy which had ever been performed at Bay View, as far as I am aware, great apprehension was felt as to the result, hence great care was taken to prepare an operating room which should be as free from germs as possible. A room, not in general use as a ward, was whitewashed with two coats, and the floor and wood work carefully scrubbed with bichloride solution. Everything was made clean. The patient was subjected to the same antiseptic preparations as have been described in the previous case, and the operation was appointed for July 22nd. The abdomen was opened by an incision two and a-half inches in length, two fingers inserted and the tubes found bound down and inflamed. After some difficulty the right tube was detached and brought up. This was about the size of the little finger, having at the end a bulbous cyst, which did not communicate with the canal of the tube. On the left side the tube was very red with its fimbriated extremity, villous and fungous looking ; some fluid was also within this tube. The ovary was normal. The broad ligaments were transfixed and tied in two halves. I irrigated pelvic cavity with hot boiled water and closed abdominal wound in the usual way. There was no shock and no nausea or vomiting and not much pain followed. Flatus passed per anum within 48 hours, and a metrostaxis occurred during the few days succeeding the operation. The sutures were removed on the eleventh day, the union being perfect. She was given no medicine whatever. The highest temperature was reached on the evening of the next day, 100°; the greatest frequency of the pulse was 96. In this case the right ovary was not found, and she has had her menses several times since. She experienced relief from the pelvic distress for awhile but is again complaining of abdominal pain, which I believe to be pure hysteria.

CASE III.—*Hydrosalpinx and Salpingitis, with Cysts of the Broad Ligament. Laparotomy. Recovery.*—M. S., white, age 24, native of Virginia, unmarried, has had one child. Complains of pain on both sides of pelvis, which she has had for three months, causing her to be almost bed ridden. Is very tender over the ovaries. Under ether the right tube and ovary could not be felt but the left could. After careful inquiries I found that she did suffer and that her suffering was not put on, hence I consented to perform laparotomy for diagnostic purposes, to be followed by removal of the tubes or ovaries if they should be diseased. Operation performed August 3rd, 1889. The patient had been prepared for operation in a similar manner to the preceding cases.

Ether narcosis. The incision went through the left rectus muscle. The peritoneum was opened and two fingers introduced when the right tube and broad ligament was found to be enlarged, adherent and covered with fibrin. With difficulty they were brought up and doubly ligated. The tube was large enough to introduce the thumb and filled with fluid. There were also numerous cysts of the broad ligament. The left tube was inflamed, its fimbriated extremity much everted and the ovary small. These were tied and cut off, the pelvic cavity thoroughly flushed with hot water and the wound closed in the usual manner. No shock at all. The woman suffered some subsequently and was very restless, requiring anodynes. Owing to her interference with the dressings they had to be renewed on the fourth day. The case pursued an almost afebrile course on the morning of the third day, the temperature being normal. The sutures were removed on the twelfth day, when the union was found to be perfect. She left hospital on September 18th, and I have not heard from her since.

CASE IV.—*Right Ovary Enlarged. Imbedded in a mass of Peritonitic Adhesions. Tube Occluded. Laparotomy. Recovery.*—Miss H., age 29, was healthy until about four years ago when she caught cold while menstruating, and a severe attack of peritonitis developed, which kept her in bed for nine weeks. Subsequently her health was impaired and she was unable to continue her occupation as a teacher. She had several attacks of pelvic trouble during the next few years, and began to suffer severely at her periods, and to have an aching heaviness in the right side. In October of this year, she sent for me during a violent attack at a menstrual period, and again two weeks later, when she had great pain, which compelled her to remain in bed several days. I saw this time any exercise would be followed by pelvic distress, causing a throbbing sensation in the right side. She is single, has never had a child, nor is there the slightest reason to suspect any venereal origin to her troubles. A vaginal examination under chloroform revealed a considerable hardness on the right side of the uterus, the uterus being virginal and normal. Nothing abnormal could be felt on the left side. An operation for the removal of this painful lump was advised and accepted. The patient was admitted to the Hospital of the Good Samaritan and laparotomy was performed in a private room on October 28th. The usual preparations of patient were made. She took chloroform very badly, and ether was substituted with no better success, and it was at least an hour before she could be sufficiently anæsthetized to proceed. A hypodermic injection of morph. sulp. gr. ¼ had been previously administered, but whether this was the cause of the difficulty in the anæsthetization I am unable to say. The abdomen was opened through the right rectus muscle, the parietes being thick and muscular. The uterus was imbedded in a mass of old peritonitic adhesions, and at first the right ovary and tube could not be distinguished, but after breaking up adhesions they were detached and brought into view, ligated and cut off. The ovary was at least twice as large as normal and contained a large blood cyst, probably the result of a recent menstruation. The tube was occluded, but contained no fluid in its cavity. The left ovary did not seem to be diseased and was not removed. Hot water irrigation was resorted to several times, which was not only useful in cleansing the parts, but floated the intestines out of the way and allowed space for working. It also restored the pulse to a considerable degree. The patient collapsed, and it became necessary to finish the operation more rapidly and less carefully than usual, and it is probable that some antiseptic precaution was neglected at the time, as the sequel will show. Hypodermic injections of whiskey were given, and external heat applied, and the patient put to bed. She has actually an exceedingly irritable stomach and vomits excessively upon any provocation. Nausea and vomiting soon set in, lasting without intermission for four days, so that it was impossible to give her any nourishment during this time. The vomiting was finally checked by the administration of cocaine muriate gr. $\frac{1}{4}$ every hour. She still had indigestion, and any food soured and caused tympanites and tormina of the bowels, requiring morphia, hence it was a week before any food could be assimilated. The bowels were moved on the fifth, and again on the seventh day. The reaction from the shock was followed by fever $101\frac{1}{2}°$, falling to $98\frac{3}{4}°$ on the fourth day. On the evening of the fourth day slight fever and pain set in, and the next evening the temperature reached $102°$. She was believed to have a localized peritonitis, but on the evening of the eighth day the temperature reached $103\frac{1}{2}°$, and the next morning two stitches were withdrawn and pus was observed to ooze through the stitch holes, the lower part of the incision being opened a considerable quantity of foul smelling pus and air bubbles escaped. The wound was washed out with bi-chloride and the temperature rapidly fell below $100°$. This favorable condition, however, only lasted about 48 hours, when the temperature again began to creep up, and I was confronted with the question whether the abdominal wound ought to be opened or not. I was very loth to do this, and hesitated several days, but when the morning temperature on the fourteenth day reached 102° I decided to delay no longer. Giving her a few whiffs of bromide of ethyl, I succeeded in passing my finger into the pelvic cavity, and upon introducing a glass drainage tube pus at once appeared. Probably an ounce of ill smelling pus was removed and the cavity cleansed, and by night the temperature had fallen to 99⅜°. This case has taught me the important lesson that it is safer to re-open the peritoneal cavity than to allow febrile symptoms to continue without exploring the pelvic cavity. Fearing the tube did not drain sufficiently well, I flushed the pelvis with a quart of warm salicylic (1-1000,) solution, which completely cleansed the abscess cavity. Although this case gave me enormous anxiety, I have learned a valuable lesson in regard to the propriety of re-opening the wound and exploring the pelvis, which I can never forget. She is now convalescent and sitting up, but it is too soon to express any opinion as to the end result of the case.

There are but few more remarkable examples of erroneous doctrine, which have been copied from one text book to another and transmitted from teacher to pupil for many years than that of "pelvic cellulitis." Inflammatory troubles within the female pelvic cavity are sufficiently common and are dependent upon many causes, among which are arrested menstruation, injuries, the effects of labor or abortion and gonorrhœa. These different affections present symptoms which are more or less common to all, as pain, tenderness of the abdomen, and more or less fever and frequently exudation around uterus and other pelvic organs which have been regarded, until recently, as infiltrations of the pelvic cellular tissue. The pathology of these affections was carefully and correctly worked out about forty years ago by Beruutz and Goupil, but the results of their investigations were either not accepted or had been forgotten when the modern theory of pelvic cellulitis gained universal credence. It was supposed that the pelvic cellular tissues was a tissue of excessive irritability, and that injuries of the uterus were especially liable to be followed by cellulitis, due to a sympathetic involvement of the connective tissue. For some years a few observers have maintained that the cellular tissue was not involved primarily in these inflammatory troubles, but if at all secondarily. The sequence of events, then, in a pelvic inflammation due to abortion or gonorrhœa, or even operations on the uterus, is an inflammation of the uterine mucous membrane septic in character, which by direct continuity extends to the Fallopian tubes producing salpingitis and frequently peritonitis by direct infection. Salpingitis is undoubtedly recovered from in some cases, generally leaving the tubes and ovaries adherent to each other or to some portion of the pelvic wall and with corresponding interference with their functions. If, however, the inflammation is virtually septic there is likely to be an intense salpingitis, with peritonitis, and ovaritis, with exudation, and the production of pus in the cavity of the tube causing pyosalpinx, the ovary also frequently is converted into a pus sac, and it may be that the cellular tissue is involved secondarily, but the exudation is intra-peritoneal and not outside of the peritoneal cavity. Pelvic cellulitis as a primary affection, either does not exist or it occurs so infrequently that its existence need not be considered. How, then, can we explain the symptoms which were formerly supposed to be due to pelvic cellulitis? In mild cases the symptoms may be caused by salpingitis or localized peritonitis, whilst in severe cases there is an intense inflammation of all these tissues and organs, generally with the production of pus. Sometimes the Fallopian tubes are distended with pus, serum or blood until they can be felt through the abdominal walls as sausage-shaped bodies connected with the uterus. With this change of view in regard to the pathology of pelvic inflammations there has come corresponding change in regard to treatment. Whilst it is proper in the mild cases to attempt to secure a cure by rest, the use of hot vaginal injections or the application of iodine ; when the exudation is large, crowding the uterus out of place or fixing it as if in plaster of paris, such treatment is worse than useless, as valuable time is lost thereby. Laparotomy and the removal of the diseased structures is the only rational procedure, and fortunately it is attended with mar-

velous success.   Whilst this is so, no one should be blind to
the difficulties which may be met, and the physician who
essays the removal of these inflammatory masses should
combine the attributes of a surgeon and a specialist.   These
operations are usually difficult and the dangers are not a few,
amongst which are hæmorrhage, the laceration of the bladder
or rectum, or injury to a ureter.   The work must be done
with the finger to a large extent, without the aid of vision,
and the breaking up of adhesions must be effected as gently
as possible.   Bleeding may be generally arrested by sponge
pressure or by flushing the cavity with hot water.   When pus
has escaped into the peritoneal cavity a thorough irrigation
with hot boiled water and a careful cleansing of the parts must
be performed, and it is safer to introduce a glass drainage
tube.   In cases in which no pus and no extensive oozing surface is left, drainage need not be done.   The patient should
have no food until the flatus has passed per anum, and for
the first twelve to twenty hours only a little hot water should
be sipped or cracked ice at intervals may be allowed.   Later
small quantities of milk, beef-tea, etc., gradually increasing
the quantity until ordinary diet may be allowed in from seven
to ten days.   The bowels should be moved by enema about
the third or fourth day or a laxative may be given per os if
nausea or vomiting have ceased.   Morphia ought not to be
administered if it can be avoided, as it arrests peristalsis and'
causes tympanites.   Sometimes it must be given if the pain
is very severe.

CASE V.—*Supra-Vaginal Hysterectomy for Multiple Uterine
Myomata.   Recovery.*—M. C., colored, aged 33 years, unmarried, nullipara, has been complaining for a long time of
profuse menstruation.   She suffers much in the lower part of
the abdomen and pelvis, and has been incapacitated from
working since last November.   In consequence of her ailments she was admitted into University Hospital last spring,
and submitted to laparotomy for the purpose of having the
ovaries removed.   As these organs could not be found the
wound was closed and recovery from the operation ensued.
She again attempted to work but her increasing infirmities
compelled her to desist and to seek further treatment.   She

accordingly entered Bay View Hospital and came under my notice in July of this year. She was at this time almost bed-ridden, feeble, sometimes having fever, frequently exhibiting nervous phenomena, bordering on hystero-epilepsy, and suffering with pelvic and abdominal distress. The abdomen was somewhat enlarged and upon palpation a large mass of uterine fibroids could be felt, pressure upon which was very painful. The bowels were usually loose and the urine contained some albumen. Taking into consideration the age of the patient and the great improbability of any improvement, I proposed hysterectomy as the only treatment which was likely to afford her any relief. As she had been through one laparotomy she was naturally reluctant to submit to another, but after due consideration decided in favor of hysterectomy. She was kept under observation for a while, and her request to be allowed to go to town to attend to some personal concerns, was granted. The visit to the city was followed by fever and increased pain, suggesting peritonitis. These symptoms abated in a few days, and the operation was set for August 14th. On the day before a purgative was given and enema on the morning of the operation. The patient had a general bath given her and then the pubes and vulva were shaved and the abdomen scrubbed with soap and water, then washed with ether and disinfected with sublimate 1-1000 and a compress moistened with 2½ per cent. carbolic solution was kept on the belly until the operation. The room had been whitewashed with two coats and the floor and wood work scrubbed with sublimate solution. Everything was clean. The instruments used had been previously boiled and cleaned, and previous to using them they were placed in 2½ per cent. carbolic acid solution. Sublimate 1-2000 was used for sponges, hands and external wound, but only plain hot boiled water was allowed to enter the peritoneal cavity. The water was kept boiling in the room by means of a little gas stove.

Ether narcosis. Urine drawn. The incision was a little to the right of the old incision, and it would have been better had I excised the cicatrix, as it subsequently prevented complete union. The tumor was adherent along the line of the former incision and had to be cut loose with scissors. The

incision was about six inches in length.   The uterus was lost
in a mass of fibroids of various sizes, making a large tumor,
which was brought through the abdominal opening without
much difficulty.   During this time a pelvic abscess in front
of the uterus was ruptured and flooded the peritoneal cavity
with pus.   This was immediately washed out with water and
the pelvis cleansed.   The broad ligaments and tubes were
doubly ligated on each side of the uterus and sewed between
the ligatures.· The ovaries were not found.   A rubber cord
was thrown around the cervix and a strong compression
clamp applied above it.   The body was now cut away without any hæmorrhage taking place.   The pedicle was short
and thick but could be brought out at the lower angle of the
wound.   The pulse of the patient was good most of the time,
but flagged once and was restored by hot irrigations.   The
parietal peritoneum was sewn to the pedicle in order to close
the peritoneal cavity.   Two rubber tubes were introduced
behind and in front of the uterus.   I closed the peritoneum
with separate sutures of catgut, and the abdominal incision
with silk.   The patient bore the operation remarkably well
and was put to bed with a good pulse and but little shock.
For several days subsequent to the operation the woman
suffered considerable pain, requiring an occasional hypodermic injection of morphia.   On the fifth day the dressing was
changed for the first time, as the temperature seemed to be
rising.   The gauze was stiff with blood, but there had been
but little discharge since the first day.   A small quantity of
bloody fluid was sucked out of the drainage tubes, but no
suppuration or sloughing had occurred.   There was no bad
odor about the wound.   The temperature on this day reached
its highest point, 102 4-5°, but this sudden rise was probably
due to the excitement attending the changing of the dressings, as it had fallen the next morning to 99 4-5°. .The
bowels were moved by liquorice powder and enema about
the sixth day, and owing to an offensive discharge the vagina
was irrigated about the same time.   It was necessary to use
the catheter for about a week, after which the functions of the
bladder were restored.   There was considerable hysteria and
nervousness, with cramps in the limbs for a few days also.

On the ninth day I removed the clamp from the pedicle. There had been no sloughing, but some suppuration. The drainage tubes were removed at the same time. The stitches were removed on the twelfth day, and it was found that the union was not perfect, which was probably due to the cicatricial character of the tissues through which the incision passed. The uterine stump retracted, depressing the abdominal walls and leaving a deep funnel-shaped cavity at the bottom of which the end of the pedicle gradually sloughed off, leaving a granulating surface, which at this writing has cicatrized. There was very little discharge at any time, and that sweet and apparently not septic. The temperature for the first week ranged about 99° in the morning, and 100° in the evening, falling below 99° on the eighth day. The pulse varied from 90 to 100 beats. For the first twenty-four hours a little crushed ice was allowed ; subsequently milk in teaspoonful doses every hour, gradually increased in quantity. She was allowed to sit up about the end of the third week, and on September 13th, four weeks after the operation, she viewed the sham bombardment of Fort McHenry from her window. October 16th, wound healed, leaving a deep depression in the hypogastric region. The patient has been going around the ward and wanted to go down stairs. Her appetite is voracious, and she is gaining flesh and strength.

The subject of the treatment of uterine myomata is a live one at this time and it is very important that accurate statistics of the results of the various methods of treatment should be secured. The methods practiced may be grouped under three heads : First, the palliative, second, the electrical, third, the operative or radical. In many cases the palliative method answers very well, and some excellent practitioners have always employed this to the exclusion of other measures. Amongst palliative means, rest, curetting the uterus, the application of medicaments, and the internal administration of ergot, all find a place ; but these are slow in their action, and the patient is obliged to lead the life of an invalid ; hence not very applicable to the case of one who is obliged to earn her own living. The treatment of uterine fibroids by electrolysis as practised by Apostoli of Paris, is still sub judice.

Apostoli himself, and others here and abroad make great claims for this method. The most important convert to Apostoli's method is Dr. Keith, now of London, who after most remarkable success in hysterectomy declares that removal of the uterus is unjustifiable, in view of the results obtained by electrolysts. Tait, with characteristic frankness, condemns the electrical treatment as useless and dangerous. Operators in this country do not, as a rule, look favorably upon the Apostoli method. Influenced by the statement of Dr. Keith, I recommended a trial of electrolysis in a case, which I saw in consultation early this year, but as there was no suitable apparatus in the city, it could not be carried out. I do not see how we can get around the statements of Apostoli, Keith and other reputable men, when they say they obtain better results by this method than by hysterectomy. Finally the operative or radical method must claim our attention. I do not here allude to the removal of sub-mucous tumors which can be exterpated per vaginam, but to those cases in which the ablation of the uterus is presented to our consideration. Hysterectomy is a radical, but dangerous, operation, the mortality varying from 8 or 10 to 40 per cent. It remains to be seen whether the mortality is inherently large, or whether it can be reduced by an improved technique. The impression which I derive from my reading is that the mortality is decreasing and will decrease still further. Before the question of treatment can be positively settled, carefully compiled statistics of each method must be made, and their results compared.

Dr. Thomas A. Ashby, Baltimore, then read a paper on

THE ORIGIN AND TREATMENT OF PUS ACCUMULATIONS IN THE FEMALE PELVIS.

Pus accumulations in the female pelvis are more frequent than was at one time supposed. They owe their presence to a number of causative influences. Broadly speaking, pus follows in the wake of inflammatory processes, both of local and remote origin, the inflammatory process of local origin being by far the most common. The pelvic cellular tissue is involved either primarily or secondarily, the process in each instance having its special mode of development and each pursuing its own clinical history. The older classification of pelvic inflammations, under the general term of "parametric," was coined to designate an inflammatory process, composite in its character and general in its involvement of the pelvic tissues.

Thus the metrium, the cellular and pelvic peritoneal tissues were supposed to be jointly the seat of inflammatory involvement, and the results were of graver significance than those which followed a pure and simple cellulitis. The points of difference between the different seats of the inflammatory action were determined with great difficulty, and the clinician could not always be sure whether the inflammation was parametric, or simply confined to the uterus, its cellular investment, or to the pelvic peritoneum.

In the acute stage of inflammatory action, the indications for treatment were so similar that differential points were not essential. But as the acute process subsided and its results were made manifest, it became less difficult to say whether resolution had been complete, whether adhesions had formed, and whether a pus accumulation was the resultant. This latter result at once defined the location of the inflammatory process in the pelvic cellular tissue, and the indications for treatment were more pronounced.

The old theory of parametric inflammation traced the extension of the process from the uterus to its peritoneal and cellular environments by direct continuity of tissue along the lymph channels. Thus the inflammation began as a metritis, extended to the cellular tissue, and finally involved the pelvic peritoneum.

Recent clinical and pathological studies have shown the incorrectness of these theories in numerous instances, and we now recognize the fact that pelvic pus accumulations have an entirely different origin in the larger number of cases observed, and a very different clinical and pathological history.

When Noeggerath asserted that latent gonorrhœa in the male established pelvic inflammation in the female through a specific influence, the significance of his observations was not fully appreciated. The progress of clinical study has not only sustained this view, but has extended the idea years before advanced by Bernutz that the one salient feature of pelvic peritonitis is salpingitis. This observer demonstrated by post-mortem investigations, that pelvic peritonitis was most often found in those patients who had died with the clinical history of pelvic cellulitis, the real seat of the inflammatory process having been confined to the pelvic peritoneum, associated with tubal inflammation and tubal pus accumulations.

Of thirteen cases of pelvic peritonitis, in nine, one or both tubes contained pus, in two the contained material was tubercular, and in one the peritonitis was due to cancer of the ovary. The cause of the inflammation he found due, in a large proportion of cases, to gonorrhœa, which had travelled along the uterine mucous membrane until it had reached the tubes, and here it had expended its virulence in provoking pus accumulations.

The observations made by Bernutz as far back as 1862, have been strengthened and confirmed by the clinical experience of Tait, Polk, Wylie and others, and the conclusion has been reached that tubal pus accumulations are the chief pathological conditions found in pelvic inflammations. The train of pathological events follows a most natural history, and can be observed in its successive stages until the pus tube is evolved, and even after it has ruptured into the pelvic cellular tissue and made its escape through its selected outlets. Beginning with a traumatism of the uterine mucous or parenchymatous tissues, the inflammation extends along the epithelial route to the tube, or having its origin in septic or gonorrhœal poison, the same route is followed until tubal inflammation is induced. The inflammatory action may end here by resolution, or it may go on to develop more disastrous consequences. In not a few cases the septic process passes into the abdominal cavity, where local or general peritonitis results, fatal or non-fatal in character, according to varying conditions.

In those cases in which tubal pus accumulations are observed, adhesive inflammation closes the tube at its outer and inner orifices; and the pus, finding no convenient outlet, swells the tube, until it reaches varying proportions or ruptures at its point of least resistance.

Outlets for the pus are made into the uterus, into the peritoneal cavity, or into the pelvic cellular tissue, and in accordance with the route chosen, presents a subsequent clinical history.

The progress of the inflammatory action may follow an acute or chronic course, and it is not unusual to find indications for treatment in the acute stage passed over unobserved and calling loudly for remedial measures when a chronic condition has been reached.

These conditions are observed under different forms and presenting widely different histories and characteristics. If the patient survives an acute process, she may apparently recover from the severity of the inflammatory action, yet under these apparently favorable circumstances, the tube may have been damaged, adhesions may have formed, and subsequent outbreaks may occur at any unfavorable moment. The statement has been made upon good authority that in pyosalpinx recovery can only be insured by removal of the tubes (Skene. *Diseases of Women* p. 550.) This statement, of course, has reference to a complete and final result, for it is well-known that women may go around with pus tubes, in fair degree of health, for months and possibly years, though at intervals subject to attacks of pelvic inflammation. In one of the cases which I shall subsequently report, I have reason to believe that the pus tube existed for over four years.

Nothing is so sure as that pyosalpinx may have both an acute and chronic course.

In the clinical study of pus tubes, the question of diagnosis presents numerous difficulties. When the tube assumes a sausage shape and feel, its detection is not so difficult, but when the pus sac has become largely distended and fills the

entire pelvis, pressing the uterus, bladder and rectum to the
wall, literally as well as figuratively speaking, fluctuation becomes difficult, if not impossible, the walls of the cyst are
thickened from inflammatory lymph deposit, and the pelvis
appears as hard and resisting as if the uterus and pelvic
organs were fixed with plaster of paris. This condition may
be mistaken as readily for an inflammatory induration and
adhesions as for a pus sac. Laparotomy here presents the
only correct way of establishing the true condition, as it
opens up the only successful method of treatment.

The pathological and clinical history of pelvic cellulitis,
strictly so-called, differs essentially from that described
under the head of pelvic peritonitis, but with which it has
been so often associated. In pelvic cellulitis, the inflammatory process is confined to the loose cellular tissue around
the uterus, though it may involve the uterine parenchyma
and the peritoneal layer. This cellular tissue is found in
loose meshes beneath the reflected peritoneum both in front
and behind the uterus, at the junction of the body with the
cervix. Inflammatory action is aroused in this region, both
by traumatic and septic influences. It follows in the wake
of operative procedures upon the cervix, as a result of abortion and child-bearing, where lacerations occur, and by the
introduction of specific contagia from the conditions
named.

The extension of the inflammation is direct and through
the lymph stream and not as in salpingitis, by continuity of
an epithelial membrane. The process does not differ from
inflammation of the cellular tissue elsewhere. There is first
congestion, followed by an effusion of blood serum, and later
on exudation of the higher organized constituents of the
blood. The process may stop here, resolution taking place
with an absorption of the effused material. Finally suppuration may occur, with destruction of the cellular tissue,
sloughing and pus. The pus accumulation may fill the loose
space between the uterus and its peritoneal folds and extend
until it has made an outlet through into the peritoneal cavity
or into the vagina, bladder, or rectum. Its favorite route is
through the vaginal wall, into the anterior or posterior va-

ginal fornix.   Should the outlet be ample, drainage is complete and the pus cavity closes by favorable resolution.
Where this result does not occur, the accumulation may persist and threaten life by septic absorption or by less favored
outlets for its drainage.   The pelvic tissues may become
honeycombed by small abscess cavities, and go on to develop a train of symptoms, both persistent and chronic in
character.   In the vast majority of cases, pelvic cellulitis is
an acute process, which only assumes a chronic type when
drainage has been imperfect.   It differs in this respect most
markedly from tubal pus accumulations, and enables one to
differentiate the two diseases by this historic feature.

In the treatment of pus accumulations following a pelvic
cellulitis, the indications all points to an early outlet for the
fluid.   Drainage is the one important method, and this may
be secured by aspiration, by free incision through the vagina
and in rare cases by opening the abdomen, breaking up the
abscess cavities, and free drainage through the wound, or by
making a conjoined vaginal outlet.

In those long standing cases where the inflammatory process has covered a large area, where the tissues have been
honeycombed with abscess cavities, where cicatricial tissue
is extensive, and where pus has made its escape through undesirable routes, such as the bowel, bladder and uterus,
laparotomy offers the most practical method of disposing of
the inflammatory products.   I am clearly of the opinion that
the surgeon should attempt to clean out the entire seat of
trouble and invite a closure of the excavation by cleanliness
and good drainage.   He may in this way remove the debris
of a slow inflammatory process and secure a positive cure,
where invalidism and ultimate death were in course of progress.   In my judgment, this latter method for the termination of pelvic cellulitis is infrequent and we will almost invariably find in these cases of supposed chronic abscess following a cellulitis that a pus tube exists in connection with
the trouble, either of primary or secondary origin. A laparotomy alone will determine this point, and this is the procedure *par excellence* for this condition.

It may be pertinently asked, what advantages are offered by a laparotomy? I answer, 1st. It presents the only accurate method of determining the location, extent and nature of the pus accumulation. 2nd. It presents the only method for the complete removal of the pus sac and for thorough cleansing and drainage of the region involved. 3rd. It is, comparatively speaking, a safe procedure when properly instituted. 4th. It offers the most reasonable hope of a complete cure of the patient.

With these arguments in support of a laparotomy, one might hastily conclude that the abdominal section was clearly demanded in the treatment of every case of pelvic abscess due to salpingitis. I certainly would not assume such a position as this. In my opinion, pus tubes can and do get well without laparotomy. The pus accumulation in the tube does not differ from a pus accumulation in other localities when adequate and proper drainage is secured for the escape of the pus. Should an opening remain at the uterine orifice of the tube, pus will seek an outlet by this route, or should a favorable route be chosen along the uterine wall and through the vaginal fornix, a similar result would be reached. Drainage is the one important consideration, and it is this factor which determines the gravity of the pus tube or of any pelvic pus accumulation. It is only in the exceptional case that successful drainage is accomplished without surgical intervention, and it is this fact which makes the indications for a laparotomy more conspicuous. That a laparotomy will sooner or later be demanded in the majority of cases of pus tubes, I think our growing experience goes to prove. The question of greatest practical moment, therefore, arises in determining when to attempt to remove the pus tubes and when to leave them alone. Just here professional opinion may arrange itself in two opposing ranks, neither of which is actuated by conservatism and matured reflection. One faction may hastily seize the knife and remove every pus tube which is found; the other faction may undervalue the claims of a laparotomy and allow cases suitable for this procedure to perish without an attempt at a curative measure. Both factions are wrong. The intermediate ground is safely reached if symptoms, clinical history and surroundings are carefully studied and weighed. It is just as sure that we can wait too long before doing a laparotomy, as that we can operate too hastily. In my judgment, these cases require careful study and a conscientious regard for the pronounced indications before we jump into them. Unless the inflammatory process is so pronounced and the pus so apparent and its presence so threatening as to demand prompt and decisive action, the surgeon should wait and employ palliative methods of treatment until positive indications arise. These indications are found upon a careful study of the history, symptoms and physical condition of the patient. The history of the case will present an explanation of the origin of the trouble, in traumatic or septic influences ; the symptoms will reveal severe pelvic pain, high and fluctuating' temperature, loss of appetite, night sweats, emaciation and general adynamia and cachexia ; the physical examination will reveal the area of tenderness on pressure, the character of the local swelling, the presence of the distended tube in many cases, and other positive evidences of pus cavities. When these indications are present, the time for a laparotomy has been reached and should be carefully approached without too great delay, otherwise the pus tube may rupture and routes be chosen for drainage which will complicate the removal of the tube at a later day. Success comes in the management of these cases in seizing the opportunity at the right moment and before the pus tube has established such relations to the surrounding tissues as to make its removal both dangerous and most difficult.

The two cases which I shall now relate will explain this point with more accuracy than descriptive language.

CASE I.—Annie J., æt. 27, married, was admitted into the Good Samaritan Hospital on July 27, 1889, suffering with intra-pelvic abscess of over four months duration. Her condition at this time was deplorable. She was emaciated to a mere skeleton, was greatly debilitated, with temperature ranging from 101° to 103°, quick and feeble pulse, profuse night sweats, severe pelvic pain, colliquative diarrhœa cystitis, her stools and urine largely made up of pus. Physical examination revealed a chronic pelvic inflammation and pelvic abscess, which had opened into both rectum and bladder, had burrowed through the abdominal muscles, and was about ready to open through the skin in the median line.

Previous History.—The previous history was involved in obscurity, but the following facts were obtained : She enjoyed excellent health up to the time of marriage, in February last. Shortly after marriage she had a severe vaginitis (gonorrhœal ?), which was followed by pelvic inflammation. The disease had continued until the present condition had been reached.

The diagnosis made was salpingitis, of gonorrhœal origin, resulting in pelvic peritonitis and pelvic abscess.

Treatment.—The condition of this patient was so depressed that I seriously hesitated whether I should allow her to die without operative interference, or do a laparotomy and take the chance of a result. I finally decided to open the abdomen and drain the pelvic cavity. On August 2, she was anæsthetized and a free opening made through the skin into the subcutaceous pus cavity. Pus in large quantities freely discharged through the incision. Introducing the index finger, the pelvic cavity was found honeycombed with pus cavities, walled in by lymph deposits, adhesions and disorganized tissue. Deep down in the pelvis a pus tube was found packed in between the uterus and rectum, distended with pus. It was adherent in every direction, and in attempting to enucleate it its walls gave way and pus was freely discharged into the pelvis. It was removed without much difficulty, though somewhat torn in the attempt.

The rectal opening was in free communication with the abscess cavity, and fecal matter was found in it. The abdomen was thoroughly washed and a drainage tube left in for subsequent cleaning and drainage.

The patient rallied after the operation and on the following morning her temperature had fallen to 99°, her appetite was fair, pain was absent, bowels loose, but general condition favorable.

The pelvic cavity was washed out carefully, two and often four times within twenty-four hours. Some pus, serum and

fecal matter came through the drainage tube at each washing. Her temperature never rose above 99°. She took milk
freely, suffered no pain, and had no vomiting. The diarrhœa
continued until her death, on the 8th day from asthenia.

Remarks.—The condition of this patient prior to the laparotomy gave little or no encouragement for this procedure.
It was a forlorn hope which stimulated me to attempt to do
something to relieve suffering, alleviate symptoms and save
life. Could this patient have been operated on prior to the
rupture of the tube into the rectum and bladder, and before
she had been reduced by prolonged suffering and emaciation,
her life could have been saved. The abdominal section conferred a marked relief to her and she would, in my judgment,
have recovered, if she had had greater recuperative power.

CASE II.—B. S., æt. 27, married, no children, one abortion
and one miscarriage. Abortion took place at the age of 16,
at which time she was ill for several weeks. Health fair
until the age of 19, and good from this age until 22, when she
miscarried, which was followed by pelvic inflammation. Her
health has not been good from that time until date of present
history. About the middle of August of the present year,
she took cold during menstruation, which resulted in a complete suppression, followed by pelvic peritonitis.

When admitted into the Good Samaritan Hospital, on
August 27, an examination revealed the following condition :
Temperature 103½°, pulse 100, respiration 30. Abdomen
very tender, swollen and distended. Uterus firmly packed in
pelvis and pushed towards the symphysis by a mass of exudation in Douglas's cul-de-sac. There were no appreciable
signs of pus.

Diagnosis.—Pelvic peritonitis, most probably of tubal
origin.

The treatment employed was rest, hot vaginal douches,
hot poultices over abdomen ; in other words, the so-called
antiphologistic and palliative treatment for pelvic inflammation. Under this regime the temperature fell to 100, pain
grew less severe and general condition improved.

Upon my first examination I was strongly impressed with
the necessity of making an abdominal section, but decided to

try the method above indicated until more positive indications for a laparotomy were presented. After three weeks of observation and tentative treatment the opportunity arrived which in my judgment demanded the abdominal section. Pain, high temperature and evidences of sepsis returned, the general condition grew worse, and I decided to open the abdomen for a clearer diagnosis, for drainage and for removal of the pus tube, if practicable.

On September 23, the patient was anæsthetized and the abdomen opened in the median line. Evidences of general peritonitis were soon encountered. The omentum and intestine were adherent in numerous points to the abdominal peritoneum, to the uterus, bladder and tubal cyst. The omentum was deeply injected, tumefied and covered with flakes of lymph. The small intestine presented a deep purplish hue, and in places were injected and tumefied. At other points it was bound up in loose, friable adhesions. The uterus was pressed up against the bladder, and impacted in the pelvis between the uterus and rectum was an enormously distended pus tube, over 3 inches in its diameters, adherent at every point to neighboring parts. The adhesions were for the most part easily broken from their attachment and the tube was shelled out of its position by repeated efforts. It was ruptured in this effort, and a pint or more of creamy pus was poured out through the abdominal wound. The tube was finally removed, save that portion attached to the uterus, which tore asunder from the tubal wall, leaving an opening at this point in the contour of the tube. The pelvic cavity was thoroughly washed clean after the removal of the tube and loose particles of lymph, omentum and tissue were carefully picked out. The abdominal wound was closed, save at the lower end, in which a glass drainage tube was inserted. The patient was greatly depressed by the operation, but rallied by the next morning. Nausea and vomiting were incessant. She was unable to take food until after the 7th day, and was supported entirely on champagne and Apollinaris and ice water. Milk and beef-tea induced vomiting the moment they were swallowed. The drainage tube was kept washed clean, but nothing but a small quantity of bloody serum escaped from it.   It was withdrawn on the 5th day, and a small glass stem substituted for it to keep the abdominal wound open.

Up to the morning of the 6th day, the patient had taken no nourishment except champagne.   Her emaciation and weakness were beginning to be alarming.   With a view of sustaining her, I ordered an enema of tepid milk.   This was injected slowly and carefully, and yet to my horror, on dressing the wound in the afternoon, I found milk with flakes of fecal matter coming through the opening.   In plain English, the rectum had given away and a communication established between this viscus and the intra-pelvic cavity from which the pus tube had been removed.   With a fecal abscess, the complications of the case were increased and the prognosis took a most gloomy turn.   I however washed the wound carefully, kept the patient on liquid diet, and by the third week had the satisfaction of seeing the fecal tract close spontaneously.

The patient made a satisfactory recovery, and was out of her bed by the end of the fifth week.   Her temperature after the operation never reached above 100°.   It ranged between 98½° and 99⅜°, until her recovery.

Remarks.—The two cases here related teach the importance of an early operation in these conditions.

In Case I, the patient came under my care after the pus had made outlets through the rectum and bladder, and when she had reached such a deplorable condition as to defeat the advantages of better methods of drainage.

In Case II, I came very near waiting too long before doing the laparotomy.   Out of deference to conservative methods of treatment, and in view of her general condition and at that time unfavorable surroundings, I deferred the abdominal section longer than in my judgment was prudent.   I came very near losing this patient through delay.   Whilst we may err in operating too soon, we may more certainly blunder in waiting too long for more pronounced indications.

DISCUSSION.

Dr. R. Winslow, Baltimore, remarked that he and Dr. Ashby did not differ materially in their views in regard to these inflammatory troubles within the pelvis. He did not deny that there might be a pelvic cellulitis, but he thought it occurred very infrequently. Dr. Jos. Price, of Philadelphia, who has had large experience in abdominal surgery, said that whilst it might be true that the inflammation began in the pelvic cellular tissues in some cases, it had not done so in the cases upon which he had operated, but had always been of tubal origin primarily. In these chronic inflammatory troubles pelvic cellulitis a distinct affection need not be considered. In regard to pus tubes, Dr. Winslow did not agree with Dr. Ashby that a middle course was the one to pursue, and that after the failure of other methods of treatment the tubes should be removed. The proper time to remove pus tubes is as soon after their discovery as may be practicable, provided the condition of the patient will admit of an operation. The opportunities for drainage are not good as the tube is apt to hang down and drainage through the uterus is not to be expected. A collection of pus in the Fallopian tube should be treated by removal, as thereby the whole disease is enucleated. The cases reported by Dr. Ashby and the first case of Dr. Winslow are sufficient evidence of the necessity of early operation in the cases. In one of Dr. Ashby's cases death resulted, not from the operation, but because it had been delayed too long. In the other a fecal fistula had occurred, which would been avoided if an operation had been performed sooner. In the case reported by himself an urinary fistula complicated the recovery, because the condition had not been recognized sufficiently early.

Dr. J. W. Chambers, Baltimore, was sure that want of cleanliness and gonorrhœa in the male were the two chief sources of pus accumulations in the tubes and cavity. It was a very important operation and every physician should be prepared to do it at any time.

Dr. C. Birnie, Taneytown, Md., remarked that he would ask Dr. Ashby: If you had an acute pelvic abscess opened by incision or opening spontaneously into the vagina, would you use any form of artificial drainage, and if you did what would you use and how would you secure it? Different gynæcologists, some of them eminent in the profession, recommend various ways, such as stitching the tube to the vagina, a self-retaining tube with a flange, &c.; but in his experience, and particularly in a case now under treatment, none of them were satisfactory, and in pursuance of the advice of W. F. Atlee, of Philadelphia, he had discarded them all and trusted to natural drainage. Dr. Birnie differed decidedly from Dr. Chambers when he said "every physician ought to be prepared to perform laparotomy at any time." A simple ovarian tumor, without any adhesions, was not very difficult to remove, but they were rare, and most laparotomies required a technical skill and knowledge that could only be acquired by practice, and should, if possible, be performed by those best qualified. It had been his misfortune also to lose several cases from lack of intelligent nursing, on which almost as much depended as on the operation. Willing nurses were abundant everywhere, but skillful nurses were scarce in the country. He thought that if any one without experience undertook such a case he would get hot and cold pretty often before he finished.

Dr. A. Friedenwald asked whether it would not have been advisable in the case reported by Dr. Ashby, in which a rectal fistula had been established, to have closed the fistula as one of the steps of the operation.

Dr. T. A. Ashby, Baltimore, in reply to Dr. Friedenwald, said that experience had taught him that such a rectal fistula would heal spontaneously without operation.

Dr. J. McP. Scott, Hagerstown, thought Dr. Birnie's question an important one. He thought it was important that only a skilled surgeon should do such an operation.

Dr. C L. G. Anderson, Hagerstown, said that he thought one way of warding off the dangers which would threaten women in some of these cases should each of us go prepared to perform laparotomy would be to prevent the trouble by protecting woman from man, as suggested by Dr. Chambers, or, as man is but the medium of contagion, by protecting her from her own sex.

This could only be brought about by State legislation and was one symptom or evidence why the membership of this Faculty should be so increased as to represent the entire profession in the State and thus become a force in the commonwealth.

Dr. T. A. Ashby, Baltimore, in closing the discussion, said that he did not wish to underestimate the great frequency of salpingitis as a cause of pus accumulations in comparison with the condition of simple pelvic cellulitis, but he could not accept the statement that the latter condition was so infrequent as has been claimed. The difference between the two forms of interior pelvic abscess are shown in their clinical histories. As a general rule cellulitis is an acute process and terminates favorably if proper drainage is secured. Salpingitis assumes both an acute and chronic type, the pus tube being the result of the more chronic varieties. Whilst operative surgery was largely instrumental in clearing up our knowledge of the pathology of pelvic abscess we have not reached a position which will absolutely warrant the statement that pelvic inflammations invariably begin in the tubal mucous membrane. The ovary itself may be exceptionally the seat of the pus accumulation. The treatment of pus accumulations hinges upon the location of the pus. If proper drainage can be secured without a laparotomy that method should be tried. It is not safe to assume that every case of salpingitis will terminate in a pus tube. Clinic experience will show that large accumulations of pus do take place in the tube and that successful evacuation does occur through the uterus, leading to a cure of the case. He was positive that he had recently seen two cases of this description where drainage occurred spontaneously through the uterine tubal orifice and a complete relief of the symptoms had taken place. These patients may, it is true, have subsequent returns of tubal troubles, but for the present there was decided relief and no indication, in his judgment, for a laparotomy. He would not underestimate the value of laparotomy in the treatment of pus accumulations. It is the only sure and safe method when indications are present. What he insisted upon is the exercise of proper conservatism and the avoidance of undue haste in disregard of a careful study of the case. Delay in operating in the face of indications is more fatal than haste, all things considered. He was convinced that the mortality following laparotomy was in direct ratio to the delay which permitted the process to assume such relations to neighboring tissues as to complicate its removal.

When the pus accumulation establishes faulty routes of drainage, that is through the bowel or bladder, the complication is a most serious one. With a growing experience his confidence in an early removal of pus accumulation by abdominal section was greatly strengthened. He agreed with the remarks of Dr. Birnie to the effect that trained, experienced assistants and favorable surroundings were necessary to the successful performance of abdominal section if mortality statistics are to be regarded.

Dr. G. J. Preston, Baltimore, then read

A REVIEW OF HYPNOTISM.

A wonderful revival has taken place of late years in the study and investigation of that curious and interesting psychical condition known as hypnotism, animal magnetism, mesmerism, Braidism, spiritism, etc. Probably no other subject illustrates more forcibly the strange fascination that mysticism in its broad sense possesses for the human mind. The fact that we have here a phenomenon, the nature of which is still wrapped in profound mystery, is in itself a sufficiently powerful stimulus to incite inquiry. Then, underlying this in a great many minds, there is a suspicion of hereditary superstition, a trace of the belief in magic and witchcraft which exerted such a powerful influence upon the lives of our not very remote progenitors. One of the things that strikes us curiously upon the most cursory examination of hypnotism, using the more modern term as an exponent for the general psychic phenomenon, is its great antiquity. And yet upon reflection it should not be a matter of surprise that such a peculiar and abnormal natural condition should have been noted and described by the ancients. In looking through the earliest literature on this subject, after due allowance has

been made for the play of the modern imagination, it is impossible to deny the fact that hypnotism was not only recognized but practiced in the earliest times of which we have
any record.   One potent reason why it never became generally known to the ancients was that it was inextricably
blended with their religion and practiced exclusively by the
priests.   The priest of antiquity was a curious compound.
He was the conservator of religious doctrines and traditions
and the performer of religious rites.   He was the philosopher
of the day, the poet and historian in many instances, and the
repository of all the knowledge then extant.   In addition to
these many functions he also performed that of physician,
and it is in this latter capacity that we meet with a certain
phase of hypnotism.   Just what connection there may be
between the spiritism of the seers and soothsayers of antiquity
and modern hypnotism it is hard to say, but that the two
states are analogous, if not even identical, is not difficult of
belief.   Going back to the earliest times of which we have
any record, we find undoubted evidence of animal magnetism.   The Chaldeans, who are accounted among the most
ancient soothsayers by Cicero, had three orders for the study
of magic: the exorcisers, the sages and the star-gazers.   It
was their custom to sleep in certain temples in order to acquire their wonderful gift.   They were reputed to cure diseases by laying on of the hands, by words, by light and
sound.   The ancient Egyptians were much given to the
practice of magic.   All through the Old Testament may be
found constant allusion to it.   An old French writer, who
studied the Egyptian hieroglyphics with the view of determining to what extent they practiced magnetism, and whose
testimony consequently has to be regarded with some caution, since he may have been too much of an enthusiast,
says: "Magnetism was daily practiced in the temples of
Isis, of Osiris and Serapis." (Montfaucon ; *Annales du Magnetisme Animal.*)   He goes on to say: "In these temples
the priests treated the sick and cured them, either by magnetic manipulation or by other means producing somnambulism."   Among other emblems he gives a picture representing a person standing before a bed on which the patient lay ;

his face is turned to the sick person ; his left hand is placed on his breast and the right is raised over the head of his patient, quite in the position of a magnetizer. Many other Egyptologists might be cited to show that in all probability the practice of magnetism was known among these people. Drawings have been found of great antiquity representing a person magnetized, with open eyes, and the series of representations show the patient gradually rising from his couch and standing erect before the magnetizer. Celsus opposed the miracles of Christ on the ground that the Egyptian charlatans, for a small sum of money would perform their wonders publicly, such as casting out devils and curing diseases, by blowing in the face of the person affected. Another Epicurean mentions the same thing and recalls the reproach that the pagans cast up to Christ that the temples of the Egyptians had been plundered and the secrets extracted. These citations go to show the fact that the Egyptians bore the reputation of being adepts in the art of magic.

Among the Hebrews we find frequent mention of seers, soothsayers and persons possessed with spirits of divers kinds. According to Herodotus, the Greeks derived their knowledge of magic from the Egyptians. In the temples of Æsculapius, of which there were great numbers in Greece, it was the custom to have sleeping rooms, where the patients who visited the shrine were accustomed to fall into a deep sleep. While in this condition the course of their malady and the necessary treatment was revealed to them. The ceremonies which took place in these temples have a striking resemblance, as we shall see, to the performances of Mesmer. The sick person was required to follow most rigorously certain rules which were laid down by the priests and to exercise faith in the gods. Everything was done to make an impression on their imaginations. Zealous prayers were said and songs recited, with the accompaniment of musical instruments. Plato relates that rhapsodical poets composed poems to be used in the temple of Æsculapius. Aristides mentions the fact that the dumb regained speech by drinking the magic water from the spring at Pergamus. The patients were stroked with the hands of the priests. They were then put in one of the sacred beds and made to sleep when visions and dreams came to them. When no cure resulted, as was not unfrequently the case, the fault was laid upon the patient, his unbelief or sin. It is interesting to note that Plautus states that consumptives found no relief. "They even weary Æsculapius in vain with their prayers and wishes." These special places, the oak of Dodona and such like bear a very strong resemblance to the magnetized trees of Mesmer and his followers. The Romans derived their knowledge of magic or magnetism from the Greeks, and in fact used frequently to consult oracles elsewhere than in their empire. One finds many passages in Latin writers clearly pointing to magnetism, as for example this one from Plautus : "How if I stroke him slowly with a soft and uplifted hand, so that he sleep?"

The Romans carried magic and all that pertained to it to a very great length, and their faith in oracles was not surpassed by that of any people before or since. Enough has been said to show that the germ of this psychic state can be recognized among the ancients. It is necessary to bear in mind this gross superstition, together with the fact that hypnotism, as it existed then, was entirely in the hands of the priests, and consequently a part of the religion of the people—a something sacred and not to be looked at with curious or unbelieving eyes.

As we approach the Christian era we see undeniable evidence of magnetism. Galen alludes to it and refers to the writings of Hippocrates on the same subject. During the early part of the Christian era we see a curious attitude expressed toward magnetism—now it is evidence of demoniac possession, and now a message from God. Tertullian describes one of the early prophetesses thus : "There is with us a sister who possesses the gift of prophecy ; she falls usually during divine service into ecstasy in which she has communications with angels and spirits. The reading of the sacred Scriptures, the singing of hymns and prayers give material for her visions, in which she will also describe the shape of the human soul." (200 A. D.)

During the middle ages the practice of hypnotism passed into the hands of, and was very successfully employed by, the clergy. As we have seen in its earliest beginnings it was a part of religion, but later was studied by the philosophers and used by the physicians. With the beginning of Christianity it again became a very potent factor in religion. The churches took the place of the temples of the ancients, and we see the same practices indulged in. Persons who were sick resorted to these churches or the tomb of some saint. All through the middle ages we find dignitaries of the church curing diseases by what would seem to have been hypnotic procedures. One reads of paralyzed persons suddenly falling into a deep sleep at the tombs of the saints and awakening to find themselves cured of their infirmities. While the descriptions clearly point to the hysterical nature of the diseases, they no less clearly show that the cure was by hypnotic suggestion. Of this nature was the power of the king's touch. This miraculous gift was said to have been first bestowed upon Philip the First of France and Edward the Confessor of England. While the disease in which it was especially potent was "king's evil" or scrofula, it extended to other maladies. These two sovereigns transmitted their gift of healing to their successors, and it was long practiced. Queen Elizabeth, *quoique heretique*, an old French writer naively adds, seems to have wrought many cures, and one William Tucker wrote a treatise concerning them. It is related that during the reign of Louis Sixteenth, when Richelieu was made generalissimo against the Spaniards, the Duke d'Epernon exclaimed, "What! has the king nothing left but the power of healing wens?" From the twelfth to the sixteenth century magic in general was supposed to come directly from the devil, and his satanic majesty was studied and worshipped by great numbers of sorcerers. Specific rules were laid down for invoking his aid or escaping from his malign influence. In spite of the gross superstition of this dark age the study of magnetism was slowly advancing. Marcellus Ficinus, born at Florence, in 1433, admitted that certain men were endowed with a mysterious power which they could exercise not only over their own bodies but over the bodies of others. Paracelsus a little later makes this candid statement: "The imagination can occasion disease and cure it. The confidence that one has in amulets and charms is the secret of their virtue." He proposed a very elaborate theory that man was endowed with two kinds of magnetism, one for his intellectual faculties and coming from the stars, the other for his organic functions coming from material elements. "Magic," says Lord Bacon, "is the power of the imagination of one individual acting upon the body of another."

The term magnetism came into vogue in the sixteenth century. The magnet had been used for the cure of diseases very much earlier, for it is mentioned in this connection by Pliny, Galen and Avicenna. Paracelsus declared that all the operations of nature were magnetic and spoke of the influence of the will over another by means of this power. Van Helmont, 1577, says: "It is foolish to believe that it is through the devil that one man may by his will influence others, even at a distance. Magnetism is present everywhere and has nothing new but the name." Van Helmont performed such wonderful cures by means of magnetism that in spite of his virtue and piety he was suspected of being in league with the devil and was thrown into prison. He recognized many of the phenomena of somnambulism and apparently possessed the power of passing into the hypnotic state, in which condition he declared that he saw visions and had many subjects of his research revealed to him.

Space does not permit any analysis of the epidemics of the middle ages; the dances of Saint Jean or Saint Guy, the Tarentism of Italy, the Possessions of the Nuns of St. Ursula at Aix, 1609, and of the Ursulines at London, 1632, and those of Louviers, 1642, together with the *convulsionnaires* of St. Medard and the estatics of different centuries and countries. While the underlying condition in all these emotional states is what would be called to-day hysteria, still one sees very clearly the prominent part played by hypnotism, especially the hypnotic suggestion, and the cures that were wrought in the case of these unfortunates by the priests and at the shrines owe their efficacy to hypnotism. In the numerous and elaborate records of these epidemics we find graphic descriptions of the condition of those effected, showing that the three hypnotic states were present, catalepsy, lethargy and somnambulism. The seventeenth century produced many zealous advocates of hypnotism, or as it was then called, magnetism. Robert Flood, (1638) of England, promulgated a very elaborate theory which supposed a universal magnetic influence pervading all matter. Thus when two men approached each other their magnetism was either positive or negative, from which sprang sympathy or antipathy. Somewhat later we find in the writings of Maxwell, a Scotch physician, the whole of Mesmer's doctrine in embryo. In his *Medicina Magnetica* he gives very specific directions for the practice of magnetism, and states very clearly his theory of the "universal spirit." In the preface to the book (published at Frankfort in 1679,) he says in defense of the opposition with which he was met: "We will, therefore, instigated by love, and for the public good, give the cure of six of the most difficult complaints and which the mob of physicians declare to be incurable. These are insanity, epilepsy, impotence, dropsy, lameness and continued, as well as intermitent fever." From the strength of the language employed we are led to suppose that the "mob of physicians" did not take very kindly to his method of curing the "six incurable diseases," for in one place he says: "Have we not in past ages seen the whole world, as it were, moved into furious hostility against this means of cure? Was it not by the loud expression of certain experience, which yet must be held even sacred and unquestioned, declared to be sorcery, devilish and deemed crime and folly? Valentine Graterakes, an Irishman, was very celebrated for his marvelous cures. He believed that his gift was from God and relates that the methods that he employed were revealed to him in a dream. Robert Boyle, President of the Royal Society of London, says of him: "Many physicians, noblemen, clergymen, etc., testify to the truth of Graterakes' cures. The chief diseases which he cured were blindness, deafness, paralysis, etc. He lays his hands on the part affected, and so moved the disease downward." We might suppose that many of these were

real cures by *massage* but for the fact that they were usually
instantaneous. Of course, in the last mentioned case and in
the case of many others who were celebrated for their "magic
cures," we cannot say that hypnotism, as we now understand
it, was the agent employed. The weight of testimony, however, is in favor of the fact that the hypnotic suggestion
played a prominent part. These names that have been mentioned were not those of men who would correspond to the
"magnetic healer" or itinerant medicine vender who instantly
cures the aches and pains of the bumpkins at the agricultural
fair, but in nearly every instance they were men noted for
their learning and held in esteem by their contemporaries.
It is interesting to follow the progress of magnetism in the
works of the learned Kircher Wirdig, professor of medicine
at Rostock, the great German philosopher, Jacob Bohme, and
the humanitarian priest, Gassner. The theory that they
adopted was fanciful to a degree, even for the time in which
they lived. Magnetism, derived from the light, from the
stars, from the moon, from all material things, was the grand
force of the universe, and by it all the phenomena of life and
death were explained.

We are brought now up to the time of the man who gave
a great impetus to the study of magnetism and whose name
has been so long employed to designate the whole system—
Mesmer. As we have seen, Mesmer can in no sense be called
the discoverer of this curious physical condition, for, as has
been shown, traces of its influence can be seen from the very
earliest times. As M. Cullerre, in a recent work on the subject (*Magnetisme et Hypnotism*, Paris, 1887,) says: "This
Christopher Columbus (Mesmer) of magnetism, as his ad-
mirers call him, was not even an American Vespucius. He
discovered nothing, he invented nothing. He simply put into
practice the facts that had already been discovered and described." About the middle of the eighteenth century Mesmer began vigorously to promulgate his doctrines. He
directed his attention especially to the treatment of incurable
diseases, so called. While he attracted great attention his
methods were so clearly those of the charlatan that he was
regarded with great distrust by the medical profession of

Vienna, where he was operating, and at length was requested by the dean of the Faculty to put an end to his nonsense. Justly discouraged by his reception in Germany, he went in 1778 to Paris. Circumstances greatly favored him, for there still lingered in the minds of the Parisians memories of Swedenborg and the impressions made by the miracles wrought at the tomb of *Diacre Paris* were not yet obliterated. Then, too, he claimed to cure all those who had been given up by the regular physician, a card which has been trumps so often. All Paris was in an uproar about him, and he made many converts in the medical profession. As to his doctrine of magnetism we have already seen it in the writings of many of his predecessors, and he added very little that was new. In his celebrated treatise [*Dissertation sur l'influence des planetes sur le corps humain*,] he speaks of a universal influence which exists between celestial bodies, the earth and animate beings. This influence he supposes to be a fluid penetrating all substances and subject to certain unknown laws. It manifests its influence particularly in the human body and possesses properties similar to those of a magnet, whence he calls it animal magnetism. He further states that it is exceedingly useful in enabling the physician to perceive the real nature of disease and to apply a suitable remedy, and predicts that the new science will revolutionize medicine.

Nothing could exceed the ridiculous nonsense and outrageous quackery of his seances. One need only read the descriptions of them to see that Mesmer in Paris was certainly the Prince of Charlatans. In a large room carefully covered with mattresses as are the strong cells in an asylum, and in fact it had been used for some such purpose, and which was denominated the "*Salle des Crises*," his patients assembled. The room was darkened, and any light that came in, passed through stained windows. In the centre of this hall was the *baquet*, a tub or box of wood in which were placed in a regular manner a number of bottles which were filled with magnetized water and tightly stoppered. The tub was filled with water, into which was thrown iron filings, pulverized glass or sand. From the tub projected iron triangles, or sometimes wires, and the patients laid hold of them, and formed a circle around the *baquet*. This circle had to be formed in this way. One hand holding the wire which was attached to the *baquet*, the other hand clasped that of the person next, feet, legs and thighs were closely opposed to the corresponding parts of the neighboring individuals, so that a solid chain was formed, through which the magnetic fluid could pass. Very soon the spell would begin to work, and one after another would fall in convulsions or *"crisis."* All the while music was softly playing, and Mesmer himself was accustomed to elicit minor notes in a certain key from harmonicum. After the patients were put in a suitable frame of mind the great magician Mesmer, clad in gorgeous apparel, usually a robe of some striking color, would enter the hall, and with an iron wand touched the parts of the bodies of his patients, which were supposed to be the seat of the disease.

Very soon these halls became notorious, for they were the resort of hysterical and superstitious men and especially women, and some of the orgies enacted there were said to rival description. A bitter quarrel sprang up between the advocates and opponents of Mesmer which finally culminated in a request from the government that the subject be officially investigated by the Academy. The commission was composed of a number of distinguished men, among whom may be mentioned Franklin, who was at that time American Minister to the court of France, Lavoisier and Bailly. Their report, which is a very interesting document, declared that this magnetic fluid could not be perceived by any of the senses ; that there was no fact to prove its existence, and that "this fluid without existence is consequently without utility." That the imagination was excited and herein lay the secret. There was an added report, which was not made public at that time, in which the opinion was expressed that these mesmeric proceedings were injurious to the public morals. Among the experiments made before this commission was one which was laughable. A desciple of Mesmer, Deslon, magnetized a certain tree in a garden at Passy, and a young man who was very susceptible to the influence of the magnetic fluid, was set to find the magic tree. After experiencing various sensations under two or three trees, he finally fell into convulsions under the branches of one which was twenty-seven feet distant from the magnetized apricot tree. In spite of this report from the Academy, Mesmer continued to enjoy a great popularity, and finally retired with a handsome fortune. Public interest had been thoroughly aroused however by this time, and almost every town in France had its *Societe de l' Harmonie* for the study of Animal Magnetism.

One of the most enthusiastic and distinguished of Mesmer's pupils was the Marquis de Puysegur, and to whom is due the discovery of magnetic somnambulism, as he designates it. The discovery was made accidentally, for as he was hypnotizing one of his patients he found that he could direct his thoughts and make him perform any movements at will. The fame of Puysegur entirely eclipsed that of Mesmer and vast crowds of people collected around him from all parts of France. About his time Dr. Petetin, of Lyons, observed and recorded the phenomena of catalepsy as one of the hypnotic states. The Abbe Faria, a Portugese priest, held sway for a time in Paris and exploited the newly discovered somnambulism.

At the request of Dr. Foissac, the Academy took up the subject of animal magnetism, and the admirable report of Husson, of the Hotel Dieu, was of a nature too favorable to be accepted by that body, but was ordered to be printed. [See *Rapports et Discussions sur le Magnetisme Animal*, par M. P. Foissac. Paris, 1883.] This was in 1831, and six years later the subject was again brought before the Academy and a large reward offered to any person who would successfully perform certain tests, such as reading with the eyes blindfolded, telling the contents of a closed book, etc. These severe tests completely discomfitted the advocates of animal magnetism, for the three subjects who competed for the prize made most signal failures and the Academy determined to have nothing further to do with this subject.

For a few years the subject rested, but in 1841 James Braid of Manchester, England, in a spirit of scepticism, began a series of investigations which resulted in a clear enunciation of the most valuable element of hypnotism, named Hypnotic

Suggestion. Braid absolutely discarded the fluid theory of Mesmer and others, and showed that the condition was brought about by the fixation of the attention absolutely, for a time, upon some object, either presented to the eye or heard by the ear. In this condition, with the attention riveted on some object, the imagination is at the mercy of any passing influence, and the unreal is accepted with no more hesitancy than in a dream. So far he was on solid ground, but unfortunately the doctrine of phrenology was rife at that day and he incorporated it into his system, alleging that by touching certain "bumps" the faculty of which they were the seat would be called into action; the subject being hypnotized. He also remarked that very curious fact that the mental state of the person hypnotized could be altered at will by giving to the body expressive attitudes. Braid also made use of hypnotism as a therapeutic agent. About this same time, and apparently independently, Grimes, in America, promulgated the doctrine of "electrobiology." He was followed by Drs. Phillips and Dods, the latter delivering a series of lectures on the subject before a committee of Congress in 1850. The work of these last mentioned observers threw no special light on the subject, as they covered the ground, so carefully gone over by Braid. In 1858, Dr. Azam, of Bordeaux, confirmed the discoveries of Braid, and observed especially the phenomenon of hypnotic anæsthesia. Velpeau and Broca made a communication to the Academy of Sciences on the use of hypnotism for surgical operations. Many other communications of like nature had been furnished by surgeons, the most important of which was that of Esdaile,, a surgeon in the hospitals at Calcutta, who wrote to Braid that he had performed six hundred or more capital operations during the hypnotic sleep.

Professor Lasegue in 1865 published his experiments on hysterical subjects in whom he readily provoked capalepsy.

In 1875 M. Ch. Richet made a careful study of the condition of somnambulism and of the production by the will of the operator, of any variety of hallucination, together with the curious fact of the modification of personality. In 1879 M. Charcot began the study of hypnotism, and his genius put it upon the most scientific basis it had as yet occupied. By confirming the facts and collecting and arranging the observations of earlier workers in the field he has given us a clear statement of the subject and a convenient classification of its different states.

The object of this paper being to review the field, space will not permit any discussion of the moot questions and allows only a rather brief summary of the present status of hypnotism. When we come to consider the nature of hypnotism, we are launched upon a sea of boundless speculation. Rumpf has proposed the theory that the state of hypnotism is brought about by vascular changes in the brain, Preyer that an oxidizable substance is formed by the cells of the cortex of the brain when specially active, Brown-Sequard that inhibition plays a prominent part, and so we might go on at great length. The explanation of the hypnotic state, if it may be called an explanation, which seems to us most satisfactory is the following: By certain procedures our attention, to use a loose term, carrying with it volition, is riveted upon a certain object or idea, thus leaving our other intellectual and physical apparatus free. Every one is perfectly familiar with this condition of abstraction. When occupied with an object or idea one responds to external stimulation, as brushing away a fly from the face for example, or may answer questions rationally but automatically. We withdraw, as it were, the will from its work of general direction and supervision and concentrate it upon some single thing. One is made to look intently at some bright object and told not to let the mind wander from it. Soon the muscles of the eyes become fatigued, the eyes gradually close, and the suggestion of sleep is strongly made. Just as in the dreams of natural sleep certain cells are functionally active and no selective or controlling influence is exercised over them, and images and events which in our waking moments would be monstrous are accepted without protest, so in the hypnotic state with volition off duty, so to speak, or more exactly detailed for special duty remote from the scene of action, suggestions enter the mind freely, hallucinations are easily provoked and the unreal is received and acted upon as real.

That some of the old superstition concerning hypnotism still lingers in the ordinary mind is evidenced by the frequently asked question whether the power to induce this state is not a peculiar one and resident only in certain persons? As has been shown, the individual himself really is responsible for the condition, the hypnotizer merely aiding in the matter of suggestion. The more decidedly and imperatively suggestions are given the more apt are they to be received and acted upon, and there is room here for some display of tact. Then, too, if the operator begets confidence it becomes easier for him to aid in the production of hypnotism, and the oftener he hypnotizes the same individual the easier it becomes. Beside this there is no more virtue in one person than another.

When we turn our attention to the question, what kind, and what proportion of persons are capable of entering the hypnotic state, opinion is considerably at variance, Charcot and the school at the Salpetriere maintaining the view that the condition in its true form is to be seen only in hysterical persons, or at least in those of a nervous temperament. Bernheim and the Nancy school hold that hypnotism can be induced in perfectly healthful individuals. The difference, which is an important one, being whether this is an abnormal condition, a sort of nervous disease, or is it simply a normal modification. The weight of evidence, it seems to us, point decidedly in favor of the former hypothesis. The best subjects are usually women, and drawn from the class of "nervous temperament," that is having a nervous system highly organized and more or less unstable. In favor of this view we find Charcot, Paul Richer, Dumontpallier, Magnin, Ball and Chambard. On the other hand Bernheim, Liebeault Bottey and others contend that the hypnotic state is merely a normal modification. The question needs yet more investigation and hinges on two points, one being the meaning of "nervous temperament," the other the classification of hypnotism which is adopted, of which we shall speak in a moment. As to the proportion of persons who can be hypnotized, the testimony of observers is at great variance, ranging from 15 per cent. by Durand to 30 by Bottey and 95 by Bernheim and the Nancy school, this difference depending, as above, on the classification adopted. "Generally speaking, the persons who most easily enter into the hypnotic state are illiterate persons, docile spirits, those accustomed to obey, as soldiers and domestics." This statement, which is from Bernheim, must be taken with a great deal of allowance, for if we lean to the idea that persons of a nervous temperament are most easily affected, we are more apt to find them in higher social planes than the classes mentioned above by Bernheim. This much may be said, that it is a *sine qua non* that the person to be hypnotized must be able to concentrate the attention and keep it so fixed for a certain time. It is almost impossible, for this reason, to hynotize the insane.

The methods of inducing hypnotism now in vogue are very simple, and the fantastic paraphanalia and elaborate system of "passes" of Mesmer and his school have fallen into disuse among all scientific workers. It is simply necessary to have a quiet room, not too many inquisitive observers, and the cooperation of the subject, and anyone of the following methods may be pursued. Fixation, either by holding some bright object close to the subject's eyes, and in such a position that the muscles of the eyes will be most readily fatigued, or by the operator requesting the subject to regard him steadily, thus fixing the eyes by the gaze. Again, many subjects may be hypnotized by simply holding the eyelids closed and maintaining a slight pressure upon the globes. Persons easily hypnotized may be thrown into the state by listening to a watch or to any monotonous sound. In some instances very susceptible persons are almost immediately hypnotized by some sudden sound, as is done in the Salpetriere by striking a gong. Space does not permit any elaboration of these well known procedures. It is always advisable to make use of suggestion, such as telling the subject that his eyes are getting heavy, that he is going to sleep, and finally to give the command in an imperative manner. Some patients who have been often hypnotized by the same individual need but to be told to sleep. Many different modes of classifying the various stages of the hypnotic state have been proposed, but the one given by M. Charcot is certainly the most scientific and serves as a basis for all the others. He divides the hypnotic state into three stages—catalepsy, lethargy and somnambulism. Catalepsy is the first condition, induced either by fixation or, often in very sensitive subjects, by a sudden noise. The characteristic of this condition is immobility. If the limbs be put in certain positions they will remain fixed for a long time. It is wonderful, and a proof of the genuineness of the condition, that the subjects will keep the arms extended without any tremor for twenty or thirty minutes, a thing impossible to feign, or at least extremely difficult. The eyes are wide open, the expression impassive. We find no hyperexcitability of the muscles that is so prominent a feature in the other states, and there is a general cutaneous anæthesia. If the eyes of the cataleptic be kept closed for a time the state of lethargy is produced. The eyes closed, the head sunk on the breast and every evidence of profound sleep. The limbs, when raised, drop back as if paralyzed. There exists complete insensibility of the skin. In this condition one may observe the phenomenon of muscular hyperexcitability. By pressing on certain muscles or on the motor nerve controlling them a strong contraction results, so strong that it is impossible to overcome it by force, and the only way to restore the muscle is by exciting its antagonist. For example : If the biceps has been excited and the arm flexed, the only way to overcome this flexion is by exciting the triceps. If the eyes are opened the condition of catalepsy is re-established. The other state, somnambulism, may be produced independently, as when the subject is put to sleep by suggestion, or it may be obtained by making slight tric-tion on the top of the head of an individual in the state of lethargy. There is complete insensibility of the skin to pain. The muscles are excited to contraction, not by deep pressure, or by touching the motor nerve, but by the lightest excitation of the skin, and contractions are overcome by slight additional friction. In this condition all the senses are very much heightened and the cerebral faculties share this excitation. In this condition the subject is an automaton, obeying the will of the operator. On awakening there is no recollection of what has passed. From any one of these three states the subject can be awakened by the operator calling on him to wake, or by lightly blowing on his eyes. Such is the classification of M. Charcot. It is as M. Cullere says, an ideal classification, which, unfortunately, has many exceptions.

Liebault gives six stages, the earlier one being a light somnolence, and the conditions of catalepsy and somnambulism are not differentiated. Bernheim follows Liebault and adds three other stages, making nine in all. Space does not permit any discussion of these different classifications, but it may be said in passing that the fact that Bernheim and his school include those light somnolent conditions under the general term hypnotism may explain the high per cent. (95) of hypnotizable subjects which they have obtained. This school denies the fact of muscular hyperexcitability, so strongly insisted upon by Charcot, saying that it is simply a phenomenon of suggestion.

Many observers unite in saying that it is not possible to draw any sharp distinction between the different stages, and that the various phenomena which have been mentioned, occur without any regular order.

Charcot has described several minor, or intermediate states, among which may be mentioned a very mild form of lethargy and a condition which he calls the state of "charm" or "fascination," the important feature of these two states is that, unlike the regular and fundamental states mentioned above, the subject remembers, upon awakening, all that has passed.

The phenomenon of hypnotic suggestion has been known and practiced, as we have seen for a long time. Any one who has seen experiments with hypnotism, especially by the professional mesmerist is familiar with the routine performances of making the subject go on a journey to the moon if desired, changing their personality, inducing hallucinations of every form, This phenomenon, in a good subject, is limited only by the imagination of the individual making the suggestions. In the lethargic and cataleptic state only a limited exercise of suggestion is possible, such as presenting a pen to a subject, who will immediately begin to write, and the curious experiments, seen in the cataleptic condition, of placing the hands in some suggestive attitude, when the face will assume the corresponding expression. For example if the hands are put in an attitude of defence, the face assumes a frown, if in a beckoning attitude, a smile overspreads the features, and so on. The state of somnambulism is the one *par excellence* in which to make suggestion. This feature of hypnotism is too well known to require any description. It has been found possible in the case of hysterical individuals, and those who have been hypnotized very often, to influence them by suggestion in the waking state, and the subject is one of interest and requires more investigation.

The most interesting feature connected with hypnotic suggestion is the fact that it is possible to suggest to a subject who is hypnotized, some action to be performed after awakening. This curious phenomenon has been studied by many observers, and many interesting facts brought out. A person in the somnambulic state, is told, "To-morrow, at a certain hour you will do a certain thing." When the appointed time comes the individual without being able to give any reason for his action, does what had been suggested the day previous. This suggestion has been found to persist for weeks, and Bernheim mentioned a case in which more than two months elapsed between the making of the suggestion, and the performance of the act suggested. A very nice legal question comes in here, for it has been proved that it is possible to suggest murder, theft and the like with such force that a subject might really put the suggestion into operation. For example: a hypnotized subject is told that a certain person has greatly wronged him, and easily pursuaded to put poison in the food or drink of such a person. Some harmless powder is made to play the part of the poison, and it is administered with a skill worthy of a poisoner of the middle ages. In his most interesting work *On the Medico-Legal Aspect of Hypnotism*, M. Gilles de la Tourette has thoroughly explored the possibilities of criminal suggestion, and shown the necessity of a law upon the subject, and it has been found necessary in France to place a legal restriction about the employment of hypnotism, or at least to recognize it in the code.

Many curious instances of auto-hypnotism might be mentioned, as the case related by Braid, who sent one of his assistants into another room to hypnotize a subject, and upon coming to him again found the subject awake, and the assistant profoundly hypnotized. Another writer mentions a young girl who would fall into this state by gazing at herself in a looking-glass, and instances might be multiplied indefinitely.

Of the value of hypnotism it is not the purpose of this article to speak. Suffice it to say that its value has been largely overestimated, both in the early days and at the present time. Its psychological value is worth something, for it allows the student of mental philosophy to study the action of the mind under peculiar circumstances. Its value in the cure of disease is not great and is confined almost, if not quite entirely, to certain hysterical conditions. It has had this good effect, that it has shown how much it is possible to accomplish over the body by the influence of suggestion. One cannot speak with very great confidence of the experiments related by certain observers, of causing a blister on the skin by a postage stamp, which the subject believed to be blistering ointment, yet certain well known names vouch for it, and photograph of the blisters thus produced are given. Still more incredible are the experiments performed by M. Luys and others, of suggestion at a distance. Near the hypnotized subjects are held small phials containing different drugs, and the various effects are thus produced : drunkenness from alcohol, sweating from pilocarpin, and the like. It is impossible to believe that there was not some suggestion made as to the effect desired to be produeed, for as we know the senses of the subject in the somnambulistic state are much heightened, and sounds and odors which would escape the notice of an individual in the waking state, are perceived by them. Such phenomena as the transfer of anæsthesia from one side of the body to another by the magnet, and of hypnotizing one individual by placing a magnet between him and a person in the hypnotic state, are clearly, as M. Bernheim has pointed out, matters of suggestion. Probably, though by no means certainly, hypnotism may be useful in certain mental conditions which lie on the borderland of insanity, such as hypochondria, melancholia, mental hysteria and the like. It was thought at one time, that it would be very useful in the treatment of the insane, and great things were expected of it, but M. Voisin of the Salpetrieres, who has taken the lead in these experiments, told the writer recently, that he had only met with a small number of cases that had been cured or relieved by this means, and that from the nature of the case it was exceedingly difficult to hypnotize the insane, or to make any lasting impression on them even were they hypnotized. In conclusion the writer would state again that it has not been his intention to discuss the various theories of hypnotism, nor to describe at length its different phases, but simply to briefly review the subject from the early days down to the present time, and show its evolution, as it were, from a mystic superstition to a well recognized psychic state.

DISCUSSION.

Dr. Joseph T. Smith, Baltimore, said : The subject which has been brought to our attention by Dr. Preston is one that it is well for us to pass in review at this time. He has gone over the whole ground thoroughly, and we simply rise to say that the conclusions to be drawn are that it should receive no encouragement at our hands. Whatever the theory of the changes it causes in the brain are, certain it is that the functional activities of the organ are interfered with and most of them suppressed,—an abnormal condition. As we are a body of men whose purpose it is to develop to the fullest extent the bodily powers, we should raise our voice in condemnation of the use of hypnotism in any form. Those who have ample facilities and make a special study of the brain and functional activities may resort to hypnotism to aid them in solving some of the problems which present themselves, but it should be unreservedly left in their hands. We read with much interest a book by Frederick Bjornstrom on this subject in the hope, partly, of finding that in some diseased conditions, especially hysteria, its quieting influence might be of benefit, but without success. In so far as we now know no good results in diseased conditions have been wrought by hypnotism. Indeed, much harm has resulted and time and money wasted for a something which should be relegated to the realm of witchcraft and sorcery where it properly belongs. All our influence, we believe, should be exerted to banish all forms of sorcery and superstition which, even in this enlightened day and age, are far too prevalent.

After the reading of the above paper, Dr. S. T. Earle from notes, which he subsequently decided not to "fill out," interested the Faculty on the subject of *The Principal Methods of treating Hemorrhoids.*" The subject was further discussed by Dr. Wm. H. Perkins, of Hancock, Md..

The following paper, in the absence of the author, Dr. J. J. Chisolm, Baltimore, was read by title.

Persistent Headaches, and How to Cure them.

Scientific truths disseminate themselves very slowly. The well tried and thoroughly proven have to be often discussed and are as frequently forgotten before they take root. They then give evidence of the fruit which they should have early borne. In this category is placed the medical and now well established fact that among the many causes of most persistent headaches eye faults are perhaps the most common ; and yet, as a rule, they are the last to be recognized.

Headaches are acknowledged to be one of the most constant effects of systemic disturbances. It is present in all of the active inflammatory diseases and in most of the chronic ones. When any of the important organs of the body get out of order the head suffers. The stomach, the kidneys, the liver, the uterus—all of them can produce headache. We know with what readiness the emptying of an impacted bowel will clear up head discomforts. The mistake made by physicians is to believe these to be the exclusive causes of headache.

Many of these sources of trouble to the head are fortunately readily found, and some of them are very easy of detection. But there is a very large number of head discomforts in which no acute inflammatory conditions exist to explain the disturbance of this sensitive centre. The general health of the individual is good. No one organ seems to be out of order. The digestive apparatus is in perfect condition. The kidneys are sound, with normal urine. If there be a uterus, its presence is known only at the catamenial period. Yet the head is not comfortable. That omnipresent cause of general disturbance, malaria, is invoked to account for the frequent complaints. It is found without seeking for it, and it is exorcised by frequently repeated doses of quinine. Relief comes temporarily under this treatment, with rest, as it would under any other, but the cure is only of short duration.

Where the malarial theory fails, some other has to be sought. Too close confinement to the house or to business is suspected, and fresh air with exercise enjoined. Good at once shows itself from this course of hygiene, but the head discomforts will return. Then comes a bright thought on the part of the troubled family physician in his efforts to find a satisfactory cause for his patient's sufferings. He calls the trouble neuralgia. Under this name the patient is often willing to suffer, obtaining temporary relief by taking quinine, morphia, antipyrine, the bromides, or some allied drug. Finally, it slowly dawns upon patients, that when they took medicines or open air exercise, *and stopped work*, relief came, but that when they resumed their occupations of reading, writing, or sewing, these being the every day employments of the majority of the population in cities, that their heads would ache. They then, from their own observations, propose the question to their medical adviser, whether in some way the eyes may not be responsible for much of the trouble which they have so long suffered? Once the discovery is made, the cause and effect can be constantly traced. They soon find out that they can read, write, or sew themselves into a headache. This sequence is so common that it ought to have been detected at a much earlier stage of the treatment.

The degree of discomfort is always in proportion to the *nervous temperament* of the patient. A safe rule for a physician to follow, is to look to the eyes as a common cause of head disturbances when the frequent headaches of a patient are not produced by some tangible disease. As a cause of headache, eye trouble should always precede malaria, neural · gia, and such commonly attributed but very obscure sources of disorders; and this, even when the painful symptoms temporarily yield to quinine, iron and arsenic Unfortunately, when the fault in the eye is paining the head, and is secondarily disturbing the whole body, the eye itself does not necessarily take on congestion, and is not even always painful, so that the casual observer can see in it no cause for trouble.

Many persons know that under the continued use of the eyes the head aches, but the seat of pain need not necessarily be in the eyes themselves. Fortunately in the majority of cases it is the pain in the eyes that precedes the pain in the head. If this sequence always existed, there would be less trouble in making a correct and early diagnosis.

Some patients will give as their case history, that up to a certain time they had, as they supposed, the strongest of eyes. They overworked them and now they will stand no work. Since the first break-down in their sight a very few minutes of reading, writing or sewing causes the eyes to water and burn, and produces a brow stricture, with eye pains. If the work is persisted in the pain extends to the temples, then to the top of the head and even to the back of the neck. Some refer all the pains to the top of the head, while the back of the head and the neck annoys some the most. In a few even the stomach becomes upset, and nausea follows, not because the liver or the brain is diseased, but as reflected disturbances from the over-taxed eye muscles.

Nature does wonderful work. The function of any organ is a marvel far beyond our comprehension, and the eye is one of the most intricate parts of the body. While we are lost in admiration over its wonderful mechanism as an optical instrument, we are also aware of some of its imperfections. We find many human eyes far from perfect. In communities advanced in civilization a perfect eye is rather the exception. Nature may start them right but school abuses soon upset them. Near-sightedness is becoming too common an eye trouble: It has as its fruitful source the present forced education of the very young. In these days there is no play time for children. Lessons in school and studies out of school absorb more than the daylight hours.

Brain work is known to be more exhausting than hand work, and young eyes cannot submit to this constant application without injury.

There is a society protecting children from cruel treatment. It prohibits their employment in factories. The factories which should head the list as most abusive to their well-being are the schools as they are now conducted.

The average citizen would restrict his idea of muscular labor to the hands alone, not knowing that eye work is a perpetual muscular labor, and of a very fatiguing character. When a person is reading, sewing or writing, the small but important eye muscles are as hard at work in their way as the arm muscles would be in sawing wood. They are as capable of being fatigued, and when fatigued suffer pain. This pain need not be restricted to the over-worked muscle. It draws into nervous sympathy contiguous parts of the body, and causes the so-called neuralgias of the head. An extremely common expression daily received from patients is that they have so much neuralgia that it makes their eyes pain them. When explained properly it means they have so much eye strain that it makes neuralgia in the head first, and then pain in the eyes.

All eye faults, and we use this term as distinct from eye diseases, do not cause headache. By eye faults I mean a faulty form of the eye-ball, a deviation from the perfect type, by which easy focusing of the dioptric media to form clear pictures on the retina is interfered with. Good sight means an eye which can make sharply defined pictures on the retina for brain interpretation. If this be done without effort the machinery runs smoothly and without discomfort, even if kept up by the hour or by the day. There is a large class of clear, perfect looking eyes with apparently excellent sight, but which give way under the continued use which our every day affairs demand. These eyes would never show their

faults were they not pressed by continuous labor. They resemble a flaw in the wheel of a railroad car, which can and
has run for many years at a 30 mile rate and seems as good
as ever, but when driven at a 60 mile speed goes to pieces.
. The trouble with such eyes began when additional work was
put upon them and they have given trouble ever since.

The true headache eye is known as an astigmatic one, from
the Greek word astigma, not a point, which means that a
point of concentrated light is not being clearly made on the
retina by the focusing apparatus. This astigmatism is usually
a fault in the cornea, although it may be more rarely produced in the lens, or might even be from irregularities in the
surface of the retina itself. It disturbs the making of sharp
retinal pictures and demands on the part of the eye muscles
more work than nature intended, to effect a given purpose.
Should we simulate the cornea to the glass which covers the
face of a watch we can readily understand how the glass may
be so mashed out of shape by lateral pressure as not to fit
the perfect rim into which it should adjust itself. In examining such a faulty glass we will find that the curvatures are
not uniform in all directions ; also that in the direction of the
mashed surface the curvature is greater than in the opposite
or true surface of the watch glass. The cornea is in this
manner distorted into astigmatism. When the two meridians
of curvature at right angles to each other, are taken they are
not found uniform. They should, in good eyes, represent
curved surfaces, all of which are made by one radius. Unfortunately in astigmatism there is a different radius for each of
the two curved surfaces.

The fixed law of optics makes the curvatures of a transparent surface responsible for the local strength or condens-
ing power of such a surface. When in an eye these corneal
surfaces all correspond, light passing through them on its
way to the retina is bent uniformly toward one point which
is called the focus. That brings out on the retina a sharp
picture made up of microscopic points of light. If, however,
these corneal surfaces are not uniform, the parts corresponding to these varied curvatures, each acting as a lens, will produce two foci of light, both not being at the same level. The

perfect part of the cornea will make its image in bright luminous points on the retina as a screen.   The imperfect part in
unfocused luminous rings will cast shadows over the brighter
points and will, more or less, blur them.   Then comes intui-
tively an effort on the part of the eyes themselves to correct
the faulty focusing and make the whole picture bright.   This
is a muscular effort and has to be repeated for every picture
that is made on the retina.

It is easy to calculate how many of these distinct pictures
are made in reading or writing, as nearly every letter has to
have its own and exclusive photographic impression.   The
brain must register this before it is effaced, so that the retina
may be ready for the succeeding letter.   To those who have
never tried the experiment, it is very startling to discover
how small a part of a word we clearly see.   Shut one eye and
look at a word containing six letters.   To see all of them
sharply you will find the eye moving from one side of the
word to the other, proving that the six small letters can not
all be focused sharply simultaneously.

When a well shaded eye adapts itself for reading, there is,
as it were, a steady contraction of the accommodating muscles,
a very easy condition to sustain for long periods.   With an
astigmatic eye a new adjustment of the muscular apparatus
has to be made for every picture, a species of perpetual
motion, which can not avoid producing fatigue and consequent pain, both in the eyes and in the head.   Each surface
has to be separately focused by the eye muscles upon the
retina, because the two can not be focused together.   To
keep the elasticity of the lens in a perpetual state of activity,
focusing first for one corneal meridian and then for the other,
demands incessant activity of the intra-ocular muscles.   This
tax is especially demanded when the eye is exercised for near
work, the more especially under bad illumination.   For an
astigmatic eye all work is more or less an effort, and night
work by artificial light is especially fatiguing.   The work of
the ciliary muscle in astigmatic eyes may be likened to the
irregular squeezing of an object by the hand.   A well shaped
cornea focuses all light passing into the eye by one effort,
just as the hand seizes and holds an object by the uniform

pressure of all the fingers. No fatigue ensues upon this simple muscular activity. If, however, the fingers do not all clasp simultaneously the object, the thumb and second finger holding it for an instant, and then the other fingers, these groups relaxing and contracting at the rate of so many times a minute, fatigue must result. If these irregular muscular hand movements were persisted in, pains would appear in the fingers, and extending up the arm, would cause an aching of the whole limb.

The source of sensation for the intra ocular eye muscle is branches of the fifth cranial nerve, the great nerve of sensation for the whole head. It is a law of the human economy, that when one branch of a sensitive nerve is excited, all the branches might exhibit sympathetic irritation. From the anatomical distribution of the ophthalmic branch of the fifth nerve to all parts of the scalp, we must expect these so-called neuralgic pains to accompany eye irritations. Therefore the irregular action of the eye muscles in astigmatic eyes is one of the fruitful sources of this head disturbance. Then will also come into play nerve reflexes, intricate and far spreading, and not restricted to the head alone. Some complain of dizziness, giddiness, irregularity in walking; others, of heart irritation, chest constriction, and of nausea. These various symptoms come on as the immediate sequel of eye work. With the very sensitive, these uncomfortable results appear when the eye has been used for only a short time; with others only after long and continuous application.

When, however, the eye finally breaks down, the irritability persists even when no close eye work is done. With this condition, reading for even a very few minutes causes pain. The eyes are sensitive to light, and more or less persistent headache results. The irritation, excited through the little use of the eyes in the day, may last through the night, so that the patient is never freed from these disturbances. With some, these head disturbances are so constant, from the ordinary uses to which the eyes are put, no eye injection accompanying them, that it is not surprising that the diagnosis is obscure, and that physicians are led astray. I daily see such cases; they report themselves the victims of perpetual

neuralgias, or of malarial saturation, or of brain troubles, because the head aches so ; or they believe themselves dyspeptic and bilious, because of nausea. Often they have had
years of medical treatment, with only temporary relief.

For such headaches, and they are very common, there are
but two remedies. The natural remedy is to abandon all use
of the eyes, and by so doing not excite the irregular fatiguing muscular contractions, which the use of astigmatic eyes
require. Simple and effective as this remedy is, it is impossible of application. No one, in these days, can make this
sacrifice, and give themselves to idleness. The only remedy
then left us is to correct the excessive and irregular action of
the interior eye muscles. This is accomplished by the use
of cylinder glasses. When carefully selected, properly
mounted, and constantly worn, at least for near work, they
make all the corneal curvatures act as if uniform in their
focusing power. By wearing proper glasses, the eye machinery runs smoothly, and headaches of year's continuance
disappear as if by magic.

A hypodermic injection of morphine can not more promptly
check pain than does the putting on of proper glasses relieve
headache. Relief is often immediate with the putting on of
cylindrical spectacles, and it becomes permanent under their
continued use. Often, during the first consultation, patients
remark how restful the glasses make the head, and how the
old sensations of discomfort come back the moment the
glasses are removed.

Quite recently an intelligent lady, 26 years of age, from
a distant city, could not recall a single day for years,
when she was free from headache. Very often she had to
seek comfort in bed, in a dark room. Her case was one of
irregular nearsightedness, or, as it is termed, "myopic astigmatism." When the proper glasses were adjusted, the beauty
and comfort of seeing was a revelation, which she expressed
by face as well as by words. She wore the glasses prescribed, and for the first time in her remembrance she enjoyed the comfort of freedom from pain. The giddiness in
her case was so annoying and her gait so unsteady at times,
that she found no pleasure in walking. With the correction

of the eye irregularity, came a steadiness of tread delightful to enjoy. I found that the nose bridge of her spectacle frame was a little too narrow, and suggested that the optician open it a little. For three days she had been living a life of luxury, going where she pleased, reading all she wanted, and with perfect bodily comfort. At my suggestion she visited the optician to have the frames properly bent. Awaiting the correction of the frames, in the store, she was forced to go without her spectacles for ten minutes, and her headache promptly returned. As she said to me, "You may imagine my anxiety to get my precious glasses back again, and how I enjoyed them from the moment I put them on."

Astigmatic eyes I see and correct every day. All astigmatic eyes under continued use cause eye and head pains, headaches more or less persistent being a constant accompaniment of such faultily constructed eye-balls. *Properly selected and properly adjusted cylinder glasses will relieve such headaches.* I therefore cure persistent, long lasting, very annoying and more or less severe headaches, every day, by prescribing glasses. With very few exceptions, all of the patients have been under medical treatment, some for very long periods. With these patients, nearly every organ of the body, *except the right one*, has been falsely accused of creating and keeping up the head disturbance. Mercury has been given to many of them for supposed liver torpidity. Iodide of potash has been swallowed by the quantity for the purpose of correcting some obscure syphilitic taint of which there is no history. During the many years of suffering quinine has been prescribed, to the extent of ounces to break up imaginary malarial impressions. The temples have been leeched and blistered, and the head neuralgias have been vigorously but unsuccessfully fought by a host of active remedies. Pessaries have been worn because the uterus was supposed to be in some mysterious way connected with the head trouble. Often it has occurred when the physicians' long list of remedies is nearly exhausted, that a friend of the patient has suggested that the constant headaches of one of her acquaintances was cured by the wearing of glasses, and perhaps in this case benefit might equally come. In this indirect way patients finally get relief.

The object of this paper is to draw the attention of physicians to the fact that constant headaches, even when not connected with imperfect vision, may be caused by faultily constructed eyes. Also, that when such is the case, medication is of no avail in obtaining permanent relief. Tonics to the enfeebled, by increasing muscular strength, may temporarily or partially relieve the discomfort. It does not remove the cause, and therefore a tonic cannot cure. Also that rest for such eyes, when pain in the eyes accompany the headache, effects no permanent good. The trouble remains to annoy as soon as the eyes are again put to use. *There is but one way to rest such badly shaped eyes, viz.: correct the fault by properly adjusted glasses.*

There are thousands of young persons in our midst who are now impatiently resting their eyes for weeks and months at a time, under medical advice. Some are kept from school, a serious break in their education, and others can illy spare their absence, from various occupations. All are taking physic to enable them to escape from annoying headaches which come on whenever they apply themselves. All of these long suffering and much-abused patients need some one to suggest to them the well established fact that, although the eyes do not visibly inflame, they are a common cause of head discomforts, and that this fact in their respective cases demands recognition. This advice properly should come from the family physician, and should not be accidentally obtained from unprofessional sources.

Having transacted some routine business, at about 4 P. M., after congratulatory and valedictory remarks by the officers and by several physicians of Hagerstown, *this most successful semi-annual meeting* of the Faculty was adjourned *sine die* by the President.

. Among the most prominent physicians from the counties present were Drs. A. S. Mason, C. B. Boyle, T. W. Simmons, N. B. and J. McP. Scott, E. M. Schindel, Andrew J. Jones, J. B. McKee, O. H. W. Ragan, Wm. Ragan, N. R. Shade, J. L. Steffy, E. A. Wareham, A. B. Mitchell, and C. L. G. Anderson, of Hagerstown; C. D. Baker, Rohrersville; E. Tracy Bishop, Smithsburg; W. M. Nihiser, Keedysville; W. H. Perkins, Hancock; V. M. Reichard, Fair Play; S. K. Wilson, Boonsboro'; John H. Koons, Ringgold; John M. Steck, Chewsville; Albert G. Lovell, Benevola; E. O. Manakee, Union Bridge; H. S. Herman, State Line, Pa.; J. J. Coffman, Scottland, Pa., and John Montgomery, Chambersburg, Pa.

WILLIAM B. CANFIELD, A. M., M. D.,
Acting Recording Secretary.

MINUTES.

Special Meeting.

HALL OF THE FACULTY,
St. Paul and Saratoga Streets.
THURSDAY, JULY 11, 1889.

The Medical and Chirurgical Faculty of Maryland taking action on the death of Dr. Oscar J. Coskery, the President, Dr. A. Friedenwald, called the Faculty to order and in a fitting enconium announced the object of the meeting.

Dr. I. E. Atkinson moved that a committee be appointed to draw up resolutions expressive of the Faculty's esteem for their deceased member, and deep sense of loss realized in his death. Thereupon the following committee was appointed:

Drs. I. E. Atkinson, George H. Rohe and E. C. Baldwin.

They presented the following resolutions, which were adopted:

WHEREAS, in the death of its late colleague, Dr. Oscar J. Coskery, the medical profession has been deprived of one of its most esteemed members and the State one of its most useful citizens, it is fitting that the Medical and Chirurgical Faculty of Maryland should express its high appreciation of his valued character as a physician and a man. It is therefore

Resolved, That this Faculty, recognizing its loss, and desiring to pay its tribute to the memory of its departed member, recalls with melancholy satisfaction the many virtues of

Dr. Coskery, his high sense of personal honor, his professional enthusiasm and intelligence, his untiring industry, his manly independence, his unselfish devotion in ministering to suffering, his moral excellence. It is amply sensible of the loss it has sustained, but is consoled by the reflection that, though called early from this sphere of usefulness, its deceased member had already achieved the lofty reputation that is the reward of a well spent life. It is also

Resolved, That a copy of these resolutions be transmitted to the family of the deceased.

> I. E. ATKINSON,
> GEORGE H. ROHE,
> EDWIN C. BALDWIN.

Remarks were made in commendation of Dr. Coskery's character as a man, christian, physician and teacher of surgery by Dr. I. E. Atkinson, Dr. George H. Rohe and Dr. Kloman.

A motion prevailed to present a copy of the resolutions to the bereaved family, after which the Faculty adjourned.

> GEO. THOMAS, M. D.,
> *Secretary, pro tem.*

Special Meeting.

HALL OF THE FACULTY,

JANUARY 3, 1890.

At a special meeting of the Faculty, called to commemorate the death of Dr. G. Ellis Porter, the President, after announcing the object of the meeting, appointed Drs. John Neff, Eugene F. Cordell and John C. Harris a committee to draft resolutions. They submitted the following:

WHEREAS, We have learned of the death of our worthy fellow member, G. ELLIS PORTER, M. D., which occurred December 30, 1889, at Lonaconing, Md., and

WHEREAS, We desire to give expression to our feelings of sympathy and respect,

Resolved, That in the death of Dr. Porter the Faculty has lost one of its most distinguished members and the community is deprived of a most skilful physician and surgeon.

Resolved, That we deplore the death of our colleague, who has been taken from his sphere of labor in the fulness of a ripe experience and at the period of his greatest usefulness.

Resolved, That our sincerest sympathy be tendered his family, bereft of one so faithful and beloved, and that a copy of these resolutions be spread upon the minutes and sent to the family of·the deceased.

> JOHN NEFF, M. D.,
> EUGENE F. CORDELL, M. D.,
> J. C. HARRIS, M. D.

After eulogistic remarks were made by many of those present, the Faculty adjourned.

> G. LANE TANEYHILL,
> *Recording Secretary.*

Special Meeting.

HALL OF THE FACULTY,

JANUARY 5, 1890.

At a largely attended meeting of the Faculty called this day to take action in regard to the death of Dr. C. O'Donovan, Sr., a prominent member of the profession, the President, Dr. Friedenwald, after commendatory remarks, appointed Drs. W. T. Howard,

G. W. Miltenberger and W. C. Kloman, a committee to present appropriate resolutions. They submitted the following:

WHEREAS, It has pleased the Almighty Ruler of the Universe to remove from us our lamented *confrere*, Dr. Charles O'Donovan, Sr., in the full maturity of his professional fame and usefulness, therefore, be it,

Resolved, That while we humbly bow to the fiat of the Supreme Will, we desire to signalize our sense of the many noble virtues and manly qualities of our deceased friend and associate. Dr. O'Donovan was characterized by every virtue that adorns and ennobles an honest man and a faithful and skilful physician. Always frank and generous in his relations alike with the profession and the public, he was endeared to a large circle of both, and no one among us could have passed away more sincerely lamented.

Resolved, That we tender our warm sympathies and sincere condolence to his bereaved family in their irreparable loss.

W. T. HOWARD, M. D.,
G. W. MILTENBERGER, M. D.,
W. C. KLOMAN, M. D.

After extended eulogistic remarks were made by Drs. Howard, Miltenberger, Harris and others, the resolutions were unanimously adopted. The resolutions were ordered to be spread on the minutes and a copy to be sent to the family of the deceased.

G. LANE TANEYHILL,
Recording Secretary.

Annual Meeting.

The Ninety-Second Annual Convention of the Medical and Chirurgical Faculty was called to order at 12.30 P. M., Tuesday, April 22nd, by the President, Dr. A. Friedenwald; 213 physicians being present.

The proceedings were opened by prayer by Rev. J. J. G. Webster, of Baltimore.

The President delivered his Annual Address on the subject, "*The Modern Hospital*," which was referred for publication.

Dr. Joseph Smith, the Corresponding Secretary, read his Report, which was, on motion, received and referred for publication.

Dr. W. F. A. Kemp, the Treasurer, read his Report, which, on motion, was referred to the Executive Committee for auditing and report.

Dr. J. E. Michael, in the absence of the Chairman, Dr. G. H. Rohe, read the Report of the Executive Committee, which, on motion, was accepted and referred for publication.

Dr. L. McLane Tiffany, through the Assistant Secretary, Dr. Robert F. Wilson, read the Report of the Examining Board, in which they recommended the unprecedented number of seventy-two candidates for membership in the Faculty.

The report was accepted and the names ordered to be listed on the bulletin board.

On motion of Dr. Taneyhill, the following resolution relative to the Report of the Examining Board was unanimously adopted :

That the membership Committee be, and are hereby instructed, to have *printed* 200 lists of the *candidates for membership*, to be distributed on Wednesday, in order that the Faculty may the more expeditiously vote on the same.

Dr. B. B. Browne, Chairman of the Library Committee, read his Report, which, on motion, was accepted and referred to the Publication Committee.

Dr. G. Lane Taneyhill, Chairman of the Publication Committee, read his Report, which, also, was accepted, and, on motion, referred for publication.

Dr. E. F. Cordell, Chairman of the Memoir Committee, read his Report, in which reference was made to the deaths in the past year, of Drs. O. J. Coskery, G. Ellis Porter, C. O'Donovan, Sr., and J. C. F. Mathieu. The report was accepted and ordered to be printed.

On account of the absence of the Chairman, the reading of the Ethics Committee's Report was postponed. Similar action was ordered in the case of the Report of the Curator.

On motion the order of business was suspended and the Faculty heard the encouraging Report of the Special Committee on "*Increasing the Membership of the Society*," as read by its indefatigable Chairman, Dr. T. A. Ashby.

Among other satisfactory announcements the Committee informed the Faculty that they have reason to believe that the increase this year in membership will be over 100. The report was enthusiastically adopted and referred for publication.

Dr. B. B. Browne, as Chairman of the Nurses Directory, read the Report of the Registrar, Dr. A. K. Bond, in which it was shown that the Directory had not only been a success in management, but a considerable source of revenue to the Library of the Faculty. The report was accepted and ordered printed.

On motion the reading of the reports from *Sections* was postponed until Wednesday, after the delivering of the oration.

On motion it was ordered that the Faculty meet daily at 12 M., and adjourn at 4 P. M., unless otherwise ordered.

The Chairman of Membership Committee announced that the members of the Faculty from the counties would be the guests of the city members at a banquet in this hall on Thursday, April 24, at 8.30 P. M.

On motion the Faculty adjourned.

G. LANE TANEYHILL,
Recording Secretary.

HALL OF THE FACULTY,
WEDNESDAY, April 23, 1890.

The Faculty was called to order this day by the Presiding Officer, Dr. A. Friedenwald, 327 physicians being present.

The minutes of previous meeting were read and approved.

The Annual Oration was delivered by Prof. Joseph Taber Johnson, M. D., Ph. D., of Washington, D. C.

On motion of Dr. W. T. Howard, a vote of thanks was tendered Prof. Johnson for his timely oration, and a copy requested for publication.

On motion the order of business was suspended.

The Treasurer was directed to read the names of those members who, having paid their dues, were entitled to vote for the candidates recommended by the Examining Board. Drs. R. W. Winslow and L. E. Neale were appointed tellers. Subsequently Dr. Winslow announced that all the candidates for membership had been elected.

The following is the list:

L. F. Ankrim, Robert Bond, S. B. Bond, J. B. Baxley, Jr., Joseph Clum, W. S. Blaisdell, F. C. Bressler, C. Birnie, J. E. Bromwell, H. J. Coffroth, Frank M. Chisolm, J. H. Christian, W. P. Chunn, J. M. Craighill, M. A. R. F. Carr, R. G. Davis, G. E. Dickinson, J. W. Funck, Geo. A. Flemming, John S. Fulton, Harry Friedenwald, A. B. Giles, Isabel K. Godfrey, N. R. Gorter, E. C. Gibbs, H. H. Goodman, H. B. Gwynn, W. S. Gardner, J. M. Hundley, J. W. Humrickhouse, H. S. Herman, W. F. Hines, H. L. Hilgartner, E. M. Hartwell, C. Hampson Jones, C. C. Jacobs, J. T. King, N. G. Keirle, S. A. Keene, W. F. Lockwood, A. S. Mason, A. H. Mann, Jr., C. O. Miller, S. K. Merrick, Russell Murdock, W. E. Mosely, Wm. H. Norris, H. C. Ohle, Wm. Osler, J. J. Pennington, I. E. Prichard, Hunter Robb, O. H. W. Ragan, M. Rowe, R. L. Randolph, J. B. Saunders, J. M. Spear, Norman B. Scott, John McP. Scott, Alan P. Smith, Jno. T. Spicknall, W. D. Thomas, W. J. Todd, J. C. Van Marter, Jr., W. W. Virdin, Hiram Woods, Jr., Mactier Warfield, E. R. Walker, R. B. Warfield, E. J. Williams, J. Jones Wilson, Charles P. Ziegler.

The Examining Board, through Dr. Henry M. Wilson, recommended the following named candidates for membership in the Faculty, viz.:

J. W. Branham, C. L. Buddenbohn, G. H. Chabbot, Wm.
D. Corse, Alice T. Hall, Wm. N. Hill, Henry M. Hurd, Thos.
M. Lumkin, Arthur Mansfield, Winton M. Nihiser, M. Laura
E. Reading, John H. Rehberger.

On motion the Committee on Ethics was allowed
to report at a subsequent hour at this convention.

Dr. G. F. Bevan, Chairman of the *Section on Surgery*, read his report. Additional papers from the
same Section were read by Drs. J. W. Chambers and
S. T. Earle. The paper of Dr. Bevan was discussed
by Dr. William H. Welch, and, on motion, the three
papers were accepted as the report of the Section,
and referred to the Publication Committee.

Dr. George J. Preston, Chairman of the *Section
on Obstetrics*, read his report. An additional paper
from the same Section was read by its author, Dr. R.
M. Hall. The papers were accepted as the report of
the Section, and referred to the Publication Committee.

Dr. G. H. Rohe, Chairman of the Executive Committee, reported that the following "*Volunteer Papers*"
would be read by their respective authors at the time
allotted in the order of business :

1st. "*One hundred consecutive cases of labor in
the Maryland Maternite, with comments on the methods practised in that institution.*" By Drs. George
H. Rohe and W. J. Todd.

2d. "*The Lung Disorders of the prevailing Influenza.*" By Dr. A. Kerr Bond.

3d. "*Nitrogen in Medicine.*" By Dr. W. R.
Monroe.

The Executive Committee reported that they had
examined and audited the accounts of the Treasurer

for the past fiscal year, and found them correct, thereupon that officer's report was accepted and referred to the Publication Committee.

On motion, the Faculty adjourned, to meet at 12 M. Thursday, April 24.

> G. LANE TANEYHILL,
> *Recording Secretary.*

HALL OF THE FACULTY,
THURSDAY, April 24, 1890.

The Faculty was called to order by the President, Dr. A. Friedenwald, 290 persons .present. The minutes of the previous meeting were read and approved.

Dr. L. E. Neale read a paper, and exhibited a specimen, from the Section on Obstetrics; it was discussed by Dr. R. M. Hall, and the paper referred to the Publication Committee.

The Examining Board through Dr. H. M. Wilson at this juncture, made a supplementary report, in which they recommended for membership the following candidates:

Wm. M. Barnes, E. Dorsey Ellis, Henry F. Hill, Edwin E. Jones, J. Randolph Page, W. C. Sandrock, W. R. Shaw, Thos. H. Buckler.

Dr. Jno. C. Hemmeter from the Section on *Anatomy*, *Physiology* and *Pathology*, read a paper from said section, which on motion was accepted and ordered to be printed.

Dr. P. C. Williams, Chairman of *Committee on Ethics*, informed the Faculty that their report was completed; on motion it was determined that the Faculty meet in "*Special Session*" on Friday, April

25th, at 11.30 A. M., to receive the report of the Ethics Committee.

Dr. E. F. Cordell from the Section on *Materia Medica and Chemistry*, acting as Chairman of said Section, read the report which was discussed by Drs. P. C. Williams, J. D. Blake, C. Hampson Jones, J. J. Chisolm, H. C. Wood, Jr., I. E. Atkinson, W. R. Monroe, J. W. Chambers, L. McL. Tiffany, G. H. Rohe, Chas. G. Hill, J. H. Branham and J. E. Michael. The report was on motion accepted and referred to Publication Committee.

Dr. C. G. Hill of the Section on *Psychology and Medical Jurisprudence*, read a paper from said section, which was accepted and ordered to be published.

The balloting for candidates for membership, resulted in the election of the following:

J. W. Branham, C. L. Buddenbohn, G. H. Chabbot, Wm. D. Corse, Alice T. Hall, Wm. N. Hill, Henry M. Hurd, Thos. M. Lumpkin, Arthur Mansfield, Winton M. Nihiser, M. Laura E. Reading, John H. Rehberger.

On motion the Faculty adjourned to meet in "*Special Session*," at 11.30 A. M., Friday, 25th April.

G. LANE TANEYHILL,　　　.

Recording Secretary.

HALL OF THE FACULTY,

APRIL 25, 1890.

The Faculty met at 11.30 A. M., in "*Special Session*" as per resolution, to receive the report of the *Committee on Ethics;* the President, Dr. Friedenwald, was in the chair, and a large number of members present.

Dr. P. C. Williams for the Committee, reported that the charges against Dr. J. H. DeWolf, had been sustained, and that the Committee now make the report to the Faculty; the report was accepted for discussion, after which a motion to expel the offending party prevailed, and the President immediately announced the sentence of the Faculty as ordered by the Constitution.

The regular order of business was resumed, the President in the chair, 209 physicians present. The minutes of the previous meeting were read and approved.

Dr. Randolph Winslow of the Examining Board and for the board, recommended the name of Dr. Philip Brisco, of Port Tobacco, Calvert county, Maryland, for membership.

Dr. J. J. Chisolm, from the Section on Ophthalmology, Laryngology and Otology, read a paper, which was on motion accepted and ordered to be published.

"*Volunteer Papers*" having been called for Dr. A. Kerr Bond, read a paper on "*The Lung disorders of the prevailing Influenza*,"—It was accepted and referred to the Publication Committee.

Dr. Geo. H. Rohe, read a volunteer paper on "*One hundred consecutive cases of Labor in the Maryland Maternite with comments on the methods practised in that institution*," the paper was discussed by Drs. J. H. Branham, L. E. Neale and others, and accepted and referred for publication.

Dr. W. R. Munroe, read a volunteer paper on "*Nitrogen in Medicine*," which was accepted and referred for publication.

On motion the order of business was suspended, and the election of officers ordered for the ensuing year, the result was as follows :   .

President.—Dr. T. A. Ashby.

Vice-Presidents.—Drs. Geo. H. Rohe and J. McPherson Scott.

Recording Secretary.—Dr. G. Lane Taneyhill.

Assistant Secretary.—Dr. Robert T. Wilson.

Corresponding Secretary.—Dr. J. T. Smith.

Reporting Secretary.—Wm. B. Canfield.

Treasurer.—Dr. W. F. A. Kemp.

Executive Committee.—Drs. P. C. Williams, S. T. Earle, A. Friedenwald, J. W. Chambers, and R. Winslow.

Examining Board of Western Shore.—Drs. C. H. Jones, B. B. Browne, Wilmer Brinton, J. E. Michael, L. E. Neale, J. D. Blake and J. H. Branham.

Examining Board of Eastern Shore.—Drs. B. W. Goldsborough, G. T. Atkinson, A. H. Bayley, J. K. H. Jacobs and W. F. Hines.

Under unfinished business Dr. E. F. Cordell, Chairman of the committee on "*Revision and Publication of the Pharmacopœia of the United States,*" reported progress, and the committee was continued another year.   The same gentleman announced, upon call for the report on National Formulæ of Unofficial Preparations—that the report had been read at a previous meeting, and would appear in the *Transactions.*

The resignation of Dr. J. F. Perkins, removed, was read and accepted.

On motion of Dr. I. E. Atkinson, the following was adopted :

WHEREAS, an effort is being made, with a reasonable expectation of success, to establish in Patterson Park, a Botanical Garden, which as an educational and ornamental feature of permanent improvement, will be most desirable,

Resolved, That this Faculty, recognizing the science of Botany in its important relation to the Medical Sciences, heartily favor the effort, and hereby endorse its importance as a valuable aid to medicine and pharmacy.

A communication from the American Medical Association on Uniform Medical Legislation in the United States was read by the Secretary, and on his motion, was referred to the Executive Committee, with discretionary power.

Dr. B. B. Browne, Chairman of the Library Board, submitted the following as a change in the Library Laws, it was adopted and ordered to be incorporated in the "Rules."

City members retaining books longer than two weeks, and county members longer than four weeks, shall be subject to the following fines, per week, viz.: 10 cents for the first week; 20 cents for the second week; 30 cents for the third week, and 20 cents per week for every week thereafter. Such fines shall be appropriated exclusively for the benefit of the Library.

On motion it was ordered that if the Publication Committee think it expedient, they be and are hereby empowered to have printed 1000 copies of the revised Constitution and By-Laws, incorporating all amendments to date.

Dr. Taneyhill, the Secretary, announced that in consequence of soliciting circulars, which he had sent to many druggists throughout the states, every allotted space in the "*Pharmaceutical Exhibition Hall*" had been taken, and that he had collected $145.00 net, from the exhibitors, which he was ready to turn into the treasury.

On motion of Dr. Joseph T. Smith, the following resolution was unanimously adopted:

Resolved, That we extend to Dr. Christopher Johnston, Sr., our sincere sympathy in this his hour of sickness, and trust that ere long, he will be fully restored to health, that he may go in and out among us, aiding us with his advice and counsel.

On motion of Dr. B. B. Browne, the following was adopted :

Resolved, That at the Annual Convention *an executive session* be held on Wednesday the second day of the Convention at 8 P. M., that at this meeting the Reports of all the Committees shall be read, miscellaneous business shall be considered, and the election of officers take place.

As germane to this resolution, it was suggested, that if approved by the Executive Committee, the Recording Secretary might prepare a programme of the business and papers to be read at the meetings of the Faculty.

On motion Dr. W. T. Howard was requested by the Faculty to write out an extended obituary notice of our late colleague, Dr. Charles O'Donovan, Sr., and that the same be incorporated in the report of the Memoir Committee.

On motion the sum of $10.00 was ordered to be paid by the Treasurer to the janitor, as an extra compensation for services.

The President directed the Secretary to read the following list of his appointments of Standing Committees, Sections and Delegates for the ensuing year:

STANDING COMMITTEES.

Library.—Drs. I. E. Atkinson, T. Barton Brune, B. B. Browne, Wm. H. Welch, G. Lane Taneyhill.

Publication.—Drs. G. Lane Taneyhill, W. F. A. Kemp, John G. Jay, Geo. J. Preston, Randolph Winslow.

Memoir.—Drs. E. F. Cordell, D. W. Cathell, W. Stump Forwood, T. B. Evans, John R. Quinan.

Ethics.—Drs. Chas. H. Jones, Thomas S. Latimer, Jos. T. Smith, Christopher Johnston, Sr., H. M. Wilson.

Increasing the Membership.—Drs. T. A. Ashby, S. T. Earle, G. Lane Taneyhill, Wm. Lee, G. W. Hemrickhouse, W. F. Hines, J. H. Branham, Geo. H. Rohe, J. W. Chambers.

Curator.—Dr. L. F. Ankrim.

SECTIONS.

Surgery.—Drs. L. McLane Tiffany, J. W. Chambers, Randolph Winslow, John McP. Scott, John D. Blake.

Practice.—Drs. Wm. Osler, Jos. T. Smith, Samuel C. Chew, David Streett, W. F. Hines.

Obstetrics.—Drs. J. E. Michael, Thomas Opie, W. E. Mosely, Wm. S. Gardner, Robt. T. Wilson.

Materia Medica.—Drs. I. E. Atkinson, R. H. P. Ellis, J. L. Ingle, Chas. G. W. McGill, H. M. Salzer.

Sanitary Science.—Drs. Geo. H. Rohe, E. M. Hartwell, Jackson Piper, E. G. Waters, John Neff.

Anatomy and Physiology.—Drs. H. Newall Martin, J. H. Branham, Herbert Harlan, Geo. J. Preston, John C. Hemmeter.

Psychology and Medical Jurisprudence.—Drs. Richard Gundry, John Morris, Wm. Lee, Chas. G. Hill, John S. Conrad.

Microscopy, &c.—Drs. Wm. T. Councilman, C. Hampson Jones, N. G. Keirle, A. K. Bond, Wm. B. Canfield.

Ophthalmology, Laryngology and Otology.—Drs. Russell Murdock, Hiram Woods, J. H. Hartman, J. W. Humrickhouse, Wm. T. Cathell.

DELEGATES.

American Medical Association at Nashville, Tenn.—I. E. Atkinson, B. B. Browne, T. Barton Brune, John D. Blake, Wilmer Brinton, Samuel C. Chew, E. F. Cordell, J. J. Chisolm, T. B. Evans, Samuel T. Earle, L. M. Eastman, A. Friedenwald,

R. H. Goldsmith, John C. Harris, John C. Hemmeter, Chas. H. Jones, C. C. Jacobs, J. A. Keene, W. F. A. Kemp, T. S. Latimer, Lee J. McComas, R. L. Randolph, David Streett, G. Lane Taneyhill, R. H. Thomas, E. G. Waters, E. R. Walker, Arthur Williams, P. C. Williams, Randolph Winslow, Whitfield Winsey.

DELEGATES TO STATE MEDICAL SOCIETIES.

West Virginia.—L. McLane Tiffany, Geo. H. Rohe, Chas. H. Ohr, H. H. Beidler, J. H. Branham.

Virginia.—I. E. Atkinson, Thomas Opie, James G. Wiltshire, Joseph E. Claggett, H. P. C. Wilson.

North Carolina.—Geo. J. Preston, J. E. Michael, Wm. H. Norris, W. C. Van Bibber, Jno. R. Winslow.

Tenth International Congress at Berlin.—G. Lane Taneyhill, Jno. Whitridge Williams.

To the Pharmacopœial Convention.—E. F. Cordell, I. E. Atkinson, T. B. Brune.

The thanks of the Faculty were tendered the officers, and the President declared the 92d Annual Convention of the Medical and Chirurgical Faculty adjourned *sine die.*

G. LANE TANEYHILL,

Recording Secretary.

REPORTS.

REPORT OF CORRESPONDING SECRETARY.

BALTIMORE, April 22, 1890.

The Medical and Chirurgical Faculty of Maryland:

GENTLEMEN:—Your Corresponding Secretary has the honor to report that he has discharged the duties of his office to the best of his ability, and he trusts it has been done to the satisfaction of the members.

In addition to the usual notices of the meeting inserted in the Baltimore papers and in view of the increased interest in the Faculty throughout the State, it was thought best to give notice of this meeting in some of the State papers outside of the city. Notices were published in the *Kent News, The Hagerstown Mail, The Easton Ledger,* and *The Centreville Observer.* All of which is

Respectfully submitted,

JOSEPH T. SMITH,

Corresponding Secretary.

REPORT OF TREASURER.

Mr. President and Members:—The report from your Treasurer at this, the 92nd Annual Convention of the Medical and Chirurgical Faculty of Maryland, will bear careful analysis by some of our members. It is our painful duty to report a larger deficiency than last year, which is made up of various items, not the least of which is the amount that must be reported as dues from members in arrears—$415.00. It is to be noted that the amount reported as collected this year is $205 less than last. Another factor is the income from rental received from local societies. However, one item which adds $38.69 to our expenses will repay in the near

future. This amount was expended in the interests of the
Semi-Annual Meeting held in Hagerstown during the last
fall. It has already secured the application for membership from fifteen physicians in the counties, and I have the
pleasure to report that they (these fifteen,) have paid their
initiation fee and the Chairman of Board of Examiners for the
Western Shore is ready to report upon them. One more
item I would make prominent. The Library Board has,
during the last year, received all its share of dues from members—the Treasurer having paid to them $569.60 from dues,
and the sales and fines at library amounting to $1.91, making
in all $571.51, which is less than the amount received during
the year ending April 23, 1889. In view of these facts, Mr.
President, I take the liberty to read the following resolutions
adopted three years ago bearing directly upon the rights of
members. They are as follows:

Resolved, That the Treasurer is hereby instructed, annually, until
otherwise ordered, to mail on April 1 a printed statement of indebtedness to all members who are delinquent, stating the year of delinquency, and informing such members that by the Constitution, unless
payment be made before the fourth Tuesday of April, they are temporarily deprived of the privileges of the Faculty, among which are
voting, eligibility to office, and appointment on standing committees,
sections, or as delegates to any convention.

Resolved, That the Treasurer is hereby instructed, annually, until
otherwise ordered, to hand up to the presiding officer at the adjournment of the third day's session a revised list of delinquents, resignations, deaths, and dropped for non-payment of dues, of members, in
order that the President may be enabled to complete a proper list of
appointees for the ensuing year.

The pleasant things are not to be forgotten. The committee appointed three years ago to collect subscriptions to
meet the deficiency remaining from publication of the Medical Annals, have this year paid $70, which was the amount
remaining on subscription reported to the Faculty in 1887,
1888 and 1889.

The Library Board will report its donations and give a
detailed account of its workings. They will mention that
they received the amount just named, $571.51.

Our gains during the year were by acquisition of the following new members: B. M. Hopkinson, Alex. L. Hogden,

Nathan R. Smith, George R. Graham, John D. Blake, Anne L. Kuhn, H. J. Berkley.

Our losses by death were : Chas. O'Donovan, Sr., G. E. Porter, Oscar J. Coskery, and C. Ferdinand Mathieu ; by resignation, F. T. Miles and W. A. Moale ; by non-payment of dues, C. C. McDowall, J. M. Bordley, John Barron, S. W. Free, John R. Quinan and J. M. Williams.

Our receipts and expenditures appear in the following table :

RECEIPTS.

From Initiation Fees,	$ 70 00
Delegates' Fees,	18 00
Rent of Hall and Telephone,	236 50
Advertisements,	75 00
Pharmaceutical Exhibit,	115 00
Amount from Committee on Deficiency,	70 00
Dues of Members,	1,167 00
Sales and Fines at Library,	1 91
	$1,752 91
Deficiency,	231 97
	$1,984 88

DISBURSEMENTS.

By Advertising Ninety-First Annual Convention,	20 10
Chairs for same,	15 00
Janitor for the year,	70 00
Gas, " "	20 50
Incidentals, Ice, Appl. and Pr.,	38 15
Payments to Library Board,	569 60
Sales and Fines at Library to the Library Board,	1 91
Rent of Hall,	600 00
Rent of Telephone,	72 00
Printing Transactions,	324 51
Stamps to mail same,	21 00
Directing and Mailing same,	10 00
Corresponding Secretary,	14 21
Reporting Secretary,	15 00
Commission for Collecting Dues,	27 80
Semi-Annual Meeting at Hagerstown, Md.,	38 69
Treasurer's Expenses,	31 50
Deficiency Reported at Last Convention,	94 91
	$1,984 88

Our assets are shown in the following table :

Amount to Credit Building Fund,	. . . . .	$ 192 00
Library and Fixtures Estimated,	. . . . .	7,500 00
Dues from Members in Arrears,	. . . . .	415 00
Rent from Local Societies,	. . . . .	25 00

In closing this report your Treasurer would mention that he has already received the initiation fees and forwarded the applications of forty-seven candidates for membership at this meeting. This is the result of the work of the Committee on Increasing Membership. Your Treasurer can but fondly indulge the hope that now, as the fee is to be $5, the members will promptly pay, and whilst it is his duty to speak encouragingly of the future, he must say to all such as are in arrears that the old dues of $8 per year are still owing by all who have not paid to the close of the year ending April 21st, 1890.

Respectfully submitted,

W. F. A. KEMP,

Treasurer.

REPORT OF EXECUTIVE COMMITTEE.

Your Committee respectfully report that during the year their duties have been light, little beside the regular routine business of the Faculty having been brought before them for decision.

The Committee authorized the Treasurer to pay the janitor the sum of ten dollars for extra services rendered during the last Annual Convention of the Faculty.

Dr. G. W. Miltenberger, resigned from the Committee on Ethics, and the vacancy was filled by the election of Dr. J. W. Chambers.

Dr. H. Clinton McSherry, resigned the Chairmanship of the Section on Ophthalmology, etc., and C. G. W. McGill, the Chairmanship of the Section on Surgery. The vacancies were filled by the election of Dr. Herbert Harlan and Dr. C. F. Bevan. Drs. McSherry and McGill, were retained as members of their respective sections. The Recording Secretary was authorized to rent the rooms of the Faculty to the Maryland State Veterinary Society, at a rental of fifty dollars per annum.

At the request of Dr. T A. Ashby, Chairman of the Special Committee on Increasing the Membership, the Executive Committee authorized the holding of a Semi-annual Meeting at Hagerstown, and authorized Dr. Ashby to draw on the Treasurer for fifty dollars, or so much thereof as was necessary, to cover the expenses of that meeting. The Committee take great pleasure in stating that this meeting was an unqualified success, and its results calculated to restore the Faculty to its pristine influence; a more extended report of the proceedings at the Semi-Annual Meeting will doubtless be presented during this Convention by the Committee presided over by Dr. Ashby.

At the request of the Baltimore Medical Association, who urged their inability to continue paying the rent they had hitherto paid for the use of the rooms of the Faculty, the Executive Committee reduced the rent to the Association to fifty dollars per annum.

The Committee take great pleasure in announcing that Dr. Joseph Taber Johnson, of Washington, has consented to deliver the annual address at this meeting, upon the subject "Abortion, and its effects."

GEORGE H. ROHE, Chairman.
B. B. BROWNE, M. D.
J. W. CHAMBERS, M. D.
J. EDWIN MICHAEL, M. D.
P. C. WILLIAMS, M. D.
ROBT. T. WILSON, M. D.,
Sec'y to Exc. Committee.

REPORT OF THE BOARD OF EXAMINERS.
WESTERN SHORE.

Mr. President and Members:—The Board of Examiners for Western Shore have considered the applications of the following named members of the medical profession, and recommend their election.   The names of the applicants have, in accordance with the constitutional provision been placed on the bulletin board.   This list of 72 names is the largest, we understand, that has ever in the history of the society now nearly a hundred years old—been presented ; we are informed by friends of candidates that many other names will be offered each day of the convention.   The Society, more especially the *Committee on Increase of Membership*, may well be congratulated on this consummation which has long been devoutly wished; and the Examining Board makes no invidious distinction when it acknowledges what a majority of the members are aware of, namely, that the most indefatigable worker among those who have brought about this welcome "increase in the family," is Dr. Thomas A. Ashby.

The names of the candidates hereby offered are as follows :—

L. F. Ankrim, Robert Bond, S. B. Bond, J. B. Baxley, Jr., Joseph Blum, W. S. Blaisdell, F. C. Bressler, C. Birnie, J. E. Bromwell, H. J.Coffroth, Frank M. Chisolm, J. H. Christian, W. P. Chunn, J. M. Craighill, M. A. R. F. Carr, R. G. Davis, G. E. Dickinson, J. W. Funk, Geo. A. Flemming, Jno. S. Fulton, Harry Friedenwald, A. B. Giles, Isabel K. Godfrey, N. R. Gorter, E. C. Gibbs, H. H. Goodman, H. B. Gwynn, W. S. Gardner, J. M. Hundley, J. W. Humrickhouse, H. S. Herman, W. F. Hines, H. L. Hilgartner, E. M. Hartwell, C. Hampson Jones, C. C. Jacobs, J. T. King, N. G. Keirle, S. A. Keene, W. F. Lockwood, A. S. Mason, A. H. Mann, Jr., C. O. Miller, S. K. Merrick, Russell Murdock, W. E. Mosely, Wm. H. Norris, H. C. Ohle, Wm. Osler, J. J. Pennington, J. E. Prichard, Hunter Robb, O. H. W. Ragan, M. Rowe, R. L. Randolph, J. B. Saunders, J. M. Spear, Norman B. Scott, John McP. Scott, Alan P. Smith, Jno. T. Spicknall, W. D. Thomas, W. J. Todd, J. G. Van Marter, Jr., W. W. Virdin, Hiram Woods, Jr., Mactier Warfield, E. R. Walker, R. B. Warfield, E. J. Williams, J. Jones Wilson, Charles B. Ziegler.

All of which is respectfully submitted,

SAMUEL C. CHEW, M. D.,

Chairman.

REPORT OF THE LIBRARY COMMITTEE.

Mr. President and Gentlemen of the Faculty :—The Library Committee has the honor to report that it organized, and elected Dr. Wm. B. Canfield, Secretary; Dr. A. K. Bond was re-elected Librarian on June 1st, Dr. H. R. Winchester was elected Assistant Librarian, we were enabled by this means to keep the Library open from 12 M., to 7 P. M., daily, three hours longer than formerly, and we are gratified to find that this new departure has given such general satisfaction to those members of the Faculty who make constant use of the Library.

As a portion of the Librarian's salary is paid out of the funds derived from the Nurses Directory independent of the amount ($46) which was turned into the Library fund, we may state that nearly the whole amount paid as salary to the Assistant Librarian, was received from the Nurses Directory.

The number of volumes in the Library at the last Annual Report was 6474.

During the current year 246 volumes have been received, making the total number on our shelves on the 31st day of March, 1890, 6720. Of this number we are indebted to Dr. A. Atkinson, for one, Dr. I. E. Atkinson, 3; Dr. W. B. Canfield 11; Dr. T. B. Brune 1; Dr. Frank Donaldson 1; Dr. B. B. Browne 29.

One hundred volumes of journals have been bound during the present year, and 1 volume (Heisters Surgery) rebound.

One hundred journals are received and placed upon the tables.

Collections of journals and pamphlets have been presented by Drs. Christopher Johnson, I. E. Atkinson, E. F. Cordell, Jos. G. Wiltshire, Wm. B. Canfield, Randolph Winslow and B. B. Browne.

Nine portraits of eminent medical men have been presented by Dr. Robert T. Wilson.

We have received in exchange from the University of Erlanger 118 Theses; University of Giessen 24 Theses; University of Goettingen 26 Theses; University of Strasburg 73

Theses. The weekly Health Reports of Baltimore City have heen regularly received.

All volumes in the Library of a later date than 1870, have been arranged in separate cases, so as to be more readily examined by members.

A table has been provided, upon which are placed certain interesting ancient books.

A box has been placed in the Library for the purpose of receiving such suggestions as members my wish to make to the Library Committee.

A large number of valuable monographs and reprints have been carefully arranged and indexed for ready reference.

The following new books have been purchased out of the Library Fund.

Transactions American Gynecological Society, 1889.

Billing's Medical Dictionary, 2 Vols.

Lawson Tait Dis. Women, Vol. 1.

Loomis' Practice of Medicine.

Payne's Pathology.

The Committee would offer the following suggestions :

1st. That more shelf room be provided for the Library.

2nd. That members be urged to send to the Library, monthly collections of current journals which they do not desire to keep : in this way a useful duplicate series of journals might be formed.

3rd. That the fines be made the same for all journals and for all bound volumes without reference to size. There is no reason why a larger fine should be attached to a folio of little value than to a duodecimo of great value.

The funds placed at the disposal of the Committee were as follows:

One-half dues as required by Constitution.

Received from the previous Committe,   - $ 8.66

   "   "   "   Treasurer,   -   -   -   569.60

   "   "   "   as fines and dues,   1.91

   "   "   "   Nurses Directory,   -   -   46.00

                                         $626.17

The expenses have been   -   -   -   -   622.12

Leaving a balance of   -   -   -   -   - $4.05

The Registrar's Report on the Nurses' Directory is appended.

All of which is respectfully submitted,

B. B. BROWNE, M. D., Chairman.

T. B. BRUNE, M. D.

W. H. WELCH, M. D.

G. LANE TANEYHILL, M. D.

W. B. CANFIELD, M. D.

REPORT ON THE NURSES DIRECTORY.

To the Library Committee :

GENTLEMEN :—The Directory for Nurses has now upon its roll 46 nurses, 5 male and 41 female. Four of these (one male and three female,) devote themselves entirely to massage. It will be observed that the roll is considerably smaller than that given last year. This does not indicate a decline in the usefulness of the Directory, but rather a decided improvement, as no nurses have been retained on the list except such as are worthy of perfect reliance and are willing to conform accurately to the rules. Only a few of the nurses who " picked up " their knowledge of nursing are retained, and these, only when strongly recommended by our most careful practitioners.

Of the 42 nurses (excluding massage) 24 have received training in good hospitals, and 3 others have taken lectures upon nursing, 6 have received certificates from the Maternite, and 2 from the Free Lying-In Hospital of this city. Several hold diplomas from reputable Training Schools. As one object of the Directory is to raise the standard of nursing in this State, it is interesting to note that during the last three years, more than 12 young nurses trained in hospital, have by the aid of the Directory, established themselves here. These are among the most intelligent, capable and attractive nurses in the city.

That all calls for nurses have not been successfully met is due, not to any fault in the Directory, but to the fact that no school for training " general and surgical " nurses has been graduating nurses in Baltimore.

When the new schools lately established begin to send out graduates into the community, an increase in our registry may be expected. The "massage" service in the past year has been very satisfactory. Ignorant "rubbers" have been carefully excluded from it.

In conclusion, it may be stated that there are indications of increased confidence in and appreciation of the work of the Directory among both physicians and laymen. The falling off in the receipts for the year is due to the fact that the demand for nurses was very slight during part of the year, and greater than could be met during the rest of it. The following is the financial exhibit:

Total Receipts, - - - - - - - - - $137.19
General expenses, $31.19. Salary $60.00, - - - - 91.19
Balance turned over to Library Committee, - - - $46.00

Respectfully,
A. K. BOND, M. D.,
Registrar.

REPORT OF PUBLICATION COMMITTEE.

Mr. President and Members :—Your Committee of Publication, at its first meeting, in May, 1889, elected Dr. C. O'Donovan, Jr., as Secretary, and contracted with Mr. John B. Kurtz to publish the regular number of *Transactions*—500—which, although delayed by the fact that several members were tardy in returning their proofs, were issued early in October, 1889.

Copies were mailed to all of the State Medical Associations and to many libraries and medical journals throughout the world, resulting in an increase of our very valuable "exchange list."

The Transactions of 1889 as a volume, compared favorably with its predecessors, and the demand for extra copies and for re-prints evinced the popularity of our publication. This popularity could be readily increased were your Publication Committee not hampered with the vexatious experience of being compelled to wait on those few negligent and thoughtless authors who retain both manuscript and proof an indefinite time. It is self evident that the sooner our Transactions are published after the adjournment of the Convention, the more popular will they be. Some State Associations, Georgia for instance, will not allow a paper to be read by title or otherwise at its Conventions until a complete copy shall have been placed in the hands of the Secretary for publication in the Transactions. Your Committee will not, on this occasion, ask that similar legislation be enacted in Maryland, but express the earnest hope that their laudable efforts be heartily and cordially aided in the coming year by prompt responses by authors when requested to return proof.

All of which is respectfully submitted,

G. LANE TANEYHILL, M. D., Chairman.
W. F. A. KEMP, M. D.,
GEO. H. ROHE, M. D.,
RANDOLPH WINSLOW, M. D.,
C. O'DONOVAN, Jr., M. D.

REPORT OF MEMOIR COMMITTEE.

Memoir of Oscar J. Coskery, M. D.

Dr. Oscar J. Coskery was born in Baltimore, March 23rd, 1843, the son of a well-known physician. Having attended several private schools, he entered the University of Maryland, where he obtained his medical degree in 1865. He rendered service in the medical department at Fortress Monroe and Hampton, Va., before his graduation. In March, 1865, he was an Acting Assistant Surgeon, and from April to September of the same year Assistant Surgeon, U. S. Volunteers. After that he returned to Baltimore and entered on practice. In 1870 St. Joseph's Hospital was established in the eastern section of the city by the Sisters of St. Francis, and he became its first medical officer. He always took great interest in the work of this institution, with which he was connected for twelve years. In 1873 he was elected Professor of Surgery in the College of Physicians and Surgeons of this city, but resigned the position after one session. In 1876 he was re-elected to the same chair and retained it from that time up to the period of his death. For several years prior to the latter event he suffered from a laryngeal affection, accompanied by frequent slight hemorrhages. Occasionally his cough and hoarseness compelled him to abandon lecturing for a time. He at last succumbed to pulmonary tuberculosis, on the 5th of July, 1889, at the age of forty-six.

Dr. Coskery was small in stature, with light hair and blue eyes. He was a hard student and an enthusiastic devotee to his profession. He possessed a quick mind and a remarkably retentive memory. He allied himself particularly with the English school of surgery, and exhibited a strong tendency to conservatism. He spoke rapidly, but never inconsiderately. His papers were prepared with care and exhibited evidences of a painstaking and judicious sifting of his experience. As a lecturer he is described as being systematic, luminous and practical. He was a warm friend, a devoted husband and kind father, a consistent member of the Roman Catholic Communion, a sympathetic and devoted physician. His death took place at St. Joseph's Hospital, whither he had been moved in order to escape the noise on Calvert street, where he resided. It seemed appropriate that he should thus end his days in the institution, to whose success he had devoted so large a share of his professional life.

Dr. Coskery was a frequent contributor to the medical journals and to the Transactions of this Society. Many of us remember with a sad interest his last appearance, one year ago, at our Annual Meeting, when, with hoarse voice and labored breathing, but with an eye undimmed in lustre and a bosom swelling with just pride, he told us how he had trephined the skull of a patient and evacuated a collection of pus, whose presence and position were only ascertainable by a careful study and correct interpretation of symptoms, based upon the laws of cerebral localization.

Memoir of G. Ellis Porter, M. D.

Dr. G. Ellis Porter was born near Frostburg, Md., July 9th, 1830. He was a descendant of John Porter, of Gloucestershire, England, and was one of fifteen children. He received his early education at Tyrone, Penna., and at the academies at Uniontown and Connellsville. He began the study of medicine with Dr. James M. Porter, of Frostburg, Md., in 1848, with whom he remained eighteen months. Having studied also a short time with Dr. L. Lindley, of Connellsville, Penna., he entered Jefferson Medical College, where he remained three years, receiving his diploma in 1853. His first practice was in association with his former teacher and relative, Dr. J. M. Porter. In 1856 he went to Lonaconing, Allegany County, Maryland, the field mainly of his future life and labors. Here he built up a large practice, having no opposition up to the beginning of the war. In the struggle between the North and South he took strong sides with the former, and made the opening speech at a mass-meeting held at Lonaconing in response to President Lincoln's call for men. A company was raised, of which he was elected captain. He was appointed major when the Second Maryland Potomac Home Brigade was organized, and in 1862 was promoted to a lieutenant-colonelcy. In 1864 he was appointed Assistant and Post Surgeon in charge of the Hospital at Cumberland. After the close of the war he returned to Lonaconing and resumed practice. For the last two years of his life he was in bad health from some spinal affection, but the immediate cause of his death was typhoid fever. He died December 30th, 1889, aged fifty-nine. Dr. Porter paid especial attention to surgery, and being located in the midst of the coal-mining region of Maryland, he had a large experience in this branch of his profession. He published several articles relating to it in the *Medical and Surgical Reporter*, of Philadelphia. He was President of the Allegany County Medical Society in 1876, and Vice-President of this Faculty in 1880. He always took an active part in politics, and was elected to the State Legislature in 1871. He was a member of the Masonic Order, Independent Order of Odd Fellows, and Knights of Honor. He was also an earnest member of the Presbyterian church. He had a well stocked library of the best books, and was a man of fine literary tastes. He left a widow and three children. His remains were interred in the family vault at Frostburg.

Memoir of Ferdinand C. Mathieu, M. D.

Dr. Ferdinand C. Mathieu was born in Salingen, Prussia, and studied medicine at the Universities of Bonn and Wurzburg, graduating at the latter. He came to Baltimore in 1870, and here acquired a large practice among the German-speaking population. He died at his residence in East Baltimore, on the 7th of January, 1890, after a three days' illness, from pneumonia, in the 42nd year of his age, leaving a wife and five children.

———

In Memoriam of Dr. Charles O'Donovan.
By W. T. Howard, M. D.

Dr. Charles O'Donovan was born in Baltimore on September 20th, 1829, and died December 23d, 1889. He was the oldest of three sons of Dr. John H. O'Donovan, for many years one of the leading physicians of this city. In his early years Dr. O'Donovan attended the school of Michael Power, one of the last and most famous of the old-time Irish school masters, whose curriculum was thoroughly classic, and who believed that the rod should not be spared. It was here that Dr. O'Donovan laid the solid foundation of that thorough education which stood him in good stead later in life.

That he was a faithful student is proven by many tokens from his master, always inscribed, "Presented to his respected pupil, Charles O'Donovan, by Michael Power," an honor that was rarely bestowed. From this training school he went next to St. Mary's College, on Paca street, now the Seminary of St. Sulpice, but at that time one of the very few seats of learning about Baltimore, and the one having by far the highest reputation.

His record there was marked by close application and by brilliant success in all the branches taught.

It was not the intention of Dr. O'Donovan's father that he should study medicine, and Charles, before the completion of his course at St. Mary's, was compelled to give up studies most congenial to him and to enter a store in preparation for a mercantile life. Here he remained until 1848, constantly fretting at the minor details of a distasteful occupation, and longing to get back to his studies, with a view of ultimately studying medicine. In two years he had completed his course, and graduated with distinction, being the valedictorian of his class. He entered at once at the University of Maryland School of Medicine, giving close attention to his studies, and living, for a part of the course, in the Hospital, at a time when the life of a resident student was no sinecure, Baltimore's great surgeon, Dr. N. R. Smith, being in the habit of going through the wards at 6 A. M. every day, and requiring many things that students now neglect. From this institution Dr. O'Donovan received his diploma, in 1853, and entered at once into regular practice with his father. From the commencement of the work he gave his life to it, never allowing any pleasure to seduce him from the strict performance of his duty to his patients, caring nothing for his own comfort so that they should be relieved, happy and contented. Thus he labored uneventfully until February 3rd. 1859, when he married Henrietta, the youngest daughter of Hugh Jenkins, the head of the house of Hugh Jenkins & Co., whose coffee fleet were regular packets between Baltimore and the Brazilian ports. Of this union were born four sons and three daughters, of whom all survive except one son.

Broussais said: "The real physician is the one who cures; the observation which does not teach the art of healing is not that of a physician, it is that of a naturalist."

As a physician Dr. O'Donovan had, in a marked degree, the necessary faculty of observing nature—he was a naturalist. But the mere naturalist is of little worth either in the relief of suffering or the cure of disease. From habits of thought and action, he looks upon the animated human being endowed with all the warm sympathies and important relations and duties of life, as the anatomist looks upon the dead body —only as an object of scientific examination and analysis. Dr. O'Donovan was a naturalist in the highest and truest sense, in that he keenly observed nature in all its phases. But he was much more. He was an intelligent, practical physician and a tender, earnest, sympathizing friend in the

families of this city, rich and poor, to which, in daily minis-
trations, his large business called him, and which he attended
with equal assiduity and fidelity. The mere scientist was
there lost in the prompt and efficient use of known truths
and remedies, and of those happy expedients, indeed, often
for which there may be no remembered or recorded experience, but which, in some men, amid the sufferings, the emergencies and the responsibilities of the bed-side, seem to be
the inspiration of difficulty and the genius of success. If it
were possible, in contemplation, to separate the good physician from the good man, we should find in Dr. O'Donovan
personal qualities of the highest order and of the most attractive kind. He was upright and honorable in all his dealings
with his fellow-man ; he was generous and charitable to a
degree ; he was true to his friends ; he was manly and faithful
in the performance of every duty ; he was genial by nature,
and kind and affable to all ; he was a gentleman in all respects,
and especially in his professional relations and conduct, an
essential necessity always, grown, unfortunately, into a distinction. He was an earnest and devoted christian, and over
the whole career, alike of the physician and the man, shone
the pervading illumination of an honest faith, exemplified in
an honest life. Such a man was an honor, not only to his
profession, but to the community in which he lived, and long
will his loss be deplored with sincere sorrow, and his memory
be cherished with affectionate regard and admiration.

All of which is respectfully submitted,

EUGENE F. CORDELL,
Chairman.

REPORT OF SPECIAL COMMITTEE ON UNOFFICIAL PREPARATIONS.

BALTIMORE, April 22, 1890.

Mr. President and Fellow Members:—The Committee to
whom was referred " *The National Formulary of Unofficial
Preparations,*" beg leave to make the following report :

The work in question, a copy of which has been placed in the hands of the Committee for examination, was prepared by an editing Committee of the American Pharmaceutical Association, enlarged by the addition of one member from every State Pharmaceutical Association in the United States and Canada. Its object is to supply standard formulæ for a large number of medicinal agents, not represented in the United States Pharmacopœia, but in constant use by physicians all over the country. Many of these preparations are of great value and very popular with the profession, and it is in the highest degree desirable that some standard should be decided on for their preparation, in order that they may be uniform, and their composition well known. At present, a druggist has often to keep a dozen forms of the same agent when one would suffice. We may name one agent pepsin— *not yet introduced into the Pharmacopœia,* but contained in this work, as showing the need of such a standard as is here attempted.

To quote from the Formulary:

"The mission which this work is to fulfill can only be properly accomplished by the co-operation of the medical profession. It is, therefore, of the greatest importance that the members of this profession, throughout the country, be made acquainted with the existence, contents and objects of this book, and that, if the same be approved by them, as is confidently expected, they will consent to accept the preparations made in accordance with the formulæ contained therein, instead of designating any special maker's product." The American Pharmaceutical Association now turns the work over to the medical profession, and asks that it shall be sanctioned by the various medical bodies throughout the country. Being satisfied of the need and expediency of such a work, and having as far as we have been able to examine that before us, been satisfied that this fulfills the requirements, we recommend that the Medical and Chirurgical Faculty of Maryland, do endorse and approve of "The National Formulary of Unofficial Preparations," and that the Secretary of the American Pharmaceutical Association be informed of this action. We may add that we find that the work has been introduced entire into the last edition of the United States Dispensatory.

Respectfully,

EUGENE F. CORDELL, M. D.,

Chairman, for the Committee.

REPORT OF COMMITTEE ON INCREASING THE MEMBERSHIP.

Mr. President and Members :—The Committee on Membership, in submitting a report of its work during the past year, is greatly encouraged by the results which have been obtained.

Early in October a circular was prepared and mailed to over 1500 physicians in this State. This circular recited the claims of the Faculty upon the profession of Maryland, and urged the importance of larger membership and more thorough interest in the purposes of the organization.

Acting under the instructions of the Faculty, arrangements were made for a Semi-Annual Meeting in Hagerstown, and a Sub-Committee acting under this Committee, took the matter in charge and successfully conducted the meeting. A programme of the scientific work arranged for the Hagerstown meeting, was published and widely distributed throughout the State, and to the journals throughout the country. In this way the meeting was thoroughly advertised.

The profession of Washington county, and of Western Maryland, heartily and energetically took up the matter and extended a most cordial and hospitable welcome to the members of the Faculty in attendance.

The Semi-Annual Meeting was in this manner, made an assured success, and its results are now apparent to all, not only were a large number of new members received through this meeting, among the physicians of Western Maryland, but interest and enthusiasm were aroused in the purposes of the Faculty, which are pregnant with lasting good to the organization. The profession of Hagerstown and Washing-ton county, not only received the Faculty with open arms, so to speak, but realizing the benefit of organization and professional corporations, organized a local medical society, which is now on the road to efficient and permanent work

The meeting at Hagerstown, demonstrated most conclu-sively to your Committee, that the Semi-Annual Meeting is a most important feature of this organization, and should be perpetuated at every hazard. As a means of enlisting the interest of the profession of the State in the work of this Faculty, it is simply indispensable. It presents the most ample opportunity for communication and intercourse be-tween the profession of the state and of the city, by bringing them together upon terms of self interest and of individual contact. Good will then result to the country practitioner and to his city brother by a better understanding and appre-ciation of their respective points of culture and professional training. Both classes will be stimulated to better work and to more harmonious action in professional organizations. Your Committee has been gratified with the generous re-sponse which has followed the action of the Faculty in low-ering its membership fee and annual dues. Over one hun-dred new members will be added to the Faculty's roll-call during the present year through this liberal action.

These new members not only represent many of the younger members of the profession, but many veterans in service. A more creditable addition to the strength of the Faculty, both in intelligence and in high standing, could not be made with-out diminishing the resources of the Faculty, its policy draws to its support a most valuable ally of new recruits. Nor will this work end here, your Committee is fully persuaded that if the liberal policy the Faculty has inaugurated of go-ing after the profession of the state, and of interesting the many worthy men, not now members, in the purposes and aims of this state organization, in less than five years its membership will embrace the larger portion of the most re-spectable physicians in Maryland in its ranks. Instead of 300 members, the Faculty will have a membership of 1200 out of the 2000 physicians engaged in the active practice of medicine in the State.

If such a culmination of things is not to be desired, let those speak who can show its undesirability, but if this Faculty is in the right path and in the pursuit of its highest objects in this work of organization, then let it follow up its present advantage and move ahead in this valuable work.

Your Committee would therefore recommend a continuation of a Committee on Membership, not in present composition, but in form and purpose, that this work may go on during the ensuing year. It is the unanimous verdict of this Committee that the Semi-Annual Meeting should be held during the coming month of November, in one of the larger cities of the Eastern Shore, subject to the selection of the Committee, and that an appropriation of fifty dollars should be made to defray the expenses of this meeting and such other work as the Committee may inaugurate in the execution of its plans.

All of which is respectfully submitted,

T. A. ASHBY, M. D., Chairman.
WILLIAM LEE, M. D.
THOMAS B. EVANS, M. D.
SAM'L T. EARLE, M. D.
CHAS. H. JONES, M. D.

PRESIDENT'S ADDRESS.

THE MODERN HOSPITAL.

By Aaron Friedenwald, M. D.,

Professor Ophthalmology, College Physicians and Surgeons of
Baltimore.

I have selected for the subject of the address which I have
the honor to deliver on this occasion, "*The Modern Hospital.*"
It has suggested itself to me in contemplating the significance
of the two new hospitals which have been established in this
city since last we met.

The Johns Hopkins Hospital, which had been in process
of construction quite a number of years, and whose completion the profession and the public were anxiously looking
forward to, was opened on the seventh day of May, 1889,
and has since then been in successful operation. The New
City Hospital, occupying the site of the City Spring, on Calvert street, was formally opened on the 23rd day of December, 1889. The acquisition of these two hospitals has marked
a great advance in the history of Baltimore in regard to its
humane institutions. The work that has been done by them
has amply demonstrated how greatly they were needed. The
former, the consummation of a most munificent foundation,
has shown to what successful results large sums may be devoted in the study of the most approved plans in hospital
construction, while the latter called into being by a religious
order, beginning its work without any means, has taught how
much can be accomplished with a comparatively moderate
amount of money by a judicious and economical plan of
building. Both institutions have taught most valuable lessons, which will surely be utilized in the building of hospitals
hereafter in our city, (for it is safe to predict that it will not
be so very long before others will be needed,) as well as in
others that will be erected elsewhere. With the progress in

the science of hospital construction, the methods will undoubtedly become more and more simplified. Much has already been accomplished in this respect, and no small amount has been contributed by the experience in military hospitals in our own country during the civil war.

In speaking of the "Modern Hospital" we must have before our mind's eye the hospitals in our time which have fulfilled or which will fulfill the full demands of the most advanced knowledge of Hygiene, and which will at the same time exhibit a simplicity of construction which will enable them to be administered on an economical basis. Furthermore, it should be fully expected that the best medical attention should be furnished to those suffering from disease and seeking relief within their walls. Important as the conditions just referred to are to the modern hospital, an efficient humane nursing is being more and more looked to as a factor in the successful management of these institutions. And lastly the patient who enters such a hospital should be spared the mortification of possibly being looked upon as a common pauper when his needy condition is due to his illness alone. In a word, the modern hospital should offer bountifully all that is made possible by an advanced science and by a refined humanity.

The hospital has a much older history than it is commonly credited with. When we consult this history we learn that it has not emanated from any single civilization. In times remote and in lands far distant from each other when, as is generally supposed, barbarism had considerable supremacy, the hospital was not unknown. The civilization which has done most to develop the hospital, to perfect its methods and to extend its usefulness, cannot claim to have originated it. While it must be accorded to christianity that the hospitals as they existed through these many centuries owed their existence to its influences, it is but due to recognize that in still earlier times there were peoples differing greatly from each other in faith, not knowing each other, who saw the helplessness of the sick, felt for them and provided places in which they could be cared for.

In a book, the Mahawanso, edited by George Turnour, (Ceylon, 1837, vol. 1, p. 66 to 196,) we find recorded that King Pandukabhayo, who reigned in Ceylon 437 B. C., founded a hospital in his capital city, Anaradhapura, beside other sanitary establishments. His successor, Dutthagamini, who died 137 B. C., had a list of his benevolent acts read at his death, in which there is enumerated : "I have constantly maintained hospitals at eighteen different places and supplied medicines through medical practitioners."

The Hindoos provided hospitals not only for man but also for animals. 1.

In a collection of heroic poems "Shah Nameh" on the ancient histories of Persia, it is stated that from the earliest times the fire worshipers were obliged in accordance with their laws to supply suitable establishments for their indigent sick, and that the King was in duty bound to provide gratuitously the best medical treatment for the inmates. 2.

The origin of the hospital has been traced as far back as the temples of Aesculapius, at Titanus, 1134 B. C. In alluding to this Dr. John Watson, in his "Anniversary Discourse before the New York Academy of Medicine," says : "As asylums these temples bore no inapt resemblance to the hospitals and infirmaries of modern times, into which some of them were ultimately converted. The temples of Aesculapius, Cos and Tricca, according to Strabo, were always filled with patients and along their walls were suspended the tablets upon which were recorded the history and treatment of the individual cases of disease."

The oldest Buddhist accounts of hospitals in the inscriptions of Piyadasis or Acokas, reach to the middle of the third century B. C. According to Virchow it is probable that the first larger christian hospitals which developed in Asia Minor and Persia own their origin somewhat to Buddhist influence, for Buddhism pushed forward to the west at an early date and at the beginning of the christian era had already reached Kabul and Bacterien. 3. The edicts of Buddhism in regard

1. Alexander Burns, Journ. of the Royal Asiatic Soc., 1834, No. 1, p. 96.
2. Hospitals Boylston Prize Essay of Harvard Univ., 1876, by W. Gill Wylie, M. D.
3. Virchow, Ueber Hospitales and Lazarette, Berlin, 1869.

to hospitals were cut upon rocks during the reign of Asoko, who died 226 years B. C. One of these bearing the date of 220 B. C., can be read to-day. It enjoins that hospitals shall be established on the highways of travel, and that they shall be provided with medicines and instruments and skillful physicians at the expense of the State. 4.

The Spaniards found on their arrival in Mexico that the Aztec civilization had amply provided for the treatment of the sick and for the care of disabled soldiers in hospitals in their principal cities. 5.

According to these data we are forced to conclude that the hospital had been regarded as a public necessity, that human suffering had received that warm sympathy which provided means for its relief among many nations, long before the time we were wont to believe that the hospital had had its beginning. It is quite probable that the methods of these ancient institutions were so crude that although inaugurated by the holiest sentiments they did as much harm as good. We are to some extent warranted in assuming this when we contemplate the fearful mortality which stands against the account of hospitals of even a much later date. The hospitals in Europe had a most varied development. We have found that the hospitals of the Hindoos and Persians had their origin in religion, so did these owe their existence to the Church.

In the early centuries, pilgrims began to direct their way toward Jerusalem. About the middle of the seventh century, near the time that the Orient inaugurated its pilgrimage to Mecca and Medina, thousands undertook pious journeys from France, England and Germany to Rome. On all the roads leading to that city provision was made to extend shelter and food to these wayworn travelers. At every monastery, near many mountain passes and in the vicinity of the larger bridges crossing impassable streams, houses were erected in which these strangers were hospitably received. These houses were under the management of religious orders. They were too limited in their capacity to offer any pro-

---

4. Hospitals, by W. Gill Wylie, M. D.
5. Prescott, Conquest of Mexico, vol. 1, p. 48.

longed residence to those who sought their shelter, and were therefore not intended for the sick and in exceptional cases only did these obtain admission. It is fair to assume however that they had much to do in offering the incentive to the erection of hospitals in later times.

But long before this period hospitals had been established. They were spoken of "in the Council of Nice, A. D. 325, as institutions well known and deserving support and encouragement." 6. Although we find no mention of any special hospital existing at this time in Europe the language quoted above is conclusive in this regard. The Hotel Dieu in Lyons was established in 542 by Childebert I, at the instance of the Archbishop of Sacerdos. 7 This hospital was also termed Xenodochium, and was under the supervision of laymen, but was transferred to the care of the clergy six hundred years afterward.

The rage of leprosy, which continued up to the fifteenth century, must be regarded as a most potent factor in promoting the growth of hospitals. The condition of its unfortunate victims was most pitiable. Not only did they suffer from the effect of the disease, the most dreaded of all of that time, but besides the cruelties inflicted upon them by the disease itself they had to submit to cruelties from their fellowmen. The diseased were removed from the home of man, excluded from religious assemblies and completely ostracized in every way. But finally there was mercy in store for them too. Men imbued with religious spirit began to care for the unfortunate ones. Prominent among these was the Bishop of Cæsarea, who built a town of small homes before the gates of the city for the reception and care of the sick of all kinds, not excluding those suffering with leprosy. These establishments warmed up the spirit of benevolence, which led to the organization of similar institutions all over Christendom till these were counted by thousands. They had been instituted in large numbers in the south and west of Germany in the seventh and eighth centuries. At an early date, possibly even before the crusades an order of knights was

6. Dr. Toners Contributions to the Annals of Progress in Medicine.
7. C. F. Heusinger, Ein Beitrag zur ältesten Geschichte der Krankeuhauser im Occidente.

organized, originally consisting exclusively of lepers, the
Knights of St. Lazare, whose object it was to care for lepers
and subdue the unbelievers. Called to Europe by Louis
VII of France, in 1149, the order established a large number
of leper-houses, which subsequently became known as Lazarettos. The order reached Germany by way of Hungary.
Eventually this order did not escape proscription and could
only maintain a foothold for itself in Savoy. It still continues
there, enjoying the highest esteem, and still charging itself
with the care of lepers. 8. When the scourge had nearly
reached its extinction in the middle of the sixteenth century,
the leper-houses lost their significance. Many were converted into institutions for the care of the aged and infirm,
and a few continued as hospitals. The term Lazarettos was
subsequently often employed to designate hospitals devoted
to the care of those suffering from contagious diseases.

During this time there were but few cities of importance in
Europe that had not a hospital of some kind. A great many
of them have been forgotten. They had but a local interest,
often ended their careers and left no record for future
times.

The Hotel Dieu, of Paris, was founded about the year
600, somewhat more than half a century later than its name-
sake in Lyons. It is probably the oldest hospital in Europe
now in use.

In England the first institution for the care of the sick was
established by Lanfranc, Archbishop of Canterbury, in the
year 1070.

In regard to the more important hospitals of Germany,
Berlin seems to have acquired them before any other city,
the Hospital of the Holy Ghost and St. George's Hospital
having been erected in 1070 and 1208 respectively.

The famous hospital at Milan, with a capacity for over
2,000 patients, was opened in 1456, and is still used for its
original purpose, and is regarded as a remarkable building at
the present time.

---

8. Cibrario Precis historique des ordres Religieuse et Militaires de St. Lazare, et de
St. Maurice et apres leur reunion. Lyon, 1860, p. 10.

It is rather surprising, when we consider the fact that war had been almost incessant, to find no account or provision being made for military hospitals prior to nearly the close of the sixteenth century. A hospital established through the influence of Ambrose Pare, at the siege of Metz, in 1575, seems to have been the pioneer in this class of humane institutions. 9. Indeed previous to the time of this great surgeon there seems to be no evidence that surgeons were considered necessary to military organization. An English author, describing the disregard of sick and wounded soldiers in the British army as late as the 16th century, states that "the poorer soldiers, when seriously wounded, were discharged with a small gratuity, to find their way home as best they might, a fact founded on the economical principle that it costs more to cure a soldier than to levy a new recruit." 10. In connection with the early development of hospitals, a brief allusion to what took place in America may not be uninteresting. Quebec is credited with having had the first hospital after this continent was settled by Europeans. It is said that a small hospital was established in that city as early as 1339. 11. In 1658, a hospital [consisting of five houses in 1679,] was organized on Manhattan Island for the benefit of sick soldiers and for the West India Company's negroes. 12.

Among the notable acts of Benjamin Franklin, it stands to his credit to have lent a helping hand to Dr. Thomas Bond, who originated the movement, the outcome of which was the Pennsylvania Hospital. This hospital obtained its charter in 1751, used temporary buildings till 1759, and completed the present building in 1805. We may judge of its importance in early times by the fact that 435 patients were admitted into it in 1775. The New York Hospital was destroyed in 1775, when it had hardly been completed. It was first built mainly through the exertions of Dr. Samuel Bard and Dr. John Jones, professors in the medical school of King's College. It was rebuilt in 1791.

9. On the Establishment of Army Hospitals, by Edward A. Crane, M. D.
10. Sir L. D. Scott's "British Army."
11. J. Beeknan, Centennial Address, N. Y. Hosp., 1871.

Hospitals have largely been found very deficient, both in their construction and in the mode of their administration regarding the sanitary requirements of the sick, hygiene being quite a new science.

It has been reserved for our time to give a more due consideration to guarding the sick against the danger which in addition to their disease they may be exposed to from these sources in the institution in which they seek relief. The conditions which created the demands for hospitals in their early development in Europe were of so urgent a nature and the distress of those seeking them was so great that any place seemed good enough for their reception.

Beside the humane spirit which provided the hospital for the benefit of the unfortunate ones, they served to no small extent the purpose of pest houses, to which communities looked for safety from infection. These fears were very often well grounded, very often they rested on superstition alone. How much the sick would injure one another when crowded together in unsuitable building did not apparently attract much attention. The old methods were not questioned at all for a very long time. At last, though, light began to break in. Men began to inquire whether the fearful death-rate of these institutions was due to the character of the diseases which .prevailed there and therefore unavoidable or whether there was not something by which the sick were surrounded which intensified their diseases and increased their dangers. Reference to a bit of history in connection with the Hotel Dieu in Paris in the 18th century will furnish an appalling account. The following spectacle is described as having been presented in that institution during this period. Two or three patients afflicted with small pox, or several surgical cases, or four women in the parturient state were assigned to *one* bed. A large proportion of the beds were made at that time expressly to afford room for four patients and sometimes as high a number as six were packed in one. In the Salle St. Charles and Salle St. Antoine there were 139 beds for four patients each, (many of which contained six,) and only 38 beds intended for one person each. The law forbade the hospital authorities to refuse admission to any one, without regard to the number that might already have been received. There is no acconnt of such crowding together of the sick in England, but there was sufficient to have caused a disastrous amount of erysipelas, hospital gangrene, and surgical fever,—and puerperal fever up to a very recent time. The same story would have to be told of the hospitals of Germany and of other countries.

Although warning voices were raised against this state of things about the middle of the 18th century and the great importance of allowing ample breathing space and of providing for proper ventilation had been advocated, it took a full century before these points received practical consideration in hospital construction. Boerhaave taught early in the 18th century and dwelt forcibly on the vitiation of the air in hospitals where many patients were crowded together, and on the value of securing an ample supply of fresh air for the sick and wounded. 13. Among his pupils there were four who did good service in suggesting improvements in the sanitary management of military hospitals; they were Sir John Pringle, Gerard Van Swieter, Donald Munro and Richard Brocklesby.

Among the earliest writings on hospital reform we find the valuable contribution of Dr. Jno. Jones whose name has already been mentioned in connection with the origin of the New York Hospital. In a work published in 1775 entitled "Plain Concise Practical Remarks on the Treatment of Wounds and Fractures," he added a short Appendix on Camp and Military Hospitals. Dr. W. Gill Wylie commenting on the advanced views presented in this book, says that "they antedate by more than ten years any other publication we have been able to find." The terrible death rate experienced by the French and British armies during the Crimean War was the impetus to secure the first great advance in the methods of constructing hospitals for the sick and wounded. Michael Leyy, sanitary inspector of the French army in the Crimea, proposed in 1854 simple wooden barracks raised from the ground and provided with ridge ventilation. 14. It

13 W. Gill Wylie Hospital, p 27.
14. Report of the proceedings of the Sanitary Commission dispatched to the seat of War in the Rast, 1855 and 56.

was in the good work growing out of the experience of the Crimean War that the name of Florence Nightingale has been immortalized.

The valuable knowledge that was gained from the observations of that period was practically and most successfully applied in the grand hospital system that was organized during the late civil war. From this time onward it has been the constant concern of those connected with the management of hospitals everywhere to improve their construction and to get rid in every way of the dangers that have heretofore beset their inmates. Statistics have been studied carefully and quite valuable conclusions have been reached. Sir James Simpson has shown that the deaths from amputation in the various London hospitals ranged from 36 to 47 per cent., while the same operations in country practice gave a death rate of only 18 per cent.

St. Bartholomew's Hospital,	366 deaths per 1000	
London Hospital, Whitechapel,	473	" "
Guy's Hospital,	382	" "
St. Thomas' Hospital,	388	" "
Nine London Hospitals,	411	" "
Royal Infirmary, Edinb.	'433	" "
" " Glasgow,	391	" "
Eleven Large Metropol. Hospitals,	' 410	" "

The statistics furnished from Lying-in Hospitals show similar results. Dr. Lefort collected statistics of 888,302 cases delivered in lying-in asylums and of 934,781 attended at home ; the deductions from these are that in hospitals 35 per 1000 die, while at home there are only 4¾ deaths to the 1000.

Baron Meydell, chief of the sanitary department of St. Petersburg has found that in the larger lying-in hospitals in which 2000 women are confined yearly, there is a death rate of 40 per cent. in those in which 1000 are delivered only 25 in 1000 die ; in institutions in which 400 are attended not more than 20 in 1000 die and in small hospitals having from 2 to 3 beds of which there are 11 in different parts of the city, giving accommodation to 1600 cases only 9 in 1000 die, while those confined in their homes including the poorest and most wretched, show a mortality of only 5 in 1000. 15.

The additional danger which surgical cases and women in the lying-in state encountered on entering a hospital was long recognized. There seemed to be no remedy for this, especially in the case of the poor who were driven by their need for help into these institutions. Hospitals were simply regarded in connection with these cases as necessary evils. As astute an observer and as high an authority as Virchow in every thing that relates to medical science said,—as late as 1861. "We know that in many cases hospitals increase the danger of the condition of those consigned to their care, and it should be made the object of practical science to limit their use as much as is possible, especially in the treatment of the wounded and of those in the lying-in state." 16. The simple wooden barracks which were adopted as offering the best form for military hospitals, during the late civil war, demonstrated conclusively the great advantage of a plentiful supply of fresh air in the hospital ward. These buildings were so arranged that every individual ward was a building standing by itself, so that the light and the air could not be readily excluded. It was this experience which first put the pavilion system that had already been adopted in Hospital Laraboisiere in Paris to a most extensive test and from which it has grown more and more in favor. In the construction of hospitals to-day, whether the pavilion system is adhered to or not,—the primary precaution for the benefit of the sick, satisfactory ventilation and perfect drainage are not likely to be neglected. Any dereliction in this regard, in the light of our present knowledge cannot be regarded but as culpable. Much however as may be justly claimed for the introduction of scientific ventilation in the modern hospital it is principally through Antisepsis that the advanced character of the modern hospital has been attained. It is not long since the surgeon before performing an operation or assuming charge of the wounded was more or less haunted by the additional

15. Report du Congress International d Hygiene et de Gauvage, Brussels 1876 vol. 1, p 226.
16. Ueber den Fortschritt in der Eutwickelung der Humanttats anstalten, Versamlung Deutscher Natur forscher und Aerzte 1861. xxxv.

danger the patient incurred on entering a hospital which were ascribable to the direct hospital influences, and not seldom would he persuade the patient to be treated in a more favorable environment. Antisepsis has changed this radically and now the hospital is regarded as the safest place where the more important surgical cases can be cared for. In regard to the treatment of lying-in women antisepsis has proved an equal if not a still greater blessing. Puerperal fever which was the terror of the institutions into which these patients were received, and to check the spread of which our art had proved utterly powerless, is fast vanishing and from all recent appearances will occur much more seldom in these institutions than in private practice. The statistics of the Vienna lying-in department will fully justify this assertion. During the year 1823 there was a mortality of $7\frac{1}{2}$ per cent. which gradually rose till it reached a death rate of 15 per cent.; in 1842 every 6th or 7th case in this department died of puerperal fever. The reform which Semmelweis suggested was introduced in 1847, and the mortality was reduced to 1-3 per cent. Under the precautions enforced by recent methods of antisepsis the rate of mortality fell to $\frac{3}{4}$ per cent. in 1882 and since this time it has been claimed that the disease has almost entirely disappeared. In the new Hospital of Prague the death rate has been reduced to less than $\frac{1}{4}$ per cent.

The hospital of to-day under these changed circumstances makes quite a different impression upon the general public than in former days, when it partook more or less, whether it continued to bear the name or not, of the character of the Lazaretto. Heretofore it was to a great extent made use of only by those who either having no homes of their own, or being destitute of the means which might have secured for them the proper treatment elsewhere had no choice left. It is now pretty well known that there are many conditions in which a patient can be better provided for in a hospital than in his own home. Persons in moderate circumstances, would often be prevented in cases requiring special skill, of obtaining the best treatment, unless they could enter a properly equipped hospital either at a small cost or gratuitously.

The humane character of the hospital has been greatly enlarged for it is not now restricted in its beneficence to those in abject poverty.

There is one important factor entering in the combination which makes up the character of the modern hospital which is asserting itself more and more every day. The very best administration, the most faithful and skilled medical staff can provide but for a part of the requirements of such an institution. The patient needs beside all that these can offer,—the services of a kind, an efficient, an intelligent, a faithful nurse. To be qualified for such a service demands primarily a devotion to the calling. No other motive would be strong enough to yield the self sacrifice which its duties exact. Religious orders have long provided for this want. The noble work which the good women have accomplished, who having renounced the pleasures of this world under religious vows to devote their lives to the service of the sick, embraces a record of heroism which at once challenges our admiration and our gratitude. The good sisters who have been the pioneers in this humane work, will certainly not be the last to accept the improved methods which a new experience may develop in the service to which they have consecrated their lives. In recent years a class of refined and intelligent, women not bound by vows but inspired by the most humane sentiment have entered into the service of the sick. Schools have been established in connection with hospitals, which have afforded them the means of acquiring the theoretical knowledge and the practical experience necessary for such a vocation. This has at once proved a new blessing in the service of the modern hospital and given dignity to a calling which too often has been regarded as of a servile character. We may now begin to hope that the day is past when the kind offices to the sick will be entrusted to the ignorant or unfeeling nurse who has no interest in the work but in the wages that it brings,—nor to the convalescent who is expected to render some service for the benefit which he has received.

It is highly gratifying to notice the increasing liberal and humane spirit that both our city and our state have lately manifested in the conception of their duty towards the indigent sick. There was a time when the consciences of the authorities was fully satisfied with the service that was done for them in the city and county alms houses, far as these fall short of hospital requirements. It has at last been acknowledged in a substantial manner by the appropriations that have been made, that the city and the state have a duty towards those who need help, but do not deserve to be placed on a level with the common pauper.

ANNUAL ADDRESS.

ABORTION AND ITS EFFECTS,

BY JOSEPH TABER JOHNSON, A. M., M. D., PH. D.,

OF WASHINGTON, D. C.

Professor of Gynæcology, University of Georgetown, &c.

Mr. President and Members of the Medical and Chirurgical Faculty of the State of Maryland.

It will be difficult for me to interest the members of this ancient and honorable Faculty, especially after such men as Billings, Wier Mitchell, Goodell, Osler and Welch have entertained and instructed you by their eloquence and wisdom.

Statistics of libraries and museums, the vagaries of the nervous system, the dangers and duties of the hour, the infectiousness of disease, and the license to practice, are all subjects which are full of interest and have been ably presented. I presume the committee expected me as a gynæcologist to discuss some topic in this branch of medicine or in abdominal surgery, and I fully intended to do so, but when I began to write it occurred to me that only a small proportion of the membership of a State Society would be especially interested in a special topic, and I shall therefore make no apology for introducing a subject which—though not of a very savory odor, yet, is of great interest to every member of the profession whether he be a specialist or a general practitioner—young or old—professor or student. I shall ask your attention, then, without further preface or delay to *The importance, the alarming frequency, the wickedness*, and to some of the *effects of procured abortion.*

All writers upon obstetrics and gynæcology admit and deplore the frequency with which the immature fœtus is expelled from the uterus.

The importance of the subject is proven by the attention given to it and to its effects, in our text-books. Thomas has an entire volume upon abortion now in press, and soon to be published, the advance sheets of which I have been kindly allowed to read. Writers upon domestic economy, upon vital statistics, upon the natural increase and decrease of our population, upon law, theology and medicine, all vie with each other in attesting the importance and wickedness of forced abortion, and all so far as they mention this point agree that it has not only been distressingly frequent in the past, but that it has been steadily upon the increase.

So much do I believe this to be the case—and so far reaching are its effects upon the health and morals of our people, that I hazard nothing when I declare that this subject is *one* of the most, if not *the* most important question before our profession to-day.—Questions of drainage, sewage—quarantine—vaccination—antiseptics, are all important in the prevention of disease, and have doubtless saved thousands of lives, but they all sink into insignificence in comparison with the importance of the subject under discussion. I believe that statistics might be adduced if time, and your patience would permit, to show conclusively that more lives are annually sacrificed by the unnecessary and intentional destruction of the human fœtus than are saved by all these agencies combined.

The recognized and described causes of abortion show that it occurs once to every five labors, and that 90 per cent. of all married women have at least one miscarriage during their childbearing life.—These are frequent enough to excite the sympathy and invoke the aid of the profession, in their prevention so far as possible—but I refer now more especially to that larger class, where there is a violent and premature expulsion of the product of conception, independent of its age, viability or normal formation, where it is artificially induced and intentional, and where it is not necessary for the safety of the mother and would not otherwise have occurred.— Some of the legislatures of our older States have been so alarmed at the lessening of their population that they have appointed committees to investigate into the causes thereof, and Dr. Nathan Allan, of Mass., in his report upon this subject, said, "that the native American stock of that State seemed to be dying out."—He mentions small towns and cities where the only increase in the population was among those of recent foreign origin, and that in those cities and districts mostly populated by native American families, there were recorded more deaths than births. That one hundred years ago it was rare to see families of less than six children and frequently there were ten—now it is rare to find as many as three, and often only one or none at all.

Grave apprehension was expressed in this report made more than twenty years ago, for the results which seemed sure to follow.

These results have been more than realized in that State. These foreign children have become of age and are now voters.

The same influences have been at work during this generation as in the last in an increased ratio, and to-day the proud city of the puritans, cultured Boston, has become almost, if not quite an Irish and a Catholic city, rejoicing in the possession of a mayor by the classic name of O'Brien. So long ago as 1857, the American Medical Association became aroused on this subject, and at its meeting in Nashville in that year, appointed a committee of eight prominent and able men to report upon criminal abortion, with a view to its general supression. A report was made in May of the next year at Louisville, which with the resolutions accompanying it, were unanimously adopted. At a subsequent meeting, a popular prize essay was authorized by the Association in which the wickedness of the crime should be set forth, its frequency condemned, and its injurious effects fully explained ·so that any woman could easily understand. The essay accepted was written by Dr. H. R. Storer, of Boston, and was entitled, "Why not, or a book for every woman." A very large number were printed, and were placed for sale in the book stores throughout the length and breadth of the land.

Medical, secular and religious journals commented favorably upon the essay, and the frequency and criminality of abortion was clearly set forth, and its perpetrators were severely denounced. I have thus far and from official testimony endeavored to show the importance of my subject, and the views which were held by the highest Medical body in the land upon its importance, and the great need which existed over thirty years ago for its suppression. It has also been shown that at last two States in our Union had become so alarmed over the decrease in the American element of their population, that legislative action was taken for its discovery and prevention.—Very interesting and instructive reading may be found in the reports of Dr. Nathan Allan, of Lowell, and Dr. Snow, of Providence, upon this subject.—From the same sources which proved to Dr. Storer and the American Medical Association, the frequency of this crime we can now gather greatly increased and multiplied testimony that this wanton, unnatural, unnecessary and basely wicked destruction of fœtal life has not only not been suppressed in obedience to unanimously passed resolutions, but that it constantly has been, and is now, largely upon the increase in our country, and for that matter throughout the entire civilized world. This crime is not indigenous to any location, section, climate or continent. Its perpetration is as world wide as are its murderous and otherwise injurious effects upon those engaged in this unholy warfare. Storer showed in 1866, from indisputable evidence, that abortion and still births were twelve times more frequent in some of our cities than the worst statistics had ever shown to exist in Paris or Vienna. From the same reasoning we cannot believe that a better condition exists in those cities now, on the contrary, we are forced to the conviction that unnecessary abortions are made to occur in a greatly increased ratio, and that the country districts, usually the most pure and upright in their morals, are not far behind the cities in proportion to their population, in their destruction of fœtal life. American families have not increased in size, and no facts exist to prove that the fecundity of men and women has in any way been lessened by the advances in christian civilization.

The evidence of physicians could be adduced if necessary to demonstrate these facts.—Vital statistics might be quoted to show that in the true American stock in some parts of our country, the ratio of deaths over the births has steadily increased.—The published number of maternal deaths from this malpractice does not appear to be decreasing. •

The arrests and trials for abortion while they may in a very faint degree, indicate its frequency, do on the other hand, and in a very emphatic manner demonstrate the laxity of morals and the law, in permitting so many of the guilty to escape their just punishment.—The obstacles to conviction, the difficulties of proof, the inefficiency of the law as well as the evident lack of a strong desire to convict on the part of all those engaged in these trials. may explain the fact, "that of the thirty-two arrests and trials of abortionists, reported by the Attorney General of the State of Mass., in a period of eight years, not one single conviction resulted." Englemann, says, "Abortionists every where are known—In the larger cities of this continent as well as Europe, they achieve a wide spread fame—are well known, and yet rarely, if ever convicted. It is a notorious fact that these worst of criminals almost invariably escape, and even in the States of Germany, where the laws are strict and rigidly enforced, where the crime of abortion is punished by imprisonment of from four to twenty years, that eminent teacher of medical jurisprudence, J. L. Caspar, says that "of all the many accused, never a one was condemned, and in no one case was the crime proven." They are sheltered by the words of the law and the sympathy of the community."* In many cases the arrest and trial is not for the crime intended. The intention is—and of a necessity must always be, to kill the fœtus ; this being done in the dark like other deeds of evil, there are no witnesses, and the crime usually escapes public notice, unless a bungler in the art, should at the time injure or destroy the mother also.—There is little or no trouble in securing conviction then, for malpractice—but the indignation of the virtuous public—and the majesty of violated law are only then aroused and invoked because the unskilful manipulator killed two human beings instead of one.—It is for the crime against the mother which

*Article on Abortion, Peper's System of Medicine.

was not intended, but which unfortunately and accidentally happened that the criminal is brought to trial.

A story is told of a wicked and unjust judge in the early days of the wild and woolly west, who in pronouncing sentence upon a man proven guilty of seduction—a crime which is the twin sister to abortion, stated to him that it was not so much for committing the wicked deed that he sentenced him to hard labor in the common jail, but it was for allowing himself to be caught in the act, and making so much public scandal and family exposure.

Another reason given by Storer in his book before referred to, for his belief in the frequency of abortion is the pecuniary success of known abortionists and of the venders of abortion producing nostrums, and again, the experience of physicians, on account of direct and frequent applications made to them to commit this crime, and in the immediate and multitudenous after effects which they see in their daily practice, upon its unhappy victims.

The evidences from these quarters, if they were convincing twenty years ago, have surely lost none of their force and convincing qualities with the lapse of time.

The public advertisements of known abortionists in our news papers and some religious journals, are more public and more numerous now than they were then, and the public display and ready sale of abortion producing nostrums by our druggists is confessedly upon the increase.

A generation ago these facts were all so fully and completely proven by the able committee of the American Medical Association, and set forth in popular language in its prize essay for distribution among the women of our land—that no effort was ever publicly made to gainsay or disprove any of the positions taken.—They were all admitted and deplored— the effect for a time was salutary—and its author received letters innumerable from good people, and from mothers made happy by the possession of healthy offspring, whose habit it had previously been to resort to abortion.

The public conscience was aroused and quickened, and the promoters of the move in the Association no doubt congratulated themselves, that they had accomplished a great good for society and the State, for morals, law and religion.— Secular, medical and religious journals approved, clergymen preached, and a sense of security probably settled down upon the virtuous public, that another growing evil had been boldly met, the battle against it successfully waged and the victory won; but the sequel in this generation proves that it was no more of a victory than was gained over his creditors by the impecunious Micawber, when he gave them his note of hand, and thanked the Lord that his *debts* were *paid*.

There is no longer any doubt from a consideration of all evidences before relied upon to prove its frequency, that abortion is now fully as frequent as it ever was in this country, and that it is alarmingly on the increase; not only is this believed to be true of the cities, but the remotest country districts seem to be affected also.

The excuses given are the same now as then—and the wickedness of the act, is, and always will be the same.—In one respect our otherwise noble profession is sadly at fault; it has not acted up to the courage of its convictions.

Of a necessity it must be, and I believe that it is unanimous in the knowledge and belief that the fœtus is just as much alive at one period of its intra uterine existence as another. It must be alive or dead all the time—if alive, it is just as much a crime to kill it in the first month of pregnancy as in the ninth month, or after it is born. Our text-books all teach, and our profession holds that the spark of life is infused at conception, and we must believe with Percival, that "to extinguish this first spark of life is a crime of the same nature both against our Maker, and society as to destroy an infant, a child or man."

Many otherwise good and exemplary women who would rather part with their right hands, or let their tongues cleave to the roof of their mouths than to commit a crime, seem to believe that prior to quickening, it is no more harm to cause the evacuation of the contents of their wombs, than it is that of their bladders or their bowels.—The law itself is largely upon their side in this most important question.—The penalties affixed to this crime being slight before quickening and vastly insufficient afterwards.—Before a woman is quick with child, abortion being considered simply as a misdemeanor, after quickening as a felony, and only is the child considered sufficiently alive to be killed, in the eye of law which ought to protect it, when it has been entirely born, and is separated from its mother and living an independent existence.

The experience of every physician is that good women as well as bad are committing this wrong in utter ignorance of the fact that it is a crime. They will boldly argue the question and will fully admit its wickedness after they can feel the motion of the child. They condemn its destruction as a cruel murder after quickening, and would no more be guilty of embruing their fair hands in its innocent blood, after they could feel it move, than they would be accessory to the destruction of their living children. The fault of our professsion is that this belief exists at all. If we really believe in accordance with the evidence and teaching of our science that the fœtus is alive before quickening, it must be our fault if this dense ignorance longer exists in the minds of our people, and that it so hinders the proper and just administration of the law. If the child is alive as we believe and teach in the first, second and third months of pregnancy just as much as it is, in seventh, eighth and ninth, then its destruction must be as wicked in one month as another. If the murder of an unarmed man in the dark and behind his back is deemed by all good people as a dastardly and cowardly act, and if the murder of innocent and unprotected children is loudly denounced the world over, what language can be sufficient to express our disapprobation and contempt for those heartless and soulless miscreants, who are in the most wholesale and cowardly manner killing countless numbers of children, who are not even protected by the law. Those who are engaged in the wicked perpetration of abortion should no longer be able to shield their crimes behind this cloak of real or pretended ignorance.

There is no household in the land or in the civilized world which is not more or less permeated by the influence and teaching of the noble science which we practice, and this ignorance of the law of life, or of the fact of life before quickening, could, if we were sufficiently alive to its importance, be utterly done away with, and wiped off the face of the earth, in a single year.

Otherwise good women would no longer boast of the number of fœtuses they had "gotten rid of"—and they would no longer teach their sisters how they could accomplish the same "innocent" feat,—when it is known and universally acknowledged that to extinguish the first spark of human life is a crime of the same nature, both against our Maker and society, as it is to destroy an infant, a child or a man—then and not until then, will abortion cease to be a common occurrence, and good men and women become ready to assume the responsibility of their own deliberate acts. The luxuries of life—the demands of fashionable society, the dislike of children—the expense of their maintenance and education, questions of taste—indolence—and convenience, can no longer be pleaded as an excuse for the committal of a cowardly, dirty, contemptible, bloody and wholly unnatural crime.

When wholesome laws are enacted and enforced, which will punish not only the principals, but all the aiders and abettors and accessories to this crime, the same as they do other murders, then its commission will be confined to those who, to carry out their wicked purposes are willing to defy any and all laws in spite of the disastrous consequences which they invite and invoke to follow—lawyers and judges need enlightenment upon this subject as well as women. They should learn that we do not, and cannot discriminate between one month and another when the fœtus is more or less alive, that quickening amounts to nothing—we all know that some women quicken as early as three, or three and one half months, and others not until six—and some not at all, and who will arise and say that in these late cases of quickening, the fœtus is not just as much alive as in the early ones, and just as much entitled to the protection of the law. That life is not infused at quickening we are all agreed. The fœtus then being as much alive before quickening as after, the popular belief and convenient ignorance on this point, it becomes the

duty of our profession to correct.   The pregnant woman receives a great many *hints* as the signs and symptoms accumu-
late and corroborate each other, that a live and growing
fœtus is developing in her uterus, but she now waits for a decided kick before she will believe that the fœtus is alive.
This kick is waited for anxiously by the woman as well as
the law, to announce that the child is sufficiently formed for
its destruction to constitute even a misdemeanor.   It must
kick very decidedly and unmistakably for several months
before its killing constitutes a felony, and as some judges
have held, should it be knocked on the head with a hammer,
or strangled with ribbons after its head is born, but before it
is wholly delivered and separated from its mother, it is not
sufficiently alive in the eye of the law for its killing to constitute murder.

Having drawn attention to the importance, frequency and
wickedness of procured abortion, I beg in conclusion to remind you of some of its effects upon the morals and the physical well being of those engaged in this nefarious practice.
By those who in their hearts consider it wrong to destroy the
unborn child, there must be an undermining of the moral
nature, which will show its effects in many other directions
than the one under discussion.   But of this phase of the subject I will leave others to speak.   In one respect however, it
deeply concerns us as well as its unhappy victims.

The remorse which comes to some, over the killing of their
unborn children, occasionally develops into melancholia and
in suicide or terminates in the madhouse.   Many a woman
has lost her life by the addition of this depressing element to
the slighter forms of septicæmia following a procured abortion.

Thus Tardiew reports that of 116 cases of criminal abortion, collected by himself in Paris, 60 died outright, and
many had a lingering convalescence, while out of 234 cases of
abortion occurring from various causes and treated by Physicians in the Rotunda Hospital in Dublin, only one died—and
the cause of death in her case, was from mitral disease of the
heart.   Lusk in his classic work on obstetrics, says that
death in consequence of criminal abortion is especially fre-

quent. Yet of the many cases who enter Bellview Hospital for treatment, whose histories he has found in the record books of the hospital, all have ended in recovery. Cases of induced abortion in their desire to avoid notice and publicity, frequently fail to properly care for themselves, they get up and about too soon, while the uterus is still large and heavy and thereby lay the foundation for future suffering and the life of an invalid.

Hirst in Mann's System of Obstetrics, p. 316, says, "criminal abortions with the additional risks of septicæmia from the unskilful use of instruments, and the probability of infection from unclean hands and implements, would show a surprisingly high rate of mortality, if it were possible to collect accurate statistics—which for obvious reasons it is impossible to do."

Again, Engelmann says, "woman requires skilled aid in labor, the physiological termination of pregnancy; more necessary still is this in the premature pathological interruption of this condition in abortion."

Benninger reported 21 cases of tetanus following abortion in the British Gynæcological Journal in 1888.

Charpentier, in his great work, published three years ago, says, "the prognosis of abortion for the mother is grave— for even if life is rarely compromised, health frequently is ;" He adds further, that "the prognosis is most unfavorable in cases where the miscarriage is the result of criminal manipulations."

The American Editor of this work says in a note, "miscarriage is fraught with more danger to the woman than labor at term—because as Goodell aptly puts it, the process is like plucking immature fruit."

The occurrence of abortion takes the uterus at a disadvantage. It is immature—it is not ready to expel its contents— Its contracting powers are not developed, and its contractions are imperfect after, as well as before, the act.

The membranes are especially adherent and frequently, if not always, some portion of them is retained after the premature expulsion of the embryo. The decidua is soft, enlarged and its bulky remains easily form the nidus for the development of germs for the future production of septicæmia or memorrhagia.

Traumatism is frequently present, inviting the absorption of septic germs, and if blood poisoning in a grave form is fortunately escaped, cellulitis,—salpingitis, ovarian or pelvic abscess is liable to develop.

Subinvolution and its resulting increased size and weight of the uterus often makes the life of the woman a burden from the endometritis, salpingitis—endocervicitis and the various uterine displacements which naturally follow as a painful train of symptoms. These are all rendered more probable from the embarrassing necessity for keeping up appearances and diverting attention and suspicion from their real cause.

These effects of abortion when it occurs from natural causes and when treated by skilful physicians, are difficult enough to avert—and are only prevented by rest in bed, good nursing and continued and careful preventative measures; when they occur however, as they so often do, in boarding houses and hotels, and among those women who desire great secrecy to avoid exposure and shame, these attentions are either not sought or permitted. The mental state added to the physical condition has proved too great a strain for many an erring woman.

Remorse of conscience has been the last straw which has driven some of these unhappy victims of their own error and folly to suicide or insanity, convalescence is generally prolonged from these causes and the patient has many weeks and perhaps months, if not years of invalidism, in which to regret the error of an illspent hour.

The free dispensaries and charity hospitals afford innumerable examples of broken constitutions and ruined lives, which have had their sad beginning in an improperly treated abortion.

It is the usual explanation given by a majority of the frequenters of the gynæcological clinic that the displacement or inflammation of the uterus for which the sufferer applies for relief, that her symptoms dated back to an abortion, three, five, or ten years ago.

Many of the cases now operated on for otherwise incurable pus tubes, or chronic inflammatory disease of the ovaries, date all their troubles back to a neglected abortion. These sufferings are not all confined to the charity patients in the lower walks of life. They are as common as is the custom of abortion itself; no one rank in society appropriates them all.

The experience of gynæcologists the world over will confirm the statement, that a majority of the patients that we are called upon to treat in our offices, or in the fine residences of their fair owners, are the outcome of abortions or of the preventative measures used against conception.

This latter subject was fully exposed and discussed not long ago by a distinguished writer and teacher from a neighboring city, in an address upon "the danger and duties of the hour" before this body and upon this platform.

This discussion of my subject forms a very appropriate appendix to his masterly oration, and my chief regret is that your Committee selected no better man to bring before you the danger and duties of the hour, so far as they relate to this still more important subject.

It is an every day occurrence for ladies to consult busy gynæcologists in our larger cities in regard to symptoms which upon inquiry, are found to date back to an unfortunate abortion.

It would be quite within the limits of truth were I to state that two-thirds of the work of the gynæcologists of this age finds its chief cause in the evils discussed upon this platform by Dr. Goodell and myself. It is a sad commentary upon the christian civilization of the age—but the experience of honest workers in this department of our science, I believe would corroborate the truth of this saddening statement.

Our sadness however is somewhat lessened when we are able to state also that the causes which we lament are among those which are demonstrated as preventable. If many err through ignorance, we may here find a glorious opportunity for the exercise of the law of prevention.

Much has been said of late of the greater mission of our science in the prevention than in the cure of disease.

How can a better field of labor be found than in the direction I have indicated. Where and how can medical men save more lives or prevent more suffering than by teaching women the dangers of abortion, and thus saving their bodies and perhaps their souls from ruin in this life and the life to come. In this exercise of our great mission we may be sure of the approval of our own consciences, of the co-operation of the Great Physician in the prevention of much sin and sorrow, and of the final judgment of "well done thou good and faithful servant."

Report of the Section on Surgery.

HYDATID CYST OF THE LIVER (SUPPURATIVE.) OPERATION, AND RECOVERY OF PATIENT.

By Charles F. Bevan, M. D., *Chairman.*

A casual reading of the standard text-books leaves one with the impression that hydatid cysts are rather of common occurrence. It is true none of the authorities express in figures or percentages, the frequency with which the affection is encountered ; and yet almost all alike speak of it as though the malady were an everyday affair. That the disease is of more frequent occurrence in some countries than in others there can be no doubt. In Iceland, Australia, and in some parts of Germany, it seems to be met with rather frequently, while in this country it is of very rare occurrence. The examination of more than 300 bodies, personally conducted, failed to reveal a single example. The records of the College of Physicians and Surgeon's dissecting room, over 1,500 examinations and the post mortem records of the City Hospital, 250 more, make no mention of the malady.

Osler, *Am. Jour. Med. Sci.*, Vol. 84, 1882, collected the records of 61 cases from museums, journals, transactions and private sources. He says, "Unfortunately we cannot say positively how many of these cases were truly American, *i. e.*, originated here, and how many were imported, but in 16 it is stated that the patients were Europeans. In the majority the nationality was not given, but in all probability at least one-third of the cases were imported, leaving only about 40 cases."

The rarity of the affection and the satisfactory result of the treatment justify me in calling your attention, therefore, to the following case.

Case.—Fred. Bersenbruch, a native of Oldenberg, Germany, 44 years of age; occupation, farmer; a resident of this country for the past eight years; was admitted to the City Hospital, October 25th, 1889, He gave the following account of himself: Has been working on a farm, and for several months has been clearing the land of stones, many of which he carried for some distance, bearing the weight against his right side. In March of 1889, he was seized suddenly with pain in the right side, back of the abdomen and chest. This pain, at first acute, subsided in a few days, without treatment. In May, a swelling was noticed by him in the right hypochon-driac region, which has since increased in size and become painful on pressure. From this time on to the date of his admission to the hospital, there has been a slow but progress-ive loss of weight, until now he is more than 40 pounds below his average weight. Disturbance of the digestive organs, vomiting, constipation, diarrhœa and dysentery, he reports as being of frequent occurrence. In July, he was taken with chills and fever, and was confined to bed for two weeks.

Examination showed a tall, cadaveric looking man, of sallow complexion, much emaciated and great feebleness. Digestive organs in fair condition. Kidneys good; pulse 80; respiration 28, shallow, coarse, and fine mucous rales over both lungs; temperature 97° F.; weight 125 pounds; abdomen much enlarged—a tumor apparently of the liver, smooth, elastic, with an obscure sense of fluctuation. The following measurements will give some idea of the altera-tion:

I.   Level of the 6th rib (in front:) right side, 19 inches; left, 17⅝ inches.

II. Level with apex of ensiform cartilage; right, 20¼; left, 18 inches.

III. Level with a point midway between ensiform cartil-age and umbilicus. Right side, 19¾ inches; left, 16¼ inches.

Dullness extends to the right nipple above, and below to within 1 inch of a horizontal line drawn through the umbilicus. In the median line, dullness extends below to within 1¼ inches of the umbilicus, and from the point upwards 3¾ inches. The area of dullness does not reach the left mammary line. The ribs are much bulged out. The swelling transmits the voice on auscultation, and vocal fremitus is clearly felt on palpation. A slight pleuritic friction sound is made out at the upper limit of the tumor on the right side. A hypodermic needle was plunged into the most prominent part of the tumor, and through it a few drops of pus were withdrawn.

October 26th, had a chill; temperature 102° F., pulse 120.

October 27th, temperature, 8.30 A. M., 98° F. 3 P. M., slight chill; temperature 103° F.

From this date to the time of operation the morning temperature would be slightly above normal, 99°--100° F., with a chill and evening rise of temperature to 102°--103½° F., the febrile condition lasting throughout the night.

On November 1st, 1889, under chloroform, with full antiseptic precaution, though done in the amphitheatre, the aspirator was introduced into the most prominent portion of the tumor. Only about one ounce of purulent matter was withdrawn, when the fluid was found to choke up the needle. This fluid, under the microscope, showed an abundance of the hooklets so characteristic of the echinococcus. An incision was now made some 3 or 4 inches long; to the right of the rectus muscle, obliquely downwards and outwards. When the peritoneum was reached it was found to be non-adherent to the liver. Accordingly, iodoform gauze was packed into the wound, absorbent cotton and a bandage applied, and the patient was put back in bed. Four days later, under chloroform, the dressings were removed. Satisfactory adhesions had been produced and an incision 3½ inches long was made into the liver and into the cyst, evacuating 1½ gallons of purulent fluid. The fluid contained myriads of transparent globules, varying in size from a pea to that of a small orange. When the sack had been well emptied, I thoroughly scraped with my hand the whole interior of the cavity, which extended to the right as far as the posterior border of the liver,

and to the left nearly as far as the end of the left lobe. The
cavity was then thoroughly washed out with a hot bichloride
solution 1--5000, a large drainage tube was inserted and the
edges of the cyst were then stitched to the skin and the remainder of the wound closed up around the tube. The
patient, more dead than alive, was then placed in bed, and
surrounded by hot bottles, etc. Reaction occurred in a few
hours. For three days the temperature remained normal,
but it rose to 101° F. on the fourth day, at which time the
dressings were removed, the cavity washed out with a warm
carbolized solution, and the patient was redressed. The
stitches were removed on the eighth and tenth days.

November 28th and 30th, the temperature reached 100° F.,
but fell at once to normal, on carefully washing the cavity.
During December, his convalescence was rather slow, his
digestive powers feeble and cough very troublesome. January 12th, 1890, he had an attack of the grippe, temperature
reaching 104° F., and slowly dropping to 99° F. The attack
decidedly aggravated the bronchial catarrh which had been
so annoying, and by January 20th, a circumscribed pneumonia of the lower part of the right lung was clearly made
out. He was able to be out of bed by the first of February,
and has slowly but steadily improved. The cavity has greatly
diminished, and now holds less than half an ounce (3 drachms.)
He has gained 21 pounds, walks everywhere he pleases, and
is desirous of resuming his occupation on the farm.

History.—Hydatid disease has been more or less under
observation from the earliest of medical times. Hippocrates
describes certain tumors, watery in character, which modern
writers accept as referring to the echinococcus. "The echinococcus," says Heller, (Ziemssen, Cyclop., Vol. III, p. 557,)
"was, however, first recognized in 1766. In 1782. Pastor
Groze discovered that the scolices were tape-worm heads."

The relationship between the echinococcus hominis and
the tænia echinococcus of the dog has been very extensively
studied and proven by experiment. Kuchenmeister, von
Siebold, von Beneden and Leuckart, in 1852, have shown
this in the most convincing manner.

The tænia echinococcus seems to be one of the parasites infecting the intestinal canal of the dog, and indeed of the whole genus canis, with great frequency.

The echinococcus, which is merely the larval state of the tænia echinococcus, is voided with the animal's dejecta, and falls upon the ground. It may find its way into running water, springs, etc., and from such a source obtain the easiest mode of access into the stomach; or, if deposited on vegetable matter, cabbage, lettuce, celery, etc., these foods, unless thoroughly cleansed, may become the carriers of the larva to the body.

When within the alimentary canal of man, the embryo begins a process of migration, and from the intestinal tract may wander to any part of the body. Every organ of the body, bones and muscles has been recorded as invaded by them. By far the largest number of cases occur in the liver. Bocker (Dissert. inaug., Berlin, 1868,) found the echinococcus 33 times amongst 4,760 dissections made at the Berlin Pathological Institute; 19 times in 3,042 males, 14 times in 1,718 females; and of these 33 cases, 27 were found in the liver alone, or in the liver and other organs together. The ductus communis choledoches is believed to afford the most direct and easiest route to the liver.

Pathology and Symptoms.—When the echinococcus reaches an organ, it begins the process of development, and may ultimately attain very large proportions. In those affecting the liver, the rapidity of growth depends somewhat on the depth at which they are situated. Rarely indeed are they found on the surface of the organ. Tait, whose operative experience is larger than that of any one else, makes the emphatic statement that the cyst "is always embedded in the substance of the liver, and to reach the cyst considerable thickness of the liver tissue has generally to be gone through. The tissue of the cyst is in immediate contact with the liver tissue, which it excavates into a form and shape to suit itself" (*Edinburgh Medical Journal*, 1889, p. 408.) As with most other tumors the general direction of growth is toward that in which the resistance is least. The displacement of relations to neighboring organs is often extreme. The increase in size of the growth, while not rapid, is believed to be continuous. The tumor may spontaneously cease to grow, and retrograde changes take place, or by an external injury, as a blow on the abdomen, or by ulceration into a bile duct, the death of the parasite may be produced *Pepper's System*, Vol. II, p. 1103.

Hydatid tumors of the liver are usually described as being smooth, of irregular outline or contour, and highly elastic. By palpation, the sign called hydatid purring, which is simply the transmission of an external impulse through the various large and small daughter cysts to the hand, may be elicited. This sign was not present in the case here reported, though carefully looked for. The purring or vibration has been considered as pathognomonic. I have noted, however, quite a number of instances in which observers call attention to the fact of its absence. The most important and satisfactory diagnostic sign may be obtained by the use of the aspirator and the discovery in the fluid withdrawn of the characteristic hooklets of the scolex. In fact, the aspirator is about the only really reliable method at our disposal for diagnostic purposes. Hydatid tumors of the liver give rise to no pathognomonic signs. Their presence may be suspected in such cases as tend to enlarge in the direction of the diaphragm, when by the ordinary methods, pleural effusions are excluded and the enlargement is clearly referable to the liver ; or when the growth extending downwards, enables the examiner to detect the presence of a smooth, elastic, irregular-shaped tumor, clearly connected with the liver. From hepatic abscess for practical purposes, differentiation is not required ; but here, too, the employment of the aspirator will enable one to arrive at correct conclusions.

Treatment :—While various plans and divers drugs have, from time to time received commendation, it is highly probable that none have been of really curative power. Errors of judgment are just as numerous here as in most other diseases. The fact is very few cases of hydatid disease are recognized during life, because the cysts give rise to no pain or annoyance, and rarely to the interference with the function of the organ ; hence most of our knowledge has been derived from pathological studies. Cure is known to have occurred, when by the process of ulceration an exit from the cyst has been provided either into the stomach, intestinal canal, pleura, or best of all into the integuments ; and death too is reported when important blood-vessels have been opened, or when the general peritoneal cavity has been invaded.

The simplest mode of procedure has been to puncture with a trocar, evacuating the fluid ; the improvement in this method due to the aspirator, has been followed by a corresponding increase in the number of reported cases. There is a reasonable doubt, however, whether the method has been so successful as the reports seem to indicate. The mere withdrawal of the fluid lessons the size of the cyst, reduces the effects of pressure upon surrounding parts, but does not diminish the reproductive power of the mother and daughter cysts left behind. Moreover, it has been frequently followed by suppuration in the cyst with a resulting sepsis ; and in still other instances fatal leakage into the general peritoneal cavity has occured

Electrolysis, as a method of cure has received some decided attention. In the Medico-Chirurgical Transactions of London 1871, Mr. C. Hilton Fagge and Mr. Arthur E. Durham, reported 8 cases successfully operated upon by the method. The procedure is not devoid of danger, however. since needles are introduced into the cyst, and leakage into the peritoneum with fatal results has followed. Dr. Murchison (Clinical Lectures on Diseases of the Liver,) reports 3 deaths in 46 cases tabulated due to paracentesis, but the deaths which result from suppuration induced by the operative procedure, or from peritonitis are not enumerated. The most satisfactory results have occurred from more elaborate surgical procedures, made possible by the modern method of wound treatment. The earliest record of operative work upon the liver, is the celebrated case of cholecystotomy done by, I am proud to say, that very distinguished American surgeon, the late J. Marion Sims, in 1878. The operation was, however, suggested as possible, by Jean Louis Petit. In this case the gall-bladder, greatly distended, contained many gall-stones, and the physical condition of the patient was such as to make the operation truly a last resort. Sims, having cut down upon the distended bladder, opened it, emptied it, and stitched its edges to the integument. His patient lived 8 days. After relating the post mortem condition, Sims sums up the lesson derived from this case in the following language: "In dropsy of the gall-bladder, in hydatid tumors of the liver, and in gall-stones, we should not wait till the patient's strength is exhausted, nor till the blood becomes bile-poisoned, producing hæmorrhage; but we should make an early exploratory incision, ascertain the true nature of the disease, and then carry out the surgical treatment that the necessities of the case may demand."

This advice of Sims' bore fruit at an early period. In August, 1879, Mr. Lawson Tait, F. R. C. S., LL. D., etc , successfully carried out the brilliant proposal of Petit and Sims, by operating for the removal of gall-stones, opening the gall-bladder and stitching its edges to the integument. In the *Edinburgh Medical Journal*, volume XXXV, 1889, 305--401, Mr. Tait reports 55 cholecystotomies with 52 recoveries; 17 cases of hepatomy 11 of which were for hydatid cyst, with 15 recoveries, and 17 cases in which an exploratory incision was made for diagnostic purposes, with 16 recoveries.

Mr. McEddowes reports a case of cyst of the liver, operated upon by incision, stitching edge of cyst to integument, followed by drainage and recovery. (*British Medical Journal*, 1884. Volume I, p. 410.)

Mr. E. Atkinson, (*British Medical Journal*, 1885, volume II, p. 873,) reports a case of cyst of the liver, treated by incision; edge of cyst stitched to the peritoneum and integument. Patient recovered.

Mr. E. H. May, (*British Medical Journal*, 1886, volume II, p. 17,) reports a case of hydatid cyst of liver. Peritoneum when reached was found non-adherent to liver; the wound was packed with carbolized gauze, and five days later adhesion having occurred, the incision was prolonged, liver and cyst incised, edges stitched to integument, drainage and subsequent washings resorted to. Patient recovered. Mr. May, relating the case says his patient, a lady, was especially fond of dogs, and had a pet lap-dog constantly about her. He wisely makes no further comments.

Mr. Wm. H. Bull, F. R. C. S., Edinburgh (*London Lancet*, volume II, 1888) reports a case operated upon by abdominal section October 9, 1887, under the impression of its being an omental tumor; when abdomen was opened, he found a hydatid cyst of the right tube of the liver. This was incised, stitched to integument, and drained. Recovery followed.

Mr. Henry Morris, (*London Lancet* volume I, 1889,) reports four cases operated upon with three recoveries and one death. In two of the four cases related, the operation was undertaken under the impression that the growths ·were ovarian tumors.

Knowsley Thornton, (*British Medical Journal*, volume II, 1886, p. 902,) reports two cases cured by operation, and Marsh, in the same journal also relates one successfully treated.

R. F. Weir, (*N. Y. Medical Journal*, volume XLI, 1885, p. 311,) reports a case of hydatid cyst treated by *small* incision and evacuation of the contents of cyst; edges stitched to peritoneum and skin; patient died. Autopsy revealed defective drainage as the probable source of the sepsis.

J. T. Whittaker, (*Philadelphia Medical News*, volume XLIX 1886, p. 75,) case of hydatid cyst of liver; after trying aspiration several times unsuccessfully, suppuration was induced; an operation was then performed by Dr. Connor. Small incision, edges stitched to peritoneum and skin. Death followed.

Including the present case, I have been able to gather the records of 25 cases occurring in the practice of English and American surgeons with but four deaths; 22 of these cases with two deaths are reported from English sources. Of the three American cases the one here presented seems to have been the only successful one. The following conclusions seem warranted by a study of the cases.

1st. Early operation, if possible before suppuration occurs; if not the sooner thereafter the better.

2nd. The division of the operation into two stages, as recommended by Volkmann, for such cases as fail to show peritoneal adhesions.

3rd. Free incision ; thorough evacuation and cleansing of the sac, with special attention to the drainage.

DISCUSSION.

Dr. Wm. H. Welch, in referring to Dr. Bevan's paper, said he had seen about half a dozen cases of hydatid cyst of the liver in this country. The books give the impression that the disease is of everyday occurrence. It does occur. He had found it in a number of pigs, and in three instances he traced the disease and found that two of the pigs got it in this region. It comes from dogs. He had examined the intestines of a large number of dogs, but had not found the tænia echinococcus. This is not wonderful, for it is very minute. Most of those are when the dog has been fed for it. The two points in diagnosis are that it is possible to make a diagnosis by the microscopical examination of the fluid withdrawn, containing the membranes and characteristic hooklets. Also, it is possible to arrive at a very probable diagnosis by a chemical examination of the fluids, which usually contain no albumen.

FOUR CASES OF PUNCTURED FRACTURE OF THE CRANIUM. ONE CASE OF PENETRATING PISTOL-SHOT WOUND OF THE CRANIUM.

BY J. W. CHAMBERS, M. D.

Mr. President and Gentlemen :—The progress of knowledge in the matter of cranial surgery, and the keen interest in the attempt to institute operative procedures for injuries to the cranium and its contents, are the bases for my venture to report in the following paper, the limited series of cases of injuries to the brain, that have come under my personal care during the past six months.

I have to report four cases of punctured fracture of the cranium, and one penetrating pistol-shot wound of the cranium, all terminating in recovery.

Case I. Penetrating pistol shot wound of the cranium. Ball within cranial cavity. Drainage. Recovery. I. H. Male: colored. Brought to City Hospital, Sept. 11th, 1889, at 5 P. M., suffering with a pistol-shot wound, (32 caliber) in the left temporal region. He walked from station house to hospital, (a distance of two squares) assisted by a police officer. Was not suffering with any marked shock. Patient was at once placed in bed, and the necessary care given by the house physician, Dr. Smith. The head was shaved, thoroughly cleansed with soap and water, then washed with 1-2000 solution of bichloride of mercury. A pad of absorbent cotton soaked in a solution of bichloride, was placed over the wound, and the patient was given ¼ grain of morphine. No further treatment was given until the next morning. Sept. 12th, 10 A. M., patient irritable and restless, can with difficulty be sufficiently aroused to answer questions, and readily relapses into a semi-unconscious condition. Temperature 99°, pulse 100, respiration 20. Pupils contracted, but respond to light.

Reflexes increased. No paralysis or twitching of muscles.
The patient was given ¼ grain of morphine hypodermically,
chloroformed, and placed upon the operating table before the
class. The point of entrance of the ball was 1¼ inches behind and ¼ inch above the external angle of the eye. This
wound was freely enlarged, and a corresponding wound of
the cranium exposed, which proved to be a very abrupt punctured fracture. The edges of the bone next the angle of the
eye being quite perpendicular. The amount of depression
was ⅓ inch, driving a small central piece of bone into the
cranial cavity. The ½ inch trephine was used, and the broken
fragments of bone removed, leaving an opening 1¼ by ¾ of
inch in extent. The dura mater was perforated, covered by
a clot of blood, very tense, and bulged into the opening. Pulsation was absent, on slitting up the dura, an ounce of clotted
blood, and broken down brain tissue welled up. After washing away this substance with a gentle stream of warm 1-4000
solution of bichloride, a grooved director was gently passed
into the bullet tract, which extended into the brain 4½ inches
inwards, obliquely backwards, and upwards. The ball was
not detected, and as there were no symptoms to indicate its
probable location, no further search was made. A rubber
drainage pipe was inserted four inches into the wounded track
of the brain, and a hot solution of 1-4000 bichloride injected.
The wound of the soft part was accurately brought together
around the drainage tube, and secured by five silk sutures.
After well dusting the wound with iodoform, a large pad of
borated cotton supported by a bandage applied with considerable pressure, completed the dressing. The patient rallied
from the anæsthetic in an hour's time, and was able to answer
questions intelligently. Took milk and ice freely, and was
free from pain. On the evening of the day of operation,
there was some restlessness and slight vomiting, the result
of chloroform. The subsequent history of the case is comparatively uneventful. The wound was not disturbed until
the 14th, after operation, when it was found to be perfectly healed throughout, except at the point of the drainage
tube. Not the slightest irritation was visible at the point of
sutures. They were removed, the drainage tube withdrawn

two inches and cut off. The dressing was renewed October 7th, and the drainage tube entirely removed. The wound rapidly healed, and the patient was discharged from the hospital cured, October 27th. I saw him a few days ago, and he was to all appearances in perfect health.

CASE II.—A case of punctured wound of the skull, trephined ; recovery.

John E. Gurns, a blacksmith, aet. 28, was admitted to the City Hospital, Nov. 5th. While engaged in an election fight, he was struck on the head with a brick, making a Y-shaped scalp wound, about two inches in length, situated rather below and behind the middle of the left parietal bone. The head was shaven, cleansed with soap and water, then washed with a solution of bichloride of mercury. A large pad of absorbent cotton soaked in a solution of bichloride, was placed over the injured part, and retained by a roller bandage. Patient put to bed and given morphia sulphate, $\frac{1}{3}$ grain hypodermatically. The man was but little affected by the injury after its immediate effect had passed off, which lasted one hour and had no idea of its serious nature. He rested well during the night. At 11 A. M., November 6, sixteen hours after receiving the injury, the patient was again given $\frac{1}{3}$ grain of morphia hypodermatically, and chloroformed. On freely enlarging the scalp wound, a V-shaped fracture of the parietal bone was exposed, with its center depressed $\frac{1}{4}$ inch. The sides of the fracture sloped evenly towards the central and most depressed point. A half inch trephine was used, and several fragments of bone removed. They, with the button, left a space where a bone was wanting 1½ by 1 inch. The dura, covered by a thin blood-clot, bulged into the wound and pulsated. The clot was thoroughly washed away with a hot solution of 1-4000 bichloride of mercury. This started fresh bleeding from one of the middle meningeal arteries, which was controlled by passing a threaded needle under it and ligating. The wound was well washed with a solution of bichloride, cat-gut drainage used, dusted with iodoform, and closed with silk sutures. A large compress of borated cotton, supported by a rather tightly applied roller bandage, completed the dressing. The amount of shock was very slight.

Was placed on a light diet. Wound redressed November 18th, twelve day after the operation and stitches removed. A linear cicatrix remained to mark the site of the wound. The temperature was normal throughout the convalescence, and no signs of constitutional disturbance whatever were present, unless an accelerated pulse, which was noted during the recovery of all cases reported, might be so considered. The patient was discharged on the 22nd day of December—to use his own words—"feeling as well as he ever felt in his life." The local and constitutional progress of this case could not have been more favorable. When I saw him the other day, four months after the injury, he told me that he had enjoyed perfect health continuously since his discharge from the hospital.

CASE III.—A case of depressed fracture of the cranium. Trephined. Recovery. Wm. Grump, aet. 17, white, laborer, fell from elevation of thirty feet, was picked up in an unconscious condition. Rapidly regained consciousness, so that when brought to the City Hospital one hour afterwards, he answered questions slowly but intelligently. On examination there was found to be a lacerated wound of the anterior part of the left parietal region of the scalp. The head was shaven, and thoroughly cleansed with soap and water, then washed with a solution of 1-1000 bichloride of mercury. A pad of absorbent cotton wet with a solution of 1-2000 bichloride was bandaged over the wound. Four hours after the accident, the patient was given a hypodermic injection of morphia, and chloroformed. On enlarging the scalp wound, a depressed fracture $2\frac{1}{2}$ by 2 inches of the anterior portion of the parietal bone was observed. The $\frac{1}{2}$ inch trephine was used. The depressed bone elevated, and several fragments removed. The dura mater bulged into the wound, was covered with a large blood-clot, and pulsated. The removal of this clot gave rise to a severe hæmorrhage from a lacerated branch of the middle meningeal artery. This hæmorrhage was, with considerable difficulty, controlled by passing a ligature around the branch, by means of a specially curved needle. The wound was then washed with a solution of bichloride, cat-gut drainage used, and dusted with iodoform. A large pad of borated cotton, retained by a roller bandage completed the dressing. The patient was severely shocked, but in two hours rallied to a complete recognition of his surroundings. Was ordered a light diet, and no drugs to be used unless especially indicated. At 6 P. M., the day of operation, the temperature was 100°, pulse 98. Patient rested well during the night and at no other time during his stay in the hospital, did his temperature range above 99°. On the removal of the dressing, the 14th day, the wounded soft parts were found to have entirely healed, except a small amount of granulation at the lower angle of the wound. The stitches were removed, the parts dusted with iodoform, and a pad of borated cotton again applied. Patient left the hospital Jan. 2nd, fully recovered from the effects of his injury.

CASE IV.—A case of punctured fracture of the skull. Trephined. Recovery. W. L. Denby. æt. 47, white, male, occupation that of a bricklayer. Fell December 27th, fifty feet from a scaffold. Was immediately brought to the City Hospital in an unconscious condition. On examination, a V-shaped wound of the scalp, just above the left frontal eminence, and half an inch to the left of the median line was observed. Also several abrasions and scratch wounds. The head was shaved, the wounds thoroughly washed with an antiseptic solution, dusted with iodoform, and covered with borated cotton. The patient was then placed in bed. For the next few hours he was very restless, and still unconscious.

At 6 P. M. on the day of accident the temperature was 100°, the pulse 68. 11 A. M., December 28th, (the day following accident), the patient was fully conscious, but complaining of headache. While answering all questions intelligently, he had no knowledge of what had passed since the accident. There were no symptoms of compression present. Being still in doubt as to the real nature of the injury of the head, a second examination of the scalp wound was made, and the fracture detected. The patient was immediately given a hypodermic injection of morphia, chloroformed, and placed upon the operating table. On enlarging the scalp wound, the punctured portion of the bone was thoroughly exposed. This fractured portion was found to be starred and depressed.

The trephine was used, the depressed portion elevated, and several fragments removed. The dura mater had been punctured, and was covered with a considerable blood clot. Upon washing away this clot, quite a free hæmorrhage ensued from an injured vessel of the dura, which was ligated. The wound was washed with a hot solution of bichloride, cat-gut drainage used, dusted with iodoform, and scalp brought together with silk sutures. A pad of borated cotton, retained by a tightly applied roller bandage completed the dressing. The patient was very little shocked from the operation. At 6 30 P. M., December 28th, the temperature was 100.5°, pulse 85. There was no headache. He felt comfortable, and was resting well. December 29th at 8 A. M., the temperature was 100°, pulse 80, and resting comfortably. At no subsequent time during his stay in the hospital, did the temperature range above 99°. The dressing and sutures were removed on the 15th day, as the wound was entirely healed. The general condition of the patient was good. He left the hospital entirely well, January 31st.

CASE V.—A punctured fracture of the skull. Trephined. Recovery. W. H. aet. 35. White. Male. Occupation that of ship-carpenter. Fell fifteen feet down hatchway of a vessel. I saw him in consultation with Dr. C. P. Strauss March 23rd, four hours after the occurrence of the accident. On examination found an irregular lacerated wound of the scalp, over the superior posterior portion of the parietal bone, leading down to a punctured fracture of same, also a Colles's fracture of the left fore-arm. The patient was dull and heavy, and answered all questions in monosyllables. The temperature was 99°, pulse 60, and full. After shaving the head, thoroughly cleansing it with a solution of chloride, a hypodermic of morphine was given, and the patient chloroformed. The ¼ inch trephine was used, and a number of fragments of the bone removed. One of these having punctured the dura mater and pia mater, giving rise to a severe hemorrhage from a wounded vessel of the pia mater, a ligature was passed around this vessel by means of a specially curved needle, all hæmorrhage controlled.

The wound was washed with a 1-4000 solution of bichloride, cat-gut drainage used, dusted with iodoform, and covered with a large pad of borated cotton, held in place by a snugly fitting roller bandage. The patient was considerably shocked after the operation, but rallied during the next four hours. There was some vomiting from the chloroform. The dressing was removed on the 7th day, and as the wound was found to be healed, the stitches were removed. Twenty days after the operation, the patient was well and about in his room.

The small number of cases which I have brought before you, are not expected to definitely settle any conclusion in reference to brain, or other injuries to the skull. For with exception of the first case related, there is but little doubt but that the brain largely escaped any very severe primary injury. There is however, one fact on which I should like to lay stress ; viz. : that the operation of trephining is not a dangerous one. The operation of trephining should be done, not so much for the elevation of the depressed bone, but for the removal of a foreign body, which may at any moment light up an inflammation of the delicate structures beneath which, although readily started, is difficult to arrest.

To the general surgical rule of immediate reduction, which is so universally accepted for all fractures of other bones, there is no sound surgical reason for making the bones of the head the exception to the universal rule of immediate reduction.

RECENT ADVANCES IN RECTAL SURGERY.

By Sam'l T. Earle, Jr., M. D.

I would like to call the attention of the Faculty to some of the advances in Rectal Surgery within the last few years.

In the first place to the treatment of that most common of all rectal complaints, hæmorrhoids. It has been very gratifying to note the decline in the use of that timid and scarcely half efficient means of dealing with these troubles that was so generally in vogue only a few years ago. I refer to the hypodermic injections of medicinal substances, and the substitution therefor of vigorous, radical, and I may say, perfectly safe operative measures. One word more about the treatment by hypodermic injections. Judging from the recent reports in the Journals of the number of cases treated by this means by several western physicians, one would think they had found it very satisfactory ; or they may think it premature in me in pronouncing such a measure almost obsolete at this day. Whatever may have been the success they have met with in its use, it has been almost the universal opinion of all eastern physicians, and most of those in the Northwest, who have given it any thing like a fair trial, that it is a very unsatisfactory, uncertain, and unscientific means of dealing with this trouble ; and in thirteen cases death has followed its use (these cases have been collected and reported by Andrews in his recent work on " Rectal Surgery.") It has in consequence been almost entirely dropped by them.

While the operative measures that have been in vogue for more than a century passed, (I refer more particularly to the old method of ligating,) have been radical in their results as a rule, they have been far from being free from danger to life; Whereas under almost any of the most approved methods of operating at the present day, such results are very rare indeed.

The most decided advance in the operative measures that have been recently advised for the treatment of these troubles has been that accredited to Dr. Whitehead of England, and generally called by his name. It is certainly the safest, most efficient, and radical operation, or measure that has ever been recommended for their relief. While I do not recommend its adoption in all cases, nor that of any other single operation, yet in aggravated cases, especially those in which there are both external and internal hæmorrhoids, or considerable tumefaction around the anus in conjunction with internal piles, think it is by far the best measure that can be used. It is scarcely worth while to describe it here, or refer in any way to the manner of performing it, as it has been so frequently, and fully described, also so thoroughly criticised within the last few years. I cannot agree with a prominent American rectal surgeon in the objections he offers to its adoption, that it is very difficult, tedious and bloody to perform, and see no reason why it could not be performed in a moderately short time with a little practice. Dr. Halsted of The Hopkins Hospital does what might appear to be a modification of this operation in the class of cases I have mentioned above, but which he has had in use for the last ten, or twelve years, and therefore antedates Whitehead's operation by several years. In this operation, instead of stitching the skin and mucous membrane together all around the anus after removing the fringe of pile bearing tissue as recommended by Dr. Whitehead, he passes two deep, burried catgut sutures, one on either side of the rectum, beneath the tissue to be removed up through the mucous membrane to prevent its retracting after being separated from the skin. The cut surface is allowed to heal by granulation. The mucous membrane is kept sufficiently drawn down by the sutures to prevent contraction taking place. I have done this operation with excelent results. All bleeding vessels are ligated, and would suggest that the same be done in Whitehead's operation, instead of relying upon torsion as recommended by him.

Dr. C. B. Ball in his excellent work on " The Rectum and Anus," speaks of a new clamp introduced by Dr. Coates, senior surgeon to the Salisbury Infirmary, for performing the clamp operation without having to resort to the Paquelin Cautery. It is well worth our notice, being a very simple and ingenious instrument, with which good results should be gotten. It is composed of two pieces of stout wire, round in shape, hinged at one end, whose surfaces nearly approximate when brought together; from the inside of one projects some five or six needles which pass through holes in the corresponding blade when the two are brought together, (the manner in which it is used) the catch forcepts being applied, the pile is drawn down, and the clamp closed upon its base; a few fine catgut sutures are then applied beneath the clamp; and the pile is cut off. The blades of the clamp are now opened for a short distance, the needles which have transfixed the base of the pile to prevent its retraction. Any vessels requiring it, are now ligated, and as soon as all bleeding is stopped the clamp is removed, and the sutures tied. In this way a cleanly incised, and evenly brought together wound is substituted for the charred and open wound of the usual clamp, and cautery operation, and of others. Although I have never operated with this form of clamp, yet it occurs to me to be an excellent procedure in those cases where the ordinary clamp and cautery operation is expedient, having also another advantage over the latter of being perfectly free from the danger of hæmorrhage. I hope to give it a trial soon. Unquestionably the most decided, bold and efficient step in rectal surgery within the last few years has been the recent operative procedure recommended for aggravated cases of prolapse of the rectum by Mikulicz, then successfully practiced by Dr. Frederick Treves, Surgeon to, and Lecturer on Anatomy at the London Hospital, as shown by his report of three successful cases in the London Lancet for February and March, 1890; also by a successful case operated on by Dr. Halsted of the Hopkins Hospital, which I had the pleasure of seeing in March, 1890. These have been the only cases I have seen reported; there may have been others. In brief the operation, which has been fully described by Mr. Treves in the London Lancet for Feb. 22nd and March 1st, 1890, consists in the total excision of the prolapsed rectum from just above the sphincter, through the entire prolapsed portion. If the peritoneal cavity is opened into, as sometimes happens and did in one of Mr. Treves cases, the opposite serous surface are to be carefully stitched together, then, after the remainder of the prolapse has been excised, the opposing ends of the rectum are brought together, and held in position by sutures passed through the mucous, sub-mucous, and muscular coats. Even in some bad cases of prolapse, only the mucous membrane comes down, as in two of the cases reported by Dr. Treves, one of which protruded four, and the other five inches; the same condition also existed in Dr. Halsted's case. When such is the case of course it is only necessary to excise the protruding mucous membrane, which simplifies the operation very much, and renders it much less dangerous to life. The results as stated both as to life and permanent relief have been most excellent. Such a procedure is only recommended in very aggravated cases, which are most likely to occur in adults, and after other simpler methods have failed. When we consider the past inefficient methods of dealing with these aggravated cases, and the distressing condition of the subjects of it, we may well congratulate ourselves that science has at last succeeded so well in remedying the evil.

Report of the Section on Practice of Medicine.

THE NATURE AND TREATMENT OF HYSTERICAL PARALYSIS.

By George J. Preston, M. D., *Chairman.*

Hysterical paralysis is one of the most prominent and characteristic members of the group of symptoms to which has been applied the general term, hysteria. Among English-speaking people, as is well known, this disease does not exist with the frequency nor severity that is seen in other nations. But even if this fact be taken into full consideration, it is remarkable how unwilling English and Americans, lay and professional, have been to award it a place among bona fide diseases. The laity of these countries even now, and unfortunately a considerable proportion of the medical profession also, regard hysteria most unqualifiedly as a feigned disease and the hysterical subject as an out and out malingerer. The very term is one of reproach, so that in this country the physician is generally obliged to retire behind such euphemisms as "functional," "nervousness" and the like, when speaking of the disease. I have seen a mother's face express almost as much indignation when I told her that her daughter was hysterical, as it would have done had I said "your daughter is a fool," or "she is a liar." The word hysteria, cannot, of course, be defended upon philological grounds, since, like so many other ancient terms in medicine, its primal significance has utterly faded. The uterus was supposed to be the seat of this affection, and, more than this, was thought to wander over the body at will, a state of affairs that the gynæcologist and obstetrician of that day must have seriously objected to. To-day we understand the term, hysteria, to comprise a fairly definite group of symptoms, and it is rather to be regretted that such a stigma of disgrace is attached to it, that we are hardly able to use it without running a risk of being misunderstood.

Of all the diseases classified as functional, hysteria probably represents the purest type, and to this fact is due the very frequent misconception of its nature. On the one hand, the extent and severity of the symptoms would seem to point to organic disease; this mistake, of course, is most common with the laity. While on the other, the patient's inconsistency and the contradictory nature of the symptoms not unfrequently lead to the mistaken and unfortunate diagnosis of malingering, or a vicious disposition.

The great fundamental fact underlying this frequent misconception of the nature of hysteria is obvious ; we do not understand the intimate relations and working of the brain.

We recognize with perfect ease a functional disease of the stomach, for example, for we know how the stomach digestion is carried on, and what and where the fault is when it occurs. With the brain, however, it is very different ; we simply see the results of the work, and are compelled to fall back, in great measure, upon theory to explain how such results have been attained. Experimental physiology, however, and pathological records in the light of this work, have given us so many indisputable facts, and so many pregnant suggestions, that we may be said to have now what scientific men are fond of calling a good working theory. The limits of this paper do not admit of even allusion to the many ingenious, amusing, or absurd theories which have been propounded to explain the nature of hysteria. What may be said concerning the nature of hysterical paralysis will hold good, with certain modifications, in the case of most of the other prominent hysterical phenomena.

In the first place, hysterical paralysis is almost certainly of cortical origin. As we shall see when we consider its symptomatology, the preservation of the reflexes, of electric reactions and of nutrition, all point most strongly to the cerebral cortex as the origin. Yet, we must look beyond the motor regions of the cortex. A patient with most marked hysterical paralysis will, under certain conditions, use the paralyzed members as freely and forcibly as if nothing were the matter. If such a patient be hypnotized, for example, and the hypnotic suggestion strongly made that the paralyzed member has recovered strength, the patient will use it freely. Or, if the patient be profoundly etherized, the paralyzed part will be forcibly moved when the effects of the anæsthetic are wearing off. In both instances, the patient may remain perfectly well or may relapse into the former condition. Or a sudden fright, the most common example, may cure instantaneously a paralysis that has existed for years. These and like examples seem to me to prove that the cortical motor cells are not effected, even functionally, for the agents which effect the cure are applied in each instance, not to the cortical motor area, but to the higher volitional centers.

Now, in all the more complicated movements, leaving out, of course, such simple, practically automatic ones as walking for example, the stimulus to the motor centers come from certain higher brain centers. To illustrate; we may be reading and have suggested by what we read a desire for food or drink, and we decide upon the character of the object desired and when and how it can be obtained, and then those motor cells are stimulated, which produce the movements necessary for the attainment of our desires. What the nature of this stimulus is, how a pure volition sets into action certain muscles is to us, as it was to the philosophers of ancient times, a mystery. We can only say that in certain regions of the brain, say the frontal area, there are cells which are probably the centers of the higher mental processes; a volition originating in these cells possibly from acquired knowledge or experience, together with certain deductions drawn from such facts finds its agents in the motor cells and communicates with them ; in other words the frontal cells are stimulated and in turn stimulate the motor. We know from the histology of the brain cortex that the relationship between the cortical cell in different parts of the brain, in fact between ganglion cells throughout the whole central nervous system is very intimate. Now suppose the connection between the frontal and Rolandic region be broken ; we would still have reflex action, but no voluntary movement, according to our theory. Suppose, again, that the cells in the frontal region, the higher centers, were exhausted, were no longer able to send a stimulus of sufficient strength to provoke a discharge in the motor cells; we would have the same conditions as above; reflex preserved, nutrition of muscles preserved, certain involuntary or purposeless movements preserved, and all decidedly voluntary purposive movements lost. This, as we shall see later, will conform to the symptomatology of hysterical paralysis. Now as to the causes that might bring about such a condition in the cells of higher mental functions. We know that repeated calls upon nerve cells exhausts them. We see this illustrated in many ways. Long continued mental exertion will bring about a condition of exhaustion such that all further attempts at mental work are useless until the cells have rested, recuperated. Practically we know from recent work in this direction (Hodge) that continued stimulation of a ganglion cell by the electric current produces a condition of vacuolation, and actual loss of protoplasm in the cell. Now what are the most potent causes in the production of hysteria? Space permits the mention of only the most prominent. Bad training in childhood, over indulgence, sudden fright, change from a luxurious to a humble mode of life, sexual excesses, religious excitement, such and like conditions are the strongest etiological factors in the production of hysteria. Hard regular mental work is rarely an exciting cause. It is abnormal mental stimulus, just the sort of causes to produce most readily, exhaustion of the higher centers. In addition to this physiological element, certain general conditions contribute to the production of this affection. Any state of the system which lowers the general nutrition, must exert a strong action upon the nerve centers, so we see hysteria often in the course of certain general conditions as tuberculosis and gout. Undoubtedly anæmia plays a prominent part in the production of hysteria, as does possibly vaso-motor spasm of reflex origin. We see that the higher centers are in such a condition of exhaustion, or perform their functions so feebly that under ordinary circumstances they are unable to stimulate the motor cells to a degree sufficiently high to produce in them a motor discharge. When these higher centers are suddenly and powerfully stimulated, as by some unexpected emotion they may in turn stimulate the motor centers sufficiently to produce normal voluntary motion. The pathogenesis of hysterical paralysis according to the theory proposed, might be expressed thus : certain abnormal stimuli, or usual stimuli acting to an extraordinary degree, produce in the higher centers a condition of exhaustion such that these higher centers are no longer able to stimulate the lower or motor centers to a degree sufficient to produce a discharge.

Did space permit, certain other well known phenomena of hysteria, such as anæsthesia, contractions and the like, could it appears to me, be sufficiently accounted for on the hypothesis given above.

Hysterical paralysis may come on gradually, the affected parts becoming progressively weaker, or suddenly following a violent hysterical seizure. In this latter class of cases it is necessary to make a differential diagnosis between the hysterical manifestation which precedes the paralysis and true apoplectic coma. This is usually not difficult, though occasionally cataleptoid states may bear a rather close resemblance to apoplexy. In this connection may be mentioned those cases of what Charcot galls traumatic hysteria. An hysterical individual receives a slight injury, which is followed by marked and sometimes prolonged paralysis. I have seen a number of cases of such injury or other painful affection leave behind an hysterical paralysis, as a case recently under my care, in which the patient had a gonorrhoeal rheumatism affecting one leg, genuine at first, but afterwards passing into a condition of hysterical paresis, with pain on movement.

The varieties of hysterical paralysis are many ; probably the most common is paraplegia. Hemiplegia is not uncommon, particularly following marked hystero-epilepsy. A number of cases of paralysis of all four limbs have been reported. Another curious form is that known as alternate paralysis, affecting the arm on one side and the leg of the side opposite. A very well marked case of this latter variety is to
· be found in the writings of Hippocrates. Then we may have

monoplegia, or even paralysis of groups of muscles only. With any of these may be associated certain other phenomena, particularly hysterical aphonia ; also certain visceral paraly- ses, bladder, rectum, æsophagus, etc.   In most instances we find, in addition to the motor affection, derangement of sen- sibility, more or less pronounced.   The paralyzed side will often be found to be anæsthetic, and this is particularly true of contractions, which so generally accompany the paralysis. These complications were well illustrated in a case seen in Baltimore county not long since.   The patient, a woman about 35 years of age, gave a history of paralysis, of a para- plegic type, which had existed for seven or eight years.   The right leg was powerless, the leg flexed almost at a right angle with the thigh, and the whole right side completely anæs- thetic.

Hysterical paralysis may be of all grades, from a slight paresis or hardly appreciable loss of power to absolute ina- bility to move the part.   Most commonly we see paralysis of certain movements of the limb only.   For example, in hys- terical paraplegia the patient will be totally unable to walk, and yet when lying down may be able to move the legs with freedom, and to exert a considerable amount of force in vari- ous directions.

The all important question is the differential diagnosis.   It is exceedingly important to bear in mind the fact that hys- teria is very apt to appear in persons who have an organic lesion of the nervous system, central or peripheral.   I have seen very marked cases of hysteria, with contractions, paraly- sis, etc., in the course of multiple sclerosis and other cord lesions.   The fact that a patient has some organic disease of the nervous system predisposes to hysteria.   The danger is that the unquestioned and obvious hysterical symptoms may distract the attention from the symptoms of organic diseases present, or that these latter may be included along with the former under the diagnosis of hysteria.   Such mistakes in prognosis are not frequently made in this way.   Then again the mimicry of hysteria is often so perfect that most careful observers are deceived.   We have seen that it will not do to

rely upon the general hysterical condition which may be
prominent in any individual case. Of course this is of great
value, and should be always sought for ; yet the very generally accepted ideas concerning the hysterical state may prove
a stumbling block. It is by no means necessary to have pronounced emotional instability. A person may have hysterical
paralysis, and yet show very few or perhaps no distinct symptoms of mental hysteria, except the weakened volition, and
this is often not brought out by superficial examination. It
becomes necessary then to distinguish between organic and
hysterical paralysis upon other grounds than the mere recognition of general hysterical symptoms. One prominent difference is in the seat of the paralysis. We often see parts affected in hysterical paralysis that would require an almost
impossible organic lesion to account for. We may have an
arm on one side and leg on the opposite, or all four limbs
affected. A very irregular paralysis should always be looked
at with the idea of its being hysterical, unless certain marked
organic symptoms show themselves, as in cases of widespread
neuritis. Then a very characteristic symptom of hysterical
paralysis is its tendency to shift its position, the part first
affected recovering, and paralysis appearing in another place.

In hysterical hemiplegia it is to be noticed that the face is
almost never attacked, and also that the gait of such a patient
differs from that of an organic hemiplegia ; in the latter instance the patient looks at the affected limb and at the floor
when walking, and the paralyzed limb is swung outward,
making the arc of a circle ; in the case of the hysterical hemiplegia the patient never, or rarely looks at the affected limb
or at the floor, and the boot is dragged without any attempt
at rotation. In hysterical paraplegia, as has been mentioned,
the limbs can often be freely moved when the patient is in the
recumbent position. Monoplegias and partial paralyses of
hysterical origin imitate closely those from cortical disease.
They are usually less complete, and their mode of onset is
different.

The important points to be observed in making differential
diagnosis between organic and hysterical paralysis are that

in the latter, knee-jerk is never lost and, generally, slightly exaggerated, the nutrition of the muscles as a rule, is preserved, and the electro-contractility practically unaltered. One symptom that I regard of great negative value is the absence of ankle clonus in those cases in which it should be found, were the cases of organic origin. Certain authors claim that this symptom may be present in hysteria, but genuine ankle clonus must be certainly very rare in purely hysterical cases. The very useful association of anæsthesia with hysterical paralysis is a symptom of importance. It is very common to find hemi-anæsthesia associated with hemiplegias and also paraplegias of hysterical origin. It is rare to find any affection of speech in hysterical paralysis, other than aphonia, which is very common. This is due to a greater or less degree of paralysis of the vocal cords, which as shown by the laryngoscope, is always bilateral. The cords do not approximate each other sufficiently. Other forms of paralysis of hysterical origin, such as paralysis of the œsophagus, rectum and bladder are met with, but are of rare occurrence.

It is well to bear in mind that even after the diagnosis of hysterical paralysis has been correctly made, it does not always follow that the case can be speedily cured, for now and then, cases are met with that resist all treatment. Then it is not improbable, as in the oft quoted case of Charcot, that what was originally functional has become organic. Cases of undoubted hysterical paralysis have been reported, in which after a time there has been muscular atrophy. It is often well to put the patient through a course of tonics. There is often enough anæmia to call for iron. A combination that I have found useful, though it probably undergoes some chemical substitution, is bromide of potash and tincture of the chloride of iron. In the pronounced cases the bromides alone are not of much value except as soporifics. One of the most formidable obstacles met with in the treatment of these case, especially if the patient be a young girl, is the girl's mother, and it is frequently necessary to begin the treatment on her. It is very hard to persuade the average mother that the symptoms are functional merely, and she will often spoil months of careful treatment by a few injudicious words. For this reason it is sometimes absolutely necessary to take the patient away from home for treatment.   As has been pointed out, the cause of hysterical paralysis is probably in the higher brain centers, consequently efforts at cure must be directed toward these centers.   The plan of threatening and frightening a patient out of her unfortunate condition will be successful in only a very small per cent. of cases.   They are told so often to exercise their will power, the very thing they cannot do, that they get sick of the very word and utterly discouraged with their failures.   In a small number of cases a cure may be affected suddenly, sometimes accidentally, sometimes intentionally.   In these cases it would seem that the higher centers were not greatly exhausted, and needed only some unusual stimulus to set them in action again.   This may be done by anæsthetizing the patient deeply, and as the effect of the anæsthetic is wearing off make them walk or use the paralyzed part.   The same thing may be better accomplished in good subjects by hypnotism.   Many of these sudden cures like sudden conversions are extremely liable to lapse into their former condition.   We have learned a valuable lesson from the many experiments that have been made with hypnotism in the line of systematic suggestion.   This it seems to me is the secret of success in the treatment of many of these cases.   In this way the will power is gradually led back to its former commanding position.   While the brilliant results of the plan of treatment advocated and practised by Playfair and Weir Mitchell are in part due to enforced rest, feeding and passive exercise, without doubt an important element is the suggestive one, the gradual cultivation and strengthening of the higher volitional centers.

The first step in the treatment is to make the patient feel that the physician has absolute control of the case, that there is no appeal from his decision.   It is usually not a difficult thing to gain the confidence of your patient, and this confidence should never þe abused.   It is a very bad plan to deceive such patients, or to hold up a threat, which the patient knows full well will never be put into execution.   If possible the physician should never take a position from which he is likely to be compelled to recede.   After proper attention to general or special conditions, that is to say tonic treatment if necessary, relief of dyspeptic or uterine trouble the patient should be put upon a system of rigid training. As has been said this is often impossible at home. Food, sleep, exercise, &c., should be ordered regularly, and the order strictly enforced. If the patient cannot sleep the required time she should remain quietly lying down. Then the special treatment to the affected part should be vigorously applied, and in the most suggestive manner. The paralyzed member should be exercised daily, or better twice a day by moderately strong Faradic currents, systematic massage applied and the patient encouraged to use the affected part. Such attempts should be encouraged, and the suggestion constantly made that improvement is going on. Sometimes it will be necessary to isolate the patient from all friends, at other times pleasant company and some mental occupation will succeed best. In all cases the efforts should be persistent. If an hysterical patient improve decidedly and then fall back, it is like a person who had climbed to a considerable height up a ladder, the higher they are when they fall, the harder the fall will be. Some of the worst cases I have ever had to treat are those that have improved a good deal and then slipped back. Often it would seem that the rigid discipline and the tedium of the treatment, force the patient to relent, but the fact is that the will-power is gradually stimulated in this way, and what seems like the discontinuance of a farce, is in reality a successful effort to set the mental machinery to work again. Usually the cure comes about by slow degrees : first, a vigorous attempt to move the paralyzed part ; then slight irregular movements which increase sometimes very slowly, sometimes quite rapidly to perfect motion.

In hysterical aphonia the strong Faradic current, either in the form of a wire brush, or if neccessary a laryngeal electrode will rapidly bring about a cure. The following case will illustrate the plan to be pursued : Miss M., general hysteria and almost absolute loss of voice. It was necessary to put the ear close to her mouth, and then many words were lost. Articulation was indistinct and slow. I impressed on her the effect that the battery would accomplish for one or two visits before applying it, speaking confidentially of the cure. I then applied an uncovered electrode to the outside of the larynx and used a painfully strong current, urging her to speak, and steadily increasing the strength of the current. After a few applications her voice came back naturally, though she had not spoken aloud for probably two years, and in the year or more that has intervened since I saw her, she has had no return of the trouble. ·

In conclusion I would call attention to the great value of hydro-therapy in the treatment of these conditions. It is well to begin with a very slight douche of moderately cold water to the spine every morning, and increase it until the patient can take a pitcher full of cold water down the spine or a general cold sponging. The cold water should not be applied to the head. The plans which have been found most useful in the treatment of the various forms of hysterical paralysis have been here only briefly indicated, space not permitting any elaboration of them. The intellectual condition and mental habits of each individual patient must be carefully studied before any intelligent treatment can be employed. It is very necessary that the physician who is called upon to treat this class of diseases should cultivate, if he do not already possess, the virtue of patience, that he should be sure of his diagnosis, and confident of the success of his mode of treatment.

Report of the Section on Obstetrics and Gynæcology.

THE REMOVAL OF SUB-MUCOUS AND INTRA-UTERINE FIBROID TUMORS BY ENUCLEATION AND TRACTION, WITH THE REPORT OF TEN CASES.

By B. BERNARD BROWNE, M. D., *Chairman.*

Various methods have been resorted to for the removal of these tumors. Separation of the pedicle by means of the ecraseur is the procedure recommended by most authorities. Thomas, Barnes, Skene and Tait recommend the ecraseur, while Emmet advises enucleation, and was the first to draw attention to the aid given by the expulsive efforts of the uterus in the removal of these tumors.

It would scarcely be necessary to state that there is no indication for the use of electricity in intra-uterine and intra-vaginal fibroids, if Apostoli had not carried its use so far as to apply it even in such cases.

The objection to the ecraseur is, first, the difficulty, or almost impossibility of applying the wire high enough up so that no portion of the tumor or pedicle be left behind in the uterus, there to undergo decomposition and develop septicæmia; and secondly, the danger of drawing in a portion of the uterine wall, and cutting it off, along with the tumor. This accident would be almost certain to occur if partial inversion existed at the time of applying the wire loop.

That these objections to the use of the ecraseur are valid and not imaginary, it is only necessary to refer to the literature of the subject.

By enucleation and traction both of these dangers are avoided, and if partial or complete inversion should occur [as in one of the cases which 1 shall report,] no danger need be apprehended, as this complication is easily managed by the method which I will suggest.

The following cases are related as bearing upon this method of operation.

CASE I.—Francis W., colored, aged 30, had had a very offensive discharge and profuse menorrhagia for six months before I saw her. The diagnosis of epithelioma had been made.

Upon examination, I found a large tumor filling up the vagina. The sound passed around the tumor up to the fundus where the pedicle was attached. The condition was found to be a sloughing fibroid. Disinfecting washes were used and the patient put under an anæsthetic. By continued traction, the tumor was gradually pulled down outside of the vulva ; at the same time, the uterus was partly inverted. The pedicle was now enucleated and the uterus reinverted. The tumor weighed 18 ounces. The patient made a good recovery.

CASE 2.—Miss S., aged 28, white, had been suffering with menorrhagia for several years. Upon examination, the cervix was found to be somewhat patulous ; the introduction of the sound into the cavity of the uterus excited profuse bleeding. Under an anæsthetic, the cervix was thoroughly dilated, and the finger introduced into the cavity of the uterus, which was found to contain a pedunculated fibroid about the size of a small orange. By pressure over the uterus and traction upon the tumor, it was gradually drawn through the cervix, and the pedicle was then enucleated by the serrated curette.

CASE 3.—Mrs. T., aged 30, married 11 years ; no children. Was seen by me in consultation. For three months, she had had very profuse flow at each menstrual period, and had lost so much blood that she remained in a state of complete collaps for 24 hours after each flow.

The uterus was found enlarged, and measured 7 inches in depth. The cervix was elongated and not patulous. Tupelo tents were inserted for the purpose of preliminary dilatation ; on the following day, they were removed, and complete dilatation accomplished with Sims' large dilator and Hanks' hard rubber dilators. Upon introducing the finger into the cavity of the uterus, a large sub-mucous fibroid was felt ; the lower corner of the capsule had ruptured, and a point of the tumor was projecting through this into the cavity of the uterus. In order to liberate the tumor, the mucous covering was slit up with long scissors, and by traction and enucleation the tumor was first drawn into the uterine cavity and then into the vagina. It had no pedicle, but was attached all around by its capsule. Weight, 14 ounces. The hæmorrhage in this case had begun at the time of rupture of the capsule.

CASE 4.—Mrs. M., aged 35, had been bleeding for several months. A bloody tumor was projecting into the vagina, and upon examination, over the abdomen a hollow indentation was found in the fundus. The diagnosis of inversion of the uterus had been made. Upon examining through the rectum, a much larger mass was found than would have been the case in inversion ; besides, the mass was much harder than in inversion. The sound passed in on the right side and could be felt through the abdominal wall. The conditions here were very similar to those of inversion, but they did not correspond entirely. I concluded to pull the presenting tumor through the vulva so as to see the orifices of the Fallopian tubes, and if it proved to be inversion, and could not be returned by taxis, I intended to cut through the posterior surface of the fundus, dilate the constriction with a dilator passed up through the opening in the fundus, and then replace the uterus as in a case reported by me some time since [*N. Y. Med. Jour.*, Nov. 24th, 1883.]

CASE 5.—Mrs. C., aged 33, white, married 7 years, has never been pregnant, has had severe dysmenorrhœa and metrorrhagia for several years. Her abdomen has become much enlarged in the past year ; the cervix was elongated and conical, with a narrow os uteri. The uterus was found to be much enlarged, and upon dilating the cervix, a large fibroid tumor, with sessile attachment, was found in the cavity

of the uterus. Complete dilatation of the cervix was obtained before any effort was made at removal, then several
pairs of large vulsella forceps were introduced into the tumor.
Traction was made first with one pair and then with another;
at the same time, pressure was made over the abdomen by
an assistant. After a considerable amount of traction, the
tumor commenced to separate from its attachment. At this
stage, Thomas' serrated scoop was passed up to the fundus,
and by gentle pressure and leverage, the tumor was partially
enucleated and drawn through the cervix. At this stage,
two large corkscrews were screwed into the tumor, and complete removal of it thereby accomplished.

CASE 6.—Mrs. K., colored, aged 36, married, no children.
Has had menorrhagia for several months, also a very offensive watery discharge during the intra-menstrual period.
Upon examination, a large fibroid was found, partly projecting into the vagina. Expulsive uterine pains had been going
on for two or three weeks before I saw her; these commenced after the administration of fluid extract of ergot,
which had been given to check the hæmorrhage. An
anæsthetic having been administered, the uterus was thoroughly dilated, traction was made upon the tumor by several
pairs of vulsella forceps, which were inserted into it at different points, pressure over the uterus was also made at the
same time, and in about a half hour the tumor was enucleated,
the uterus contracting firmly behind it.

This case resembled, very much, No. 1.

CASE 7.—Miss F., aged 31, white, has had dysmenorrhœa
and menorrhagia for 18 months. Abdomen considerably
enlarged. Upon examination the uterus was found to be an-
teverted, the cervix was conical and elongated, the cavity of
the uterus measured six inches. As it was impossible to obtain sufficient dilatation at one sitting, the cervix was dilated
moderately with a small dilator and plugged with three tupelo
tents; these were allowed to remain in for 24 hours; upon
their removal the cervix was softened and dilatable and upon
inserting the index finger a tumor could be felt projecting
into the uterine cavity and attached at the anterior portion of

the fundus.   By traction with volsella, leverage with Thomas' serrated scoop and pressure over the abdomen, the tumor, the size of an orange, was readily enucleated from its attachments and removed, the uterine surface being left almost as smooth where the tumor had been attached as at any other portion.

CASE 8.—Miss F., aged about 26, had been perfectly healthy until about one year before I saw her. During this year the first half, she had profuse menorrhagia and lost so much blood that she was obliged to remain in bed several days each month, then all flow ceased for about six months, and suddenly again, profuse hæmorrhage began, and had continued for about a week in spite of all the usual remedies which were used to check it.   At this time I saw her with her physician who had already detached a portion of a tumor projecting through the os.   After dilating the cervix very thoroughly the tumor was seized and enucleated by traction and pressure over the uterus.

CASE 9.—M. D., colored, aged 35, married, one child 13 years old, has had menorrhagia for the past three years. About six months before I saw her, she felt a lump in her abdomen which was tender and painful.   About four months after she first felt it, it suddenly disappeared and at the same time she had violent bearing-down pains, which continued at intervals until I saw her.   Upon examination I found the vagina completely distended by a large tumor apparently as large as a fœtal head.   As usual in such cases where the tumor has passed partly into the vagina, the lower portion had commenced to undergo disintegration.   With the patient under an anæsthetic several pairs of vulsella forceps were inserted into it so as to make traction from different directions at the same time.   Finding it immovable, two large sized cork-screws were screwed into it; by the aid of these, with an assistant pressing down on the tumor from above, it was gradually drawn outside of the vulva and the pedicle enucleated with Thomas' serrated scoop.   There was very little bleeding, and the woman left the hospital well, in two weeks after the operation.

CASE 10.—V. H., aged 34, colored, one child eight years old, has had menorrhagia for two years. Uterus enlarged and extended, cervix not dilated, uterus measured six inches. Upon dilatation a fibroid tumor as large as an orange was felt attached to the fundus. She was sent into the hospital, and the tumor was removed by traction and enucleation.

Interference through the vagina with tumors that are entirely sub-mucous should be delayed as long as the condition of the patient will admit. Electricity and ergot frequently do good where menorrhagia is excessive. The uterine contractions excited by the agents also tend to rupture the capsule and force the tumor partly into the uterus cavity as in case 3. When the symptoms occasioned by sub-mucous fibroids necessitate surgical interference, it is generally safer to deal with them as in the interstitial variety, by removal of the uterine appendages.

In conclusion I offer for your consideration the following summary;

1st. By traction and enucleation we get the benefit of normal uterine expulsive power.

2nd. We do not incur the risk of amputating a portion of the uterus, or of cutting off a portion of the tumor and leaving it in the cavity.

3rd. We leave a clean intra-uterine surface.

4th. We have a perfect means of diagnosis between a projecting fibroid tumor and inversion of the uterus.

FIBROID TUMORS COMPLICATING PREGNANCY.

By Reverdy M. Hall, M. D.

Under the term "fibroid tumors of the uterus," we may have fibromata, fibromyomata, myomata, etc., indicating the relative predominance of fibrous or muscular tissue. These may be interstitial, sub-peritoneal, or sub-mucous. The intra-uterine growths being frequently polypoid. Their most common site is said to be the posterior wall of the body, fibromata of the cervix being rare. Out of 74 cases of fibroids in the non-pregnant woman, it was found there were only four in the cervix. Sims found only 2 in 114 cases. They usually occupy the posterior lip of the cervix and rarely involve both lips. Apart from the changes which pregnancy and parturition cause in myomata, they may become hypertrophied, atrophied, fatty degenerated, vascular, etc. In consequence of being vascular, œdema, congestion, infiltration, extravasation or gangrene may follow this vascular dilatation. Each of these conditions may affect the general health and cause peritonitis usually circumscribed. Myomata do not offer an insurmountable obstacle to pregnancy. Fecundation is not impossible, but there is a connection between sterility and the presence of these fibromata; while sterility may be a direct cause of the development of fibroids nearly all specialists think fibroids cause sterility. The changes in the shape, situation and cavity of the uterus, and the altered relations between the ovary and tube are mechanical obstacles to fecundation. Fibroids are more common in married, than in single women, since out of 1634 women, 1192 were married, and 442 single; or, nearly 3 to 1. Fibroid tumors are very common among colored females, for out of a large number of colored women whom I have examined all who had tumors, excepting those who had cancer, had fibroids. They are also very frequent among sterile women, for Sims found 119 cases of fibroid in 605 sterile women. The chances of fecundation are very much lessened by the presence of fibroids;

for, of 1,554 women observed by various writers, 476 or 1 in
305 were sterile.   Myomata being composed of tissues identical with that of the uterus, it is not strange that they are
modified by pregnancy, but fibromata, fibro-myomata and
myomata undergo different changes; these changes depend
upon their seat, the more intimate their relations to the uterus,
the more they will share in the physiological phenomena
which take place in that organ and the more closely they
partake of the nature of the uterus, the more pronounced
will be the changes.   Fibromata, the tissue of which is
denser and more compact are less affected than myomata.
Fibroid tumors increase in volume during pregnancy, and
after delivery undergo an involution analagous to that of the
uterus.   The entire disappearance of a myoma is said to be
rare.   In many cases these tumors become flattened, so that
they can not be felt during pregnancy; this being observed
in interstitial myomata.   The placenta may be inserted on
the fibrous growth itself or on the lower segment of the
uterus.   Pregnancy may pursue its regular course even in
case of multiple fibroids.   Abortion and premature labor result about 1 in 4 cases.   If the tumor be outside of the true
pelvis, it rises with the enlarging uterus and only affects the
pregnancy by its pressure.   The myoma may undergo morbid changes which affect the general health.   If the tumor
is intra-uterine it grows simultaneously with the fœtus; if
located between the pelvic wall and the lower two-thirds of
the uterus, these tumors whether sessile or pediculated are
the most dangerous of all as regards pregnancy, especially
if in the posterior wall.   Hæmorrhage is not common since
it accompanies the sub-mucous variety.   The tumor may,
during pregnancy, compress the fœtus and cause abortion.
The location of the fibroids is of more importance than the
number and size.   If the tumor is situated at the cervix it
may, by its size alone cause dystocia.

If the tumor is sub-mucous, it is pediculated, and if it is
situated in the inferior segment of the uterus it will often be
expelled before the fœtus.   If the tumor is situated higher
up, delivery may be more difficult, and we may have to use
forceps or perform craniotomy.   If the tumors are interstitial,

and occupy the lower segment of the uterus, they often cause
serious difficulty.   If they are higher up in the uterus, they
rarely cause any difficulty.   If they can be pushed up in the
pelvis in front of the child, they often ascend above the presenting part, and thus allow its passage, or they are so softened and flattened out by the fœtal part that they offer no
obstacle to delivery.   Here the size of the tumor, although
it is an important element, it is not the principal one, since
it is rather the situation of the growth with reference to the
pelvis.   Large sessile, sub-peritoneal tumors with broad
bases are especially apt to ascend during labor, caused by
uterine contraction, the dilatation of cervix and the escape of
the waters.

When the membranes rupture, the walls of the uterus, retract, the longitudinal fibres contract, and the lower segment
of the uterus is drawn up.   Unfortunately, this ascension of
the tumor does not always take place, whence arises insurmountable obstacles which may render Cæsarean section
necessary.   But aside from the difficulties attributable to
fibroid tumors, mal-presentations of the fœtus are much more
frequent in pregnancies complicated with fibroid tumors.   In
a number of cases reported by various authors the majority
were not normal presentations.   Breech presentations are regarded as the most favorable in cases of fibroid tumors and
vertex the most serious.   A case is reported by Dr. Charpentier in which the os was partially dilated, the fœtal head
could be felt; the head was perforated, but the child could
not be extracted, and the woman died undelivered.

I had a case some years ago, in which the woman, though
pregnant, presented a large interstitial fibroid at the lower
segment of the uterus; I had delivered her with forceps
about two years previously; then no fibroid was perceptible.   At the latter pregnancy no advancement of the
head would take place on account of the fibroid; and in consultation with another physician we tried in vain to deliver
with forceps.   We waited for a few hours hoping that nature
would possibly bring relief, but she died undelivered in the
course of a few hours.

On the 25th of September, 1889, I was sent for to see Mrs.
J., age 38, primipara. She was suffering severe pains in her
abdomen ; she stated to me that she had missed her sickness
about the middle of May, 1889. Upon examination her abdomen was very much enlarged, somewhat tender and tym-
panitic. A tumor sub-peritoneal was discovered above and
to the right of the pubis. It was painful and very tender to the
touch. Upon examination per vaginum another large tumor
was found at the lower and posterior segment of the uterus.
There was no bleeding from the tumor ; she stated to me
that she had been examined by a physician some years previously, who told her she had womb trouble but did not
indicate its character. During menstruation she had had no
immoderate flow, it lasting three or four days. On account
of the pain I administered morphia, and as she had considerable nausea and sometimes vomiting, I gave her small doses
of creasote and bismuth. The pains were not of that character which indicated the pains of labor, neither was the os
dilated by them ; they seemed to be of a colicky nature
owing to a large amount of flatus within the bowels, and
possibly some localized peritonitis around the tumor. She
also suffered from dysuria. I continued in attendance upon
her throughout the month of October and at times the pains
and tenderness were so great as to compel me to use hypodermic injections of morphia to give relief. Believing that
the case would be a very difficult one at the time of labor, I
called in Dr. B. B. Browne at this time. He verified my
diagnosis and remarked it would be well to watch the case
as the time of labor approached. According to her testimony
I need not expect labor until between the middle and last of
February. On Tuesday, December 10th, I was summoned
to her hurriedly about 1.30 P. M., and found her in labor,
with the os well dilated, the cord prolapsed and the head
above the brim. Pains were pretty severe. I immediately
hastened for a consultation and as Dr. Browne was not in at
that hour, I called in Dr. Chunn. I related to him the history of the case. The fibroid had flattened itself and had
risen somewhat in the pelvis. A little later in the day I
called in Dr. Browne ; from his previous knowledge of the

case he was enabled to take in the situation at a glance. We accordingly chloroformed her. The pulsation of the cord had ceased; this was at 4.30 P. M., no signs of life could be detected in the child. Dr. Chunn placed and kept her under the influence of the anæsthetic. Dr. Browne applied Tarnier's forceps to the head which was above and immediately over the pubis, whilst I made pressure downwards and backwards upon the head. All efforts to dislodge the head from its position were futile. After having tried for a considerable while, the attempt to extract by forceps was abandoned and then he attempted to perform version, which after considerable labor and trouble he was enabled to do. The after-coming-head gave no trouble. There was born a well developed male child at full term about five hours after labor had fully set in.

The father of the child stated to me after the labor was completed, that its mother was mistaken in regard to her period of confinement, as her last menstruation had ceased in March instead of May. After labor, the womb contracted properly, and both tumors could be distinctly felt —the one above the pubis on the right side and sub-peritoneal, and the other in the lower and posterior segment of the uterus. The mother came out from under the influence of the anæsthetic well and did nicely for the following three days, when peritonitis developed itself, and after an illness of five days, she died on the eight day after confinement. As the time of labor approached, we had intended to hold another consultation in order to determine whether it was best or not to suggest to the family the necessity of a Cæsarean operation, and if so, to watch the case more closely, and make preparation to perform the same, believing that the interests of both mother and child demanded it. I believed, from the history of the case, we had ample time to consider the case. I was not able to ascertain the time of quickening; the abdomen continued very much swollen, and I was led to believe that her normal confinement would take place in February, but as it was, her natural period ended in December, of which I was not aware until after delivery. I had ceased to visit her for several weeks previous to her confinement. The illness from which she suffered in September and October was no doubt due, in part, to a circumscribed peritonitis in the region of the sub-peritoneal fibroid, and after delivery that circumscribed peritonitis developed into a general peritonitis, which caused her death eight days after confinement.

DISCUSSION.

Dr. B. B. Browne, in referring to the necessity of Cæsarean section, referred to by Dr. Hall, said that the idea was to perform the section, but as the pulsation in the cord had ceased such a thing was out of the question. Still, it was well to keep such cases in view, and be ready for the operation to be done at any time.

Report of the Section on Materia Medica and Chemistry.

THERAPEUTIC PROGRESS DURING THE PAST YEAR.

By Eugene F. Cordell, M. D., *Chairman*.

There have been no great additions to our therapeutical resources during the past year. Nevertheless, good work has been done in demonstrating the falsity of extravagant claims made in the case of several new remedial agents, and in establishing the exact value of those with which we were previously made acquainted. Interest still centres in the class of (a), antipyretic-analgesics and (b), hypnotics. Perhaps the most important contribution of the year is an agent belonging to the former class, viz.: exalgine or methylacetanilide.

Exalgine (ex, algos) derives its name from the most important of its characteristics—its power of relieving pain. It is one of the four isomeric methyl derivatives of acetanilide, and occurs in needles, or long, colorless, tablet-like crystals, sparingly soluble in cold water, quite soluble in hot water and in water to which a little alcohol is added; it is without taste or smell. Its chemical composition is $C_9H_{11}NO$. Physiologically, it is closely allied to acetanilide and antipyrin; its effects on the sensorium are, however, more marked, while its antipyretic powers are less, depressing the temperature $1-3°$ C. The dose is 4–6 grains two or three times a day. All forms of neuralgia are said to be benefited by it, including visceral neuralgia, and it sometimes relieves where antipyrin and antifebrin fail. It antagonizes convulsive symptoms and checks polyuria. It produces no gastro-intestinal irritation, rash or cyanosis, but occasionally causes slight vertigo and tinnitus.

The system becomes habituated to its use. In fatal doses, it appears to paralyze the respiratory centre. It is eliminated by the kidneys, diminishing markedly the urinary secretion.

Dujardin-Beaumetz, in discussing the agents of this class (the antipyretic-analgesics,) classifies them according to their value and properties as follows :

1st, Antipyrin : soluble ; but little toxic ; causing scarlatiniform eruption, sweats and collapse, even in small doses ; diminishing the activity of the brain and cord ; especially useful in migraine and the congestive neuralgias ; anti-choreic.

2nd, Exalgine : second only on account of its relative insolubility ; never producing an eruption ; to be given in moderate doses, as four grains twice or thrice a day, in capsules, or preferable in solution, as with tincture of orange-peel, syrup and water.

3rd, Phenacetine : third on account of its great insolubility ; this, however, an advantage, rendering it non-toxic ; to be given in capsules, seven and a half grains once or twice a day, in neuralgia.

4th, Acetanilide : placed last not because less powerful, but because of cyanosis, which is calculated to frighten the patient and attendants, but is not harmful ; may be given for months or years without other effect than a passing bluish discoloration of the face and mucous membranes ; very active ; very cheap ; requiring a large quantity of alcohol to dissolve ; best given in capsules, five or ten grains, thrice daily.*

It is thus seen, from the estimate of this distinguished therapeutist, that these four important new remedies possess remarkably similar characteristics, which makes it hard to gauge their relative value.

Bardet, of Paris, cautions us to be sure, in using exalgine, to get the genuine article, which may be known by melting at 214° F., since isomeric bodies are being sold under the same name, which are therapeutically nearly inert. ‡

---

*Therapeutic Gazette, Dec. 15, 1889.
‡Therapeutic Gazette, Sep. 15, 1889.

Another antipyretic brought recently into prominence is *pyrodine*, one of the numerous derivatives of coal-tar, a white, crystalline powder, sparingly soluble in cold water, without odor, and nearly tasteless.   It is a powerful antipyretic and analgesic, and is given in the dose of twelve grains or less, once in 18–24 hours.   Its use is accompanied by profuse sweating, and if continued a few days, by a toxic effect on the blood—hæmoglobinuria.   It cannot therefore, be regarded as a safe remedy for use, and we shall probably hear little more of it.§   Its active principle, hydracetine, has also been employed with similar results.

Thallin once a prominent antipyretic, has also proven to be a pronounced toxic agent, and has been relegated to obscurity.

Among hypnotics, *sulphonal* has continued to exact a large share of attention and research.   When it was first introduced to the notice of the profession, great hopes were entertained that at last an ideal hypnotic had been found.   For a time the reports were almost without exception favorable, but as time wore on they became less and less so, and it can now be said that this agent has fallen much below the position which it occupied when we last met.   In noting the accumulating unfavorable evidence, the editor of the *Therapeutic Gazette* (Dec. 15, 1889,) says : "The testimony as to the inconveniences, and indeed almost the dangers attending the use of sulphonal, is so rapidly accumulating, that it is evident its field of usefulness is becoming greatly restricted." Among the drawbacks to the use of the remedy are its expensiveness, its insolubility, the uncertainty of the dose and effect, the slowness of action, the persistency of the hypnotic effect, cumulative action and unpleasant and even dangerous sequelæ. Among the toxic effects reported are vomiting, faintness, tinnitus, vertigo, headache, muscular ataxia, tottering gait, excitement, delirium, delusions, cyanosis, pulmonary congestion, collapse.   These ill effects were usually seen most after large or repeated, but also sometimes after small, doses, and death has followed a moderate dose.   It is difficult to avoid

§Dr. Lafleur, of the Johns Hopkins Hospital, has confirmed the unfavorable report of this agent.—Johns Hopkins Hospital Reports

the conclusion from the contradictory reports that there must
be great variation in the composition of the drug, and that
toxic principles must be present in some preparations and absent in others.   To a considerable extent, doubtless, the ill
effects may be obviated by restricting the dose.   Ordinarily,
this should not exceed ten or fifteen, or, at most, twenty
grains, and remembering its cumulative effects and the slowness of its elimination owing to its insolubility, in case of
repetition the dose should be diminished.   In practice among
the insane, however, all experience proves that less than 30
grains is useless.

Choralamide is a combination of chloral and formamide,
occurs in colorless, odorless crystals, which have a faintly
bitter taste, are readily soluble in water, and still more so in
alcohol.   It is given in 15–45 grain doses, is pleasant to take,
and cheap.   Its effects are manifested more slowly than those
of chloral, but it is claimed to be free from the depressing
effect upon the heart and circulation exhibited by the latter.
It is not free, however, from unpleasant after-effects, and frequently fails to produce hypnotism.   The estimate of its
utility varies.   Lettow found it eminently satisfactory in 74
per cent. of his cases; with Fürbringer and Robinson it failed
in 46 per cent., and at the Johns Hopkins Hospital, where it
was used under Professor Osler's direction in 50 cases, the
following results are reported (Toulmin):

Total number of doses administered	186
Undoubted hypnotic action in	86
Negative results in	85
Results uncertain in	15
Ill effects (headache, mental confusion, or derangement,) in	16*

Somnal is the name given to a mixture of alcohol, chloral
and urethan, by Radlauer, a druggist of Berlin, who claims
that in 30-drop doses it produces a quiet, deep and natural
sleep, commencing half an hour after administration and lasting six to eight hours.   But Liebreich† states that the inventor

---

*Johns Hopkins Hospital Bulletin, Feb. 1890.
†Therapeutische Monatshefte, Dec. 1889.

does not know the composition of the agent and that his claims are fallacious, and Robinson (assistant of Prof. Fürbringer,) finds that it exerts a hypnotic effect only in about 30 per cent. of cases, besides having a very undesirable, and occasionally even dangerous, secondary action on the heart.

Amylene hydrate has established for itself a place scarcely inferior to sulphonal. It acts rapidly, producing a sleep of some six to twelve hours duration. The respiration, circulation and digestion are not notably affected. On account of its irritating character, it should not be given by the mouth when there is gastric disorder or nausea. It may, however, be given by the rectum. Because of its disagreeable taste and odor, it is not suited for use by fastidious patients and children. Slight toxic effects are sometimes observed, as headache, nausea, oppression about the chest, etc. The dose is 30 to 45 grains, and it is best given in capsules, or in mixture flavored by licorice.

Urethan is a mild and uncertain hypnotic in the dose of 30-60 grains. It is very soluble in water and its taste is not offensive.

Professor Leech‡ gives the following order as representing the hypnotic power of the several drugs mentioned and paraldehyde : 1, sulphonal ; 2, amylene hydrate ; 3, paraldehyde ; 4, urethan. None of these, he states, equal chloral hydrate in certainty of action, although either of the first two may succeed where the latter has failed. None of these agents are adapted to the insomnia due to pain.

The search for an antiseptic which shall be efficient, and at the same time harmless, continues. *Creolin* is the latest agent claiming our attention from this direction. It is derived from creosote, but its composition has not been determined ; its antiseptic power is probably to be ascribed to phenol : it contains scarcely a trace of pure carbolic acid. It is non-volatile, readily forms an emulsion with water and is not poisonous. Dr. Spaeth and others took daily eight grammes for a length of time without local or general bad consequences. A patient of Dr. Kortüm drank by mistake sixty grammes in a five per

‡British Medical Journal, Nov. 1889.

cent. solution without experiencing any bad effects. It is lubricating, non-corrosive even when pure, does not injure clothing, and can be washed out of material without leaving a spot. Among other advantages claimed for it are, that it is a deodorizer, parasiticide and styptic, easily distinguised by color and smell, and cheap, the price being about one-fourth that of carbolic acid. A two or three per cent. emulsion is employed for external use. We are cautioned against imitations, and Pearson's preparation is said to be the best. Further observation is needed to establish the exact value of this preparation.*

"By very simple processes, most individuals, at least of some races, and many individuals of all races, can be thrown into a condition of preverted consciousness, in which they are automatisms, controlled by the will of the operator, insensitive in such portions of the body as he declares are devoid of feeling, sensitive when he declares sensation exists, physically, morally, seemingly in all respects an *alter ego* to the man who commands them." † This state is known as *hypnotism*, from its resemblance to natural sleep. Now it has been found that this state may be utilized in the relief of various ailments not only functional, but also structural, among which are included menstrual troubles, rheumatism, gout, constipation, diarrhœa, general debility, paralysis, especially infantile, cramps from over-use, etc. It is principally in France that hypnotism has been practiced, and almost miraculous results have been claimed there from it. The method of treatment is simply by suggestions made to the patient during the hypnotic state, as for instance, that she would not have her customary pain during her approaching menstrual period. I will not lengthen this report by a recital of the wonderful results that have been secured by this method. There can be no doubt that they have been actually secured, but there is some doubt as to the connection of the suggestion and the result. It is in the neurotic class of patients that hypnotism alone is possible, and Charcot asserts that there is a very close relation between hypnotism and hysteria. Now we are

*See Deutsche Medicinische Zeitung, July 1889.
†Therapeutic Gazette, Sept 1889

well aware of the power of mental impressions over the subjects of this protean malady.   Hypnotism is therefore probably only faith-cure under another name.   In this connection two cases exhibited at the clinic of Professor Wood, of Philadelphia, have an important bearing.   One was a case of almost complete paraplegia, the other had suffered from incessant tremor of the right hand, exactly simulating paralysis agitans; both were doubtless hysterical in character.   Both were rapidly cured by hypnotism without any suggestions whatever being made during the hypnosis.   Professor Wood commented upon the want of control experiments in the elucidation of this subject.‡   In this connection it is of interest that hypnotism has been abandoned at Professor Charcot's clinic and that Meynert, of Vienna, refuses to employ it, because it weakens the will, which in neurotic subjects it is desirable to strengthen.   Virchow and von Ziemssen also oppose it. From extensive personal experience, the latter finds its influence only transient even in slight functional disturbances, and that it is powerless to mitigate the severe neuroses—epilepsy, chorea and paralysis agitans, to say nothing of deep-seated organic disturbances.   Its power for harm too is great, since it may convert a slight hysteria into a "grande hysterie," as noted by Charcot; and finally it may possibly place in the hands of unscrupulous persons the power to commit crime without the possibility of their detection.   So far we seem to have escaped a visitation of this therapeutic vagary, but it is almost too much to expect that a country and people whose imitative faculties are so good as ours will remain altogether inhospitable to this novelty.

During the year an important addition has been made to the therapeutics of spinal diseases, especially of locomotor ataxia, viz : *suspension.*   By means of Sayre's apparatus, patients are suspended every other day, so that the toes just touch the floor. At first the treatment lasts only a half-minute, but after eight or ten séances it is prolonged to three minutes. The treatment is said to be harmless, but should never be entrusted to the patient or his attendants alone.   Of eighteen cases of pronounced tabes with 400 séances extending over a

‡Therapeutic Gazette, January 1890.

period of four months (Charcot,) fourteen were benefited, eight remarkably. The good effects were evidenced by immediate improvement in the gait, by disappearance of Romberg's symptom, by a lessening or cessation of vesical troubles and lightning pains, and by return of sexual power. The patellar reflex, however, did not return, and the pupil symptom persisted. These results have been confirmed by Dujardin-Beaumetz and Bernhardt. So far, no cures have been reported ; still, in an affection with so hopeless a prognosis as locomotor ataxia and with the paucity of resources at our command, we may well welcome this addition. A semi-suspension has also been practiced with good results. This consists in making the patient take hold of the top of a door and lift his feet off the floor.

Of the utility of *electricity* as a therapeutic agent, there can be no doubt, but that fashion has much to do with its popularity there can be also little question. It is a good and harmless divertisement for patients and satisfies them that the physician is not neglecting them. With the rich, it is a fruitful source of income to the profession. Static electricity may be ignored, the galvanic and faradic currents answering all the purposes of the physician. The galvanic current may produce chemical changes, which according to their degree, may be either stimulant or destructive ; the interrupted, or faradic current, promotes functional activity. As a therapeutic agent, the use of electricity is limited, extending only to the treatment of the neuroses and the symptoms of organic disease. So good an observer as Dr. M. Allen Starr, of New York, declares that after its constant use for ten years he has been disappointed in the results. Dr. L. C. Gray, in discussing which pole should be used in faradism, says, that notwithstanding the chemical, physiological and sensory differences between the negative and positive poles, he has never been able to satisfy himself as to their therapeutic differences, and he lays down the following rule : When one pole does not agree, try the other, and if that does not agree, stop using electricity. This simplifies matters very much.* In connection with this subject, I may call attention to the fact that Bal-

---

*New York Medical Record, April 6, 1889.

timore excels at this time in the manufacture of electric batteries.   The advantages of the Barrett dry-cell batteries are
doubtless known to you all, and it is only to be regretted that
the manufacturers by their exorbitant prices have placed
them beyond the reach of so many of the profession.

In 1888, Surgeon-Major E. Lawrie, the resident surgeon
in Hyderabad, India, applied to the local Government of that
province for the appointment of a commission to investigate
the action of chloroform, on the ground that the views entertained in the profession of the action of this anæsthetic were
erroneous.   A commission was accordingly appointed, and
as a result of their investigations they reported that "chloroform may be given by inhalation with perfect safety, and
without any fear of accidental death if only the respiration be
carefully attended to throughout."   This conclusion was
naturally received with suspicion and doubt, and a second
commission was appointed to repeat the experiments on an
enlarged scale, and Dr. Lauder Brunton, the eminent teacher
and pharmacologist was added to it.   The conclusions of the
second Hyderabad Chloroform Commission have just been
published and deserve our careful study.   Four hundred and
thirty experiments were performed upon different animals—
dogs, monkeys, goats, and horses, and we may epitomize
their most important conclusions as follows :—The recumbent position is essential.   Absolute freedom of respiration
should be secured.   An apparatus should not be used.   The
administrator should avoid giving the vapor in too concentrated a form at first.   As soon as the eye-ball can be touched
without exciting winking, the operation should be commenced.   As a rule no operation should be commenced until
full anæsthesia is secured. *The administrator should be guided
entirely by the respiration*, any interference with which, however slight, should cause an immediate cessation of the anæsthesia.   In embarrassed respiration, pull the lower jaw forward to raise the epiglottis, and practise artificial respiration.
If respiration stop, lower the head, draw forward the tongue
and practise artificial respiration.   Atropia should not be
used before the anæsthesia, but alcohol may be useful. "*The
commission has no doubt whatever, that if the above rules be fol-*

*lowed, chloroform may be given in any case requiring an opera-
tion, with perfect ease and absolute safety so as to do good without the risk of evil."*§

These results are so completely subversive of our previous
views regarding chloroform anæsthesia, that it is hardly to
be expected that they will obtain immediate acceptance at
the hands of the profession in this country and Europe, especially since they are based exclusiveiy upon experiments upon
animals—mainly dogs. They are nevertheless, very striking
and call for renewed physiological and clinical investigation
of the subject. In this connection, the fact has been revealed
that Syme laid stress upon attention to the respiration rather
than the circulation in chloroform anæsthesia. It is also a
significant fact that the conclusions reached by the Committee are contrary to those held by Dr. Brunton previous to the
investigations in which he took part.

Among minor points to which the Section would call attention are the following : the use of glycerine enemata for
constipation, ℥ i-ii in an adult and ℥ss-i in a child exciting
reflex peristaltic action in a few minutes without pain or irritation. It is especially adapted to use in pregnancy and in
children. Messrs. Sharp & Dohme, of this city, prepare a
very beautiful suppository, which can be used in whole or
part for different ages ; it contains 95 per cent. of glycerine.

Prof. Field, of Dartmouth College, draws attention to the
extreme insolubility of the alkaloid strychnine, of which such
large use is made in the manufacture of pills and granules.
The sulphate of strychnia should always be substituted. He
recommends the following improved formula for a purgative
granule, one granule being usually sufficient to produce pur-
gation.

    ℞—Aloin.,   . .   gr. ⅛
      Strychninæ sulph.,   gr. ¹⁄₆₀
      Extr. balladonnæ, . gr. ¹⁄₁₅
      Pulv. ipecac.,   . gr. ½
    Ft. pillula i.

§Lancet.

The same gentleman refers to the overdosing with digitalis, and says that the dose should not be greater than five drops three or four times a day.*

Remarkable results are claimed by a Russian observer (Mandelstanu, of Kazan), from the use of phosphorus in rickets.   He gave it in the dose of about ⅟₁ gr. in cod-liver oil, once or twice a day.   Of 214 patients, 120 were cured and 43 benefited.   The benefit is seen after two months.†

The difficulty of finding a suitable excipient for permanganate of potash seems to be overcome by the recommendation of lanolin.   In the proportion of one part of lanolin to ten of the permanganate, the pills are said to be easy to make, to be hard, and to retain their shape perfectly.‡

Sir Alfred Baring Garrod has called attention to the value of sulphur in small doses in habitual constipation, hepatic sluggishness, piles, rheumatoid arthritis, gout, chronic muscular rheumatism, skin diseases, and pulmonary affections. He administers it in a lozenge containing milk of sulphur, 5 grains, and cream of tartar, one grain.§

Dr. Sternberg has recommended a formula for the treatment of yellow fever, which commends itself on theoretical grounds, and has also given satisfaction in actual practice. It is based upon the highly acid condition of the stomach and urine, and the probability that an acid medium may favor the development of the germ in the intestinal canal.   It is composed as follows :

> ℞.—Sodii bicarb.,   .   .   ℨiv
> Hydrarg, chlorid. cor.,   gr ½
> Aquæ puræ,   .   .   qt. j.
> M. S. ℨi⅔ every hour, ice-cold.‖

Prof. H. C. Wood states that the only remedy he has found of any service in hay-fever is cocaine, administered in the form of nasal bougies made with cocoa butter, each containing gr. ⅟₁₀ atropine and 1 gr. cocaine, to be introduced high up in the nostril while the patient is recumbent.

*Therapeutic Gazette, Dec. 1889.
†Medical Press and Circular, July 17, 1889.
‡Phar. Journal and Trans., National Druggist, July 1, 1889.
§Lancet, April 6, 1889.
  Therapeutic Gazette, Dec. 1889.

This report would not be complete without allusion to the National Formulary of Unofficinal Preparations, issued by authority of the American Pharmaceutical Association, in 1888. It is an attempt to provide an authoritative standard for the large number of drugs and formulæ which are in use by the profession, but for which the United States Pharmacopœia makes, as yet, no mention. It is an excellent work and deserves to be generally adopted. I am glad to announce that it has been recommended by a committee of this Faculty and has been incorporated into the last edition of the United States Dispensatory.

DISCUSSION.

Dr. P. C. Williams spoke of the difficulties of finding a reliable hypnotic, especially in cases of hysteria. Sulphonal is slow and uncertain, and fails in hysterical cases, although it is good in mere wakefulness. He endorsed what was said about chloroform. Do not put a patient under it too gradually. The best inhaler is a cylinder. He gives chloroform chiefly in labor, and then uses it whether the heart is affected or not. Its use prevents unnecessary strain on a diseased heart.

Dr. J. D. Blake thought the danger of chloroform was at the beginning. The nervous system should become gradually accustomed to the chloroform.

Dr. C. H. Jones thought the Hyderabad Commission had shown nothing new in its investigations.

Dr. J. J. Chisolm has fought the battle for chloroform for twenty years. The Hyderabad Commission has sustained every point he had made.　　　•

Dr. A. K. Bond thought the pupil should be watched in chloroform anæsthesia. This was more important than the pulse or respiration.

Dr. Hiram Woods said there was no use in watching these signs. Some have susceptible hearts and will die anyhow.

Dr. I. E. Atkinson thought the skill of the anæsthetizer should be taken into account.

Dr. J. W. Chambers thought the amount and method of giving it made very little difference.   Some die anyhow.

Dr. L. McLane Tiffany said neither chloroform nor ether was the best.   The medical man should confine himself to neither, exclusively, and use his judgment and discretion.

Dr. George H. Rohé thought the cases should be selected.

Dr. C. G. Hill gave chloroform at first and followed it up with ether.

This paper was further discussed by Drs. W. R. Monroe, J. H. Branham, J. E. Michael and R. Winslow.

Report of the Section on Anatomy, Physiology and Pathology.

A CONTRIBUTION TO THE THEORY OF NEURO-METABOLIC PROCESSES.

By John C. Hemmeter, Dr. Med. et. Philos.

There are many phenomena that have led to the establishing of a separate category of trophic nerves. The smallest part of the material which stimulated this classification came from physiological experiment, the largest part from clinical observation. Without intending to underestimate the value of bedside studies, results of this method cannot be reproduced at will nor under varying conditions, hence conclusions from them must be drawn with caution. In attempting a review of the experiments upon animals that have led to the conception of trophic nerves, the following results merit consideration.

According to Bruecke the pigment cells in the epidermis of the chameleon and of frogs are under the influence of motor nerves. Ehrmann has observed the direct entrance of nerve fibres into the pigment cells of the epidermis of the frog. Leydig had observed the same fact in other reptilia prior to Ehrmann. Kühne states that the cells of the cornea can be stimulated through the fibres of the corneal nerves to retract their processes. It is probable that this dependence upon the nervous system of cells distributed in tissues has been observed only in case of pigment and corneal cells, because they offer a better opportunity for study. It is plausible to presume that there are in the animal organism a large number of other kinds of cells that are under the direct imperium of nerves as is the case in the pigment and corneal cells referred to. In case the nerve fibres going to such cells are cut off or are irritated for any length of time, we might expect changes to result, which have been designated as trophic disturbances, and which up to the present time have been ascribed to paralysis or irritation of trophic nerves.

Landowsky, Maddox and Calberla have described connections of nerve fibres with so called connective tisue corpuscles, and recently E. F. Hoffmann found the same in Bruecke's Laboratory. We know furthermore that the secretory nerves of glands, when stimulated, change the chemical processes in the organ essentially and also the amount of blood flowing into them. It is therefore not impossible, that similar nerves go to other organs essentially changing and influencing the chemical processes in them and consequently also their nutrition. In the category of metabolic nerves we must also classify those very interesting nerve fibres going to the luminous organs of certain invertebrates, and whose irritation causes a luminous effect, a flashing up of these peculiar structures. Panceri has studied these phenomena in case of Philorfhœ bucephala and Max Schultze in case of Lampyris Splendidula and Kolliker and Bellesme have confirmed that the luminous organ is in connection with and under the influence of nerve fibres. One is here forced to the conclusion that a nervous influence may cause a chemical process by which a luminous effect is directly produced.

In returning to instances of neuro metabolic processes in the vertebrates we are confronted by the epoch making results of Wm. H. Gaskell and T. Wesley Mills. For when Gaskell demonstrates that stimulation of the cardiac nerves increases the conductive power of the auricular substance, so that after a partial block has been caused by divison of the auricle so that only every *second* contraction passed, after stimulation of the nerves *every* contraction passed, he gives evidence that these nerves directly influence nutrition in the cardiac muscle. Moreover, he goes on to show (McKendrick's Physiology Vol. II, P. 242) that sometimes such stimulation seemed to increase the block, in which every second contraction passed before stimulation of the right vagus and coronary nerves, while no contraction passed during stimulation. The action of the nerve stimulus is thus usually and normally shown to hasten the recovery of the conducting power of the muscular tissue, and thus facilitate the transmission of the contraction wave.   In this way Gaskell (Gaskell "on certain points in the function of cardiac muscle" Proceedings of the Cambridge Philosophical Society Vol. IV, 1882) leads the way to the valuable suggestion that the influence of the vagus (the so called inhibitory influence) is to intensify function and that it may be regarded as the *trophic* nerve of the heart, that is to say it depresses or exalts the different functions of the heart muscle as regards rhythm, contraction, tone, conduction or excitability.   In speaking of the ganglionic nerve cells of the heart Gaskell distinguishes two classes, 1st, motor and 2nd, trophic.   The vagus acts on both of these classes.   If the impulses reach the motor group the *rate* of the rythm is affected and if they reach the trophic, they affect the force of the contraction, the conduction and the tonicity. (W. H. Gaskell on the innervation of the heart of the tortoise "*Jour. of Physiol. Vol. III.*)   These are also the views of T. Wesley Mills (the innervation of the heart of the Slider Terrapin [pseudemys rugosa]—T. Wesley Mills, *Jour. Physiol. Vol. VI.*)   Thus following out the indications afforded by these and other inquiries, Gaskell has been led to the profound conception that the apparently opposite action of the fibres of the vagus and of the sympathetic on the heart is due to their influence on the nutritive processes occurring in the cardiac tissue.   It is well known that prolonged stimulation of the sympathetic nerve soon exhausts the energy of the heart beats so that they become weaker.   Gaskell observed on the contrary that while stimulation of the vagus diminishes the energy of the heart beats for a time, when the stimulation ceases, the heart beats as strongly or more strongly than before.   The action of the vagus (McKendrick) is apparently to improve the condition of the heart, so that the sympathetic may, in consequence of the stimulation of the vagus, regain some of its lost power over the heart.   Thus the last author quoted compares the action of the sympathetic fibres to that of a motor nerve in a muscle, leading to destructive metabolism, or *katabolism* while on the other hand the action of the vagus fibres to do with constructive metabolism or *anabolism*.

The sympathetic fibres excite processes of decomposition by the splitting up of complex muscle protoplasm into simpler bodies, and the vagus fibres, on the other hand excite processes of repair. The vagus fibres are therefore *anabolic* while those of the sympathetic are *katabolic*. These terms are more expressive than inhibitory and motor, because they indicate the nature of the processes in which the nerve fibres are engaged (W. H. Gaskell—"structure and function of visceral nerves"—*Jour. of Physiolog., Vol. VII*—also—"The inhibitory actions and inhibitor nerves in general." Trans. of eighth Session of the International Med. Congress, in Copenhagen, 1884.)

McKendrick raises the question. "Is inhibition an indication of Katabolism? How can this be discovered? And thereupon very ingeniously continues to examine minutely the molecular processes occurring in connection with it, and as the most convincing proofs of molecular processes in muscle are derived from an investigation of the electrical phenomena connected with them, he turns to this field of inquiry. It is well known that the action of a nerve ending on the protoplasm of muscle is to cause a katabolic change, which finds a physical expression in a fall of electrical potential at the stimulated point that is to say the stimulated point becomes negative to any other part of the muscle substance. On the other hand, an anabolic change might be reasonably expected to cause a rise of electrical potential, so that when the change occurred the part would become positive to any other part of the muscle. In the case of the heart Gaskell has shown that when the vagus is stimulated in the neck of the tortoise, and when a preparation has been made from the heart by cutting away the sinus and part of the auricles without cutting the coronary nerve, there is always an *increase of positivity*. Here the nervous influence which causes inhibition produces *positivity*, so that the cardiac muscles under the influence of an inhibitory nerve becomes positive to the quiescent muscle just as the contracted muscle becomes negative to the uncontracted (W. H. Gaskell—"Ueber die Elektrischen Veraenderungen, welche in dem ruhenden Herzmuskel die Reizung des Nervus Vagus begleiten." Beitrage Zur Physiologie. C.

Ludwigs' Festschrift also *Journ. of Physiol., Vol. VII.*) Gaskell has further shown that by stimulating the sympathetic nerve negativity of the tissue is produced (W H. Gaskell—Muscarine and Cardiac Electric Changes *Journ. Physiol. Vol. VIII*).

These results of Gaskell and others point clearly to the fact that there is in the heart muscle at least a direct functional influence of nerve fibres over metabolism.

Another fact which merits notice in considering the evidence for and against metabolic nerves, is that after suture of long divided nerves, indolent ulcers have been known to heal with great rapidity.

After section of both vagi, death results after a period varying in time as do also the symptoms with the animal.

Eichorst and Zander, have studied in pigeons the alterations produced in the myocardium by bilateral section of the vagus. They found a fatty degeneration of the heart, which the former attributed to absence of the influence of the vagus on the myocardium and by the latter to inanition—Zander founded his hypothesis on the fact that the animals constantly and progressively lost weight. Fantoni with the support of Dr. Lustig repeated these experiments in the laboratory of the Hospital of Humbert I—Fantoni tried bilateral section of the vagus and found that pulmonitis as a rule supervened. He then confined his studies to animals in whom a unilateral section had been simply made, and here pulmonary complications never arose, nor did the animals lose weight. He found distinct change as early as 48 hours after section of one of the vagi. These changes were observable macroscopically as yellowish white patches of various size, isolated and distributed especially on the two faces of the interventricular septum, the gross papillary muscles and the external surface of the heart along the sulci of the coronary arteries. On micro·scopic examination the principal features were, numerous foci of infiltration with small round cells in the interfascicular spaces gradually invading the interfibrillar spaces. The foci become rapidly diffused in the following days, the round cells become fusiform, and they form in the cardiac muscle a true netting whose meshes separate the muscular fibres from one another. From the eighth to the tenth day many of these fibres present a notable degree of atrophy. Fibres devoid of nuclei are more numerous than in previous days. In more advanced epochs (eighteenth to thirtieth day) many fibres have disappeared and are substituted by fascicles of connective tissue rich in young connective cells. The general conclusion is that the fibres of the vagus not only have a functional value but that they exercise over the heart a metabolic influence. Fantoni also informs us that bilateral section of the sympathetic gave no alterations in the heart, whilst section of the depressor gave the alterations, which have been described for section of the pneumogastric but less pronounced. (T. Wesley Mills on Fantoni's results—Montreal, 1889.

Many of the functional diseases of the heart, and even the diseases of the myocardium may be found to have disturbances in the metabolic functions of the vagus, and sympathetic as etiological factors. It is a plausible deduction from the results of Gaskell, Mills, Eickhorst, Zander and especially Putjakin (Virchow's Archiv. lxxiv,) that the heart ganglia are directly concerned in these metabolic disturbances. And we have it on authority of Osler, that changes in the cardiac ganglia, as occurring in "centres of control, probably have more to do with cardiac atony and breakdown than we generally admit. (Am. Syst. Med. Vol. iii, P. 633.)

Magendie was the first to call attention to changes in the eye, following section of the trigeminal, which began with cloudiness of the cornea, and later on led to destruction of the eyeball by suppuration. We will further on return to the consideration of these observations.

After section of the sciatic in animals ulceration of the paws have been noticed.

On cutting through all nerves that go to an extremity, changes take place which have been studied by Mantegazza, Schiff and Vulpian. Schiff found in dogs, cats and frogs, after section of the crural and sciatic nerve, that the bones on the operated side had been reduced in size after 3 months, the periostium was thickened and often consisted of several layers. In these reduced bones a diminution in inorganic constituents had taken place (Schiff Compt.—rend. 1854 P. 1050.) Kassouitz, has made the same observations (Centralbl. f. d. Med. Wiss. 1878. S. 790). Vulpian and Philipeaux, Nelaton and Obolensky observed atrophy of the testicle after section of the spermatic nerve.

Haidenhain, Bidder and Claude Bernard have recorded degeneration of the salivary glands after section of their nerves.

Schiff and Legros described atrophy of the coxcomb after section of its nerve.

Brown-Sequard observed in guinea pigs a remarkable effect which section of the sympathetic had upon the brain. After bilateral section of these nerves in the neck he found after eighteen months the brain to be much less in volume than in intact animals of the same age. More important than this experiment, is another one of the same author in which after unilateral section of the sympathetic the brain became atrophied on the corresponding side—Vulpian has partly confirmed Brown-Sequards results.

Section of motor nerves exerts a very important influence on their corresponding muscles. Aside from altered reaction of the muscles to stimulation of the galvanic and faradic current, there are changes in the muscles substance proper and in the sarcolemma which are degenerative and atrophic.

There are a large number of observations on trophic disturbances in man in connection with disease or injury to the nervous system. Samuel, Weir Mitchell, Charcot, Erb and Bowlby have given compilations of these phenomena. It is claimed that trophic disturbances have been established after disease or injury to sensory motor and mixed nerves.

After neuralgic affections the following changes have been seen and recorded. Changes in the color, number and thickness, also distribution of the hair, growing thin of the skin and disappearance of the adipose tissue. In the skin and at the eye various affections such as, erythema, erysipelas, urticaria, pemphigus and particularly herpes.

Similar appearances occur when anæsthesia has occurred in a peripheral region, as a result of interruption in the nervous conducting paths between it and the brain.

As a result of peripheral paralyses, the dermis often shows signs of atrophy ; becoming thin as paper, smooth and shining, especially at the fingers and toes (glossy fingers, glossy skin). The dermis is disposed to ulcerations and decubitus. Weir Mitchell has noticed a disappearance of hair, while Schiefferdecker regularly saw an increase. Bones atrophy and loose weight. Joints become stiff, swollen and painful. The striated muscles undergo a kind of atrophy which is in no way different from that which results from intersection of motor nerves.

In disease or injury to the spinal cord, in general the same trophic disturbances have been established as in changes of the peripheral nerves. These disturbances seem to eminate rather from the peripheral nerves than from the spinal cord itself. The cause of degenerative atrophy of muscles is a sign of protopathic progressive muscular atrophy, of amyotrophique lateral sclerosis, which the majority of authors primarily ascribe to localized changes in the nerve cells of the anterior gray horns. This view, however, has been repeatedly disputed (Friedreich and Lichtheim). The dermis may be the seat of the same disturbances under spinal trouble as those which have been mentioned under the head of injuries to peripheral nerves. (Charcot—éschare a formation rapide.) In serious traumatic lesions to the cord, Charcot· describes a rapidly spreading decubitus in cases where local pressure and uncleanliness could be entirely eliminated.

Charcot has recently called attention to very remarkable disintegration of joints which occasionally occur during the progress of tabes dorsalis and after traumatism of the cord in spontaneous myelitis.

In hemiplegia from cerebral causes rapidly developing arthropathies are recorded.

Schiff, Brown-Sequard and Ebstein, have observed ecchymoses in the lungs, pleuræ and particularly in the stomach after injury and disease of certain parts of the brain (optic thalamus, corpus striatum and pons.)

It will now be our object to investigate the extent to which this material referred to, justifies the establishing of a definite category of trophic nerves. First of all, to put this question in a clear light it will be necessary, to separate the phenomena which have been observed after section of motor and secretory nerves, in muscles and in the submaxillary glands, from the phenomena that occur in other organs under similar conditions. To approach the question of the existence or nonexistence of so called trophic nerves in muscles and glands, it would be necessary first to define the requisites which these nerves would have to comply with ; if they are to be considered physiologically a distinct class. The results of the two methods of physiology, nerve section and nerve stimulation ought to supplement each other to the effect that with destruction of the nerve action a loss of normal nutritive processes ought to occur, but with artificial stimulation, changes in nutrition ought to result that are capable of demonstration. The facts so far ascertained however do not satisfy these requisites. The disturbances in the nutrition of muscles occur far too late to be attributable to an exclusion of a direct trophic influence, and there are no facts to allow one to judge of nutritive changes following artificial nerve stimulation. So that with the facts on hand we can outside of motor nerves not ascribe, special trophic nerves to muscles. But the following principle may be laid down.

"The central nervous substance (Gray,) the peripheral fibre and the peripheral end organs do not merely represent one single functional unity of excitation but also a trophic or nutritive unity." (Sigmund.) So that all nerves are in some sense metabolic.

In the normal organism, striated muscles are exited to contraction from the nervous central organs, and the glandular tissues are stimulated to their normal activity only from these centres. In all three constituents of this apparatus, there must occur a series of specific changes, the final result of which is in the muscle, contraction, in the glandular tissue secretion. If therefore a cooperation of the three parts of this apparatus is necessary to produce changes in nutrition of a specific character, for as such we must regard contraction and secretion, then we have good reason for assuming that these three factors exert this reciprocal action also in those conditions of the organism, in which these specific trophic or metabolic phenomena are absent. This reciprocal action need not express itself in voluntary motion, nor in conscious sensation, nor in secretion nor in other changes perceptible by the senses, but simply in a definite regulation of metabolism, in a very definite relation between consumption and renewal of nutritive material. The final result of this reciprocal action can be nothing else but normal nutrition, the preservation of a definite form, of a definite chemical composition. With the dissolution of this unity of excitation (central organ, nerve and peripheral organs) the trophic unity disappears also. The processes which then develop are atrophy and allotrophy.

The trophic processes in nerves, muscles and glands separated from their centres do not cease entirely but are led into channels, that are no longer subject to the purposes of the total organism. Just as a separated muscle is only paralyzed as far as the movements serving normal purposes of the organism are concerned, but outside of that such a muscle is capable of moving itself (spontaneous paralytic oscillation) or capable of excitation although in a different manner, to the electric current.

In order to explain the disturbances that have thus far been classed as trophic we must regard the result of loss of function and abnormally increased function in (a) sensory or centripetal nerves and (b) vaso motor nerves (vaso constrictor and vasodilator.)

It seems established from the results of many investigations that the morbid appearances in the eye after section of the trigeminal as well as the changes in the gums and lips are produced by loss of sensibility and consequent absence of certain movements for protection. In a similar manner one could explain the ulcerations in other parts after eliminating the sensory nerves. Elimination of sensory nerves does not merely act by causing a loss of reflex motility in important organs of protection but also by preventing at the same time, the transmissions to central organs of reflex regulatory innervatious for local blood supply.

The intervention of vaso motor nerves in the production of certain changes in nutrition and growth can not be denied.

It is more than probable that the hyperæmia and local elevation of temperature, which follows section of vaso constrictor nerves may effect an acceleration in metabolism. But as this hyperæmia soon goes back, and the tonus of the vessels returns, this increased metabolism can not last long. On the contrary there may be a retardation of the nutritive process, as the blood vessels remain in a medium state of contraction and only oscillate in a passive manner under influence of alternating blood pressure, and never again become as expanded, as was possible under the influence of the nervous central organs. Perhaps we must also reckon here with a loss of vaso dilator innervation. The observations, to which I have referred before, concerning atrophy of erectile structures in birds can be accounted for in this way, for the nutrition of these structures is dependent upon the congestion occurring from time to time under influence of the vaso dilator nerves.

The question whether elimination of vaso motor innervations can produce imflammatory and exudative processes is difficult to answer. There is some good evidence for believing that prolonged stimulation of vaso constrictor nerves may finally give rise to an inflammatory process.

The mechanism which is here at work has been pointed out by Cohnheim (Untersuchungen uber die embolischen Processe Berlin 1872). Cohnheim discovered, that capillary regions, that had been excluded for a prolonged period from normal circulation, after a while were subject to metabolic, trophic disturbances, finally producing those phenomena that are characteristic of inflammation. Now if for example we can imagine a prolonged constriction of the arterioles as a result of disease of any part of the vaso constrictor apparatus, the defective circulation in the capillaries thus produced, may cause trophic disturbances whose final result would be inflammation. As we know that the tonus of vaso constrictor nerves, is for most part under control of sensory excitement—the inflammatory processes, in the course of neuralgias (Herpes Zooster) might here find explanation.

٭Physiology has yet no explanation for the forms of decubitus in the course of injuries and diseases of the nervous central organs. It would be too hypothetical to explain this by trophic nerves.

How could stimulation or paralysis of a nerve cause gangrenous disintegration of tissues, with which that nerve has no connection whatever, I mean with the connective tissue elements of the skin and with the cells of the rete malpighi.

Until a direct nervous connection with these cells has been established, it would be much more rational to attribute gangrenous nutritive disturbances to interference with the blood supplying tracks.

Function and nutrition are but different phrases of the same thing, the general metabolism of the body, hence all nerves are in some sense metabolic nerves (Mills.) The nutritive processes are under constant regulative influence by the nervous system, but sufficient proof for existence of so called trophic nerves pure and simple has not yet been furnished; except in those nutritive processes of a specific nature occurring in muscles and glands. Most so called trophic disturbances may find an explanation in loss of vaso motor innervation.

Report of the Section on Psychology and Medical Jurisprudence.

RECENT PSYCHOLOGICAL PROGRESS.

By Charles G. Hill, M. D.

In consenting to make the report for this Section, on account of Dr. Conrad's illness during the winter, I very much fear that I was more charitable to him than to either this Faculty or myself, thereby falsifying the old saying that charity begins at home. The brevity and poverty of the report, I must in all candor admit is due neither to the lack of progress of this branch of medicine during the past year, nor to the committee to whom was entrusted its compilation, but to your humble servant, who, under a pressure of other matters, neglected it until too late to do justice to the subject.

Gladly would recount in detail the rapid strides being made by this division of medical science, and show that *pari passu* with the others, it is steadily advancing. And nowhere else can be found a more prompt, practical and humane application of the attainments of science, than in the care and treatment of those whose higher faculties are perverted and distorted by disease. Dr. Andrew White, late of Cornell, in his "New Chapters on the Warfare of Science," speaks to the point when he says, "Of all the triumph won by science for humanity, none have been further reaching in its good effects than the modern treatment of the insane." I hold up this tangible and useful result of psychological advancement because the best standard of measurement for medical science in any of its branches is its capacity to contribute to the welfare of the human race.

But psychological progress has not been confined to the practical alone, the theoretical and speculative have also come in for their share of attention. As an instance, go with me for a moment into some of the beautiful and intricate theories, from the pen of Dr. Henry Smith Williams, of New York, on the "Molecular Dynamics of the Encephalon." Assuming, as an anatomical fact, that each pyramidal cell of the cortex cerebri is made up of fibrils, with a surrounding matrix of nitrogenous matter, and that these cells seem to be built up out of other nervous tissue, and have fibrils entering and issuing from them, and that it would seem, *a priori* probable that their structure is likewise fibrillar, therefore, without other experiment, except that the latest direct observations are confirmatory of this supposition, he proceeds to the elaboration of what is called the "vibratory theory of mind," and concludes that the "mind is an organism engendered transmutation of the forces of the environment, and as completely and rigidly dependent upon these forces as is any other effect upon its cause." He believes, in accord with the teachings of modern physics, that each and all of these forces come to the organism as forms or modes of motion, and hence may be associated in their incipiency as vibrations. These vibrations he considers of unknown form and infinite number. Says he, " Vibrations of heat, light, magnetism, electricity, and perchance a thousand other known or unknown forces, are beating upon all portions of the organism, and each one is caught up by a peripheral nerve element and transmitted to a common centre. Each channel of such transmission is demonstratably a delicate fibril, and it can scarcely be doubted that the transmutable force as it travels along this wire is still made manifest in a vibration of matter. But just what particular form of vibration is here involved is not, by any means, so easily settled. Doubtless it has many points of resemblance to electricity, but various considerations among others its comparative sluggishness, make the idea of identity untenable. Most probably it is a condition, *sui generis*, a transformation of electricity, light, heat, sound and other forces, yet in itself neither one nor the other of these. Once caught up or evolved by the peripheral nerve elements it is transmitted along well-known different tracts till it reaches its central destination in the cerebral cell. A purely physical, and, in a sense, comprehensible, vibration we follow it to this point, but here, in the midst of those highly evolved organic tissues, we are at the very border line of the material, and it seems as if, could we take one further step, we would open tangibly the nature of the spiritual. Our vibration quivers in the labyrinthine cells of the cortex, a physical vibration still ; and then, of a sudden it has flashed beyond our ken, and reappears, as if beyond a bridgeless chasm, transformed into a new entity, a sensation of consciousness. Why flashed it there ? Why must we fail to follow it? Why is it changed, nay, metamorphosed, into consciousness ?''   •

Doubtless it would be interesting to follow the learned writer further into this prolific field of inquiry,* but my object in quoting so much of his paper is to show that psychological progress is not measured by the advancements in cerebral localization, and the application of new remedies by which troublesome nervous manifestations may be tamed and subdued, but in its scope it reaches out into the metaphysical and subtle relation of mind and matter, and boldly invades the obscure and delicate realms of consciousness, will and memory.

But, to return to the practical, probably no subject has received more careful study in all its details and made more rapid progress, than that of cerebral localization. This has carried with it a better general knowledge of cerebral anatomy, psychology and pathology, and deeper research into the functions of the cortex of the brain, by the means of physiological experiment and chemical observation. The result of the late advances in cranio-cerebral topography has already been made manifest in the recent wonderful development of brain surgery—the demonstration of the possibility of locating and removing brain tumors and delicate portions of brain, constitutes one of the greatest advancements of modern surgery, and the brilliancy of this discovery shines with at least reflective light on the department of medicine which is now under consideration. It would consume too much of your

---

*Refer here to the author above quoted and to Charles Mercier.

time to attempt any detailed review of the advances in cerebral localization, and I shall confine myself to a very brief
summary of what has been recently done in this line.

The location of all mental functions in the cortex, if this
assumption needs further verification, is negatively proven by
the fact, as recently shown, that atrophy of the cortex is a
constant concomitant of an advanced mental disease. In only
six out of sixty-eight autopsies made at the Boston Lunatic
Asylum by Dr. W. W. Garnett was there lack of evidence of
some degree of atrophy of the cortex. In these six cases
the patients died of some fatal organic disease intercurrent
with the insanity. In two of these there was extensive pachy-
meningitis ; in one, external exostosis of the skull ; in one,
great anæmia of the brain, and in the last, geneal tuberculosis. In each case the patient died before insanity was fully
developed, and no doubt atrophy would have occurred sooner
or later. In *five* of the six cases there was a lesion which
affected the cortex generally, and in only one case was there
an apparent exception to the rule, and this was the case of
general tuberculosis.

Admitting that many forms of insanity are functional in
their earlier stages, and hence curable, I beg leave to insist
that a diseased mind means a diseased brain, and to emphasize the foregoing figures for the sake of those who persist in
locating nearly all cases of insanity in the uterus and ovaries
of the female, or sexual apparatus of the male. But advancements and achievements in this line by no means stop with the
location of the seat of the lesions of insanity in the cerebral
cortex. Since M. Broca, to whom is due the honor of being
the pioneer in this line of investigation, first pointed out that
the motor centres of speech were located in the posterior third
of the third left frontal convolution, more than half the cortex
has been distinctly mapped out with a score or more of
centres of movement or sensation. This has been accomplished more by physiological experiment than by the study
of lesions affecting the cortex. We call these localizations
motor and sensory centers, but they are really centres of
ideation. The mental operations are in a great part connected
with sensory and motor phenomena, and are so completely

represented in the regions described that it is hard to imagine just what functions the unassigned portions of the cortex can represent. Stimulation of this enclosure is negative in its results. Generally speaking, the anterior half of the frontal lobes, the posterior portion of the occipital lobes, and the basal surface of the two hemispheres, constitute the true "terra incognita" of the cortex, and would we not be justified in locating by exclusion, in this otherwise unaccountable region, the higher centers of mental action ?

I cannot close this desultory report without allusion to the valuable addition that has been recently made to the list of therapeutic agents, adapted to the relief and cure of mental and nervous disorders and diseases. These are divisible into three heads :

1st, Those derivatives of coal-tar, whose principal effects are to cause a lowering of the animal temperature and antisepsis.

2nd, Those of the ether series of compounds which have an anæsthetic and hypnotic action when inhaled or otherwise introduced into the system.

3rd, That important and very different group of complex organic composition—the so-called active principles of vegetable life.

The first group embracing the now well known antipyrine, antifebrine, phenacetine, etc., I will pass by as being not directly in the line of our inquiry.

To the second, or other series, we are indebted for many valuable remedies, to some of which I will briefly invite your attention. The first place on this list, I unquestionably give sulphonal, the very queen of hypnotics. The almost universal report of this agent is that its very effect is the important one of increasing and prolonging the natural tendency to sleep ; that its action is not narcotic, but purely hypnotic; that the pulse, pupils, temperature, respiration, appetite and the secretions remain practically unaffected after its daily use for indefinite periods, and that it is promptly eliminated from the system, principally by the kidneys, without irritation or detriment to these organs. It is slower in its action than chloral, but more prolonged, and its constant use does not weaken its physiological effect, nor does it produce the desire for a narcotic, that makes chloral and other drugs so dangerous. It is claimed that it does not affect the heart-action, but I believe my experience with it justifies me in going further, and saying that it does affect it, favorably. I am satisfied that it increases arterial tension, being thus beneficial to the weak and depressed patient, and I have never seen an instance of heart failure when sulphonal was freely administered. Much more might be said in praise of this wonderful agent, but I must pass on to others.

Of *chloralamid*, I cannot speak so favorably. It is generally efficacious in doses of 15 to 75 grains, but in many cases it fails entirely where chloral succeeds in smaller doses. It frequently causes severe headache, loss of appetite and drowsiness, and does not seem to possess any decided advantage over many other drugs of its class.

Urethan, like sulphonal, does not depress the heart, and is said to notably increase the amount of oxygen in the blood. It is less certain in its action than sulphonal, but has the one advantage over it of being moderately analgesic.

Paraldehyde, notwithstanding its bulky and unpalatable form, is justly growing in popularity. It is said to diminish the force and frequency of the heart's action, and occasions a brain anæmia, as occurs in natural sleep, but is still considered a valuable and safe medicine. In experiments to determine its effects, animals fed on chloral perish in about half the time of those fed on paraldehyde.

Of the third or vegetable class, I will only claim your attention for a moment to consider very briefly the several derivatives of hyoscyamus. They embrace hyoscyamine and its sulphate, and hyoscine with the hydrobromate and hydrochlorate of the same. For a thorough and interesting article on these and other hypnotics, I beg leave to refer you to a paper read by Dr. Henry W. Wetherill of the Pennsylvania Hospital for the Insane, at the last meeting of Superintendents of Asylums and published in the *American Journal of Insanity* for July, 1889. The great advantages possessed by these products, are the smallness of the dose, ranging according to the preparation from $\frac{1}{2}$ to $\frac{1}{10}$ of a grain, their solubility and hence their fitness for hypodermic medication, though they are equally efficacious when given by the mouth, and the rapidity of this action.

The experiments of Dr. Wetherill, in the paper above referred to, showed conclusively that the hyoscine is by far the most reliable and efficacious. The disadvantages are mostly due to the uncertainty of the preparations in the market, as I am satisfied from experience, that many of them are entirely inert. I have found, for instance, that the hypodermic tablets gotton from a well known drug house in this city, gave perfect satisfaction, while the same article in bulk was useless and void of effect. Hyoscine is contraindicated in advanced cardiac lesions, in grave cardiac weakness and in states of profound weakness. In mental disorders its range of general applicability seems to be almost universal, but with occasional failure, from which it is difficult to account. Individual idiosyncrasy is a term used as a shield to our ignorance of its effect on certain constitutions, or under certain circumstances.

Report of the Section on Ophthalmology, Otology and Laryngology.

THE EXCLUSION OF LIGHT IS NOT BENEFICIAL IN THE AFTER TREATMENT OF CATARACT OPERATIONS.

By Julian J. Chisolm, M. D.

Conservatism in medicine often resembles a rut, more or less deep, in which thought or want of thought can be well hidden by those who are constantly traversing this special road. We get into certain ways of doing a thing, whether these be right or wrong, useful or useless. It often needs some convulsion, a little short of a dynamite explosion, to lift us out of this well worn groove. When we get accidentally on the upper surface we observe that there are other roads to the goal for which we are striving, some smoother and more direct than one which we had so long used. We would never have discovered these, had not accident forced us out of the old well trodden path. In this category I place the orthodox, called classic, after treatment of cataract operations.

For many years but one stereotyped method has been followed by ophthalmic surgeons when everything else was changing around them. Instruments and manipulations were all being modified for the better, but the old habitual faulty bandaging of eyes remained.

This bandaging of eyes was a plan devised long ago by a leading surgeon when ophthalmic surgeons of note were few. It was adopted by those who followed his teaching and in time it became general. It was based upon the prevailing belief that absolute quiet, in the dark, was necessary for the healing of a corneal wound.

The plan selected was as follows: after the clean wound was made by the sharpest of instruments, and the opaque lens was removed from the eye, both eyes were covered by soft compresses which were well secured in position by bandaging the head. The patient was then put to bed in a room from which all light was shut out. In this dark chamber he was kept absolutely quiet, all causes for excitement being carefully excluded. In this condition of seclusion he was constantly watched for eight days. The bandages were removed daily for eye inspection by candle light, and were then replaced. At the end of eight days the corneal wound was presumed to have healed, and the bandages were no longer continued. On account of the absolute darkness to which the eyes had been submitted for so long a time, they would exhibit extreme irritability when exposed to the least light. The windows of the chamber were therefore covered by heavy curtains, until such a time as the eyes had regained some little of their former strength. Under the protection of dark smoked glasses and brow shades, light was day by day slowly admitted, until ordinary daylight could be borne. Good results came to the patient from the carefully performed operation, and under the confining treatment. It was these final good results which were so much to be desired. Hence one surgeon after another fell into this rutty method of treating such cases. The dark room with bed confinement and absolute quiet became the orthodox treatment of cataract patients. No one questioned the propriety of this course so universally adopted.

I got into the rut which my teachers had so well trodden, and for twenty-five years I steadily followed this classic method of dressing and treating my cataract patients. In hundreds of cases after cataract and iridectomy operations I followed this restraining and confining method without questioning its value. In visiting such patients at noonday a candle was a necessary and constant companion to see one's way in the dark sick room. This routine is still kept up by many; It is one of the relics which ophthalmic surgery has not yet shaken off.

The large pledget of soft lint which is secured over both eyes adapts itself to the irregularities of the socket and is supposed to exert an equal pressure over the whole front of the eye ball, keeping it quiet and promoting thereby healing. When after one week's confinement in the dark room the bandages are removed, the sensitive eyes stream with tears. This symptom is explained as the natural consequence of the operation. We expect to see this weeping of the eyes when the bandages are finally taken off after the eight days of confinement, and we are never disappointed. All eyes weep in the dark after the removal of the confining cataract dressings.

Four years ago I began to doubt the propriety of this universally adopted method of treating cataract patients. I first questioned the confiding faith in the supporting bandage. The eye after cataract extraction presented itself to me as a hollow elastic ball, with an incision made into its upper surface of one third the circumference of the cornea. As I inspected it, when the extraction operation had been completed, the lips of the wound adjusted themselves as perfectly to the opposing surfaces as to exclude detection. Here was a perfect adaptation which the closing of the lips did not disturb. If I pressed upon the centre of the cornea the wound showed a disposition to gape, which tendency disappeared the moment pressure was relieved. The question which suggested itself to my mind was this, viz.: did not the compress, secured over the eye, make just such pressure upon the prominent cornea as I had made with my instrument, and was not a tendency to disturbance created by its presence? As the patient lay upon the operating table with eyes closed, I knew that the adjustment was perfect, and the eye in the very best condition for rapid healing. If I could keep it in that condition only a few days I felt that the wound must cicatrize, and that the very best results would be secured. How to keep it so was the question. It seemed to be rationally answered by this suggestion. Keep the lids together by the careful application of light non-irritating diaphinous adhesive plaster, rather than by thick compresses and bandages.

I adopt this method of treatment: A piece of salicylated soft silk isinglass plaster, one and a half inches long and one inch wide, was placed upon the closed eye lids. It extended from beneath the brow well down upon the cheek. It was not as wide as the lids, and therefore left the angular margins exposed for the ready escape of secretions. It also permitted the instillation of eye drops, without the displacement or removal of the retaining plaster. When dampened by a little water, and its surface pressed by a spatula, in its wet limp condition, it adapted itself to every irregularity of the lid surface. In drying, it kept the lids together as if they had been an unbroken septum, and that without making irregular pressure upon the cut eye ball. The plaster being diaphinous every lash could be seen as they lay stretched out on the cheek. The eye lids could be inspected through the plaster dressing as when the compresses are removed for the daily examination under the old treatment. This seemed to be, theoretically at least, a perfect eye dressing.

My first experiments were watched from day to day with anxious care. I always found some secretions escaping, seldom enough to detach the plaster, and never enough to disturb its transparency or to interfere with the inspection. In the old treatment I daily examined the eye cloths and compresses. If comparatively clean I accepted their condition as an index of the absence of inflammation, and this without looking into the eye itself. The appearance of the adhesive strip without its removal, I found an equally good index of the condition of the eye. It does away with all eye disturbance from the daily renewal of dressings. After the eight days of watching, when the plasters were removed, I found thoroughly healed corneal wounds, in every way as perfect as when compresses had been used. The comfort to the patient under the new dressing had been very much enhanced ; no head bands to annoy or to slip or be renewed from time to time. This was an immense improvement over the old method. The adhesive plaster soon proved itself so simple and efficient a dressing that it usurped the place which compresses and bandages had heretofore held in my estimation.

Once having abandoned the so called classic method of dressing an eye after cataract and iridectomy operations, the accompaniments of this treatment, upon which so much stress is laid, were one by one modified. The first very important item to be set aside was the dark window curtains, and the closed shutters. If the closed eye from which the cataract had just been removed was not inconvenienced by the strong light of the operating room, I saw no reason why it should not continue to submit comfortably to this exposure. Now in my practice a window shade to shut out strong light is the extent of screening found needful.

The next move was to leave uncovered the eye not operated upon in which there was still some useful sight. With this eye open, in a moderately light room, patients were never for a moment in the dark. They could see to help themselves in many ways, and they appreciate immensely this modification of the old treatment.

The next attack was made upon bodily restraints. This confinement in bed lying on the back, with instructions to keep quiet, and for one or two days to chew nothing so that the movement of the jaws would not disturb the healing of the cornea. Experience had proven to me that the movements of the exposed eye did not disturb the healing of the cut one, and therefore the movement of the legs, hands and jaws, were less likely to do so. Bed treatment was therefore abandoned. As my daily experience was forcing upon me the recognition of the fact that absolute quiet was not an essential in the successful treatment of cataract extractions, my patients were allowed to move about in moderation. As time wore on and my percentage of successes steadily increased with the liberties which my patients enjoyed, I became the more confirmed in the value of my modifications in the treatment of such cases.

In the meantime the removal of cataracts without iridectomy was introduced. I with others accepted this improvement, and for the past two years have left the iris intact with pupil undisturbed. A sine-qua-non for the success of this new operation, we were told was that patients must be kept absolutely quiet, on their backs, in bed. That the least jolting would open the corneal wound and allow a piece of the iris to protrude, causing the serious complication of an iritic hernia, with ugly results. So confident had I become in the thorough support which the lids, closed by adhesive plaster, give to the eye ball and the cut cornea that I made no change in the dressings, nor in the after treatment for the new operation. My results were equally satisfactory with those who used every bodily restraint. In my early operations without iridectomy I had every now and then a hernia of the iris, but so had those who adhered to the old method of dressing with bed treatment. I could not attribute this accident to the after treatment, because it occurred where either method was carefully used. I was more disposed to explain it by some fault in the manual of operative procedure which I hoped that time, and a greater familiarity would overcome. This has shown itself to be correct. A prolaps of iris now very seldom occurs in my practice.

In cases in which there had been loss of vitrious during the extraction, my superstitious reverence for the imaginary protection of a compress and bandage made me doubt at first the propriety of trusting the eye to the adhesive strap. This feeling I have quite outgrown. Even in these cases of loss of vitrious I now rely with confidence upon the equible support of the adhesive strap as the sole and best eye dressing. If it is carefully applied it will as a rule remain on securely for many days, regardless of the escape of secretions. Should I find it loosening on the second or third day I remove the old piece and adjust a fresh one. If it does not become displaced before the fourth or fifth day, I do not find it necessary to replace it, because by this time the corneal wound is quite healed and needs no longer protection.

Now and then a case presents itself in which the very stiff out curved eye lashes will not lie smoothly on the cheek under the adhesive dressing. They tend to lift the plaster in a groove along the free border of the lid. They prevent the perfect adjustment of the plaster. It will stick well upon the smooth surface of the eye lid and also on the cheek, but remains irregularly adherent to the lashes. At first this condition annoyed me much, and I would make repeated attempts to get a fresh piece of plaster to lie more smoothly. Now I no longer regard it. Experience has taught me that should a little lid separation exist after the dressing is applied, no harm comes from it. I have had patients blind in both eyes, with one operated upon, remark, an hour after the extraction, that they could peep out of the newly operated eye and see objects dimly. No injury would come from this apparent liberty. The wounded part of the eye ball is always thoroughly covered, supported and protected by gentle lid pressure and that is all that is required for promoting the quick healing of the corneal wound.

The most striking results of this unrestraining treatment of cataract patients in light rooms is the comparative freedom from weeping which the eye exhibits when the adhesive strap is removed and the eye is permanently exposed, even as early as the fifth day. This is to me very conspicuous when I recall my own former experience, and when I examine the Hospital work of other specialists who still adhere to the dark room confinement. Red, watery, painful eyes they expect to see, and are never disappointed. In my practice such red and watery eyes form a decided exception to the rule of comparatively dry, non congested eyes. This very satisfactory condition I attribute solely to the change in the after treatment. The red watery eyes I formerly had, as specialists still have, when I kept patients in the dark for days as they do.

My present method of treating cataract extractions is as follows: I try to make the manual of operation as smooth in every particular as I possibly can, using for asepsis instruments which I had previously immersed in boiling water. I use no antiseptic liquid on eye or face of patient, or on instrument. If the surface of the eye is in a healthy condition, I do not believe that pyogenic germs have collected on the conjunctiva awaiting their opportunity to rush into the corneal wound as soon as formed. I no longer go through the useless form of washing out the conjunctival sac. I see many surgeons put a few drops of a necessarily weak germicide solution on the eye and immediately afterwards proceed to make the corneal section. If the pyogenic germs were there no harm could come to them from this very transient water bath. Bacteriologists are very much amused at the superstitious reverence of the modern surgeon who goes through this veriest form and imagines that he performs a most important duty. I have broken away from this useless habit of many, of trying to fight malignant bacteria which are not present, by the momentary use of weak germicides which can do them no injury. I adhere rigidly to cleanliness for protection. Under the anæsthetic influence of a four per cent. solution of cocaine, I make in senile cataracts a large corneal opening following the sclero corneal circle for nearly one-third of its circumference. I find that this kind of opening just where the clear cornea ends, facilitates the easy exit of the lens. Cutting across the clear cornea as is often done in the iridectomy extraction, leaves a corneal shelf which obstructs the escape of the lens. After the corneal section I introduce the cystotome and with it I thoroughly tear up the capsule over the pupilary area.

At one time I practiced opening the capsule with the point of the cataract knife as it traversed the aquious chamber. This was a brilliant manœuvre with which I was much pleased. I found that in some cases it increased the difficulties of making smooth operations. The lens would jump forward when the incision into the capsule released it. This movement would sometimes push the iris over the edge of the knife. It was not always easy to dislodge it, or to avoid injury to the iris in completing the corneal section. In some cases I was forced to make an iridectomy when I had not so intended. I have therefore given up this step for the safer method of releasing the lens after the corneal incisions had been perfected.

When the corneal wound is large enough, and is well placed at the uppermost circle of the clear cornea the pressure of a shell spoon upon the lower part of the eye ball tilts the upper edge of the lens forward and starts its delivery. The iris at first caps it, but by continued pressure the pupil expands, the iritic curtain gets out of the way, and the lens escapes through the corneal opening. There is usually some soft lens matter left which can all be coaxed out by the careful pressure of the spoon without washing out the anterior chamber by using a syringe. The pupil then regains its black color. If the speculum does not compress the eye ball the iris will most frequently, without external aid, resume its proper place within the anterior chamber. Should it show a disposition to lag at the corneal wound it is replaced in the eye chamber by a few strokes of a spatula. When one becomes familiar, by an every day experience, he no longer wonders at the liberties which, under dextrous manipulation can be safely taken with even this delicate sensitive membrane. With the spatula the iris is not only pushed back under the cornea but by sundry gentle strokes in can be smoothed out until the pupil assumes its normal size and appearance. The eye then looks as perfect as if no operation had been yet made and fingers can be readily counted by the patient. This little trial assures them of the success of the operation and gives the blind a fore taste of the good things to come.

The speculum is now removed and a few drops of a solution of eserine, two grains to an ounce of water, are put on the cornea. The object of these drops is to produce a decided and protracted contraction of the pupil. Both eyes are temporarily closed, and the eye from which the cataract had been removed is ready for its single and simple dressing. The adhesive strip is placed in position over the eye lids. If the secretions from the eye are not sufficient to make it stick, it is moistened. When stroked by the shell spoon it lies smoothly over the lid and cheek. Any excess of moisture is removed by the gentle pressure of a fold of a soft towel. In a few minutes the plaster dries. The cut eye is now shut in from all harm by having the lids permanently stretched out over it as a supporting mould. The patient can open the other eye, and without fear of injury can walk unaided from the operating room to his own chamber.

Usually the excitement of the operation is followed by some lassitude and patients prefer to lie on the bed. If they be of the more stolid kind, and prefer sitting or reclining on a couch, no objection is made to it. Operations are always performed by me after two P. M., when my morning's office work is finished. When supper time comes, by aid of the eye not covered, patients can partake of the evening meal without being fed. They are also allowed to make their own toilet at bedtime. As an aid in keeping the pupil contracted and the iris away from the corneal wound, at bedtime a few drops of the eserine solution are put at the inner canthus of the closed eye. These find their way into the eye without displacing the adhesive strip. As they often cause brow ache and some pain in the eye which might interfere with quiet sleep, a bromide or chloral mixture is given as a sleeping dose. The following morning a few of the eserine drops are again instilled and with this drop ends all applications to the closed eye. If they desire it patients get up at their usual rising hour making their own toilet. This, they do the day after the operation. The consequitive ones are spent sitting or reclining, seeing friends, if they desire it, and partaking of regular solid meals. The closed eye is inspected daily to note whether there has been much discharge of eye secretions. Also to discover if there be any tendency to displacement of the adhesive strip. Often, after the second day, the plaster at its centre, along the lid border, seems to have been liberated from the lashes, forming a loose groove, the whole length of the lid split. Experience has taught me that this does not interfere with the most perfect final results.

Day by day I watch the appearance of the lids through the diaphanous dressing. The good light in the room permits their thorough examination. By the fifth day, should there have been no evidence of suppuration, I know that the corneal wound has healed, and I remove the adhesive dressing. Sometimes I wet it before removal. At other times I detach it from the eye dry and then bathe the eye with warm water to get rid of all sticky matter, remnants of the adhesive substance from the plaster and dessicated eye secretions, the accumulation of five days collection.

As a rule when the eye is liberated in the light room it is not much injected, nor does it run much water. From this time forth it is left uncovered and unprotected. The only treatment for the recently operated upon eye is the instillation of a few drops of a four grain solution of the sulphate of atropia, for the purpose of breaking up any recent adhesions which may have formed between the iris and the lens capsule.

After from eight to ten days, when the eye no longer feels weak in the subdued light of the chamber, the window shade is partly raised for the admission of more light. At the end of two weeks patients can usually stand the full light of the open window, and can go about the house, with unprotected eye. When dismissed from the Hospital they go away without having worn smoked glasses. They are warned to keep out of the sun and to follow this simple rule as to exposure, *'any light that is not uncomfortable to the eye will not be injurious.* Those after cataract operations who find sun light not painful will not be injured by going into it. I find that a great many can go into the street with uncovered eyes and without discomfort two weeks after a cataract extraction, provided the whole treatment has been conducted in light rooms with the one eye unprotected, continuously exposed to the light.

In other words, my four years experience with the treatment of cataract patients after operation in many hundred cases shows very positively, that the weakness of eyes operated upon are not so much the result of the operation, but depend in a large measure upon the after treatment to which they are subjected. Good healthy eyes kept in darkness for one week can not stand the light when exposed to it. Eyes that have never been in the dark exhibit no such irritation.

I am glad to know that this line of treatment, so revolutionary in its nature, which originated at the Presbyterian Eye, Ear and Throat Charity Hospital of Baltimore City, four years ago, has made itself felt throughout this country, and is being adopted by some of the specialists of Europe. I hope that the day is not far off when the harsh and useless treatment, of bed confinement, in the dark, with the many bodily restraints, which have been imposed upon cataract patients will only be read about as evidences of what superstitions formerly pervaded the medical mind ; also as illustrations of the wonderful docility of patients who quietly submitted to a treatment against which they had such good reasons for rebelling.

VOLUNTEER PAPERS·

ONE HUNDRED CONSECUTIVE CASES OF LABOR AT THE MARYLAND MATERNITÉ, WITH A DESCRIPTION OF THE METHODS PRAC-TISED IN THAT INSTITUTION.

By George H. Rohé, M. D., *Director* and Wm. J. Todd, M. D., *Resident Physician.*

— .- -

The following paper is a brief description of the antiseptic precautions taken in the care and treatment of the patients before, during, and after confinement in the Maryland Maternité, Baltimore, Maryland.

To this is added a summary of one hundred consecutive cases occurring from May 3rd, 1889, to January 22nd, 1890, inclusive.

In the institution mentioned, practical obstetrics is taught to about three hundred students yearly. This, and also the bad hygienic condition of the majority of the patients admitted, and of the homes they come from, render the strictest observance of the latest antiseptic precautions necessary for the prevention of diseases peculiar to the lying-in period.

Adding to the above disadvantages, the fact that about twenty per cent. of the patients are confined within the first twenty-four hours after they are admitted increases this necessity.

Of the above named twenty per cent. perhaps one half are admitted when in the second stage of labor, hardly giving enough time to undress the patient and place her in the bed.

The patient when applying for the benefits of this charity, is encouraged to tell the history of her pregnancy. She is then taken to a vacant ward ; her breasts and abdomen are inspected; the condition of the cervix is ascertained by vaginal touch. Here the antiseptic precautions begin: The physician's hands are washed in the ordinary way in hot water, scrubbed with a nail brush, then immersed in a solution of bi-chloride of mercury of the strength of 1 to 2000, and lubricated with olive oil.

In the majority of cases, an ocular examination of the pudendum is also made.

The legs are examined for ulcers, varicosed veins, and scars of old lesions.

The pelvis externally, is measured with a pelvimeter. The diameters between the anterior superior spinous processes, the widest part of the iliac crests, and the external conjugate diameters are taken.

These figures with a memorandum of the name, age, color, nativity, number of pregnancy, and the date of the last menstruation of the patient are noted.

If her expected confinement is more than two or three weeks off, she is given a card admitting her on or before a certain fixed date, which usually allows her about two weeks in the hospital before her confinement.

This card instructs her to return to the hospital immediately upon the first symptoms of labor, if they should come on before the date fixed. It further instructs her as to what clothing to bring and what not to bring to the hospital.

When admitted to the hospital the patient is taken to the bath-room; here she is required to take a full bath under the direction, inspection, and assistance of a nurse.

If she does not have clean under-clothing, this is furnished to her; also a clean wrapper.

Corsets are forbidden during the patient's stay in the hospital.

A tight-fitting waist or jacket, with two or three rows of buttons around the waist, from which to suspend the skirts, is recommended.

Where this jacket has been tried it has proved a success and a comfort to the wearer.

One hour before breakfast each morning ℥ i sulphate of magnesia is given to the newly admitted patient.

This hygienic precaution is necessary, as more than seventy-five per cent. of the patients admitted are constipated to a greater or less degree.

During the time between her admittance to the hospital and her confinement, the patient is required to take a full bath twice a week. On the second or third day after the patient has been admitted, her urine is examined. The specific gravity and the reaction are taken, a test for albumen and sugar is also made, and the percentage of chlorides is noted.

If the sample of urine is found to be normal, a second examination is not made until the first day after labor, or symptoms are developed that would suggest an examination. Should there be any abnormality about the urine, the patient is watched closely, and the urine is tested frequently. On the eighth day after confinement, the urine is again examined.

Immediately after the beginning of the first stage of labor, the patient is given a full bath.

If this stage has progressed too far to admit of such an exertion upon the part of the patient, or the labor is likely to progress rapidly, the patient is washed by the nurse from the mammary glands to the knees.

She is given an enema to unload the bowels, followed by a vaginal douche of a solution of bi-chloride of mercury, 1-4000. This last being repeated, if thought necessary, two or three times.

The attendants making vaginal examinations are required to use the nail brush freely, with plenty of hot water and soap.

After drying the hands and forearms on a clean towel, they are immersed in a solution of bi-chloride of mercury, 1-2000. So much of this solution as will, is allowed to remain on the hands.

Carbolized olive oil is used to lubricate the fingers of the examining hand.

The above precautions are carried out before each and every vaginal examination.

It is also recommended that the space under the finger nails be filled in with soap; also around the junction of the nail and skin.

This, while being an additional precaution against the infection of the patient by the examiner, also affords protection to the examiner against any possible infection of his fingers by discharges from the patient.

Puncture of the Membranes.—It was the rule in the early part of the year to puncture the membranes when the os was fully dilated, but during the last six months it has been thought best not to interfere with the possible good they might do as a dilator, and allow the sac to rupture of itself, or to puncture it when it makes its appearance at the vulva.

During the first stage of labor, the patient is allowed to walk around the room, or remain in bed, as she may elect. During the second stage she is placed in bed and required to remain there.

It is the endeavor of the physicians to control the patient as to "bearing down."

The perineum is supported with the left hand, and the coming head is held in check by the fingers of the right hand.

All lacerations of the perineum are sewed up immediately, or within eight hours, with silk thread.

After the head is born the fundus of the uterus is followed up by the hand of the nurse. As the proper shoulder comes down on the perineum, the left hand is again placed to support it while the right lifts the head of the child upward to the symphysis pubis.

In a number of cases the shoulders of the child have lacerated the perineum which had remained intact after the passage of the head.

The child is placed upon its right side, its eyes and mouth are wiped dry with a clean soft towel.

Allowing the infant to breathe fully for one or two minutes, and the pulsation of the cord to cease, two ligatures are placed on the cord and the latter divided between the ligatures.

The attendant then places his hand on the abdomen over the fundus of the uterus.

After waiting about fifteen minutes he makes a gentle kneading motion with his fingers over the fundus; this causes further contractions of the uterus.

No traction is made on the funis; it remains on the bed as it fell after being severed from the infant.

The presenting side of the placenta is easily noticed at the vaginal orifice—this side is noted; it is then twisted so that a cord is formed of the after coming membranes which soon drop out on the bed.

The placenta is then examined. If any part is remaining in the vagina or uterus, the attendant, immersing his hand in a solution of bichloride of mercury, passes it in the vagina, or if necessary, into the uterus and empties it.

If there is any indication of hæmorrhage, ergot is given hypodermatically, but if there be no hæmorrhage, ergot is not given.

The hand of the nurse remains on the abdomen over the fundus of the uterus for fifteen to thirty minutes after the physicians leave the case in her charge.

The patient is made as comfortable as possible, and is allowed to rest twenty to thirty minutes. She is then given a vaginal douche of a hot solution of bi-chloride of mercury 1-4000.

All parts of the person that have been soiled by blood or discharge are washed; clean linen is put on the patient.

The lips of the vulva are parted and a powder of iodoform and boracic acid thrown in as far as possible, a wad of sub-limated (1-1000) jute or hemp is then placed over the vulva, then a large muslin pad.

The patient is then lifted off the confinement bed and placed in a clean and freshly prepared bed.

Twice daily for eight or nine days the patient is washed, iodoform and boracic acid powder used, a new wad of sub-limated hemp applied and the under pad changed.

The bed and body linen are changed entire at the morning bath, and the soiled clothing disinfected in bi-chloride solu-tion and boiled.

The lochial discharge is noticed particularly as to color, odor and quantity.

The pulse and temperature of the mother are taken twice a day at 9 A. M. and 7 P. M.

On the evening of the third day, or morning of the fourth day, one ounce of sulphate of magnesia is given to unload the alimentary canal. This is repeated during her stay in bed as is necessary.

The ninth day after labor, if the condition of the patient will admit, she is allowed to sit up in an easy chair three hours, divided into periods of one hour in length.

The morning of the tenth day her condition is noted before she is allowed out of bed. If favorable, she is allowed to use her pleasure as to when and how long she may rest in bed or in the easy chair.

On the 14th day, if her recovery has been complete, she is discharged, to return home or to her friends, with caution as to the care she must take of herself.

Diet of the Mother.—For the first day, toast and a soft-boiled egg with tea or coffee.

The second day, a small piece of meat is added, after this a general diet is allowed.

The Child.—The cord being properly tied, the infant is handed to a nurse, who has a warmed blanket ready to receive it.

She places it in a safe place taking care that it is lying on its right side.

A clinical thermometer is placed in the rectum and the temperature registered is noted.

After the mother has been washed and placed in a new clean bed, the infant is weighed and measured.

The occipito-frontal, the occipito-mental, the sub-occipito-bregmatic, and biparietal diameters are taken, also the occipito-frontal and sub-occipito-bregmatic circumferences, as well as the circumferences of the shoulders and hips.

The length of the infant is also noted.

While all this is being done, the greatest care is taken to keep the infant as warm as possible. Finally before turning the infant over to the nurse to be washed and dressed, a few drops of a solution of nitrate of silver of the strength of grains v to the ʒ i, are dropped into its eyes as a prophylactic measure against ophthalmia neonatorum.

The nurse taking charge of the infant, immediately examines the stump of the funis, and places a second ligature about half an inch back of the one already on. She then anoints the infant with olive oil and washes it in the usual way with hot water and soap.

The stump of the cord is then dressed with absorbent cotton dusted with iodoform.

After dressing the infant it is placed to the mother's breast.

All infants are washed and dressed twice a day, morning and evening.

All clothing is changed throughout at the morning bath, and the necessary changes of napkins are made during the day.

Cradles are provided and the nurses are expected to keep the infants in them, except when nursed by the mother.

The weight of the infant is taken at birth, and again on the third and sixth days, also on the day of discharge.

On the fourth day the diameters and circumferences of the head, as named above, are again taken.

The Bed.—In cases for demonstration, the bedstead is one made of iron, thirty inches wide, twenty-six inches high, and six feet six inches long.

A husk mattress is placed upon it, then covered with a rubber blanket, and the usual sheets, etc.

This high bedstead affords every opportunity for those that are spectators to observe the different steps of the labor and care for the mother and infant.   It gives the attending physician full control of the patient, also is a great saving to his own back, this last being no small consideration.

It is a cardinal rule, the observation of which is positively insisted upon, that during the second stage of labor a good supply of boiling water shall be near at hand ; that a clean syringe with a vaginal tube is within sight, so that if a post-mortem hæmorrhage should occur, no delay will be necessary in stopping the flow of blood.

A hypodermic syringe is also filled with fluid extract of ergot, and is near at hand.   The above precautions are taken in every case.

The placenta after being examined by the attendant to ascertain that it is intact, is placed in a vessel containing a solution of bichloride of mercury 1-2000.

After the infant has been weighed, etc., the placenta is weighed, measured and a diagram of its shape is made.   It is then replaced in the bichloride of mercury solution and then taken from the room and burnt.

The clothes, all the bed and body linen of the patient, and towels, napkins, etc., are taken immediately to the laundry. After being washed and boiled, the linen is placed in a strong solution of bi-chloride of mercury, for not less than two hours, then wrung out dry and placed on a line.

All linen that has been soiled by blood or discharges at other times is treated in the same way.

Absolute cleanliness is exacted of all in the hospital.

The nurses wear dresses of washable material.   None of the floors in the wards or confinement rooms are carpeted.

All floors and staircases are washed three times a week with water and soap.   When dry, they are washed a second time with a solution of bichloride of mercury only.

Any one visiting the dissecting rooms, or who has lately assisted at a post-mortem examination is not allowed to enter the confinement room.

The following statistics of one hundred cases confined in this institution between the dates mentioned in the beginning of this paper are added, as a contribution to the statistics of labor in American Maternity Hospitals. The tables give the figures in detail, divided into classes of twenty-five each. As a general summary, the following may be given : there were

Whites	60
Colored .	40
American .	88
German .	5
English .	2
Irish	4
Scotch . . .	1
The average age was . . .	23 years.
Oldest	40 years.
Youngest	14 years.

The most frequent time of beginning of labor was between 12, midnight, and 3 A. M.

	hrs.	min.
Average duration of 1st stage,	11	45
" " 2nd "	1	26
" " 3rd "	0	9
" " entire labor	13	21

Method of delivery of Placenta :

Credé	83 times
Spontaneous .	12 "
Manual (intrauterine) .	5 "

Result to mother :—

Perineum intact . .	58
Perineum lacerated 1st, degree .	40
" " 2nd, "	1
" not stated	
Discharged recovered .	99
Died (uremic poisoning) .	1
Ergot given in . .	24 cases
" not given in .	75 "
not stated .	1 case
Chloroform given in .	5 cases
Quinine " in .	2 "
Forceps applied .	5 times

Of the Children there were :

Males . .	52
Females .	48
Delivered living .	97
" dead	3

(Two of these were premature deliveries at 4-4½ months and 5-6 months.)

Presentation :

Vertex	89
Breech .	2
. Not stated . . .	9

Position :

Of 91 cases noted, there were

L. O. I. A. . . .	53
R. O. I. A. .	31
L. O. I. T. .	1
R. O. I. T. .	-
L. O. I. P. .	3
L. S. I. A.	2

The fœtal heart pulsations were noted 68 times. Of these the quickest was 144 beats ; the slowest was 108 beats.

(Predictions of sex based upon the frequency of heart beats were sometimes made, but not always successfully.)

The average weight of the children was 6.715 lbs. Heaviest 10 ℔s. Lightest 1 ℔.

There was a general loss in weight between birth and the third day after. The greatest loss amounted to   1 ℔.

Smallest	1 oz. av.
Average loss	6½ oz. av.

The average weight of the placenta was 1 ℔ 3⅓ oz.

The placenta was delivered with fœtal side out in 71 cases; with uterine side out in 26 cases ; in fragments in 3 cases.

The average measurements of the pelvis externally were between ant. sup. sp. processes ; 9.49 in., between widest part of iliac crests, 10.33 in., external conjugate 7.4 in.

Divided as to race :

1st 25,	White	14
	Black	11
2nd 25,	White	17
	Black	8
3rd 25,	White	15
	Black	10
4th 25,	White	14
	Black	11
Total,	White	60
	Black	40

Nativity :

First 25 Patients :

Maryland	. . . .	16
Virginia	. . . .	3
Delaware	. . . . .	1
Indiana	. . . . .	2
New York	. . . .	
Germany	. . . . .	1
England	. . . .	25

Second 25 Patients :

Maryland	. . . . .	16
Virginia	. . . .	2
W. Virginia	. . . .	1
New York	. . . .	
New Jersey	. . . .	
Pennsylvania	. . . .	1
Germany	. . . .	1
Ireland	. . . .	
Scotland	. . . .	25

Third 25 Patients :

Maryland	. . . .	14
Virginia	. . . .	2
W. Virginia	. . . .	
Ohio	. . . .	
Penna.	. . . . .	2
N. Carolina	. . . .	1
Germany	. . . . .	2
Ireland	. . . . .	2 25

Nativity.

Fourth 25 Patients :

Maryland	11
Virginia	5
W. Virginia	1
Pennsylvania	1
Ohio	1
N. Carolina	1
Nebraska	1
D. Columbia	1
Ireland	1
England	1
Germany	1

25

Nativity.

Total Maryland	57
Virginia	12
W. Virginia	4
Delaware	1
Indiana	2
New York	2
New Jersey	1
Pennsylvania	4
Ohio	2
N. Carolina	2
D. Columbia	1
Germany	5
England	2
Ireland	4
Scotland	1

100

Age of patients :

1st 25	Sum	591
	Average	23
	Oldest	30
	Youngest	17
2nd 25	Sum	581
	Average	23
	Oldest	36
	Youngest	18

3rd 25 Sum		556
	Average	22
	Oldest	40
	Youngest	14
4th 25 Sum		576
	Average	23
	Oldest	32
	Youngest	14
Total Sum,		2,304
	Average	23
	Oldest	40
	Youngest	14

Hours of the beginning of labor pains. The time the patient notifies the nurse is not taken as the beginning of the first stage; the patient is questioned closely as are those in the same ward, and this information is used to substantiate the patient's statements.

Between 12 Midnight and 3 A. M. inclusive,				40	
" 2 "	" 6	"	"	6	
" 6 "	" 9	"	"	9	
" 9 'M.	" 12 M.			3	
" 12 M.	" 3 P. M.	"		11	
" 3 P. M.	" 6 "			6	
" 6 "	" 9 "	"		11	
" 9 "	" 12 Midnight "			7	
Not stated				7	100

Duration of stage : (1st stage.)

1st 25 cases
    20 cases noted.

		hrs.	min.
Average, ...		8	35

2nd 25 cases.
    20 cases noted.

Average, ...		15	28

3rd 25 cases.
    20 cases noted.

Average, ...		15	13

4th 25 cases.
    21 cases noted.

Average, ...		7	56

Average duration of 1st stage of labor 11 hours 45 minutes.

Duration of 2nd stage.

	min.
1st 25 cases.	
Average of 20 cases noted . .	56
2nd 25 cases.	
Average of 21 cases noted . .	1.42
3rd 25 cases.	
Average of 21 cases noted . .	1.08
4th 25 cases.	
Average of 21 cases noted . .	1.02

	hrs.	min.
Average	1	26

Duration of 3rd stage :

	minutes.
1st 25 cases averaged	13
2nd 25 " "	9
3rd 25 " "	7
4th 25 " "	7

Average 9½ minutes.

Duration of 1st and 2nd stages combined : was not able to say in these cases when second stage commenced.

	hrs.	min.
In the 1st 25 cases, 4 so		
noted, average time. . . .	5	35
In the 2nd 25 cases, 2 so		
noted, average time . . .	6	42
In the 3rd 25 cases, 2 so		
noted, average time . . .	13	12
In the 4th 25 cases, 2 so		
noted, average time . . .	6	34

Method of delivering placenta.

1st 25 cases, Credé method . . .	24
By fingers in the uterus . .	1
2nd 25 cases, Credé method . . .	21
Spontaneous	4
3rd 25 cases, Credé method . . .	16
By fingers in the uterus . .	2
Spontaneous	7
4th 25 cases, Credé method . . .	22
By fingers in the uterus . .	2
Spontaneous	1
Total, By Credé method . . .	83
By fingers in the uterus . .	5
Spontaneous	12
	100

Condition of perineum after delivery of child.

1st 25 Intact	14
Lacerated to first degree . .	11
2nd 25 Intact	13
Lacerated to first degree . .	12
3rd 25 Intact, (Head enucleated twice) .	13
Lacerated to first degree . .	10
Lacerated to second degree .	1
Not stated	1
4th 25 Intact, (Head enucleated once) .	18
Lacerated to first degree . .	7
Total, Intact, (Head enucleated 3 times)	58
Lacerated to first degree . .	40
Lacerated to second degree .	1
Not stated	1
	100

Disposal of patients.

Discharged fully recovered	99
Died of uremic poisoning . .	1
	100

Died of uremia:

Delivered May 25, 4.37 A. M.

25th, 3.55 P. M. Convulsions commenced; typical hysterical; passed urine involuntarily, in large quantities.

No albumen in urine.

Convulsions were at first at regular intervals; when the clock was removed from the room they became irregular.

Patient would not swallow.

Morphia given hypodermically.

30th. Died 9.40 A. M. Post-mortem held June 1st, 11 o'clock.

Had double pneumonia in lower lobes in first and second stages; kidneys smaller than normal, flat and lobulated.

Uterus: a few clots, no membranes attached. 7½ inches long, 5 inches wide, 1⅛ lbs. weight.

Heart: Normal, with clot.

Dr. Keirle decided the patient had chronic Bright's disease, and death was caused by uremic poisoning.

Administration of drugs during labor :

1st 25.	No ergot given in . . .	18
	Over ℥ i ergot in . . .	6
	Not stated	1
2nd 25.	No ergot given in . . .	21
	Over ℥ iss	4

Of above,

Chloroform to partial anæsthesia in 2nd
stage, ... 1

Quin. sulph., grs. x, 2nd stage, . . . 2

Whiskey for shock, 3rd stage . . . 1

3rd 25.	No ergot given	20
	Ergot given, [average 45 minutes]	5

Of above, chloroform to partial anæsthesia,
2nd stage, ... 3

4th 25,	No ergot given	16
	Ergot given, [aver. ℥i] . .	9

Of above, Chloroform 1
Whiskey 1

Total, Ergot not given	75	cases.
Ergot given	24	"
Not stated	1	"
Chloroform	5	
Quinine sulph. . . .	2	
Whiskey	1	

Statistics as to infant's sex ·

1st 25 cases, Males		14
Females		11
2nd 25 cases, Males		15
Females		10
3rd 25 cases, Males		13
Females		12
4th 25 cases, Males		10
Females		15
Total : Males		52
Females		48

Position of head :

1st 25 cases.

L. O. I. A. .	13
R. O. I. A. .	7
L. O. I. T. .	1
R. O. I. T. .	
L. O. I. P. .	
Not stated .	!
	25

2nd 25 cases.

L. O. I. A.	13
R. O. I. A.	8
L. S. I. A.	2
Not stated	
	25

3rd 25 cases.

L. O. I. A.	11
R. O. I. A.	1(
L. O. I. P.	
Not stated	
	25

4th 25 cases.

L. O. I. A.	16
R. O. I. A.	5
Not stated	4
	25

Total.

L. O. I. A.	53
R. O. I. A.	31
L. O. I. T.	1
R. O. I. T.	1
L. O. I. P.	3
L. S. I. A.	2
Not stated	9
	100

Pulsation of fœtal heart between pains :

1st 25 cases. Times noted	18
Times not noted	7
Average pulsation	128
Quickest	140
Slowest	108

2nd 25 cases. Times noted   20
              Times not noted   .   5
              Average pulsation   .   .   123
              Quickest   .   140
              Slowest   .   .   112
3rd 25 cases.   Times noted.   17
              Times not noted   .   8
              Average pulsation   .   124
              Quickest   "   144
              Slowest   "   .   112
4th 25 cases.   Times noted   13
              Times not noted   .   12
              Average pulsation   .   127
              Quickest   "   140
              Slowest   "   112
Total.   Times noted   68
       Times not noted   .   32
       Average   .   .   .   125
       Quickest   .   144
       Slowest   .   .   .   108

Weight of child at birth :

1st 25 cases   168
2nd 25 "   176
3rd 25 "   .   .   .   174
4th 25 '   152
                                ———
        Total   670
Average weight   .   .   6.7 ℔
Heaviest child   .   10   "
Lightest   "   .   .   .   1

Weight of child the third day.

Of the first twenty-five, twenty-four were weighed.   160℔
Of the second twenty-five, twenty-four were weighed, 160 "
Of the third twenty-five cases,   164 "
Of the fourth twenty-five cases,
   twenty-two were weighed,   140 "
                                    ———
            Total   624 "

Average weight at third day, . 6.5 lbs
Heaviest at third day, . 9 "
Lightest, " . . . . 4¹⁄₈"
Greatest loss between weight at birth, and
 weight at third day . . .
Smallest loss between weight at birth, and
 weight at third day, . . . 1 oz
Average loss as above, . . . 6½ "
Retaining the weight at birth not gaining
 or losing, ... 1 case
Gained in weight over that at birth, . 1 case, ¼lb

Weight of infant at sixth day.

Of the first twenty-five cases, twenty-two were
 weighed 154¼lb
Of the second twenty-five cases, twenty-three
 were weighed . . . . 153½ "
Third twenty-five cases . . . . 172 "
Of the fourth twenty-five cases, twenty-two
 were weighed, ... 146¼ "

     Total 626 "

Average weight at sixth day, . 6¾ "
Heaviest weight at sixth day, . 9½ "
Lightest " " " . . . 4 "
Greatest gain in weight over weight at birth, ¾ "
Greatest loss in weight compared with weight
 at birth, ... 1⅜ "
Average gain of those that did gain, compared
 with the weight at birth, . . . 4 oz
Average loss of those that did lose, compared
 with weight at birth, . . . 5 '

Placenta Weight.

1st 25 cases total weight . . 30 lbs
  Average . . . 1 lb 3⅓ oz
  Heaviest . . 3 lb 7 oz
  Lightest . . 9 oz
2nd 25 cases total weight . 29¾ "
  Average . . . 1 lb ¾ oz
  Heaviest . 3 lbs
  Lightest . 14 oz

3rd 25 cases total weight .   .   30 ℔s
       Average   .   .   .   1 ℔ 14 oz
       Heaviest   .   .   3 ℔ 12 "
       Lightest   .   .   14 "
4th 25 cases total weight .   . '   30 ℔s
       Average weight   .   . 1 ℔ 3⅓ oz
       Heaviest   .   .   3   "
       Lightest   .   .   14 "
               Total weight   .   .   120 ℔s
       Average weight 1   ℔   . 1 ℔ 3⅓ oz
       Heaviest   "   .   . 3 ℔ 12 oz
       Lightest   "   .   14 oz

Placenta :

The side of the placenta delivered first :

1st 25 cases, Uterine side .   .   .   10
             Fœtal side   .   15
2nd 25 cases, Uterine side .   5
             Fœtal side   .   20
3rd 25 cases, Uterine side .   6
             Fœtal side   .   18
             In parts   .   1
4th 25 cases, Uterine side .   5
             Fœtal side   .   18
             In parts   .   2
             Fœtal side out   71
             Uterine side out   .   26
             In parts   .   3
                                 100

             Infants born alive   .   97
             Still births   .   .   3   100

Of the still births, the utero-gestation of two was about 4 to 4½ months, of one at about 5 to 6 months. The mothers of the first two still-born children were admitted to hospital in labor. The mother of the last still-born child had been in the hospital two days.

In case thirty, the mother was admitted to hospital in labor, delivered of a live infant, of utero-gestation of about 6½ months, which lived 2 hrs. and 7 min.

External Measurements of Pelvis between Ant S. S
Processes :

1st 25 cases, 19 patients measured	9.43 in.
2nd 25 cases, 25 patients measured	9.46 "
3rd 25 cases, 23 patients measured	6.35 "
4th 25 cases, 22 patients measured	9.72 "

Average 9.49 in.

Between widest part iliac crests :

1st 25 cases, 19 patients measured .	10.30 in.
2nd 25 cases, 25 patients measured .	10.30 "
3rd 25 cases, 23 patients measured .	10.25 "
4th 25 cases, 22 patients measured .	10.48 "

Average 10.33 in.

Ext. Conj. diam.

1st 25 cases, 19 patients measured	7.12 in.
2nd 25 cases, 25 patients measured	7.24 "
3rd 35 cases, 23 patients measured	7.69 "
4th 25 cases, 22 patients measured .	7.57 "

Average 7.4 in.

FORCEPS DELIVERIES :

Case 1479 : Labor began May 25, 1 A. M.
Delivery   "   25, 4.46 A. M.

Position of head L. O. I. P.—this fact and the history
of a former delivery with forceps of a dead infant, also that
the head had been on the perineum two hours, decided to
deliver with Simpson's forceps, child alive and discharged
with mother.

Case 1499 : Labor began Oct 1st, 1 A. M.
Delivered   "   "   7 P. M.

Head of infant would not engage at superior strait. Patient
was placed under the influence of chloroform and Hodge's
forceps applied by Prof. Rohé, forceps on the head 15 min.

Respiration and circulation of the infant was feeble. Child
was placed in a basin containing hot water, then a basin of
cold water, alternately ; with desired success.

Case 1535 :   Labor began Oct. 12, 5 A. M.
        Delivery   " 13, 1.55 P. M.

Head would not engage at the superior strait. Hodge's forceps used by Prof. Rohé. Instrument on the head 23 min.

Case 1542, 1st pregnancy :
        Labor began Oct. 1, 7.30 P. M.
        Delivery   " 2, 9.32 P. M.

Head of infant rested on the perineum for three hours, the contractions of the uterus not being of sufficient force to expel the infant.

Quinia sulph. was given, with little effect. The contractions becoming less frequent, patient was chloroformed and Simpson's forceps applied by Dr. W. S. Gardner. He had them on the head 8 minutes. Infant taken without rupture of the perineum.

Case 1549 :   Labor began Oct. 11, 12.05 A. M.
        Delivery   " 12, 6.35 P. M.

Head at inferior strait two hours. Simpson's forceps applied by Prof. Rohé. Infant delivered successfully.

THE LUNG DISORDERS OF THE PREVAILING INFLUENZA.

By A. K. Bond, M. D., of Baltimore.

About the end of 1889, the epidemic which had for some time prevailed in Europe, made its appearance in Baltimore. Manifesting its presence at first by various severe but transitory disturbances of the nervous and digestive systems, which yielded quickly to divers simple remedies, it produced in the minds of physicians the belief that its invasion of the city was a matter of little moment, and that its course could, in each individual case, be readily checked by proper remedies.

Gradually, however, the nervous and digestive symptoms have retreated into the background, and catarrhal disturbances of the respiratory tract, which observant physicians have all the while suspected to be the starting-point of the whole trouble, have come to the front.

That these disorders of the respiratory tract constitute the essential peculiarity of the epidemic, which may, therefore, be properly called an "influenza," is very probable for several reasons.

First, because they have been present in all cases. While the nervous symptoms varied greatly in different cases, and digestive disturbances could not always be detected, a disordered condition of the mucous membrane of the nose, the pharynx or the lower respiratory tract has in the experience of the writer, been always perceptible, either as a simple congestion or as a catarrhal inflammation of the membrane. In its milder form, this symptom has generally been overlooked or considered of no importance.

Second, because fatal cases have generally, if not always, exhibited signs of disease of the lungs or bronchial tubes.

Third, because the respiratory troubles, alone of all the symptoms, persisted in spite of treatment. In the very beginning of the epidemic I learned this fact and formed the habit of telling my patients that these respiratory disorders, although moderated and prevented from serious hurtfulness by therapeutic measures, would continue for a considerable period, disappearing gradually, according to their own laws. This, of course, on the supposition that the patient would continue to reside in the infected district.

Inasmuch, therefore, as these disorders formed such an important part of the disease, and inasmuch as they appeared under so many guises, and differed in some respects from the diseases of these parts with which we are familiar, I have thought it worth while to discuss them briefly in this paper, confining my attention to a limited portion of the respiratory tract—the lungs and bronchial tubes. In preparing for my task I have endeavored rather to gain a clear comprehension of the whole subject and to mark the varying importance of each symptom in different countries, than to digest all the multitudinous reports which have appeared concerning the influenza.

As might be expected, the disease-processes excited in the lower respiratory tract by the influenza were complicated in many cases by other diseases which happened to prevail at the same time, as for instance, diphtheritic, asthmatic and ordinary bronchitic affections. The disordered condition of the mucous membranes caused by the influenza-process doubtless presented an unusually favorable opportunity for the innoculation of various infectious matters.

The most serious complication of all was croupous pneumonia. I have not myself met with a case of this sort, and I do not believe that it was very often observed in Baltimore. The high death rate in certain European cities was, however, due to this complication. Professor Nothnagel (as reported in the *Lancet*, Jan. 18th, 1890, p. 173,) expressed the conviction that "the deaths from pneumonia which occurred in Vienna during the past few weeks, could not be regarded as due to influenza directly, because an epidemic of pneumonia had been observed by him before the outbreak of influenza at the end of November, 1889, which becoming more severe, attacked many patients convalescent from influenza." Again, (as quoted in the *British Medical Journal*, January 11th,

1890, p. 97,) he stated that "it was not this form (capillary bronchitis or broncho-pneumonia) of pneumonia which created alarm, but the croupous variety, which really occurred at that time more frequently than before. It might be said with certainty that there was no close or essential connection between these diseases, but a certain external influence could not be denied. This was to be understood in the following way : Influenza and croupous pneumonia were two morbid processes, entirely different in character. The latter could never develop directly out of the former. If a patient with influenza became also affected with croupous pneumonia, this was only a coincidence, the one process having prepared the soil for the development of the other." The frequency of this complication varied greatly in different localities and at different stages of the epidemic. Thus, Finkler, of Bonn (*British Medical Journal*, February 15th, 1890, p. 384,) records among 45 cases of inflammation of the lung in influenza only two cases in which the symptoms of simple typical lobar fibrinous pneumonia were present; while Dr. Guiteras of the New York Health Department, states (*Medical Record*, January 25th, 1890, p. 95,) that during the heat of the epidemic lobar pneumonia was the more frequent and deadly, attacking patients, generally men past forty, during the stage of prostration, affecting frequently both lungs, and causing very high fever; while at a later period in the epidemic lobular pneumonia and bronchitis of the smaller tubes and capillaries was more frequent and very fatal, although less fatal than the other form. It seems certain, then, that croupous pneumonia was associated with the influenza only as a complication—that it does not form an essential part of the true influenza process.

The disorder of the lungs and bronchial tubes, which is a part of the influenza process, may be limited to a mere congestion of some definite portion of the walls of the air-passages, or it may pass into a catarrhal inflammation of the lining-membranes with exudation of mucus or pus into the lumen of the air-passages, or in the most severe cases it may strike more deeply and cause some slight consolidation of the lung.

As to location, the process may be confined to a small region of the larger or smaller tubes, or it may gradually extend from the large bronchi downward to the pulmonary vesicles, or it may extend from one level of the lung to another, subsiding in one part as it develops in another. Often both sides of the chest present symptoms of infection at the same time, and it is probable that any part may be reinfected again and again at short intervals. These phenomena seem to indicate that there is a definite foreign causative agent which, settling upon some portion of the respiratory tract, passes through peculiar phases of development and decline, sometimes confining its action to its original location sometimes infecting neighboring regions.

The physical signs yielded upon examination vary according to the location and the existing phase of the disease. In some patients the process seems to be attended by very little exudation, the sounds upon auscultation indicating rather a congestion of the larger bronchial tubes with the collection in them of a small quantity of adhesive mucus ; in others, fine crepitant rales, heard only at the end of deep inspiration, mark the site of the affection. These sounds usually give place after a few hours or days to moist bronchial or sub-crepitant rales, which mark the transition from the stage of congestion to that of exudative inflammation. There is little or no interference with the normal percussion resonance. A peculiar feature of the disorder is the limitation of the rales to one lung or to a small portion of one lung. I may cite several illustrative cases which I have recently treated.

One patient went about his work for weeks with sonorous rales in the right mammary region, distinct enough to be heard by the patient himself, or by a person who placed his ear within half a foot of the chest walls. He had never been affected in this way before. Upon auscultation these rales seemed to be dry, and to be located in the larger bronchi and confined to a region but one or two inches in diameter. Gradually the part healed without any evidence of more extensive infection of the lung.

A second patient, a healthy man, exhibited only fine dry rales upon deep inspiration over a district one or two inches

in diameter in the infra-axillary region. The rales were
evidently situated near the surface of the lung, in the finest
bronchioles, or in the air-vesicles. They persisted for one
or two days, and were then replaced by small scattered moist
rales which gradually disappeared during convalescence.
There was no sign of extension from the point first infected.

The third patient, a healthy workingman, became extremely ill with what seemed to be capillary bronchitis of the
lower part of one lung. As time went by, first the middle
and then the top of the same lung became involved in the
exudative process, which affected also the larger tubes.
When the inflammation was still intense in the upper part of
the lung it was subsiding in the lower part, and gradually,
after a month or more, the whole lung was restored to health.
There was no consolidation of the affected lung, and no rusty
sputum nor other sign of croupous pneumonia. The other
lung remained healthy throughout the whole illness.

The general symptoms connected with the lung trouble of
influenza vary greatly in intensity in different cases. The increase in temperature may be slight, or may be very noticeable, but it is largely dependent upon disorders of other parts
of the body. There is often, in the affected regions, intense
and constant pain, which seems to be largely due to some
accidental neuralgic complication similar to that which is so
frequently met with in other parts of the body in this disease.
In some cases where it is very severe, there are no signs of
pleurisy ; in other cases complicated with pleurisy, it is, as a
writer has remarked, more intense than the pain of pleurisy.
The sputum may be scanty or abundant. It is white, as in
bronchitis, and may be streaked with blood, or perhaps be
purulent, but in uncomplicated cases it is probably never
rust-colored. Cough is generally present. It is sometimes
very persistent and exhausting, preventing sleep. "Sometimes," says Dr. Eade (*Lancet*, Feb. 1st, 1890, p. 230,) "the
dyspnœa has been a striking feature, disproportionate to the
extent of lung tissue affected, and occasionally becoming a
most formidable symptom. It is doubtless due to a condition of partial 'pulmonary paralysis.' "

I have myself had no opportunity for post-mortem examination of the diseased lungs. Prof. Nothnagel (quoted in the *Lancet*, Jan. 18th, 1890, p. 173,) states that "at the Vienna General Hospital, some cases of influenza were observed in which the post-mortem examination proved the presence of suppurative processes in the lungs and pleuræ which have not been observed till now in the course of any other disease; so that they are believed to be peculiar to the influenza."

As my audience is largely composed of practising physicians, and not of pathologists, I shall not attempt to discuss the results of microscopic investigation of the secretions and tissues of the affected lungs, nor to describe the many unsuccessful efforts to isolate the influenza germ.

The mucous membrane of the respiratory tract is doubtless the tissue through which the poison of influenza generally gains access to the system, and if so, disorders of these parts must precede the other symptoms of the disease. But the upper air-passages may be the first involved, and implication of the bronchial tubes and lungs may occur at some later period, either by extension downwards of the disease-process, or by a new infection from without. In some cases the lung trouble is the first, and, it may be, the only prominent indication of the presence of the disease.

The *diagnosis* of the influenza process in the lungs and bronchi is often difficult to establish with absolute certainty. During the epidemic, congestive or inflammatory disturbances in these organs may properly be ascribed to it if they are associated with the peculiar pains throughout the body, which are caused by its poison ; or, if they are very persistent and are accompanied by great depression of spirits and loss of flesh and strength—especially if they are confined to a limited portion of one lung, or spread over it in the manner already described. From phthisis pulmonalis they are distinguished by their peculiar course and by the absence of serious or permanent injury to the tissues involved.

In the *treatment*, the ordinary remedies for bronchitis may be employed with benefit. It should be remembered that we have to deal with a process which tends to self-limitation, and which is attended with enfeeblement of the patient. I have treated many persons in whom the affection caused but little inconvenience, running its course in one or several weeks, and resembling in many respects a mild double bronchitis. Tonics were given, containing cinchona and iron, and cough mixtures were taken by the patient if he was sick enough to need them. In the beginning of the epidemic, I was disposed to confine patients to the house or bed as long as symptoms of extensive bronchitis—especially if it involved the small tubes—were present. Learning from experience that these symptoms might persist for weeks, and that open-air exercise in good weather was rather beneficial, I recommended, during the rest of the epidemic, that patients should attend to their ordinary duties, short of fatigue, provided that they did not "feel sick" and had no considerable fever. Pain and cough were, in most cases, quickly controlled by fractional doses of sulphate of codeia, with moderate doses of carbonate of ammonia as a stimulant expectorant. In one case a child, two years old, with catarrh of the larger tubes, was kept awake for several nights by a cough which resisted moderate doses of codeia and bromides. Upon removal to the country, he recovered at once, gaining rapidly in general health. I lost two aged female patients with influenza bronchitis. In one, the bronchitis was very slight, but was accompanied by depression of the vital powers and loss of appetite. The other, who had been much prostrated by family worries, took to bed complaining chiefly of pains in one side of the chest. Finding a general bronchitis of the medium-sized tubes on the affected side, I had poultices applied to the part, and ordered ⅓ grain of sulphate of codeia, with 2 grains of carbonate of ammonia, in syrup of tolu, every four hours. Next day the pain had disappeared and the bronchitis was no worse. Great depression had set in, however, with nervous tossing and feverishness, intelligence being retained. Medication was now limited to large and frequent doses of brandy. The patient died next morning. In these two cases there was not sufficient disease of the lungs to seriously injure the patient, and the fever was not high, but death seemed due to the action of the influenza-poison on the nervous system.

In conclusion, I think it is well proven.

1st, That there is a peculiar disorder of the lungs and bronchial tubes due to influenza.

2nd, That it is marked by congestion or exudative inflammation of the affected surfaces, which is either limited to particular regions, or spreads slowly to adjacent parts of the air passages.

3rd, That it is due to inoculation by some foreign agent.

4th, That it is obstinate to treatment, but self-limited.

5th, That it predisposes to the inoculation of various other diseases.

6th, That as a rule, it does not permanently damage the respiratory organs.

7th, That in uncomplicated cases, death does not often, if at all, result from local interference with the functions of the lungs.

8th, That some poisonous agent is absorbed from the affected tissues into the general system, and causes a depression of the vital powers, which frequently produces death in the aged and feeble.

9th, That the best remedies are stimulant expectorants, mild opiates, tonics and removal to the country or sea-side.

NITROGEN IN MEDICINE AND SURGERY.

By W. R. Monroe, M. D.

About four-fifths of the air both by weight or measure is nitrogen, and about one-fifth is oxygen. In combination nitrogen occurs in the mineral kingdom as the basis of nitrates, nitrites, etc. It enters into the composition of almost all animal tissues, and in the vegetable kingdom it is found as a constituent of the alkaloids and the most active medicines, as well as the most nourishing foods. Organic substances are formed upon three or four ever similar elements to which other accessory ones join themselves : they are oxygen, hydrogen, carbon and nitrogen. While the most active substances are the nitrogenized, yet there are some exceptions as Gubler has shown, as, picrotoxine, duboisine, morphine, tea, coffee and cocoa.

Nitrogen is a colorless odorless gas, sp. gr. 975, soluble in water to some extent. When free it is chemically inactive and does not readily unite with other elements. It has been used as an anæsthetic supposed to be due to asphyxia from the absence of oxygen, but as the carbonic acid is constantly removed by inhalation of nitrogen, the symptoms of irritation produced by it in ordinary asphyxia are absent. Drs. Phillips and L. Johnson in their materia-medica and therapeutics published in 1882, by Wm. Wood & Co., express the opinion on the physiological action of nitrogen, that it is negative in character ; the gas will not support respiration nor combustion, and seems to act in the atmosphere as a diluting agent for the too stimulating oxygen. Steinbrick (Vienna) has lately recommended nitrogen inhalations in the first and second stages of phthisis in young persons, stating that they lower the circulation and allay nerve irritability, give great relief and sometimes cure. All observers agree as to the soporific effects of nitrogen. Mermagen says that he has seen more than one patient go to sleep while the inhalation was in progress, and that others were able to sleep for eight hours at a time: whereas, before, their night's rest had been prevented by cough and dyspnœa. The appetite is perceptibly increased, and consequently the nutrition improved.

Gubler says,—there are inhalations of gases properly so called, such as carbonic acid gas, nitrogen, compressed air; and oxygen. There are a great many springs which evolve such enormous quantities of gas, and are continually bubbling, that they have the appearance of boiling. Some contain a constant escape of carbonic acid, but it is a bad anæsthetic. There are springs which appear as if they contain the same gas, but which contain only nitrogen, perhaps under the form of entozone. The nitrogen disengaged by certain mineral waters is not useless, and there are patients who derive great benefit from breathing it. The nitrogen springs most remarkable, are those found near the village of Hoosic (Rensselaer county,) six miles from Bennington, Vermont. There are three springs within an area of four or five acres of land. The quantity of nitrogen gas which escapes under the form of bubbles is incalculable: it seems to rise from the gravel which forms the soil of the springs. Here pure nitrogen may be procured by inverted jars, amounting to a litre of gas in ten seconds.

Nitrogen is necessary for the manifestation of any energy, or any chemical change. According to Dr. Parks, every structure in the body on which any form of energy is manifested (heat, mechanical motion, chemical or electrical action, etc.,) is nitrogenous. The nitrogenous aliments are blood fibrin, muscle fibrin or syntonen, myosin, vegetable fibrin, albumin in its various forms, casein (in its animal and vegetable forms,) and globulin. Their composition, etc., are remarkably uniform; they contain between 15.4 and 16.5 per cent. of nitrogen, and may be conveniently distinguished by the common term of albuminates. They can replace each other in nutrition. The nerves, the muscles, the gland cells, the floating cells in the various liquids, the semen and the ovarian cells, are all nitrogenous. Even the non-cellular liquids passing out into the alimentary canal at various points, which so great an action in preparing the food in different ways, are not only nitrogenous, but the constancy of this implies the necessity of the nitrogen, in order that these actions shall be performed; and the same constancy of the presence of nitrogen, when the function is performed, is apparently traceable through the whole world. Surely such constancy proves necessity. Then, if the nitrogen be cut off from the body, the various functions languish. This does not occur at once, for every body contains a store of nitrogen, but it is at length inevitable. Again, if it is wished to increase the manifestation of the energies of the various organs, more nitrogen must be supplied. The experiments of Pettenkofer and Voit, show that the nitrogenous substances comprising the textures of the body determine the absorption of oxygen. The condensation of oxygen from the atmosphere, its conversion into its active condition (ozone) and its application to oxidation, are according to their experiments entirely under the control of the nitrogenous tissues (fixed and floating,) and are apparently proportional to their size and vigor; Dr. Parke's theory is that without the participation of nitrogenous bodies, no oxidation and no manifestation of energy is possible. The experiments show that the absorption of oxygen by the lungs (blood composition, and physical conditions of pressure, etc., remaining constant) is dependent on its disposal in the body, and that this disposal is in direct relation with the absolute and relative amount and action of the nitrogenous structures.

The nitrogen of the blood was first demonstrated by the experiments of Magnus, who considered this element as merely dissolved in the nourishing fluid. This opinion is generally adopted, and following the apt language of M. Longet is evolved there (in the blood) as in running waters which freely communicate with the surrounding atmosphere. According to M. M. Fornet and Setschenow, a portion of this gas also appear to be chemically combined, as in case of oxygen and carbonic acid.

M. Edwards asserts, that, an animal breathing atmospheric air also absorbs nitrogen. Absorbed nitrogen is carried wholly or partly into the mass of blood. Nitrogen absorbed is replaced by a quantity approximately equivalent of exhaled nitrogen which is derived wholly or partly from the blood. It has often been asked, how does it appear that the gas most abundantly diffused in nature, nitrogen has not been the object of more frequent investigations; How happens it that nobody has more curiosity regarding the fluid which constitutes nearly four-fifths of the atmosphere in which we live? Its consideration has been set aside with the simple expression, *unsuited to respiration*. The same answer might be given against the consideration of carbonic acid and hydrogen, from the fact that each is deprived of oxogen. But apart from the lack of the vital quality, it is evident that each of these gases exercise a special agency, and possess some degree of influence on the human organism which is proper to it. It is asserted that surgical practice has been an excellent guide and has furnished us relatively to the physiological action of nitrogen, a criterion which physiological experimentation very probably will only corroborate.

About the close of the last and the beginning of the present century nitrogen had been the subject of two monographs. The first published in 1796, in New York by Winthrop Saltonstall, 8 vo. The other by Dagroumer in Paris in 1816. Nysten, the friend and colloborater of Bichat was a diligent student upon the action which various gases, injected into the circulatory system, exercise upon the organism. He injected nitrogen into the veins and believed that from it he recognized a sedative action on the heart. He always considered it as indicated in the more acute diseases of the respiratory organs.

Demarquay says:—"We have concluded from our experiments upon animals, and, later, our studies upon man, that nitrogen is, in a manner, the mere absorbent of oxygen, and that of itself it has no active properties: further, that the irritating properties of the air, as regards wounds, recognized by Monro and Hunter, and more recently by surgeons who have made a special study of tenotomy, are due to oxygen. If these speculative views are corroborated we shall then have found in nitrogen the demonstration of one of the greatest problems which confronts the modern surgeon, that is to say, the reunion of wounds by first intention by placing them under new conditions, which will maintain, in the work of repair or adhesion, a degree of activity or excitation which will not exceed certain limits. Perhaps there will be deduced from these various studies a practical fact which avail something for the relief of the afflicted and toward the progress of surgery. Besides the attempt made by Leconte and ourselves may be readily repeated. *It is only necessary to have nitrogen.* The operation being done, the limb, upper or lower, is placed in an India-rubber apparatus, a kind of muff or boot. This apparatus properly applied, is filled with nitrogen. We have studied the employment of this gas in a double point of view ; first, from the point of view of original disease, and second, from the point of view of reunion, or rather the work of reparation of wounds. Pains inseparable from all operations performed upon an organized or living part can be quieted by this gas, while chloroform removes sensibility only momentarily, but chloroform having ceased to act, the pain, often very intense and very lasting, returns. (In all cases where pain is the result of exposure of the wound to the atmosphere, relief is complete from the application of nitrogen.) It cannot be said with certainty that the pain which follows all operations is a result of contact with the air, for in this case all subcutaneous operations, properly made, ought to cease to be painful as soon as terminated, but unfortunately it is not so. The operation finished, there remain nerve trunks which are bathed by the blood ; besides there is reaction which always follows from every operation. If then, all surgical operations involving division or cutting of tissues are inevitably painful, it remains to be determined whether it is not possible to moderate the pain. Various narcotic substances have been applied in the form of fomentations and chloroform spray used, but unfortunately, this substance applied to the tissues, and even upon the integument excites active irritation, even to the extent of blistering. Nitrogen has not this objection.''

Many experiments were made in conjunction with Leconte. which were reported by Lemoine, a prominent interne of the Hospital, which have been translated and published. A summary of these reported cases have been read with great

interest, as most of them confirm the reported value of nitrogen in the relief of pain, and hasten the healing of the
wounds. In some cases the application of oxygen, only for
a short time, alternated that of nitrogen, where healthy
granulations were desired to hasten the healing process. In
closing the report on these cases, the author says,—they are
not to be accepted as conclusions; but they warrant the
hope, that, with suitable apparatus, and with nitrogen carefully prepared, we may be enabled, first, to moderate the inflammatory re-action of wounds; second, to favor union by
first intention.

PROTOXIDE OF NITROGEN (NITROGEN MONOXIDE.)

Priestly had the honor to discover the protoxide of nitrogen, 1776. Not until 1800 when Sir Humphrey Davy became
impressed with the curious properties of protoxide of nitrogen did he make it the subject of careful investigation, of
which he published the results in a book 8 vo. 580 pages, in
London, entitled, *Chemical and Philosophical Researches,
Principally upon Nitrous Oxide and its Respiration.* Humphrey David subjected himself at one time for a week, and
at another time to two months consecutively, to the daily use
of this gas, by inhalations three times a day, and experienced
from it a decided feeling of comfort. That which impressed
him most forcibly was a general exaltation of all the functions particularly of those sensations which are manifested
by perceptions clearer and brighter than ordinary. He also
found in this gas the first general anæsthetic which had been
brought to light. He said in substance at the end of his
work,—that the protoxide of nitrogen appears to have, among
other properties, that of annihilating pain.

As a transient anæsthetic its use has become so universal,
as almost, to overshadow all other uses. It ought to be a
vital oxidizer, because it supports combustion almost as well
as oxygen itself. It is also far more soluble in water and
all aqueous fluids than the latter gas. Empirically, it is
found to allay spasm, relieve pain, relax nervous tension and
to induce a feeling of rest and exhilaration. Nitrogen monoxide is a definite compound containing two atoms of nitro-

gen in a state of chemical combination with one atom of oxygen. The usual mode of exhibiting this gas, therapeutically, is to add from 15 to 40 per cent. of it to pure oxygen; still further diluting this mixture with common air. Used in this strength it is found to add materially to the quieting and restful influence of oxygen. In all neurasthenic and neuralgic conditions, it is a valuable adjunct and synergist of oxygen. It does not seem to deteriorate with age. At a pressure of 50 atmospheres it assumes the liquid form. A half gallon flask will easily hold the equivalent of 100 gallons of the gas at its normal tension, under a pressure of one atmosphere.

The most extensive volume yet published on the medical uses of nitrogen monoxide, has been by Dr. Geo. J. Ziegler, of Philadelphia, 1865. He devoted about 16 years to the study of this agent. He indulges in an extravagant estimate of its hygienic and therapeutic value : " The effects of protoxide of nitrogen on the human system passes from a gentle acceleration of the functions to a high degree of physical and mental exhilaration. It has special tendencies to certain parts of the body, the blood, the brain, nervous system, and genito-urinary organs. Its potency is largely but not wholly derived from its oxygen, a fact proved by the peculiarity of some of its effects, which are unknown in connection with the use of oxygen alone. It both supplies essential material for organization, and promotes the general molecular, nutrient, reproductive, and dynamic operations of the animal economy. Hence it promotes the various functions of digestion, absorption, circulation, æration, hœmetosis, etc. This agent may be made an efficient substitute for alcohol, ammonia, quassia, strychnia, and others classified as stimulants, tonics, etc. It is strongly indicated in atonic conditions of the genito-urinary apparatus, such as incontinence, suppression, vesical paralysis, spermatorrhœa, impotence, sterility, dysmenorrhœa, etc.

In certain stages of phthisis it is very useful in promoting assimilation and hœmatosis, and in relieving oppression of breathing, cough and other distressing symptoms. In mild forms of glycosuria he has repeatedly seen the sæcharine element rapidly disappear under the use of protoxide of nitrogen."

As an anæsthetic, protoxide of nitrogen is unique, differing essentially from all other agents of its kind in its chemical constitution, physical properties, and physiological influences. Most anæsthetics are composed essentially of hydrogen and carbon, while this is a compound of oxygen and nitrogen. The former produce insensibility by preventing æration of and deoxidizing the blood, depressing the nervous system, stupefying the brain, and paralyzing the heart. Nitrous oxide, increases oxidation, stimulates the brain, invigorates the system, and acts as a true tonic. In a word, while chloroform and ether arrest vital processes, nitrous oxide promotes life and action.

In conclusion :—As this gas is such a safe anæsthetic, only lacking duration in its effects, may it not be possible that some skilful experimenter may yet discover some modification of it by the combination of some other element, or otherwise, that will render its action and effects so prolonged as to answer all the purposes for any operation, and thus supersede the more unsafe and unpleasant anæsthetics, as chloroform and ether.

As it has been demonstrated that nitrogen properly applied to wounds will relieve pain and induce healing by first intention, why may it not prove useful if applied to surfaces burned or scalded, in excluding the air, relieving pain, preventing suppuration, and inducing speedy healing by first intention.

Pure nitrogen can be easily and abundantly obtained from Nitrogen Springs, as those at Hoosic Nitrogen Springs in the State of Vermont. It may be used in its gaseous form, or compressed into a fluid,—can be used internally as well as externally. In painful dysentery, injected into the rectum, would probably afford great relief.

A spasmodic inclination to cough has often been checked by a brief suspension of respiration : after taking a full inspiration of air, when the oxygen becomes absorbed, the nitrogen remains in the irritable bronchial tubes acting like a hypnotic or anodyne. May it not remain for some of the younger members of the profession to immortalize themselves by occupying this important field of research that they may discover all that is valuable in nitrogen for the practice of medicine and surgery.

Rules for the Government of the Library.

Adopted May 9th and 12th, 1882.

I. The Librarian or Assistant Librarian shall attend at the Library Rooms daily, except Sunday and legal holidays. from 12 o'clock until 8 o'clock P. M., during which hours only, books and journals may be taken from the Library.

II. Each member of the Faculty, paying the annual dues, shall be entitled to take out at one time, four volumes duodecimo, two volumes octavo, one volume quarto, or one volume folio. This rule may be suspended by the written order of three members of the Library Committee.

III. City members retaining books longer than *two weeks* and county members longer than four weeks, shall be subject to the following *fines* per week, viz. : 10 cents for the first week, 20 cents for the second week, 30 cents for the third week, and 20 cents per week for every week thereafter. Such fines shall be appropriated exclusively for the benefit of the Library.

IV. No book shall be delivered to a member unless in person or to his written order. A member receiving a book shall be held responsible for it from the time of its delivery until its return to the Library.

V. A member not returning a book or books, belonging to the Library, within four weeks after the date of receiving them, shall be notified *by the Librarian* that he is incurring a fine ; and if they be not returned within three months, in the absence of satisfactory reasons therefor, the Librarian shall recover them, or if they be lost, their value, in behalf of the Faculty ; otherwise, the defaulting member shall forfeit the privileges of the Library, and shall be reported at the next annual convention of the Faculty, by the Library Committee. Should any book be injured or defaced while in the possession of a member, he shall be fined, at the discretion of the Library Committee, or, at his option, may furnish such a copy of the same work as shall be acceptable to the Committee.

VI. If any member, upon returning a book, shall find that there has been no application for it while in his possession, he may take it again for the time allowed in Rule III, but

may not take it out a third time until after the expiration of one week succeeding its return to the Library. New books may not be taken by members for more than one term of two weeks, until after the expiration of one additional week after their return.

VII. Members are not entitled to receive books from the Library until all arrearages for fines are paid.   Fines may be remitted or reduced, for just and sufficient reasons, by the Library Committee.

VIII. The Librarian shall appropriately number and stamp the books, pamphlets and periodicals, and place them in proper order on the shelves. He shall obtain and keep a correct list of the members paying the annual dues. He shall record, in a book kept for the purpose, the names of members who receive books from the Library, the titles and sizes of the books, the time of their delivery and of their return. He shall continue the catalogue of the books, pamphlets, periodicals, etc.; keep an account of all moneys received by him for fines, contributions, sales, etc., which moneys he shall pay into the hands of the Chairman of the Library Committee on the last week-day of each month. He shall report during the last week in March of each year to the Library Committee, a statement of such donations of money or of books as may have been made to the Library, with the names of the donors, as well as of such books, pamphlets, periodicals, or other valuable matter as may have come into the possion of the Library by purchase, exchange, or otherwise. He shall keep a record of all books, periodicals, etc., upon the subscription list of the Library Committee, shall keep due record of their receipt at the proper time, and shall report to the Library Committee the non-receipt of any when over-due. He shall keep on file applications for such books as may have been let out of the Library; and may make any suggestions to the Committee he may deem necessary.

IX. Under no circumstances will members be permitted to remove new books, new journals, or other recently received matter, before such time as the Library Committee shall determine.

X. Scarce and valuable books, the loss of which it would be difficult to replace, shall not be removed from the Library rooms without the approbation of two members of the Library Committee.

XI. The Librarian is empowered to sell or exchange duplicate books, journals, etc., upon such terms as may appear advantageous, upon the approval of the Library Committee.

LIST OF PRESIDENTS—1799–1889.

---------- ----

Upton Scott—1799-1801.
Philip Thomas—1801-15.
Ennals Martin—1815-20.
Robert Moore—1820-26.
Robert Goldsborough—1826-36.
Maxwell McDowell—1836-41.
Joel Hopkins—1841-48.
Richard S. Steuert—1848-51.
William W. Handy—1851-52.
Michael S. Baer—1852-53.
John L. Yates—1853-54.
John Fonerden—1854-55.
Jacob Baer—1855-56.
Christopher C. Cox—1856-57.
Joshua I. Cohen—1857-58.
Joel Hopkins—1858-59.
Geo. C. M. Roberts—1859-70.
John R. W. Dunbar—1870-70.
Nathan R. Smith—1870-72.
P. C. Williams—1872-73.
Charles H. Ohr—1873-74.
Henry M. Wilson—1874-75.
John F. Monmonier—1875-76.
Christopher Johnston—1876-77.
Abram B. Arnold—1877-78.
Samuel P. Smith—1878-79.
Samuel C. Chew—1879-80.
H. P. C. Wilson—1880-81.
Frank Donaldson—1881-82.
William M. Kemp—1882-83.
Richard McSherry—1883-84.
Thomas S. Latimer—1884-85.
John R. Quinan—1885-86.
Geo. W. Miltenberger—1886-87.
I. Edmondson Atkinson—1887-88.
John Morris—1888-89.
Aaron Friedenwald—1889-90.
Thomas A. Ashby—1890-91.

ACTIVE MEMBERS.

Andre, J. Ridgeway, 1123 E. Baltimore Street, Baltimore.
Ankrim, L. F., 4 S. Broadway, Baltimore.
Aronsohn, Abram, 712 N. Eutaw Street, Baltimore.
Ashby, Thos. A., 1125 Madison Avenue, Baltimore.
Atkinson, Archibald, 2101 Charles Street Avenue, Baltimore.
Atkinson, G. T., Crisfield, Somerset County.
Atkinson, I. E., 605 Cathedral Street, Baltimore.
Baldwin, Ed. C., 304 N. Exeter Street, Baltimore.
Barnes, Wm. M., 905 N. Stricker Street, Baltimore.
Barron, John, Govanstown, Baltimore County.
Baxley, J. B., Jr., 1531 Madison Avenue, Baltimore.
Bayly, Alex. H., Cambridge, Dorchester County.
Belt, Alfred M., 1010 Cathedral Street, Baltimore.
Belt, S. J., 314 N. Exeter Street, Baltimore.
Benson, B. R., Cockeysville, Baltimore County.
Berkley, Harry J., 1303 Park Avenue, Baltimore.
Bevan, Chas. F., 807 Cathedral Street, Baltimore.
Biedler, H. H., 119 W. Saratoga Street, Baltimore.
Billingslea, M. B., 1206 E. Preston Street, Baltimore.
Birnie, C., Taneytown, Carroll County.
Blaisdell, W. S., 285 N. Exeter Street, Baltimore.
Blake, John D., 602 S. Paca Street, Baltimore.
Blum, Joseph, 641 Columbia Avenue, Baltimore.
Bond, A. K., 311 W. Biddle Street, Baltimore.
Bond, Robert, Brooklyn, Anne Arundel County.
Bond, S. B., 202 W. Franklin Street, Baltimore.
Booker, Wm. D., 851 Park Avenue, Baltimore.
Bosley, James, 1701 Hollins Street, Baltimore.
Bowie, Howard S., 811 N. Eutaw Street, Baltimore.
Branham, J. H., 538 N. Arlington Avenue, Baltimore.
Branham, J. W., 538 N. Arlington Avenue, Baltimore.
Brawner, J. B., Emmittsburg, Frederick County.

Bressler, F. C., 1703 Bank Street, Baltimore.
Brinton, Wilmer, S. W. Cor. Preston and Calvert Streets, Baltimore.
Bromwell, J. E., Mt. Airey, Baltimore County.
Browne, B. B., 1218 Madison Avenue, Baltimore.
Brown, James, 131 W. Lanvale Street, Baltimore.
Brune, T. Barton, 1815 N. Charles Street, Baltimore.
Bubert, Charles Hy., 1926 Pennsylvania Avenue, Baltimore.
Buckler, Thos. H., Albion Hotel, Baltimore.
Buddenbohn, C. L., 602 S. Paca Street, Baltimore.
Campbell, Wm. H. H., Owings Mills, Baltimore County.
Canfield, Wm. B., 1010 N. Charles Street, Baltimore.
Carnes, Geo. H., Woodberry, Baltimore,
Carr, M. A. R. F., Cumberland, Allegany County.
Cathell, D. Webster, 1308 N. Charles Street, Baltimore.
Cathell, W. T., 1308 N. Charles Street, Baltimore.
Chabbot, G. H., 1111 E. Preston Street, Baltimore.
Chamberlaine, J. E. M., Easton, Talbot County.
Chambers, John W., 309 N. Exeter Street, Baltimore.
Chancellor, C. W., 103 W. First Street, Baltimore.
Chatard, Ferd. E., Jr., 516 Park Avenue, Baltimore.
Ghew, Sam'l C., 215 W. Lanvale Street, Baltimore.
†Chilton, Orrick M.
Chisolm, J. J., 112 W. Franklin Street, Baltimore.
Chisolm, F. M., 114 W. Franklin Street, Baltimore.
Christian, J. H., 1821 Madison Avenue, Baltimore.
Chunn, W. P., 1023 Madison Avenue, Baltimore.
Clagett, Joseph E., 108 S. Eutaw Street, Baltimore.
Coffroth, H. J., 924 Madison Avenue, Baltimore.
Conrad, John S., St. Denis P. O., Baltimore County.
Cooke, Theodore, 910 N. Charles Street, Baltimore.
Cordell, Eugene F., 2113 Maryland Avenue, Baltimore.
Corse, Geo. F., Gardenville, Baltimore County.
Corse, Wm. D., Gardenville, Baltimore County.
*Coskery, Oscar J., 624 N. Calvert Street, Baltimore.
Councilman, W. T., Johns Hopkins University, Baltimore.
Craighill, J. M., 1720 N. Charles Street, Baltimore.
Dalrymple, A. J., 2006 E. Pratt Street, Baltimore.
Dashiell, N. L., Jr., 2128 Madison Avenue, Baltimore.
Dausch, Pierre G., 1727 E. Baltimore Street, Baltimore.
Davis, R. G., 1307 N. Caroline Street, Baltimore.
Dickinson, G. E., Upper Fairmount, Charles County.
Dickson, I. N., Reisterstown, Baltimore County,
Dickson, John, 1018 Madison Avenue, Baltimore.
†Diller, Chas. H., Double Pipe Creek, Carroll County.
Donaldson, Frank, 510 Park Avenue, Baltimore.

Downey, Jesse W., New Market, Frederick County.
*Drought, A. M., Huntington Avenue, Baltimore.
Dulin, Alex'r F., 107 W. Monument Street, Baltimore.
Dwinelle, J. E., 1701 E. Baltimore Street, Baltimore.
Eareckson, R. W., Elkridge Landing, Howard County.
Earle, Sam'l T., 1431 Linden Avenue, Baltimore.
Eastman, Lewis M. 722 W. Lexington Street, Baltimore.
Ellis, E. Dorsey, 915 Light Street, Baltimore.
Ellis, R. H. P., 733 W. Fayette Street. Baltimore.
Evans, Thomas B., 121 Jackson Place, Baltimore.
Fiske, John D., 8 S. Patterson Park Avenue, Baltimore.
Flemming, Geo. A., 928 Madison Avenue, Baltimore.
Fort, Sam'l J., Font Hill, Ellicott City, Howard County.
†Free, S. M.,————Pennsylvania.
Forwood, W. Stump, Darlington, Hartford County.
Friedenwald, Aaron, 310 N. Eutaw Street, Baltimore.
Friedenwald, Harry, 922 Madison Avenue, Baltimore.
Fulton, John S., Salisbury, Wicomico County.
Funck, J. W., 1710 W. Fayette Street, Baltimore.
Gardner, Frank B., 424 N. Greene Street, Baltimore.
Gardner, W. S., 410 N. Howard Street, Baltimore.
Gibbons, Jas. E., 833 Edmonson Avenue, Baltimore.
Gibbs, E. C., 440 E. North Avenue, Baltimore.
Giles, A. B., 1340 Aisquith Street. Baltimore.
†Gleitsman, J. Wm., 117 Second Avenue, New York.
Godfrey, Isabel K., 104 E. Madison Street. Baltimore.
Goldsborough, Brice W., Cambridge, Dorchester County.
Goldsmith, Robert H., 647 N. Calhoun Street, Baltimore.
Goodman, H. H., 410 Hanover Street, Baltimore.
Gorter, N. R., 1 W. Biddle Street, Baltimore.
Graham, Geo. R., 725 Columbia Avenue, Baltimore.
Griffith, L. A., Upper Marlboro, Prince George's County.
Grimes, J. H., 102 Second Street, (Belt,) Baltimore.
Grove, B. Frank, 1321 E. Biddle Street, Baltimore.
Gundry, Richard, Catonsville, Baltimore County.
Gwynn, H. B., 724 N. Gilmor Street, Baltimore.
Hall, Alice T., 708 N. Howard Street, Baltimore.
Hall, Reverdy M., 1019 Druid Hill Avenue, Baltimore.
Harlan, Herbert, 317 N. Charles Street, Baltimore.
Harris, John C., 773 W. Lexington Street, Baltimore.
Hartman, George A., 1121 N. Caroline Street, Baltimore.
Hartman, Jacob H., 5 W. Franklin Street, Baltimore.
Hartwell, E. M., Johns Hopkins Hospital, Baltimore.
Heldman, Joel A., 254 Pearl Street, Baltimore.
Hemmeter, John C., 633 W. Lombard Street, Baltimore.

Herman, H. S., State Line, Pa.
Hilgartner. H. L., E. Baltimore Street, Baltimore.
Hill, Chas. G., Arlington, Baltimore County.
Hill, Henry F., 1001 Edmondson Avenue, Baltimore.
Hill, Wm. N., 1438 E. Baltimore Street, Baltimore.
Hines, W. F., Chestertown.
Hocking, Geo. H., Mt. Savage, Alleghany County.
Hoen, Adolph G., 713 York Road, Baltimore.
Hogden, Alexander Lewis, 1235 Lafayette Avenue, Baltimore.
Hopkins, Howard H., New Market, Frederick County.
Hopkinson, B. Merrill, 1524 Park Avenue, Baltimore.
Howard, Wm. T., 804 Madison Avenue, Baltimore.
Humrickhouse, J. W., Hagerstown, Washington County.
Hundley, J. M., 1002 Edmondson Avenue, Baltimore.
Hurd, Henry M., Johns Hopkins Hospital, Baltimore.
Iglehart, J. D., 322 W. Biddle Street, Baltimore.
Ingle, J. L., 1007 W. Lanvale Street.
Irons, Ed. P., 1835 E. Baltimore Street, Baltimore.
Jacobs, C. C., Frostburg, Garrett County.
Jacobs, J. K. H., Kennedysville, Kent County.
Jay, John G., 212 W. Franklin Street, Baltimore.
Jenkins, Felix, 400 Cathedral Street, Baltimore.
Johnson, Robt. W., 101 W. Franklin Street, Baltimore.
Johnston, Christopher, 201 W. Franklin Street, Baltimore.
Johnston, Christopher, Jr., 201 W. Franklin Street, Baltimore.
Johnston, Samuel, 204 W. Monument Street, Baltimore.
Jones, C. Hampson, 25 W. Saratoga Street, Baltimore.
Jones, Charles H., 1083 W. Fayette Street, Baltimore.
Jones, Edwin E., Pennsylvania and Wylie Aves., Baltimore County.
Jones, Wm. T., 1238 Greenmount Avenue, Baltimore.
Keane, S. A., 1010 Linden Avenue, Baltimore.
Keirle, N. G., 1419 W. Lexington Street, Baltimore.
Keller, Josiah G., 222 W. Monument Street, Baltimore.
Kemp, Wm. F. A., 305 N. Greene Street, Baltimore.
King, J. T., 640 N. Carrollton Avenue, Baltimore.
Kloman, W. C., 1519 John Street, Baltimore.
Knight, Louis W., 414 N. Greene Street, Baltimore.
Kremein, John D., 667 W. Lexington Street, Baltimore.
Krozer, J. J. R., 662 W. Lexington Street, Baltimore.
Kuhn, Anna L., 1435 Light Street, Baltimore.
Latimer, Thos. S., 103 W. Monument Street, Baltimore.
Lee, Wm., 323 W. Hoffman Street, Baltimore.
Lockwood, W. F., 201 W. Madison Street Baltimore.
Lumpkin, Thos. M., 640 W. Barre Street, Baltimore.

MacGill, Chas. G. W., Catonsville, Baltimore County.
Mackenzie, Ed. E., 325 W. Biddle Street, Baltimore.
Mackenzie, John N., 205 N. Charles Street, Baltimore.
Magruder, W. E., Olney, Montgomery County.
Mann, A. H., Jr., 934 Madison Avenue, Baltimore.
Mansfield, Arthur, 129 S. Broadway, Baltimore.
Mansfield, R. W., 129 S. Broadway, Baltimore.
Marsh, Wm. H., Solomon's Island, Calvert County.
Mason, A. S., Hagerstown, Washington County.
Martin, H. Newell, 925 St. Paul Street, Baltimore.
Martin, James S., Brookville, Montgomery County.
Maxwell, Wm. S., Still Pond, Kent County.
McComas, J. Lee, Oakland, Garrett County.
McCormick, Thos. P., 1529 Eutaw Place, Baltimore.
†McDowell, C. C., 1521 W. Fayette Street, Baltimore.
McKnew, Wm. R., 1401 Linden Avenue, Baltimore.
McSherry, H. Clinton, 612 N. Howard Street, Baltimore.
Merrick, S. K., 420 W. Biddle Street, Baltimore.
Michael, J. Edwin, 937 Madison Avenue, Baltimore,
Miller, C. O., 312 W. Madison Street, Baltimore.
Miltenberger, Geo. W., 319 W. Monument Street, Baltimore
Moale, Wm. A., 716 N. Charles Street, Baltimore.
Monmonier, John F., 824 N. Calvert Street, Baltimore.
Monroe, Wm. R., 1734 Bolton Street, Baltimore.
Morgan, Wilbur P., 315 W. Monument Street, Baltimore.
Morison, Rob't B., 827 St. Paul Street, Baltimore.
Morris, John, 118 E. Franklin Street, Baltimore.
Mosely, W. E., 614 N. Howard Street, Baltimore.
Moyer, F. G., 4 S. Exeter Street, Baltimore.
Murdoch, Thos. F., 8 W. Read Street, Baltimore.
Murdock, Russell, 410 Cathedrel Street, Baltimore.
Neale, L. Ernest, 319 W. Monument Street, Baltimore.
Neff, John, 701 N. Carrollton Avenue, Baltimore.
Nickerson, Wm. M., 700 N. Arlington Avenue, Baltimore.
Nihiser, Winton M., Keedysville.
Norris, Amanda Taylor, 871 Harlem Avenue, Baltimore.
Norris, Wm. H., 1300 E. Baltimore Street, Baltimore.
O'Donavan, Chas., Jr., 311 W. Monument Street, Baltimore.
Ohle, H. C., 1203 W. Fayette Street, Baltimore.
Ohr, Chas. H., Cumberland, Alleghany County.
Opie, Thomas, 600 N. Howard Street, Baltimore.
Osler, Wm., 209 W. Monument Street, Baltimore.
Page, I. Randolph, 1206 Linden Avenue, Baltimore.
Pennington, J. I., 804 N. Carrollton Avenue, Baltimore.
Perkins, Joseph F., 317 N. Charles Street, Baltimore.

Piper, Jackson, Towson, Baltimore County.
Platt, Walter B., 859 Park Avenue, Baltimore.
Pole, A. C., 2102 Madison Avenue, Baltimore.
Porter, G. Ellis, Lonaconing, Alleghany County.
Powell, Alfred H., 212 W. Madison Street, Baltimore.
Preston, Geo. J., 9 E. Townsend Street, Baltimore.
Prichard, J. E., 1010 S. Chesapeake Street, Baltimore.
†Quinan, John R., 1637 N. Gilmor Street, Baltimore.
Ragan, O. H. W., Hagerstown, Washington County.
Randolph, R. L., 211 W. Madison Street, Baltimore.
Reid, E. Miller, 904 N. Fremont Street, Baltimore.
Redding, M. Laura Ewing, 930 Madison Avenue, Baltimore.
Rehberger, John H., 1709 Aliceanna Street, Baltimore.
Reiche, P. H., 906 Gorsuch Avenue, Baltimore.
Reinhard, G. A. Ferd., 220 W. Madison Street, Baltimore.
Rennolds, Hy. T., 722 Aisquith Street, Baltimore.
Reynolds, Geo. B., 711 N. Calvert Street, Baltimore.
Rickert, Wm., 1841 Pennsylvania Avenue, Baltimore.
Riley, Charles H., 1113 Madison Avenue, Baltimore.
Robb, Hunter, Johns Hopkins Hospital, Baltimore.
Rohé, George H., 611 N. Calvert Street, Baltimore.
Rowe, M., Deals Island, Somerset County.
Rusk, G. Glanville, 2000 E. Baltimore Street, Baltimore.
Salzer, Henry, 613 Park Avenue, Baltimore.
Sandrock, W. Christian, Broadway and Chase Street. Baltimore.
Saunders, J. B., 819 E. Chase Street, Baltimore.
Sappington, Purnell F., Baltimore.
Sappington, Thomas, 919 N. Calvert Street, Baltimore.
Scott, John McP., Hagerstown, Washington County.
Scott, Norman B., Hagerstown, Washington County.
Seldner, Samuel W., 947 N. Caroline Street, Baltimore.
Sellman, W. A. B., 5 E. Biddle Street, Baltimore.
Shaw, W. Rutherford, 10 E. Read Street, Baltimore.
Shippen, Chas. C., 603 N. Charles Street, Baltimore.
Skilling, W. Quail, Lonaconing, Alleghany County.
Smith, Alan P., 24 W. Franklin Street, Baltimore.
Smith, Nathan R., 24 W. Franklin Street, Baltimore.
Smith, Jos. T., 1010 Madison Avenue, Baltimore.
Spear, J. M., Cumberland, Alleghany County.
Spicknall, Jno. T., N. Patterson Park Avenue, Baltimore.
Steiner, L. H., 1038 N. Eutaw Street, Baltimore.
Steuart, Jas. A., New York.
Streett, David, 403 N. Exeter Street, Baltimore.
Taneyhill, G. Lane, 1103 Madison Avenue, Baltimore.

Teakle, St. Geo. W., 702 Park Avenue, Baltimore.
Theobald, Samuel, 304 W. Monument Street, Baltimore.
Thomas, George, 550 Presstman Street, Baltimore.
Thomas, Jas. Carey, 1228 Madison Avenue, Baltimore.
Thomas, Richard H., 714 N. Howard Street, Baltimore.
Thomas, W. D., 611 N. Carrollton Avenue, Baltimore.
Thompson, W. H., 526 St. Paul Street, Baltimore.
Tiffany, L. McLane, 831 Park Avenue, Baltimore.
Todd, W. J., Mt. Washington, Baltimore County.
Van Bibber, Claude, 26 W. Franklin Street, Baltimore.
Van Bibber, John, 26 W. Franklin Street, Baltimore.
Van Bibber, W. Chew, 26 W. Franklin Street, Baltimore.
Van Marter, I. G., Jr., Rome, Italy.
Vees, Chas. H., 1210 E. Eager Street, Baltimore.
Virdin, W. W., Lapidum, Harford County.
Walker, E. R., 1703 N. Charles Street, Baltimore.
Warfield, Mactier, 719 N. Howard Street, Baltimore.
Warfield, R. B., 214 W. Franklin Street, Baltimore.
Waters, Edmund G., 1429 McCulloh Street, Baltimore.
Welch, W. H., 506 Cathedral Street, Baltimore.
White, W. W., 1101 N. Broadway, Baltimore.
Whitridge, Wm., 829 N. Charles Street, Baltimore.
Wiegand, Wm. E. 2023 Druid Hill Avenue, Baltimore.
Williams, Arthur, Elkridge Landing, Howard County.
Williams, E. J., Elkridge Landing, Howard County.
Williams, John M., Lonaconing, Alleghany County.
Williams, J. Whitridge, 900 Madison Avenue, Baltimore.
Williams, Philip C., 900 Madison Avenue, Baltimore.
Wilson, Henry M., 1008 Madison Avenue, Baltimore
Wilson, H. P. C., 814 Park Avenue, Baltimore.
Wilson, J. Jones, Cumberland, Alleghany County.
Wilson, Robert T., 820 Park Avenue, Baltimore.
Wiltshire, Jas. G., 418 W. Fayette Street, Baltimore.
Winsey, Whitfield, 1220 E. Fayette Street, Baltimore.
Winslow, Caleb, 924 McCulloh Street, Baltimore.
Winslow, John R., 924 McCulloh Street, Baltimore.
Winslow, Randolph, 1 Mt. Royal Terrace, Baltimore.
Winternitz, L. C., 25 S. Eden Street, Baltimore.
Woods, Hiram, Jr., 525 N. Howard Street, Baltimore.
Ziegler, Charles B., 920 N. Broadway, Baltimore.

HONORARY MEMBERS.

Bartholow, Roberts, M. D , Philadelphia, Pa.
Billings, John S., M. D., U. S. A., Washington, D. C.
Chaille, Stanford E., M. D., New Orleans, La.
Dunott, Thomas J., M. D., Harrisburg, Pa.
Goodell. Wm., M. D., Philadelphia, Pa.
Mallet, John W., M. D., University of Virginia.
Mitchell, S. Weir, M. D., Philadelphia, Pa.
Moorman, John J., M. D., Salem, Va.
Pepper, William, M. D., Philadelphia, Pa.
Toner, Joseph M., M. D., Washington, D. C.

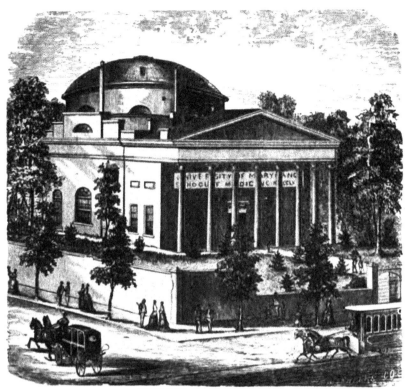

SCHOOL OF MEDICINE.

N. E. COR. LOMBARD AND GREENE STS., BALTIMORE, MD.

The Eighty-fourth Annual Course of Lectures in this institution will commence on OCTOBER 1st, 1890

FACULTY OF PHYSIC.

GEO. W. MILTENBERGER, M. D., Emeritus Professor of Obstetrics and Honorary President of the Faculty

CHRISTOPHER JOHNSTON, M. D. Emeritus Professor of Surgery

SAMUEL C. CHEW, M. D. Prof. of Principles and Practice of Medicine and Hygiene

FRANK DONALDSON, M. D., Emeritus Clinical Prof. of Diseases of the Throat & Chest

WM. T. HOWARD, M. D., Prof. of Diseases of Women & Children, & Clinical Medicine

JULIAN J. CHISOLM, M. D., Professor of Eye and Ear Diseases

FRANCIS T. MILES, M. D., Professor of Physiology, and Clinical Professor of Diseases of Nervous System

LOUIS McLANE TIFFANY, M. D., Professor of Surgery

J. EDWIN MICHAEL, M. D. Professor of Obstetrics

ISAAC EDMONDSON ATKINSON, M. D., Professor of Materia Medica and Therapeutics, Clinical Medicine and Dermatology

FERD J. S. GORGAS, M. D., D. D. S., Professor of Principles of Dental Science, Dental Surgery and Dental Mechanism

JAMES H. HARRIS, M. D., D. D. S., Professor of Operative and Clinical Dentistry

R. DORSEY COALE, Ph. D. Professor of Chemistry and Toxicology

JOHN NOLAND MACKENZIE, M. D., Clinical Prof. of Diseases of the Throat & Nose.
——— ———, M. D., Professor of Anatomy

J. HOLMES SMITH, M. D., Demonstrator of Anatomy.

For further information apply to

I. EDMONDSON ATKINSON, M. D., Dean, 605 Cathedral St., Balto., Md.

College of Physicians and Surgeons,

BALTIMORE, MD.

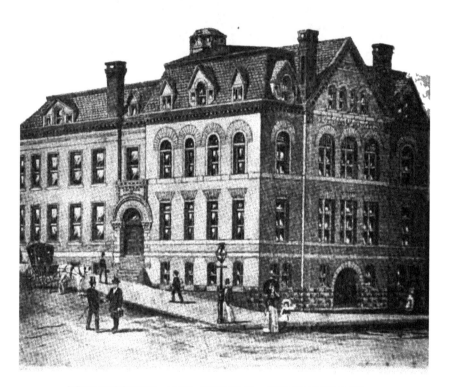

PROFESSORS AND SPECIAL INSTRUCTORS.

FACULTY.

ABRAM B. ARNOLD, M. D., Emeritus Professor of Clinical Medicine.
THOS. OPIE, M. D., Prof. of Gynæcology, and Dean of the Faculty.
THOS. S. LATIMER, M. D., Prof. of Principles and Practice of Medicine and Clinical
    Medicine.
AARON FRIEDENWALD, M. D., Professor of Diseases of the Eye and Ear.
CHAS. F. BEVAN, M. D., Prof. of Principles & Practice of Surgery & Clinical Surgery.
RICHARD GUNDRY, M. D., Prof. of Materia Medica, Therapeutics & Mental Diseases.
WM. SIMON, Ph. D., M. D., Professor of Chemistry.
GEORGE H. ROHE, M. D., Professor of Obstetrics and Hygiene.
J. W. CHAMBERS, M. D., Professor of Anatomy and Clinical Surgery.
GEORGE J. PRESTON, M. D., Prof. of Physiology, and Clinical Professor of Diseases
    of the Nervous System.

he Maryland Lying-In Asylum,

115 WEST LOMBARD STREET,

BALTIMORE, MD.

nder the Exclusive Control of the College of Physicians & Surgeons.

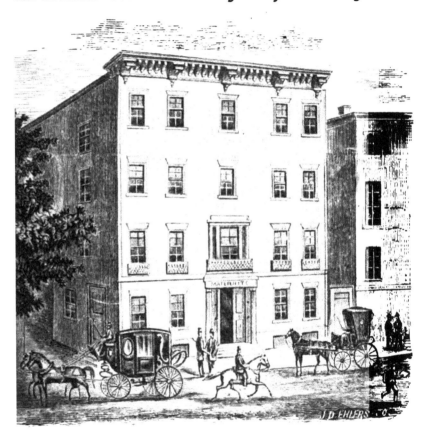

This Institution is open for the reception of patients   Indigent women of this City
 State are admitted for their confinement, and carefully attended by scientific phy-
ans and skilled nurses. Having been liberally aided by the Legislature, no cost or
 s have been spared to render it as perfect as possible in all its departments   The
lic Wards are spacious, well warmed and ventilated, and are supplied with all the
liances and conveniences which can conduce to the comfort of the paturient woman.

Board, attention by a member of the Faculty, nursing and medicines, are given free
harge to all patients in the Public Wards.

Every precaution is taken to prevent the recognition of inmates.

Private patients are furnished rooms at from $6.00 to $12 per week. according to the
 and location of the chambers.

For additional information, apply to the Dean, or S. H. Allen, M. D., House
sician.

PHILLIPS' COD LIVER OIL

EMULSION.

A True Emulsion Without Saponification.

In all essential features, it represents the highest degree of perfection in the Emulsionizing of Cod Liver Oil.

This preparation is not advertised to the public, and enjoys Professional popularity because of its high standard of excellence, uniformity and reliability.

(*A pamphlet, with formula, Photo-Micrographic illustrations, &c., mailed upon application.*)

PHOSPHO-MURIATE OF QUININE,

COMPOUND.

A RELIABLE ALTERATO-CONSTRUCTIVE,

Particularly indicated in conditions of **disturbed nutrition** and **tissue retrograde.**

An easily appropriated general tonic, promoting digestion, and safe under prolonged use.

A permanent combination of the soluble Wheat Phosphates, with Muriate of Quinine, Iron and Strychnia.

Of greater strength than the various Hypophosphite compounds.

DIGESTIBLE COCOA,
WHEAT PHOSPHATES,
MILK OF MAGNESIA.

The Chas. H. Phillips Chemical Co.

77 Pine St., New York.

We respectfully call the attention of the Medical Profession to our new preparation of Ergot of Rye

ERGOTOLE

specially made for hypodermic use by a new process; representing all the active principles of Ergot in a very concentrated form, and entirely freed from all inert and irritating constituents.

Used hypodermically it causes neither pain nor abscess, and keeps perfectly without precipitation for any length of time. It has been extensively tried in hospital and private practice, hypodermically and administered by the mouth, proving uniformly efficacious, and it has been pronounced the most efficient preparation of Ergot in use, one minim representing the full therapeutic strength of about 2½ grains of the best Spanish Ergot.

PAN-PEPTIC TABLETS.

An efficient Tonic Digestive combination of 1 grain pure pepsin, 1 grain pure Pancreatin, ¼ grain pure Caffeine with Acid Lacto-Phosphate of Calcium and Celery.

The Pepsin and Pancreatin used in these tablets possess highest digestive power and cannot fail to promptly start and accomplish the digestion of food, whilst the Caffeine by its stimulant tonic action on stomach and bowels, assists and quickens the normal disgestion and assimilation of food. The Acid Lacto-Phosphate of Calcium also contributes to the tonic action of the tablets, and aids to build up the general system, and a small quantity of that refreshing aromatic nerve stimulant, Celery, imparts a pleasant flavor and acts as an appetizer.

LAPACTIC PILLS, S. & D's.

(Aloin 1-4 gr., Strychnine, 1-60 gr., Extr. Belladonna 1-8 gr , Ipecac 1-16 gr.

An elegant and most efficient combination introduced by us and found in practice to possess superior advantages over other similar formulæ for the relief of *Habitual Constipation, Atonic Dyspepsia, Biliary Engorgement and many Gastric Disorders.*

☞Samples and special circulars on the above preparations sent to Physicians on application.

SHARP & DOHME,

Manufacturing Chemists,

ESTABLISHED 1860.   BALTIMORE, MD.

MANUFACTURERS OF

STANDARD MEDICINAL FLUID AND SOLID EXTRACTS, SOLUBLE HYPODERMIC TABLETS, SOLUBLE GELATIN AND SUGAR COATED PILLS AND GRANULES, GRANULAR EFFER-VESCENT SALTS COMPRESSED LOZENGES AND TABLETS, FINE CHEMICALS, &C

W<u>yeth's</u> BEEF JUICE.

A Liquid Preparation of the Choicest Beef, containing the Nutritious Albuminous Principles in an unaltered and soluble form.

Physicians have, for a long time, had their attention called to the fact that beef extracts, made by the LIEBIG process, are utterly devoid of the valuable and nutritious albuminous constituents of meat, as these are coagulated and filtered out in the process of manufacture. In consequence, the most advanced class of medical practitioners to-day, merely use the commercial extracts of meat as stimulants, and not for any nutritious properties they may possess. Realizing this fact, we have, after continued and exhaustive experiments, succeeded in preparing the article which we offer as WYETH'S BEEF JUICE, and for which we make the following claims :

FIRST.—That it contains all of the albuminous principles of beef in an active and soluble form. This may be proven by mixing a small portion of Beef Juice with an equal part of water in a test-tube or any convenient vessel, and gradually heating to the boiling point, when the albuminous principles will be coagulated.

SECOND.—That it contains the Hæmoglobin of the meat unaltered, as is evidenced by the bright arterial color of the preparation, and by the fact that it loses this color upon boiling, as the Hæmoglobin is precipitated with the albumen.

THIRD—That it will be found upon trial to possess the nutritive properties of the choicest beef to a higher degree than any extract of meat yet offered to the profession.

Physicians will find WYETH'S BEEF JUICE of great value as a strengthening diet in cases of convalescence, consumption, nervous prostration, and similar diseases ; also, in typhoid fever, debility, etc. Beef Tea prepared from it contains more nourishment than any other liquid preparation of meat, and, when properly seasoned, is more grateful and appetizing to the patient. Professional men who are suffering from over-work, mental anxiety, etc., will find that one-half teaspoonful in about half a glass of iced water, taken at intervals during the day, and upon retiring, will relieve fatigue,—both of mind and body.

DIRECTIONS.—In cases of debility, nervous prostration, convalescence, etc., one-half to one teaspoonful in a half tumblerful of iced or luke-warm water.

CAUTION.—As the valuable albuminous elements are rendered insoluble by extreme heat, this preparation should only be mixed with iced or LUKE-WARM water, and never with water at the boiling point.

MANUFACTURED BY

JOHN WYETH & BROTHER,

PHILADELPHIA, PA.

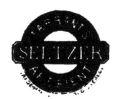

TARRANT'S

(EFFERVESCENT.)

SELTZER APERIENT,

Prepared for the use of N. Y. Physicians in 1844.

PROPERTIES.

ANT–ACID!   ALTERATIVE!   LAXATIVE!

PARTICULARLY ADAPTED FOR USE IN THE

CONSTIPATION OF PREGNANCY.

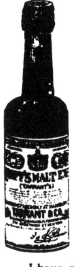

HOFF'S MALT,

(TARRANT'S)

The Standard Nutritive Tonic.

PRESCRIBED BY AMERICAN PHYSICIANS FOR 24 YEARS.

For many years I have used Hoff's TARRANT'S Extract of Malt. I find it very valuable as a nutrient and readily assimilated.

HUNTER McGUIRE, M. D.
Richmond, Va., June 10, 1889.

I have prescribed with much satisfaction for now twenty years TARRANT'S Hoff's Malt Extract. It is readily assimilated by the sick, has an agreeable taste, and I am sure is a genuine nutrient.
Louisville, Ky., Aug. 12, 1888.   D. W. YANDELL, M. D.

ALWAYS SPECIFY

TARRANT'S when prescribing MALT EXTRACT.

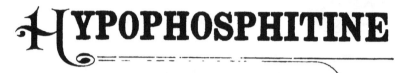

MALTINE

Is a perfectly pure concentrated extract of Malted Barley, Wheat and Oats, containing all the digestive and nutritive principles of these three important cereals, with absolutely no syrup or sugar other than that of the malt itself.

It also contains large proportions of Nitrogenous matter, Carbohydrates and Phosphates, and is, therefore, rich in bone-producing, fat-making and strengthening elements.

It possesses from three to four times the power of any other extract of malt as a natural solvent of all farinaceous food, and is an invaluable aid to a sound and healthy digestion.

Unlike other extracts of malt, it will not ferment or congeal in any climate, or at any season of the year.

Complete List of Maltine Preparations:

MALTINE PLAIN,
MALTINE WITH COD LIVER OIL,
MALTINE WITH CASCARA SAGRADA,
MALTINE WITH HYPOPHOSPHITES,
MALTO—YERBINE.
MALTINE FERRATED,
MALTINE WITH PEPTONES,
MALTINE WITH PHOSPHATE IRON, QUININE & STRYCHNIA.

We will send to any physician who will pay expressage, a case containing eight ounces, each of any two preparations that may be selected from our list.

THE MALTINE MANUFACTURING CO.
19 Warren St., New York.

LIQUID PANCREOPEPSINE.
(WM. R. WARNER & CO.)
A REMEDY FOR INDIGESTION.

Containing Pancreatine, Pepsin, Lactic and Muriatic Acids, Etc. The combined Principles of Indigestion. To aid in digesting Animal and Vegetable Cooked Food, Fatty and Amylaceous Substances.

DOSE:—A tablespoonful, containing 5 grs., Pepsin, after each meal, with an Aperient Pill taken occasionally.

Elixir Salicylic Acid Compound.
(WM. R. WARNER & CO.)
A Potent & Reliable Remedy in Rheumatism, Gout, Lumbago & Kindred Diseases.

This preparation combines in a pleasant and agreeable form:— Salicylic Acid, Cimicifugæ, Gelseminum, Sodii Bi-Carb., and Potass. Iodid., so combined as to be more prompt and effective in the treatment of this class of diseases than either of the ingredients when administered alone.

The dose is from a teaspoonful to a dessertspoonful, and increased as necessary to meet the requirements of the case.

Each teaspoonful contains five grains of Salicylic Acid.

Elixir Salicylic Acid Comp is put up in 12-oz. square bottles, and may be obtained from Druggists everywhere.

Prepared only by WM. R. WARNER & CO.

MANUFACTURING CHEMISTS,

1228 Market St., Philadelphia.   18 Liberty St., New York.

TRANSACTIONS

—OF THE—

edical and Chirurgical Faculty

—OF THE—

⇒STATE OF MARYLAND,⇐

emi-Annual Session, Held at Cambridge, Md., Nov., 1890.

Ninety-Third Annual Session

—HELD AT—

BALTIMORE, MARYLAND, APRIL, 1891.

———

BALTIMORE:
GRIFFIN, CURLEY & CO., PRINTERS,
202 E. Baltimore Street,
1891.

Officers, Committees, Sections and Delegates.

FOR THE YEAR 1891-92.

President.

WM. H. WELCH.

Vice-Presidents.

J. W. HUMRICHOUSE,   DAVID STREETT.

Recording Secretary.

G. LANE TANEYHILL.

Assistant Secretary.

ROBERT T. WILSON.

Corresponding Secretary.

JOSEPH T. SMITH.

Reporting Secretary.

WM. B. CANFIELD.

Treasurer.

W. F. A. KEMP.

Executive Committee.

T. A. ASHBY,   J. E. MICHAEL,   G. H. ROHE,
P. C. WILLIAMS,   WILMER BRINTON.

Examining Board of Western Shore.

J. W. CHAMBERS,   L. McLANE TIFFANY,   E. F. CORDELL,
HIRAM WOODS,   D. W. CATHELL,   W. H. NORRIS,
B. B. BROWNE.

Examining Board of Eastern Shore.

B. W. GOLDSBOROUGH,   G. T. ATKINSON,   A. H. BAYLEY,
J. K. H. JACOBS,   W. F. HINES.

Library Committee.

T. BARTON BRUNE,   G. LANE TANEYHILL,   B. B. BROWNE,
WM. OSLER.   S. T. EARLE.

Publication Committee.

G. LANE TANEYHILL,   W. F. A. KEMP,   J. E. MICHAEL,
H. M. WILSON,   C. H. RILEY.

Memoir Committee.

E. F. CORDELL,   J. McP. SCOTT,   G. T. ATKINSON,
C. F. BEVAN,   ALICE T. HALL.

Committee on Ethics.

L. McLANE TIFFANY.   P. C. WILLIAMS,   E. G. WATERS,
CALEB WINSLOW,   ALAN P. SMITH.

Membership Committee.

T. A. ASHBY,   B. W. GOLDSBOROUGH,   G. LANE TANEYHILL,
W. F. HINES,   S. T. EARLE.

Curator.

L. F. ANKRIM.

Section on Surgery.

R. W. JOHNSON, JOHN G. JAY, E. R. WALKER,
A. S. MASON, H. H. BIEDLER.

Section on Practice.

S. C. CHEW, F. C. BRESSLER, DAVID STREETT,
B. W. GOLDSBOROUGH, H. M. SALZER.

Section on Obstetrics and Gynæcology.

L. E. NEALE, J. WHITRIDGE WILLIAMS. HUNTER ROBB,
R. T. WILSON, ARTHUR WILLIAMS.

Section on Materia Medica and Chemistry.

T. B. BRUNE, J. W. HUMRICHOUSE, I. E. ATKINSON,
J. T. SMITH. A. K. BOND.

Section on Sanitary Science.

E. F. CORDELL, G. H. ROHE, W. B. PLATT,
E. M. SCHAEFFER, A. H. BAYLEY.

Section on Anatomy, Physiology and Pathology.

J. W. CHAMBERS, C. O. MILLER, RANDOLPH WINSLOW,
J. C. HEMMETER, J. D. BLAKE.

Section on Psychology and Medical Jurisprudence.

H. M. HURD, C. G. HILL, H. J. BERKLEY,
S. J. FORT, E. M. REID.

Section on Microscopy, Micro-Chemistry, and Spectral Analysis.

C. HAMPSON JONES, W. D. BOOKER, J. W. FUNK,
N. G. KEIRLE, WM. OSLER.

Section on Ophthalmology, Otology and Laryngology.

S. K. MERRICK, J. N. MACKENZIE, R. L. RANDOLPH,
G. W. THOMAS, HARRY FRIEDENWALD.

Delegates to American Medical Association.

JOS. BROWN, T. B. EVANS, G. J. PRESTON,
J. W. BRANHAM, A. FRIEDENWALD, J. McP. SCOTT,
WILMER BRINTON, N. R. GORTER, ALAN P. SMITH,
W. B. CANFIELD, H. HARLAN, DAVID STREETT,
E. M. CHAMBERLAINE, H. F. HILL, E. M. SCHAEFFER,
J. J. CHISOLM, B. M. HOPKINSON, W. A. B. SELLMAN,
W. P. CHUNN, C. JOHNSTON, G. LANE TANEYHILL,
JNO. DICKSON, T. S. LATIMER, S. THEOBALD,
F. DONALDSON, R. B. MORISON, W. C. VAN BIBBER,
S. T. EARLE, W. B. PLATT, ARTHUR WILLIAMS,
R. H P. ELLIS, WM. OSLER, WM. H. WELCH.

Delegates to West Virginia State Medical Society.

B. B. BROWNE, W. A. R. F. CARR, THOMAS OPIE,
J. M. CRAIGHILL, J. G. WILTSHIRE.

Delegates to Virginia State Medical Society.

J. R. MICHAEL, J. S. CONRAD, A. C. POLE,
I. R. PAGE, H. P. C. WILSON.

Delegates to North Carolina Medical Society.

C. G. HILL, W. T. HOWARD, HIRAM WOODS.
I. E. ATKINSON, R. T. WILSON.

DISCLAIMER. The Medical and Chirurgical Faculty of the State of Maryland, while formally accepting and publishing the reports of the various Sections and Volunteer Papers read at its sessions, *does not hold itself responsible* for the opinions, theories or criticisms therein contained.

To AUTHORS. Contributors to any volume of the TRANSACTIONS are requested to observe the following: 1st, Write on one side of the paper only. 2nd, Write without breaks, *i. e.*, do not begin a new sentence on a new line; when you want to begin a new paragraph, begin in the middle of the line. 3rd, Draw a line along the margin of such paragraphs as should be printed in smaller type—for instance, all that is clinical history in reports of cases, or that which is quoted, &c. 4th, Words to be printed in *italics* should be underscored once; in SMALL CAPITALS twice; in LARGE CAPITALS three times. 5th, Proofs sent for revision should be, returned without delay; authors who contemplate a temporary absence from their regular residence any time during the summer, should notify the Recording Secretary, thus avoiding vexatious delays in the delivery of proof. 6th, Authors whose papers have been "accepted" by the Faculty and referred to the Publication Committee—such papers thus becoming the property of the Faculty—are expected to place the original or a verbatim printable copy on desk of the Recording Secretary immediately after the reading of the same. 7th, The Publication Committee is instructed by the Faculty to publish no paper that has been read before a local medical society prior to the publication of the TRANSACTIONS of the Faculty. 8th, Alterations in manuscript should be limited to what is of essential importance, they are equivalent to resetting, and cause additional expense, such changes, if they exceed half a page of printed matter, as also all wood cuts, photographs and electrotypes, are invariably to be paid for by authors.

MEMBERSHIP. Applications for membership in the Medical and Chirurgical Faculty should be addressed to the Recording Secretary, Corresponding Secretary, Treasurer, or Chairman of the Examining Board, and should state name in full, post office address, where graduated in medicine, date of graduation, and by whom recommended. They must be accompanied by the *initiation fee* of five dollars: no membership dues are required for the first current year: a copy of the annual TRANSACTIONS is mailed gratuitously to each member. *Blank applications* for membership will be mailed to any address on application to the Recording Secretary or Treasurer.

CONTENTS.

Semi-Annual Meeting.

The Semi-Annual Convention for 1890 of the Medical and Chirurgical Faculty was called to order this day by the President, Dr. T. A. Ashby. The Recording Secretary, Dr. G. Lane Taneyhill, was at his desk. On motion of Dr. R. Winslow the members of the profession present were invited to seats in the convention, and to participate in the debates.

Dr. A. H. Bayley, of Cambridge, delivered the following—

ADDRESS OF WELCOME.

MR. PRESIDENT AND GENTLEMEN OF THE MEDICAL AND CHIRURGICAL FACULTY: It is with rare pleasure I greet you and extend a warm heartfelt welcome to our beautifully embowered little city, and feel most deeply the compliment you have conferred upon us in selecting this place for the meeting of the Medical and Chirurgical Faculty, being the first ever held on the Eastern Shore since its organization of nearly one hundred years ago, and will be ever born in pleasing remembrance and mark an epoch in the history of our city.

I feel and believe that the medical profession of our city and county will derive much benefit, and consequently the community at large, from the learning and experience of this representation from the old time honored Medical and Chirurgical Faculty, and may it ever flourish in strength and usefulness a proud monument to its learned and noble founders whose memories will not fade away.

Again I greet you, aye, thrice welcome and when you have returned to your homes in the beautiful and flourishing city of Baltimore, proverbial for its lovely ladies and elegant hospitalities, I hope and trust that you may have been so impressed, that recollections of our dear old Eastern Shore may linger in memory with such kindly feeling as to impel you to grace again our city with your presence.

The President, Dr. T. A. Ashby, delivered an edifying and interesting address:

THE INTERESTS AND AIMS OF THE MEDICAL AND CHIRURGICAL FACULTY OF THE STATE OF MARYLAND.

It is my honored privilege and most agreeable duty to preside over the first meeting of this Faculty ever held on the Eastern Shore. The occasion upon which we meet is one of uncommon interest and importance. We are assembled in a section of our State noted for the fertility of its soil and for the beauty, extent and productiveness of its bays, rivers and water-courses, from which come for the service of man those rich and choice products of land and water, equaled in variety and abundance by few sections of the world's surface, and surpassed by none. We meet in a community noted for the culture, refinement and hospitality of its citizens, and bearing the classic name of two great centres of education and learning—the one in old England, the other in New England—a sufficient reminder of stimulating and ennobling influences in the region of thought and ideas.

I regard this meeting as having a striking significance and appropriate existence. It may be accepted as an evidence of a spirit of progress and of growing usefulness upon the part of this ancient and honorable organization worthy of our encouragement and approbation. In the history of this Faculty, very nearly co-extensive with that of the great Commonwealth of Maryland, it has numbered, and still numbers among its membership the names of many of the most eminent members of our profession residing on the Eastern

Shore. It has received the loyal support of these men under circumstances attended with difficulties and embarrassments. We now visit their section to show them that this Faculty has a personal pride in all of her children, and is endeared to their best interests and welfare. In the organization of this Faculty, early consideration was given to the advancement of the interests of the medical profession in every section of the State. Provision was made for a general representation in its work and administration. A Board of Examiners was selected annually from the Western and Eastern Shores, and through this doorway admission to active membership was within the reach of every worthy candidate.

Our forefathers in medicine in this State who framed the machinery which now works this organization, had in view the very largest and most comprehensive idea of co-operative work, and in putting this machinery in motion designed that it should meet every professional want, and that it should consolidate the energies and aims of the profession into a strong and harmonious purpose, having in view the good which could be made to flow from a thoroughly organized professional body. For many years the system as thus inaugurated worked with rare singleness of purpose, and in practical harmony. Its principles of organization were enforced, and the interests of the profession were subserved. The Faculty maintained for many years an ascendency over the entire profession in Maryland, and so justly and successfully were its affairs conducted that its government was recognized as an authoritative source of power and influence. So long as this condition of affairs remained in force the professional *esprit de corps* was maintained, and the practice of medicine was regulated by principles of honor and high character, by a large body of physicians throughout the State. Quackery, empiricism and irregular methods were kept down and the work of the profession was conducted almost exclusively by men who enjoyed the confidence of this Faculty, and possessed its authority to engage in medical work. The Faculty was the great and only regulating body in the State, and its authority conveyed the only legal right to practice medicine in Maryland. We can well perceive that

under such a system of professional co-operation the best
interests of medicine were subserved, and that the profession
of medicine and the citizens of Maryland were secured against
those systems of irregularity which are supported and maintained by the lowest monetary considerations. Under the
old regime we of to-day can picture the pleasure and satisfaction of professional work. The association of earnest and
cultivated minds in friendly professional intercourse, the conduct of professional work along lines of manly and honorable endeavor, the exchange of those courtesies and civilities which make physicians feel like brethren in a common
and noble calling, and the absence of those sordid considerations which degrade the practice of medicine; these were the
conditions which were best maintained by such a system of
organization as I have here referred to. But aside from the
standpoint of pure ethics which this Faculty instituted and
fostered by its discipline and enlightened government, the
highest consideration was given in its system of organization
to the claims of an educational qualification and scientific
standard. The Faculty at its very outset divided its work
into sections, made provision for annual reports upon the
progress of the medical sciences in every department, gave
encouragement to a system of prize essays, original papers
and to public addresses which were designed as important
factors in the educational and scientific training of its membership. Not content with this work we find that as its membership grew, and as its resources increased, it secured its own
hall with its own means, and here laid the foundation for a
library which it still maintains, and which gives evidence of
the wisdom, unselfishness, and enlightened understanding of
its founders.

From these considerations thus hastily presented, I desire
to show that the organization which meets here to-day was
founded upon the broadest principles of professional policy
and had for its highest and purest aim, the cultivation and
advancement of the medical profession in those paths of professional work which make the humane, honorable, skilful
and learned physician.

Starting out with such a high conception of an ideal professional body, we are prepared to understand the nature of those difficulties which ever assail the work of men and institutions intent upon pure and unselfish purposes. In the scheme of the Faculty no provision was made for avarice, selfishness, and monetary irregularities. It offered no short cuts to wealth or fame, but assumed to regulate the affairs of the profession on the basis of merit and honorable industry. It aimed simply to help the earnest, ambitious, and honest worker in medicine. But as the population in Maryland multiplied, as new men came in to take the places of the old or to occupy new territory, as the race for wealth and position gave stimulus to avarice and greed, we find that the ideal body of which I have spoken, becomes tinctured with the spirit of the times, desertions from its ranks occur, its influence begins to waver, and, finally, its authority is violated and then thrown overboard. It is not pertinent to this occasion to show the various steps by which these changes were brought about. I simply refer to the result, and offer in evidence the fact that from having at one time exercised a pre-eminent authority and influence over the entire profession in this State, this authority virtually passed away. Divested of the right to regulate the practice of medicine in Maryland by a virtual surrender of its legal authority, this Faculty stands to-day clothed with the same charter under which our predecessors worked. Whilst then in one sense it has lost its authority over the affairs of the profession in Maryland, that is, in the sense of not having the legal right to license those who engage in the practice of medicine in the State, in every other respect it maintains its ancient and honorable influence, and to-day represents in its organization and practices, the high and ennobling idea of professional purity, learning and ethics, which characterized it in the past. This Faculty has never lowered its principles; it has never compromised its opinions by association with ideas or -isms derogatory to the highest standard of professional morality and ethics. For some years past it has maintained its organization upon such a high plane of work that its influence has

been directed more largely upon its individual membership
than upon the profession at large throughout the State, but
this action has been in a measure inseparable from those conditions of environment which often circumscribe the actions
of individuals as well as of institutions. We must, therefore,
look for the causes of this condition in circumstances which
are remediable, and which can be made to disappear. The
social and political upheaval in this State, which grew out of
the late civil war, the causes which led to it, and those disturbances which followed in its wake, in largest measure, account for the shrinkage in the membership of the Faculty
during the past thirty or more years, and for the character
of a local, as distinguished from a State society, which its
organization assumed.

For plain and satisfactory reasons, the annual meetings of
this Faculty have always been held in Baltimore. Its hall
and library are located there, and its chief support has come
from the profession of the city. Only in this sense has it any
significance as a local body. Its plan, scope and work are as
broad and comprehensive as the resources of medicine demand. Its membership and privileges are within the reach
of every respectable physician engaged in the practice of
regular medicine in the State.

It is practically, as well as theoretically, the only State
medical society in Maryland, and having in the past exercised
this influence over the affairs of the profession, it is now the
only organization competent to assume this relation towards
the profession of this State. I have been induced to make
these hurried considerations touching upon the past history
of the Faculty, in order that I might present in a clearer light
the present and prospective work before this organization.
As honorable as its record in the past has been, as pure and
inspiring as its traditions and principles are to-day, let us
hold fast to these things and press forward to a larger and
more important work for the future.

Two years or more ago, the members of the Faculty were
brought to realize that the usefulness and influence of the

organization were impaired by reason of the purely local character which was given to its annual meetings. An examination of its list of members revealed the fact that with 208 names on its roll call, only twenty-four of this number were non-residents of Baltimore. Here was a fact, and an explanation was forthcoming. It was self-evident that no effort had been made for a number of years past to interest the profession in the Counties in the affairs of the Faculty, and that it had been allowed to drift along in this way, adding at each annual meeting about enough new members to fill the places made vacant by deaths and resignations. It became very apparent that the aim and purposes of the Faculty, so far as the profession at large throughout the State was concerned, could only be carried out in their full design by enlisting the County Physicians into the ranks of the Faculty. A movement was set on foot and such alterations made in the constitution which would open the doorway to this recruiting enterprise. The membership fee was reduced from $10 to $5, and the annual dues for County members from $3 to $2.

The next step provided for a revival of the semi-annual meetings which formerly were held in different sections of the State in the fall season. This matter was placed in the hands of a Special Committee, which soon determined upon a plan of action. The first of these semi-annual meetings was held in the City of Hagerstown, on the 2nd Tuesday and Wednesday in November, 1889. This meeting, though held in the nature of an experiment, was most encouraging and hopeful in its results. The profession of Western Maryland gave a most cordial reception to the Faculty, and entered heart and soul in giving aid to the purposes of the meeting. As a partial result of this meeting, about one hundred new members were added to the roll-call at the annual meeting in April last, and a new impulse and zest was given to its work such as it had not experienced for years. The results upon the Faculty were immediate and practical, but these influences of the meeting did not end here. The profession of Washington County were induced to organize a local medical

society which has held bi-monthly meetings since its organization, and has an active membership of twenty-four.

As a further outcome of this meeting in Hagerstown, a
Convention of medical men from various sections of the State
was held in the City of Baltimore on the 2nd day of January
last, and there and then determined upon an act of medical
legislation which, with slight modifications, was passed by
the General Assembly at Annapolis. This act has passed
into the history of the profession of this State. This is not
a proper place and occasion to particularize in regard to its
fate. I will here say that this Faculty as such, was in no
manner responsible for the act or for the fate which overtook
it. The act originated in the Convention as above stated,
and its passage was urged by the almost unanimous sentiment of the profession in this State. Its death was brought
about by a very small and narrow professional clique which
exercised a very decided and malicious political power. A
few men holding positions of trust in the dominant political
party in this State, found in the act as passed by the General
Assembly, no position and no emoluments for a political ap-
pointee, and its destruction was not only sought but obtained.
This medical bill asked for no State appropriation to carry its
provisions into execution and to keep its machinery in motion. It undertook to make "brick without straw," a seemingly unwise and irrational act in the eyes of the lover of the
public soup house. It asked for the entire profession of the
State the right to organize a Board of Medical Examiners
composed of reputable physicians, and empower this Board
with the authority to license all physicians who might enter
upon the practice of medicine in the State, subsequent to the
passage of the act. Every necessary safeguard was thrown
around the applicant's interests providing for him a judicious
and impartial examination. The act aimed to protect the
citizens of Maryland against incompetent medical practitioners. It was unjust towards none, it was fair towards all.
We may vainly speculate as to the causes which induced his
Excellency to withhold his signature from this bill, but I
venture to say here that whatever may have been the motive

which dictated such a course of action, the decision reached by the Chief Executive of this State, was not only disappointing to a large and influential body of citizens, but was a manifest and gross disrespect to the medical profession of Maryland. It is not my desire to impugn motives or to be disrespectful towards the Governor of a great Commonwealth who is sworn to protect the rights and interests of all classes of its citizens, but I am prepared to assert here that if there was anything in this act unconstitutional or unjust, or in any way, shape, or form contrary to the best interests of the citizens of Maryland, I challenge the enemies of the bill to show it.

I have no desire to dwell upon this subject at any further length, but I wish, with your permission, to point out a lesson which this experience seems to teach. The profession of this State has enjoyed none of the advantages of an organized body for many years. Its influence, politically speaking, has been confined to a few individuals, and these men, with a few exceptions, have held the few political offices within the reach of medical men in the State. As a result of this system the profession of the State, as such, does not exercise the least influence in the selection of the men who hold these political offices; it exercises little or no influence upon matters of legislation which directly affect the physicians and citizens of the State; it rarely ventures to ask the law-makers of the State to repeal acts of legislation which bear unjustly against the business interests of medical men or to enact laws for the protection of medical practitioners in the exercise of their duties as physicians and as citizens. For years past the medical profession has gone along bearing the burden of unjust laws upon the statute books; it has placidly submitted to discriminations against its interests without an iota of resistance. When it has ventured to ask the General Assembly for appropriations, for the enactment of laws, or has attempted to exercise any preference in the appointment of its own members to places of trust, its influence has been felt in the feeblest manner. This condition of things is but the natural result of a system of disorganization which prevails in our ranks, and for which we are entirely responsible. The old adage "what is every man's business is no man's business" holds true in respect to the medical profession in Maryland.

The profession has made no systematic effort to protect its rights as a professional body. Individually we have squirmed and grown restless under grievances as plain and bare-faced as the light of day, without coming together as a body and seeking by a co-operative effort a redress for such wrongs. If one desires to know some of the burdens we carry, let me ask, what preference has a physician's account against an estate? We are less thought of than the undertaker who may gobble up an entire residue in luxurious decorations. What protection has a physician in giving testimony before the courts in a matter of privileged communication? What rights has a physician in giving evidence in civil and criminal cases? In these as in other respects he is regarded as a citizen and not in the light of a professional character. It is quite true that many of us have lived and worked under these idiosyncrasies of the law in Maryland for many years and may not feel disposed to change, but I claim here that as an organization, or brotherhood, having rights as such, we are entirely too complacent. The time has come when we should seek to better our condition, and it behooves us to put the ball in motion looking to a complete revolution of the affairs of the profession in Maryland. The senior members of the profession, whose time is absorbed in an active and lucrative professional work, may view such matters with indifference, but I say on behalf of the juniors, that there is need for reform. An active and progressive medical organization in this State is demanded alike by the spirit of the times, by the necessities of our position, and by those influences in other departments of human industry and learning which convincingly establish the importance of a system of co-operation and of associated effort. In whichever direction the eye is turned, the influence of organized labor is apparent.

The tendency upon the part of a few to trespass upon the rights of the many, is exemplified in the history of many social, political, educational and religious bodies now in operation in our country. The monopolists of the day are not exclusively confined to that class of men designated as capitalists, high tariff lords and money barons, but may be found in the less pretentious walks of life pressing now here, now there upon the rights of the many. In our own profession these influences may be felt. Individuals and institutions both in the name of science and of charity, are not incapable of wronging the many to benefit the few. Is it proper for the profession to take notice of such matters, or shall we go along on the principle, every man for himself, and permit systems, -isms, and methods of professional work to pass current for the genuine coin whilst their entire fabric is soaked with the liquor of avarice and greed? Nay more; shall we suffer our vision to become obscured by the tinsel and glitter which they parade, and our ears to be deafened by the bold professions of philanthropy and science which they proclaim? I claim that it is high time for the profession to discriminate.

If the time was ever necessary for a thorough organization of the profession in this State it seems to me that time is the present, for never before in its history has it been brought so closely in contact with systems of irregularity and unfair competition. A few medical men progress in their medical work upon terms of satisfaction and independence, but I speak for the many when I say that their efforts are illy rewarded and their work is burdened with conditions unnecessarily unjust and severe. Many of these men are powerless to help themselves, for they are the victims of a system which, as individuals, they cannot overthrow. There is help for such men in the strong arm of an organized body, which can address itself to the correction of such influences. One of the objects of this meeting is to present the claims of this Faculty as a basis for a system of professional organization so sadly needed in Maryland. In this body we have the machinery well-nigh perfect in its design and scope, and fully tested by time and experience. It represents the highest conceptions of a scientific organization having for its purpose the elevation of the professional body, the cultivation of the professional mind and the regulation of professional interests upon sound ethical principles. The question for the profession of the State to determine is, whether it will enlist under the banner of this Faculty and work out the problems which confront it, under its influence and leadership, or organize under an independent body having the same aims and purposes in view. The inexpediency of the latter proposition does not admit of argument, whilst the wisdom of the former must be apparent to all; hence I here assert that it becomes the duty of the entire profession of regular medicine in this State to come forward and give a loyal support to the Medical and Chirurgical Faculty of Maryland.

We meet this year on the Eastern Shore, as we met last year in Western Maryland, to make the profession of this section personally acquainted with the plan and purposes which this Faculty represents. We are here to show the influence which an organization can exert and to enlist your hearty co-operation in the work it has in view. We desire to establish the fact that the highest objects of professional work are connected with and promoted by an organized professional body. Whether we view these objects from the standpoint of pure science, of pure ethics or of true charity, they pay obedience to the law of organization and of co-operation. The man who leans upon himself and who does not touch his fellow associate in work at any point is robbing himself of that influence and sympathy which come from contact with mind, spirit and matter so capable of bringing life, and its noble uses, into harmony with its environments, and of softening and fraternizing man's relations with his fellow man. One of the most benevolent features of our age and civilization is the growing tendency upon the part of men in all walks, avocations and professions to take advantage of the opportunities presented for associated work. Whilst, then, experience has shown the advantages of associated work, not only upon the individual, but upon systems and principles, shall we continue to ignore such influences in our professional work and relations in Maryland, and go along as we have largely done in the past, every man for himself, or shall we come together as fellow workers under an organized leadership, and embrace the opportunities for self-improvement and development which contact and associated work can and will promote? I feel assured that the views which I have expressed will ultimately prevail and that this work will go forward until this Faculty has enlisted in its ranks every worthy member of the profession in this State.

Permit me now to refer to another line of work which should keep pace with a general organization of the profession in this State. I refer to the organization of local medical societies in the cities and counties throughout the State. The benefit of these local bodies upon the local profession is two-fold. In the first place they give a healthy stimulus and incentive to professional study and culture by encouraging the preparation of papers, the careful observation and record of instructive pathological and clinical conditions, and arouse an interest in medical work from a scientific as distinguished from a purely monetary standpoint. In the second place the ethical and personal relations of men engaged in the same work in the same community are smoother and more agreeable when such men are brought into closer contact and affiliation in an organization which has in view the good of its entire membership. The only practical difficulty in the way of the organization of such societies in different counties is the one which has to contend with the indifference and apathy of physicians towards such organizations. I hope to see the time come when the physicians on the Eastern Shore will embrace the opportunities for local organization which are clearly within their reach. There seems to me to be an urgent demand for such associated work as is here suggested. On this Peninsula, at no remote geological period redeemed from the waters of the great Atlantic and noble Chesapeake, there are present conditions of climate and soil which invite the most earnest and careful study of the physician and scientist. If this section of this State is to become, as has been suggested, the great sanitarium and health resort for the invalid class of the great Atlantic and interior States of our country, so rapidly gaining in wealth and population, there are problems in climatology, in vital statistics and in clinical medicine which the physicians of this section must work out and elaborate. These are grave responsibilities, which, as physicians and as public spirited citizens, you must assume. Nor can you long postpone the consideration of such important lines of professional duty. The work before you and the opportunities which this work suggests and presents you should eagerly embrace. In no way can you more successfully prepare for such undertakings than by the organization of local medical societies in your counties. Such organizied bodies will at once give encouragement to habits of careful observation, will suggest lines of profitable investigation, and will stimulate such an interest in the study of your climate and local conditions as will open up to the knowledge of the medical profession at large and to the general public those advantages and gifts of nature which undoubtedly are enjoyed by the inhabitants of this hospitable and favored region.

May I hope that this meeting of this Faculty on the Eastern Shore will give a helpful stimulus to the physicians and citizens of this section of our State in the direction indicated and lead to the inauguration of such practical lines of work as will show to the outside world the rich blessings of climate and soil as are here offered for the relief of human suffering and for the cure of disease.　.

On motion of Dr. S. T. Earle is was

Resolved, That the President's address delivered to-day, November 11th, 1890, before the Medical and Chirurgical Faculty at its semi-annual meeting, be printed in pamphlet form and sent to every regular practitioner of medicine in Maryland.

The first paper of the morning was read by Dr. Randolph Winslow, on

"Simultaneous Distal Ligation of the Right Common Carotid and Right Subclavian Arteries for Supposed Innominate Aneurism."

A female, partly Indian, partly Negro, æt. 38, presented herself at the surgical clinic of the Woman's Medical College of Baltimore, in the latter part of the summer of 1889. For two years she had noticed a small pulsating lump at the root of the neck, behind the right sterno-cleido-mastoid muscle. The lump increased slowly, accompanied with discomfort, oppression of breathing, more or less cough and hemicrania, and on account of these ailments she applied for treatment. Upon inspection a pulsating tumor was seen, situated at the root of the neck, just above the right-sterno clavicular articulation, and raising the right sterno cleido mastoid muscle with each impulse of the heart. The pulsating area appeared about the size of a small hen's egg. A distinct, but not very loud, bruit was heard over the tumor. There was no perceptible difference between the radial pulses, but the right carotid artery did not seem to beat so forcibly as the left. She was admitted to the Hospital of the Good Samaritan, where she was kept under observation, and the following additional facts learned in regard to her history. For a long time she has indulged to excess in the use of liquor, and has led a wild life. She has had five children, or premature births. She denied having contracted syphilis, but it is probable that she did, though there were no specially characteristic symptoms of the disease present. The urine was increased in amount, but did not contain albumen, nor did a microscopic examination reveal casts. The heart sounds were normal, except that the second sound seemed to be a little accentuated. The lungs appeared to be healthy. There was no tracheal tug, which is sometimes present when the aorta is the seat of aneurism. My colleagues upon the medical side, Profs. Cordell and Thomas, concurred in the diagnosis of innominate aneurism, but Prof. Thomas thought that the first portion of the subclavian and the arch of the aorta were also involved, as there was some thoracic dullness upon percussion. She was placed flat in bed and kept on very low diet, causing her to complain that she was being starved, and 10 grains iodide potash was given three times a day. She did not improve much under this treatment, which was continued for about six weeks. The lump seemed to become larger, and the choking, cough, oppression and headache increased. No treatment seemed to relieve these symptoms, but, on the contrary, they became worse; severe epistaxis also occurred upon several occasions. As medical treatment had not yielded any good result, it was decided to ligate the right common carotid and right subclavian arteries. A few days previous to the operation, the patient went home on a visit and returned intoxicated almost to the verge of mania-a-potu. On November 29, 1889, the patient having been antiseptically prepared, the right common carotid was exposed by an incision along the inner border of the sterno-mastoid muscle. The neck was thick, and the artery placed deeply, which rendered this part of the operation rather tedious. The vessel was ligated with stout juniper oil catgut, below the omohyoid muscle, the internal jugular vein not being seen. Immediately upon tightening the ligature the heart's action became tumultuous and irregular and the tumor harder and larger. After waiting awhile for the heart to become quieter, the third portion of the subclavian was exposed by an incision along the clavicle, the fascia being torn through and the veins drawn aside. The artery was deeply placed, but was found without difficulty, and was tied externally to the scalemus anticus muscle, catgut being used. Upon tieing the ligature the aneurism became smaller and softer, and the radial pulse immediately ceased, whilst the heart's action became more nearly natural. No cerebral symptoms supervened at any time. The arm was wrapped with cotton wool and the neck padded with the same, after having closed the wounds with catgut and applied an iodoform and bichloride dressing. Within twenty-four hours the recurrent circulation was completely established, and a very small but distinct radial pulse could be felt. The temporal pulsation never returned. The temperature reached 101.2° on the evening of the second day, falling to normal the next evening. The pulse was increased in frequency at once, varying from 115 to 150 beats per minute, and at the end of four weeks was still 100. The respiration was also accelerated for a long time. She was kept in bed on low diet for several weeks after the operation, and the aneurismal swelling seemed to diminish, but did not disappear. The wounds healed promptly without suppuration. For a while there was some numbness about the right arm, but this gradually disappeared.

I had the opportunity of examining this woman about one year after the operation, and she seemed to be cured ; the lump, pulsation and bruit had almost entirely disappeared.

I place this case upon record as a contribution to the history of the distal ligation of the carotid and subclavian vessels for the relief of innominate and aortic aneurisms. Mistakes in the diagnosis of aneurism of the innominate or aorta have been very frequent in the past, and literature teems with cases of supposed aneurism of one or the other of these vessels, in which errors of diagnosis have been made ; hence I am not sure that this woman was suffering from this affection, though the diagnosis was confirmed by expert diagnosticians.

Aneurism is always a formidable disease, and when it affects the innominate artery or the arch of the aorta its gravity is vastly greater than when more superficial vessels are attacked. This arises from the fact that the vessels are not only of great size, but from the impossibility of applying either pressure or the ligature between the heart and the tumor. Various methods of treatment have been instituted for the cure or relief of these affections, which may be classified as the medical and operative methods. Amongst purely medical measures may be mentioned the postural and dietetic, as exemplified by Tuffnell's method. This consists in the restriction of the patient's food and drink to the lowest point compatible with fairly comfortable living, and the observance of recumbency for a period of several weeks or months; this is often associated with the administration of iodide of potassium, or of tincture of digitalis. There can be no doubt that excellent results have followed these methods, either singly or combined, and a careful trial of such should always be made before subjecting a patient to an operation, if the rupture of the aneurism does not appear to be impending. There is considerable divergence of opinion in regard to the utility of the iodide of potassium in the cure of aneurism, and this diversity is explained by Dr. G. W. Balfour, (*London Lancet*, vol. 1, 1886, p. 356,) as being due to improper administration of the drug. He says the iodide should be administered every eight hours in increasing doses, guided by its action on the pulse. If the normal pulse rate is increased, the dose must be diminished. First learn the pulse rate in recumbency, then give ten grains every eight hours, increasing the dose by five grains every week, if the pulse remains normal. It causes hypertrophy of the aneurismal walls by lowering tension. Other methods of treatment are the galvano-puncture, and the introduction of wire, horsehair or catgut into the sac through a canula. These measures have not been attended with such success as to justify their frequent repetition. For many years occasional attempts have been made to cure these aneurisms by the distal ligation of one or both of the great trunks which arise from the innominate artery, with variable success. We must, therefore, study the results of the operations for purposes of comparison under the following heads :

1. Ligature of right common carotid.

2. Ligature of right subclavian.

3. Ligature of left carotid.

4. Consecutive distal ligature of right common carotid and right subclavian, third part.

5. Simultaneous distal ligation of right common carotid and right subclavian, (third portion or axillary, first part.)

6. Distal ligature of left carotid and left subclavian.

As elaborate papers have already appeared upon this subject by Dr. John A. Wyeth, of New York, in the *American Journal of the Medical Sciences*, January, 1881, and by Rosenstern, of San Francisco, in the *Archiv f. klin. Chirurg.*, 1886, p. 49, I will avail myself of their statistics to a large extent in the preparation of the following tables :

TABLE I.—LIGATURE OF RIGHT COMMON CAROTID, ALONE.

OPERATOR.	NUMBER.	YEAR.	VESSEL INVOLVED.	AGE.	SEX.	RESULT.	CAUSE OF DEATH.	KIND OF LIGATURE USED.	ANTISEPTIC.	REMARKS.
V. Mott.	1	1820	Innominate.	60	M.	D.	Secondary hæmorrhage	?	No.	Died in 20 days.
Evans.	2	1828	Innominate and root of carotid.	30	"	R.		"	"	Permanent cure, lived for 30 years, abcess and rupture of sac.
Neumeister.	3	1829	Innominate.	51	"	D.	Cerebral complication. Died on 5th day.	"	"	
V. Mott.	4	1829	"	51	"	R.	Pressure on trachea.	"	"	Died in 7 months from pressure of the consolidated aneurism on the trachea.
Key.	5	1830	" and aorta.	61	F.	D.	Cerebral anemia in a few hours.	"	"	Left carotid nearly obliterated.
Morrison.	6	1832	" and root of carotid.	42	M.	R.		"	"	Improved. Died suddenly 20 months later.
Scott.	7	1834	Innominate,			D.	Rupture of sac.	"	"	Died on 7th day.
Dohlhoff.	8	1837	"			"	Cerebral complications.	"	"	Died suddenly during some slight effort.
O'Shaughnessy	9	1840 ?	aorta.	42	"	"	Died on 10th day. Rupture of sac.	"	"	
Hutton.	10	1841	Innominate.	47	"	"	Rupture of sac into trachea.	"	"	
Ferguson.	11	1841	" and root of right subclavian.	55	"	"	On 7th day.	"	"	Death the result of operation.
Porta.	12	1842	Innominate and roots of right carotid and subclavian.	60	F.	"	No cause given.	"	"	Died in 40 hours.
Rompani.	13	844	Carotid and innominate.	70	M.	"	Secondary hæmorrhage.	"	"	Died on 21st day. Double aneurism of carotid and innominate.
Campbell.	14	1845	Innominate.	48	"	"	Suffocation from pressure.	"	"	Died in 19 days.

No.	Date	Name	Seat of aneurism	Sex	Result	Age	Cause of death	Ligature	Cured	Remarks
15	?	Vilardebo.	Double aneurism of right ca-rotid, right subclavian and innominate.	M.	D.	?	Abscess of the brain.	?	No.	Died on 21st day.
16	1855	Wright.	Innominate.	"	"	70		"	"	Lived nearly three months.
17	1859	Ordite.	"	"	"			"	"	No particulars given.
18	1860	Broadbent.	"	"	R.	50		"	"	Died in four months.
19	1860	Pirogoff.	"	"	"	?		"	"	Improved, and lost sight of.
20	?	Nusbaum.	"	"	D.		Growth of aneurism.	"	"	
21	?	Nusbaum.	"	"	"			"	"	
22	1863	Butcher.	Dilatation of innominate, an-eurism of 3d pt. subclavian.	"	"	42	Death in 88 hours.	"	"	Innominate and 1st part of subclavian enormously dilated.
23	1867	Hutchison.	Aorta, innominate and right carotid and right subclavian.	"	"	48	Death in 41 days from suffo-cation.	"	"	Also attempted to tie the right subclavian, but the vessel was not included in the ligature.
24	1867	Hewson.	Aorta and innominate.	"	"	51	Died on 10th day. Asphyxia from pressure.	"	"	
25	1875	Annandale.	Aorta.	"	R.	62		"	Yes.	Patient very much improved.
26	1877	Bryant.	"	"	D.	56	Died on 10th day.	Catgut.	"	Operation had done no good.
27	1879	Keyber.	Innominate.	"	R.	53		"	"	Improved.
28	1879	Kuster.	"	"	D.		Died in 40 hours. Œdema of lungs.	"	"	
29		Bryant.	"	"	R.			"	"	"
30		Kuster.	"	"	"			"	"	"
31	1883	Golding Bird.	"	"	D.		Died in 6 days.			Retropharyngeal abscess.
32	1884	Ferguson.	"	"	R.	38		Chro-mic gut.		Œdema of lungs. Died two years later.
33	?	Ashhurst.	Aorta,	"	"	43				No improvement.

TABLE II.—LIGATURE OF RIGHT SUBCLAVIAN ALONE.

Operator.	Number.	Year.	Vessel Involved.	Age.	Sex.	Result.	Cause of Death.	Kind of Ligature Used.	Antiseptic.	Remarks.
Wardrop.	1	1827	Innominate.	41	F.	R.			No.	Died 2 years and 2 months later.
Laugier.	2	1834	"	57	M.	D.	Secondary hæmorrhage.			Died in 1 month, bleeding from peripheral end of subclavian.
Broca.	3	1862	"	50	"	R.				Died in 6 months from gangrene of the lung.
Lane.	4	?	"	?	"	D.				Died in 8 days.
Bryant.	5	1871	"	33	"	R.		Carbol. catgut		Died in 5 years from pressure of the Aneurism.

TABLE III.—LIGATURE OF LEFT COMMON CAROTID ALONE.

Operator.	Number.	Year.	Vessel Involved.	Age.	Sex.	Result.	Cause of Death.	Kind of Ligature Used.	Antiseptic.	Remarks.
Montgomery.	1	1829	Aorta.	40	M.	R.			No.	Improved, but died in 4 months from hæmorrhage.
Tillanus or Rigen.	2	1829	"	?	"	"			"	Improved, but died in 5 months from asthma and spasm.
Pirogoff.	3	?	"	?	"	"			"	Left hospital in 2½ months very much improved.
Pirogoff.	4	?	Innomin and aorta.	?	F.	D.	Death in 3 weeks.			Hemiplegia.

Operator.	Number.	Year.	Vessel Involved.	Age.	Sex.	Result.	Cause of Death.	Kind of Ligature Used.	Antiseptic.	Remarks.
Heath.	5	1872	Aorta.	48	M.	R.	Death in a few hours from cerebral aneurism.	Catgut.	Yes	Great relief, died 4½ years after operation
Heath.	6	1874	"			D.				Right carotid had been previously obliterated.
Holmes.	7	1875	End of arch of aorta.	21	F.	R.			"	Alive 7 months later.
Barwell.	8	1877	Transverse aorta.	56	M.	"			"	Improved, and died in 4 months of kidney disease.
Dauchez.	9	1879	Aorta mistaken for carotid			"				Improved, but died in 13 months.
Hardie.	10	1880	Transverse aorta.						Carbol. silk.		Died 6 ... er. Ligature un-
Bryant.	11	1881	Innominate.			D.	Died on 19th day.	Catgut		Operation from pul ... the growth. Death ma and gangrene.
Ashhurst.	12	?	Aorta.			R.				
Heath.	13	1890		38	M.	"	Died in 2 mon.			Cocaine anesthesia.

TABLE IV.—CONSECUTIVE DISTAL LIGATION OF THE RIGHT CO . ON CAROTID, AND RIGHT SUBCLAVIAN THIRD PORTION.

Operator.	Number.	Year.	Vessel Involved.	Age.	Sex.	Result.	Cause of Death.	Kind of Ligature Used.	Antiseptic.	Remarks.
Wickham.	1	1827	Innominate.	55	M.	D.	Rupture.	Silk.	No.	Died of pleurisy—alcoholic.
Fearn.	2	1836	"	28	F.	R.	Died 4 months after last operation.		"	Greatly improved.
Malgaigne.	3	1845	"	46	M.	D	Rupture of sac 21 days, first operation.			Alcoholic.
Bickersteth.	4	1864	Aorta and innominate.	35	"	X				Died in 5 months from the progress of the disease.
Speir.	5	1874	Aorta supposed innominate.	31	"	D.	Rupture of sac on 34th day.			Speirs constrictor to carotid; 48 hours later tied subclavian.

TABLE IV.—CONTINUED.

OPERATOR.	NUMBER.	YEAR.	VESSEL INVOLVED.	AGE.	SEX.	RESULT.	CAUSE OF DEATH.	KIND OF LIGATURE USED.	ANTISEPTIC.	REMARKS.
Doughty and Mott.	6	1875	Innominate.	40	M.	R.				Greatly improved. Died of phthisis 3 years after operation.
Kuster.	7	1879	Aorta.	37	"	"		Carbol catgut.		Died three months after last operation. Wounds healed.
Adams and Treves.	8	1880	Innominate.	47	"	D.	Died 37 days after last operation; rupture of sac.	Catgut.		Carotid not obliterated. Subclavian obliterated.
Wolf.	9	1882	Aorta.	32	"	R.		Silk.		Died 5 months after last operation.
Schede.	10	?	"	?	"	D.	Secondary hemorrhage.			
Gay.	11	?	Innominate.	38	"	R.		"		Great improvement. Died 1 year later. Ligated carotid and 2 months later subclavian.

TABLE V.—SIMULTANEOUS DISTAL LIGATION OF RIGHT CAROTID AND RIGHT SUBCLAVIAN.

OPERATOR.	NUMBER.	YEAR.	VESSEL INVOLVED.	AGE.	SEX.	RESULT.	CAUSE OF DEATH.	KIND OF LIGATURE USED.	ANTISEPTIC.	REMARKS.
Hobart.	1	1839	Aorta mistaken for innominate.	25	F.	D.	Died on 16th day; hemorrhage from carotid.		No.	Common carotid tied 1 inch above origin. Subclavian in its first part.
Rossi.	2	1844	Innominate.		"	"	Died on 6th day. Left carotid and right vertebral obliterated.		"	As the left vertebral was the only vessel to carry on the cerebral circulation, he probably died of anæmia of the brain.
C. Heath.	3	1865	Aorta mistaken for innominate.	30		R.			?	Great improvement. Died from external bursting of an aortic aneurism, 4 years and 17 days p.-operation.

Name	No.	Year	Nature	Age	Sex	Result	Death / Outcome	Ligature	Cured	Remarks
Maunder.	4	1867	Aorta mistaken for innominate.	37	M.	D.	Died on 5th day; occlusion of aorta by clot.		?	Clot projected from innominate into aorta.
Hodges.	5	1868	No true aneurism.	55	"	"	Died on 12th day; exhaustion.		"	Fusiform dilatation of innominate and aorta, but no true aneurism.
Sands.	6	1868	Aorta mistaken for innominate.	43	F.	R.	Died in 13 months.	Silk or thread.	No.	Tumor diminished and visible pulsation ceased.
Jas. Lane.	7	1871	Innominate and aorta.	40	"	"	Died in about 30 days from bursting of sac.	Silk.	Yes	Improved and left hospital in 46 days. Died suddenly about 50th day.
Holmes.	8	1871	"	40	M.	"	Died on 55th day; œdema and exhaustion.	Catgut.	"	One month p.-operation galvano puncture; later sac opened with knife.
McCarthy.	9	1872	" and aorta.	45	"	D.	Died on 16th day from hæmorrhage.	Silk.	"	Bleeding from subclavian, ulceration at seat of ligature.
Durham.	10	1872	"	?	"	"	Died on 7th day; apparently shock.	"	"	Ligated subclavian first, then carotid.
Ensor.	11	1874	"	50	"	R.	Died on 65th day from rupture of aneurism.	"	"	Progressed favorably. Exposed himself and contracted rheumatism.
Weir.	12	1876	"	45	"	"	Died on 15th day from rupture of aneurism.	Catgut.	"	Pulsation returned in right temporal in 2 hours and in radial in 6 hours.
Elliott.	13	1876	"	41	"	D.	Died on 26th day; hæmorrhage from sac.	Silk.	"	Ulceration of tumor. Rupture of aneurism.
King.	14	1876	"	37	"	R.	Death on 11th day from rupture of aneurism.	Catgut.	"	Much improved. Got on spree and died of hæmorrhage.
Little.	15	1877	"	46	"	"	Death from pleurisy 3 years and 4 mos. after p.-oper'n.	"	"	Subclavian tied first. Permanently cured. Death not connected with operation.
Barwell.	16	1877	Aorta and innominate.	45	"	"	Death from broncho-pneumonia in 100 days.	"	"	Ligature of carotid, and 24 hours later, subclavian. Aneurism cured.
Barwell.	17	1877	"	57	F.	"	Death in 19 months from bronchitis.	"	"	Great improvement. Married in February, 1879.

TABLE V.—Continued.

Operator.	Number.	Year.	Vessel Involved.	Age.	Sex.	Result.	Cause of Death.	Kind of Ligature Used.	Antiseptic.	Remarks.
Barwell.	18	1881	Innominate.	48	M.	D.	Died 30 hours from the anæsthetic.	Catgut.	Yes	Patient never recovered from the ether, remained cyanosed.
Ransohoff.	20	1890	"	48	"	"	Died on 7th day; asphyxia.	Carbol. Silk.	"	Fusiform dilatation of arch of aorta, and aneurism of innominate.
Barwell.	21	1879	Aorta.	39	"	R.	Died in 15 months of a new aneurism.	Flat ox-aorta ligat're Cat.gut.	"	Great improvement, lived 15 mos. in comfort; original aneurism completely cured.
Barwell.	19	1878	Innominate.	27	F.	"			"	Great improvement. Still alive when reported.
Stimson.	22	1880	"	34	M.	"			"	Cured; Died of phthisis 21 months p.-operation. Aneurism cured.
Palmer.	23	1880	" and aorta.	50	F.	"	Died in 4 months of hæmorrhage.	Hemp. No.		Aneurism filled with laminated clot, communication between innominate and vein, opening into trachea.
Lediard.	24	1880	Aorta.	42	M.	"	Died in 11 months p-operation.	Lig. ox. aorta.	"	Great improvement. Aneurism filled with hard clot at autopsy, 11 months p.-operation.
Wyeth.	25	1880	"	42	F.	"	Died 1 year later. Acute diarrhœa.		"	Great improvement. Almost cured, but a small cavity remained. Woman addicted to drink.
King.	26	1880	Root of neck.	40	M.	"	Living when reported.	Antiseptic Silk.	"	Dismissed 8 weeks p-operation; aneurism smaller and patient free from pain.
Marsh.	27	1881	Aorta.	30	"	D.	Ruptured on 31st day.	Chr'mic catgut.	Yes	Rapid enlargement of aneurism to left post-operation.
Pollock.	28	1881	Innominate.	37	"	"	Dyspnœa.	Catgut and tendon.	"	Catgut ligature for carotid. Kangaroo tendon for subclavian.

Name	No.	Year	Type	Age	Sex	R/D	Result	Ligature	Improved	Remarks
Langley-Brown	29	1881	Innominate.	32	M.	R.		Chrm'ic catgut.	Yes	Improved. Living two years later.
Cameron.	30	1882	"	57	F.	"		Catgut.	"	Alive and well 20 months post-operation.
Lane.	31	1882	"	?	M.	"	Died in 10 months.	Carbol silk.	"	Marked relief; returned to work; died after 10 months.
v. Bergman.	32	1883	"	40	"	"		Carbol.	::	Improved; rapid healing; decrease in size.
May.	33	1883	"	40	"	D.	Died in 2 days from cyanosis	Catgut.	"	Tied axillary, 1st part and carotid.
Rosenstern.	34	1883	"	42	F.	R.		Silk.	"	Ligatures on carotid separated in 5 or 6 weeks. On subclavian in 3 months. Great improvement. Alive and at work 2½ years later.
Gerster.	35	1884	"	51	M.	"		Catgut.	"	Tied axillary, 1st part, then carotid.
Barwell.	36	1884	"	48	F.	"		Ox. aor- ta.	"	All pulsation disappeared and patient seemed cured 4 months later.
Banks.	37	1884	"	?	M.	D.	Died in 1 month. Hemorrhage from subclavian.	Kanga- roo ten- don lig.		Aneurism nearly filled with laminated fibrin.
Alexander.	38	1882	" and aorta.	48	F.	R.	Died in six months, dyspnœa	Catgut.		Some relief.
Beany.	39	?	"			"				Mentioned by Barwell in Med. Chir. Trans., 85, vol. lxviii, p. 123.
Beany.	40	?	"			"				Mentioned by Barwell in Med. Chir. Trans., 85, vol. lxviii, p. 123.
Hartley.	41	1885	Innominate.		M.					Improved; patient exhibited November 16, 1888. Aneurism extending.
Jessup.	42	?	"			D.	Hæmorrhage on 49th day.	Silk.		Reported by Mr. Ward.
Jessup.	43	?	"			R.		Catgut.		Aneurism not cured.
Jessup.	44	?	"			"		Silk.		Secondary hæmorrhage; stopped by gal- vano puncture.
Jameson.	45	?	Aorta simulating innomin'te.	59	"	"			No.	Result, 3 months freedom from pain.
Lawrie.	46	1885	Aorta.	38	"	"		Carbol. silk.	Yes	Much improved 4 months subsequently.

TABLE V.—CONTINUED.

Operator.	Number.	Year.	Vessel Involved.	Age.	Sex.	Result.	Cause of Death.	Kind of Lig-ature Used.	Antiseptic.	Remarks.
Prager.	47	1886	Innominate.	60	M.	R.	Death from bronchitis 1 year p-operation.			Hemiplegia 2 days after operation, same day slight pulse in radial.
McBurney.	48	1886	"	35	"	"		Catgut	Yes	Alive and apparently cured 18 months subsequently.
Ashhurst.	49	1886	"	42	"	"		"		Discharged 2 months subsequently.
Mynter.	50	1887	"	54	F.	"		"		Much Improved.
Heath.	51	?	"	?		"		?		Discharged improved on 31st day.
Percival.	52	?	"			"		Chrom-ic gut.	?	Marked improvement; antimony post-operation seemed to be of benefit.
Wells.	53	?	Aorta.	70	F.	"		Catgut		Apparently complete cure.
Dunlop.	54	?	Innominate.			"				Almost a cure, much improved.
Dunlop.	55	1888	"			?				Doing well when reported.
Packard.	56	1888	"	26	M.	D.	Suffocation, 5th day.	Catgut.		Aneurism the result of injury.
Meriwether.	57	1888	Aorta.	35	F.	R.		"		On 26th day no pulsation; considers her cured.
J. C. Warren.	58	1889	Innominate.	59	M.	"	Death in 3 months from rupture of aneurism.	Boiled silk.		Tied 1st portion axillary between the two portions of the pectoris major.
Winslow.	59	1889	Supposed innominate.	37	F.	"	Still living.	Catgut.	Yes	Wounds healed p-pulsation not arrested
Pettus.	60									Have not been able to come across report of this case.
Ashhurst.	61	1889	Aorta.	49	M.	R.		Catgut.	Yes	Aneurismal symptoms much improved.

TABLE VI.—CONSECUTIVE LIGATURE OF LEFT CAROTID AND LEFT SUBCLAVIAN OR LEFT AXILLARY.

Operator.	Number.	Year.	Vessel Involved.	Age.	Sex.	Result.	Cause of Death.	Kind of Ligature Used.	Antiseptic.	Remarks.
Schede.	1	?	Arch of aorta.	34	M.	R.			Yes	Great improvement, died suddenly in 6 months.
Busch.	2	1880	Two aneurisms of aorta.	45	M.	D.	Died on 4th day.		"	First part of axillary tied. Operation of no benefit.

TABLE VII.—SIMULTANEOUS LIGATION OF LEFT CAROTID AND SUBCLAVIAN.

Operator.	Number.	Year.	Vessel Involved.	Age.	Sex.	Result.	Cause of Death.	Kind of Ligature Used.	Antiseptic.	Remarks.
Wyeth.	1	1889	Aorta involving roots of left carotid and left subclavian.	48	M.	D.	Died in 72 hours.	Catgut	Yes	

TABLE I.—DISTAL LIGATURE OF THE RIGHT CAROTID, ALONE.

Number of cases, 33 ; recovered, 11 ; cured, 1; improved, 7; died, 22.

Cause of death : Secondary hæmorrhage, 2 ; cerebral complications, 4 ; rupture of sac, 3 ; pressure, 4 ; œdema of lungs, 1 ; retro-pharyngeal abscess, 1 ; doubtful, 5.

Pre-antiseptic cases, 24; recovered, 5 ; cured, 1 ; (this patient lived for thirty years after the operation,) died, 19.

Antiseptic, 9 ; recovered, 6 ; cured, 0; died, 3.

Males, 22 ; females, 2 ; unknown, 9.

TABLE II.—LIGATION OF RIGHT SUBCLAVIAN, ALONE.

Number of cases, 5 ; recovered, 3 ; cured. 0; improved, 3 ; died, 2.

Cause of death : Secondary hæmorrhage, 1 ; not stated, 1. One patient lived 3 years, one 2 years and 2 months, and one only 6 months.

Males, 4 ; females, 1.

TABLE III.—DISTAL LIGATION OF THE LEFT COMMON CAROTID, ALONE.

Number of cases, 13 ; recovered, 10 ; apparently cured, 2 ; improved, 7 ; died, 3.

Cause of death : One case from hemiplegia in three weeks, one from cerebral anæmia in a few hours, and one from pulmonary œdema and gangrene.

Pre-antiseptic cases, 4 ; recovered, 2 ; died, 2.

Antiseptic, 9 ; recovered, 7 ; apparently cured, 2 ; died, 2.

Males, 6 ; females, 2 ; unknown, 5.

TABLE IV.—CONSECUTIVE LIGATION OF RIGHT COMMON CAROTID AND RIGHT SUBCLAVIAN, THIRD PORTION.

Number of cases, 11 ; recovery from operation, 6 ; cured, 1 ; improved, 4 ; died within 40 days, 5.

Cause of death : Rupture of sac, 4 ; secondary hæmorrhage, 1. Spier's constrictor was used in one case to carotid, and 48 hours subsequently the right subclavian was ligated. The patient died 34 days later from rupture of the sac.

Males, 10 ; females, 1.

TABLE V.—RESULTS OF SIMULTANEOUS DISTAL LIGATION OF THE RIGHT COMMON CAROTID AND RIGHT SUBCLAVIAN, THIRD PORTION, OR AXILLARY, FIRST PORTION.

Total cases, 59 ; recovered from operation, 43 ; apparently cured, 16 ; improved, 20 ; died, 16.

Antiseptic, 53 ; recovered, 41 ; apparently cured, 16 ; died, 12.

Pre-antiseptic, 6 ; recovered, 2 ; died, 4.

Ligature material, silk or thread, 20 ; recovered, 10 ; died, 10.

Cause of death : Hæmorrhage, 4 ; cerebral anæmia, 1 ; occlusion of aorta, 1 ; exhaustion 1 ; shock, 1 ; asphyxia, 1.

Catgut, 26 ; recovered, 20 ; apparently cured, 8 ; died, 6.

Causes of death : Hæmorrhage, 0 ; rupture of sac, 2 ; anæsthetic, 1 ; cyanosis, 1 ; suffocation, 1 ; dyspnœa, 1.

Ox aorta, 4 cases ; 4 recoveries ; apparently cured, 3.

Males, 34 ; females, 16 ; unknown, 10.

Amongst these cases are included one in which the first portion of the right subclavian was tied, death resulting on the sixteenth day of hæmorrhage, and three in which the vessel was tied below the clavicle (first portion of axillary, English, third portion of subclavian, German); with one death on the second day from cyanosis, and two recoveries.

TABLE VI.—LIGATIONS OF LEFT COMMON CAROTID AND LEFT SUBCLAVIAN OR AXILLARY.

Consecutive, carotid and subclavian.—Number of cases, 1; recovered, 1, improved, 1.

Carotid and axillary : Number of cases, 1 ; died on fourth day.

Simultaneous carotid and subclavian : Number of cases, 1 ; died in 72 hours.

Males 3 ; females, 0.

The cases here tabulated are not supposed to be all that
have been operated on, but they are all that have been accessible to me for purposes of study and comparison, and they
are sufficient in point of numbers for the elucidation of the
main features involved. I have not attempted to tabulate
separately the results of operations for the relief of aneurisms of the arch of the aorta, but have included aortic and
innominate aneurisms together. This would, perhaps, not
have been the best procedure, but as the mistakes in diagnosis have been very numerous, and usually only discovered
upon post-mortem examination, it is probably not a matter
of much moment. A noticeable feature in this inquiry is
the very much greater proportion of aneurisms affecting the
male sex than the female ; of the 98 cases in which operations
were performed, and the sex recorded, 76 were male, and 22
female. This is in accordance with the well known law that
aneurism is most frequent in the male sex, which the elder
Gross attributes not so much to the more laborious occupations of men as to the fact that women are not so prone to
arterial degenerations. A glance at the histories of these
cases also shows a very large proportion of habitual topers ;
and the fatal result in not a few cases is directly traceable to
the evil effects of a debauch. The ages of those subjected
to operation varies from 21 to 70 years, which classified in
decennial periods is as follows : From 21 to 30, 5 cases ; 30
to 40, 22 cases ; 40 to 50, 34 cases ; 50 to 60, 19 cases ; 60 to
70, 5 cases ; over 70, 4 cases.

We will see by reference to the tables that the simultaneous distal ligation of the right common carotid, and the
right subclavian arteries has been performed much more frequently than any other operation for the cure of these
aneurisms, and with a much larger proportion of recoveries,
72¾ per cent., as compared with 54½ per cent. in the consecutive distal ligation of the same vessels. Distal deligation
of the right common carotid alone gives a percentage of recoveries of only 33⅓, whilst the ligation of the right subclavian alone, which has only been performed five times, gives
a proportion of 60 per cent. of recoveries. The left common
carotid artery has been tied thirteen times for aortic aneurism,

with a proportion of recoveries of nearly 77 per cent., and with very great improvement in the patients, but this operation is only applicable to aneurisms affecting the summit and left extremity of the arch of the aorta. If we analyze the cases more carefully we shall find that the results have been materially modified by the introduction of antiseptic methods. As we cannot state definitely in every case whether the operation was conducted upon antiseptic principles or not, we will have to satisfy ourselves by referring to those cases which occurred before 1871 as pre-antiseptic, and those since as antiseptic operations, and we will find a most remarkable difference in the behavior of the two classes of cases. In the antiseptic simultaneous ligations of the right carotid and subclavian, the recoveries amount to 77⅓ per cent., in the pre-antiseptic cases only 33⅓ per cent. recovered. In the antiseptic distal ligation of the right common carotid artery, alone, the proportion of recoveries was 66⅔ per cent.; in the pre-antiseptic, 20¾ per cent. In the antiseptic distal ligation of the left common carotid, 77¾ per cent. recovered ; in the pre-antiseptic, 50 per cent. The best permanent results are also found to belong to the simultaneous distal ligation of the common carotid and subclavian of the right side, though Mr. T. Holmes thinks that about all the good which is obtained is to be had from ligation of the carotid first, and if necessity should occur, subsequently, the subclavian. Very interesting questions are raised in regard to the action of different kinds of ligatures when applied to these large vessels.

The early operations were performed without antiseptic precautions, and silk or hemp ligatures were used. This involved a more or less tedious convalescence, with suppuration, in those cases which recovered ; and not unfrequently death from secondary hæmorrhage occurred, upon the separation of the ligature. Of the operations performed within antiseptic times, for the ligation of the right common carotid and right subclavian, simultaneously, in 14 cases silk or thread was used, with 9 recoveries and 5 deaths, only one of the deaths, however, being from secondary hæmorrhage. In 26 cases catgut was used, with 20 recoveries and 6 deaths, none of the fatal cases resulting from secondary hæmorrhage. In 4 cases the flat ox aorta ligatures were used, all recovering; and in 2 cases kangaroo tendon was the ligature material, both terminating fatally. The number of observations recorded is too small for making any special generalization, but they are suggestive. There can be no doubt that a person is more exposed to the danger of secondary hæmorrhage when a non-absorbable ligature is used, than when catgut or other absorbable material is made use of; but silk is more easily and effectively sterilized than any animal material. On the whole, however, an absorbable material secures more favorable results, and the question is more in regard to the particular animal tissue to be used, and the shape of the ligature. Barwell has especially eulogized the flat ligatures made from the aorta of the ox, and they have given satisfaction wherever used. His idea in introducing these ligatures was that the coats of the artery would not be cut through by the broad, tape-like ligatures, but that the circulation would be effectively shut off for a sufficient time to allow consolidation of the aneurism, and the ligatures would then be absorbed, leaving the artery simply closed by a diaphragm, where its walls had been in contact. Whilst good results have resulted from the use of this ligature, it is doubtful whether it possesses any advantage over ordinary stout, round catgut, and it seems to me to be pretty well proven that the best and safest way of occluding an artery is by constricting it with sufficient force to divide its inner coats and thereby cause complete severance of the continuity of the vessel. I think, therefore, that properly prepared catgut is the most available as well as the best ligature material to be used in these cases. Kangaroo and other tendinous ligatures are too difficult to obtain for general use, and do not seem to me to present any commensurate advantage. In one case Mr. Speir successfully occluded the right carotid artery with his "constrictor," and 48 hours later tied the subclavian. This was essentially a simultaneous operation, but is not included in the table of simultaneous ligations. If it were not for the fact that the use of a catgut ligature leaves but little to be desired, a further trial of Speir's "constrictor" might be made with advantage.

In looking over the causes of death, I find 7 cases in which the fatal result is definitely attributed to secondary hæmorrhage, and of these four in which the vessel was tied with silk or hemp, and one with kangaroo tendon. Bursting of the sac, either internally or externally, is by far the most frequent cause of death, occurring in from 10 days to 4 months after the operation. This is the natural tendency of all aneurisms, and it is remarkable that the sudden strain which is thrown upon the sac by the ligation of the great vessels coming from it, does not more frequently cause its rupture. Amongst the causes of death, we find "cerebral complications" occupying quite a prominent place. This is not to be wondered at, considering the sudden anæmia which is produced by the ligation of the common carotid, which, however, quickly passes off. In some cases several of the trunks leading to the brain have been previously obliterated, and the ligation of one of the remaining vessels produces such a degree of anæmia as to cause death. The ligation of the subclavian alone would naturally be supposed to favor cerebral embolism, but in the 5 cases in which the right subclavian has been ligated alone, no such result followed. Pressure symptoms belong to the natural history of aneurism, and we find that many succumb after operations to pressure on the trachea, bronchi or lungs, producing cyanosis, dyspnœa and asphyxia, or œdema and gangrene of the lungs. In one case death is said to have been caused by the occlusion of the aorta, by a clot which projected from the innominate; this occurred on the fifth day *post-operationem*. One death is attributed to post-pharyngeal abscess, which was probably the result of infection at the time of the operation. In conclusion it may be stated that simultaneous distal ligation of the right common carotid and right subclavian artery, in its third portion, has not, *per se*, a very high rate of mortality, when performed antiseptically, with an absorbable ligature; and that in a large proportion of cases great benefit will follow, whilst in a small proportion of cases a permanent cure will be obtained.

DISCUSSION.

Dr. R. W. Johnson thought that in 1871 very few antiseptic operations were performed, and even now surgeons do not always operate antiseptically. It is not a point of election whether you do a distal or a proximal ligation. The strong pulsations of the heart are apt to break through the weak arterial walls. He also thought that the absorbable ligature was by far the best.

Dr. Winslow said that most men mentioned were those who operated since antisepsis was introduced, and it was fair to presume that they used it.

The second paper was read by Dr. S. T. Earle on "*The use of Electrolysis in Stricture of the Rectum.*" The paper was, on motion "referred" to the Publication Committee, after discussion by Drs. W. S. Gardner, Geo. J. Preston and others.

THE USE OF ELECTROLYSIS IN STRICTURE OF THE RECTUM.

I would like to call attention to the report of three *cases of benign stricture of the rectum treated by electrolysis,* and make some general remarks upon the subject.

Electrolysis as first announced by Nicholson and Carlisle in 1800, is the process by which a compound body, in fusion, or solution, is decomposed by passing through it, an electrical current of sufficient strength to overcome the chemical affinity between the component molicules. Dr. Geo. H. Rohe, in a recent article on "The Electrolytic Decomposition of Organic Tissues," says :

"In electrolysis of organic tissues, there are probably several processes to take into account. In the first place, it is extremely likely that the water of the tissues with certain salts, acids, and other compounds in solution yields to the disruptive power of the current, and hydrogen with other electro-positive ions are set free, or combined at the negative electrode, while oxygen and negative ions are separated at the anode,

"But while this liberation of atoms and molecules takes place at the terminals of the battery, what is going on in the track of the contrary processions of ions between the electrodes? In other words, is there any interpolar action of current, and in what does it exist? In my opinion, there is of necessity a loosening, or shaking up of the interpolar compounds which results variously, according to the vitality of the tissues. If the current is of moderate strength and the tissues have the normal degree of vital resistance, the molecular disturbance will probably result merely in an improvement of nutrition, in accordance with the general biological law that moderate stimulation produces increase in nutrition. If the current is of excessive strength, there will probably be some breaking up of the compounds which may affect nutrition unfavorably.

"Actually, we know really nothing of the interpolar effects of electric currents in organic tissues. In inorganic compounds, with their simple and stable organization, the electric current may not produce any interpolar change, although the theory of Clausius rather favors the view that interpolar decomposition occurs. But in organic compounds, with their more complex and unstable composition, we can readily understand that the continual re-arrangement of molecules under the influence of electrolytic constriction may so disturb the harmonious relations of the molecules as to render decomposition more easy. If the tissues are normal, recovery and repair of slight defects may promptly follow; but in the case of pathological products—inflammatory infiltrations, new growths, serous effusions, etc.,—it stands to reason that a molecular disturbance of some extent, or continued for some time may produce such a modification of nutrition in the tissues as to promote its regressive metamorphosis. That this actually takes place, I firmly believe, although I am unable to give an exact demonstration of the process. I am also strongly of opinion that in many pathological products, or tissues a retrogressive change begun under the influence of an electrolytic current is kept up after the immediate action of the current has been discontinued."

I have made this very liberal quotation because it expresses so well the present theory on electrolysis.

Dr. Robt. Newman, of New York City, claims with good reason to have been the first to use electrolysis in the treatment of rectal stricture in 1871. In the same article, he refers to its use in 1872 by Dr. Beard; in 1873 by Dr. Groh, of Olmutz; and in 1875 by Dr. Leute. While the results obtained even in these early days of its application to such purposes seems to have been satisfactory to those using it, in spite of the very weak currents used, and the want of means for measuring the amount they did use; we can confidently look for much better results with our recently improved methods of generating and applying the current; our means for measuring quite accurately the amount we use, and from the greater strength of current we now employ.

It is very important to have a battery capable of furnishing the amount of current necessary to accomplish the desired results; and as a means for ascertaining that fact, we should also have, and use it at each sitting, a reliable galvanometer for measuring the amount of current used. There are so many batteries on the market, that one is so likely to be led astray by the many advantages claimed for each, I should by all means advise that every one should inform himself upon the subject before undertaking it, and know exactly what he needs, and make his own selection of the battery that will best meet his requirements. For brief and concise information on the subject, I would refer the reader to "*Lockwood on Electrical Measurements;*" "Massey on *Electricity in Gynæcology and Practice,*" and Engelman on "*the use of Electricity in Gynæcological Practice.*" I would briefly state we need a battery that will not polarize quickly, one of sufficient electro-motor force to overcome all resistance; and one of sufficient current strength to give from 100 to 125 milli-amperes of current after all resistance has been overcome. This has been the amount of working current I have found necessary to accomplish the desired results in these cases, and is as much as the patient can bear without an anæsthetic. After having tried several of the most approved batteries I have found by far the most satisfactory to be one composed of from thirty to fifty cells of the Leclanche pattern, it is also reasonable in price, (one of the most approved varieties of that pattern, having recently cost me sixty-five cents a cell.) It is not portable however— an objection that can be laid at the door of all batteries I have ever seen capable of doing efficient electrolytic work. It requires very little attention; the cells are joined up in series, and are connected with a switch board where you can turn on the desired number of cells. I have a Wait and Bartlett milli-ampere metre, which I think is fairly accurate.

Four sizes of metallic electrodes, conical in shape, and varying in size from one, to three and three-eighth inches in circumferance are all that I have found necessary for practical purposes. These are used as the negative electrodes inside the rectum; while a large piece of absorbent cotton net in a strong solution of salt is used under the positive electrode on the skin of the buttock, if the stricture is low down in the rectum, but just over the pubes if high up.

I would like to say a word in passing of the decided effect of the salt solution in assisting to overcome the resistance of the skin. As an instance, when using twenty-six cells with the cotton under the positive pole wet with water, I only got twenty-five milli-amperes of current; without any other change than merely wetting the cotton under the positive pole with a strong solution of salt, I got one hundred milli-amperes from thirteen cells. In treating these cases I let each sitting last for ten minutes, twice during each week, if the case is aggravated; once, if mild.

Sometimes when there is much irritation of the rectum, the currents of the strength mentioned above may increase the irritation, as will be seen in one of the cases which I here report, when the strength and frequency of application have to be lessened.

Mrs. H., white, æt 30 years. I first saw her January 25th, 1888, with Dr. Rohe, who kindly sent her to me. Had difficulty in having evacuations from her bowels for seven or eight years. Has a history of syphilis contracted about fourteen years ago. Was treated two years previous to coming to me for stricture of the rectum, first by gradual dilatation; then by linear proctotomy, which was not followed by subsequent dilatation as it should have been, and consequently was left in a worse condition after, than before the operation. At the time I saw her she rarely had any but very fluid stools, and when moulded were very narrow and flat, and caused excruciating pain.

On examination I found the sphincters only partially closed the bowel, having the scar resulting from the linear proctotomy between their cut ends. About one inch above the site of the external sphincter was a very tight stricture—so tight that it would admit little more than the ordinary probe; there was a large indurated mass, about the size of a small lemon, in Douglass cul-de-sac; the anterior wall of the rectum was very much indurated; there was a constant discharge of a muco-purulent fluid from the bowel; and she sufferred very much from dysmenorrhœa, and during the act of copulation.

January 30th, 1888, commenced dilatation of the stricture by electrolysis, using from ten to fifteen cells of "Barrett's Chloride of silver battery." The first negative electrode used to pass the stricture, was only a little thicker than a match, which passed with comparative ease after the current had been turned on for several minutes. At the same sitting I finally succeeded in passing another electrode one inch in circumference, but only after allowing the current to pass through it for several minutes while being gently pressed against the stricture. I continued the current until it passed back and forth through the stricture with perfect ease.

January 31st, the patient reported that the pain, which was not very much, caused by the treatment the day before had soon subsided, and she had two almost painless actions that morning without the aid of a laxative.

Feburary 6th, 1888, passed an electrode one and a half inches in circumference. From this date on to April 23rd, 1888, I gradually increased the size of the electrodes until I passed one on this date that measured two inches in circumference. Her condition began to improve with the use of electrolysis; the muco-purulent discharge gradually grew less; painful menstruation got very much better; stools were passed with less and less pain, and the neoplasm in Douglass cul-de-sac gradually disappeared.

May 27th, 1888, there are some indications of ulceration of the mucous membrane of the nose, associated with constant headache. Up to this time I intentionally avoided all constitutional treatment. I now put her on Iodide of Potash, which controlled the headache, and relieved the nasal symptoms in a few weeks. I continued the electrolysis at varying intervals, from once in two weeks to as often in several months, until November, 1889, since which time I have not used it.

October 29th, 1890, I saw and examined her; she has no trouble at all with her bowels; there is no discharge of muco-purulent matter from the rectum; evacuations are regular, although if loose they cannot be controlled on account of the old scar from the proctotomy. On examination, I find no sign of the old neoplasm in Douglass cul-de-sac; the induration in the anterior wall of the rectum is also gone, and there only remains of the old stricture a narrow band about an inch above the normal site of the anus, symmetrical in shape, and perfectly dilatable to the size of the finger; it really acts in part, the place of the sphincter, which only does partial duty.

Mrs. E., white, æt 45 years. Has a history of ulceration high up in the rectum, commencing in the fall of 1887, which got so much better before coming to me that it was not mentioned. . She presented herself to me January 23rd, 1889, suffering very much from a growth, about the size of an English Walnut, on the side of the anus which had been very much irritated from hypodermic injections into it of carbolic acid. After its removal, this growth was unfortunately mislaid and could not be examined carefully, but from its dense character and general microscopical appearance, I am quite sure it was a fibroid. I also removed at the same time from the wall of the rectum on the same side, a considerable amount of dense fibrous tissue that extended up the wall for about two inches. I removed all I could feel. This tissue was examined at the Pathological Laboratory of the Johns Hopkins Hospital, and pronounced benign in character. The case went on to do well, and when nearly healed, the patient returned to her home in Washington. I subsequently learned from her (in June, 1890,) that she never got entirely well, but several months after her return home symptoms of ulceration made their appearance again in the form of a muco-purulent discharge, tenesmus, pain, and frequent stools.

These symptoms continued to grow worse up to the time of her return to me in 1890, when she was suffering very much.

On examination I found the rectal walls very generally infiltrated; the calibre very much narrowed, and about three inches above the anus a very narrow constriction, which would only admit the end of a small electrode, about one fourth of an inch in diameter. For several weeks I made applications to the inside of the rectum of a solution of argenti nitras gr. viii: to Aq. zi., and ordered a solution of boracic acid to be injected night and morning, but these did not do any good.

June 14th, 1890, commenced treatment by electrolysis, and have used it since then on seventeen occasions. After several applications her symptoms began to improve decidedly; the pain and tenesmus grew less; the discharge decreased very much, and she soon began to have moulded stools.

November 10th, 1890, has some return of the irritation about the rectum, due, I think in the first place to a long walk taken about two weeks ago, and subsequently kept up by the use of too strong currents in applying electrolysis; a precaution that has to be looked out for in the varying conditions of the parts. On examination I find the condition of the rectum has improved very much; the infiltration having almost entirely disappeared; the stricture reduced to a narrow band of constriction and very flacid, and the skin at the verge of the anus has lost the unhealthy, œdematous appearance it formerly had. The case gives many promises of a perfectly satisfactory termination.

Mrs. M., white, domestic, æt, 40 years, presented herself September 10th, 1890. Has had a muco-purulent discharge from her bowels for several years; with pain and tenesmus attending the act of defecation, the latter symptom only appearing recently. On examination I found a fistulous opening about one and a half inches to the left of the anus, the discharge from which contained fœcal matter. On introducing the finger, it met with a dense constriction about one inch above the anus, which would not allow the finger to pass. A probe passed through the fistulæ, penetrated the rectum just above the lowest part of the constriction and could be felt with the finger. I laid this fistulous tract open, together with the lower part of the constriction, I could then pass my finger into the constricted part of the rectum and found the constriction to exist as far up as I could reach with my finger; the walls of the rectum were very much infiltrated. There is no history, nor symptoms of syphilis, or dysentery; no special trouble with either of her two labors; the last of which occurred fourteen years ago. The discharge has no peculiar odor.

October 1st, 1890, commenced the use of electrolysis, using it twice each week for ten minutes at each sitting, and used one hundred milli-amperes of current each time.

November 9th, 1890, is very much better, the discharge having grown less, almost entirely ceasing at times, and then returning slightly; the infiltration of the walls of the rectum has almost disappeared, and the stricture is very flacid. I attribute the rapid progress in the improvement of this case to the uniformly large currents I have been able to use. This case also promises to be a great success for electrolysis.

DISCUSSION.

Dr. Winslow asked if the cases had been under observation long. The cure cannot be maintained too soon after the operation.

Dr. W. S. Gardner referred to one case noted in which an electrode no larger than a match could be introduced, while after a short time Dr. Earle claimed to introduce an electrode one inch in diameter.   Was this electrolytic action or simply dilatation ?

Dr. Earle said that one case that was operated on two years ago was practically well now.   As for the electrode, he said that often an electrode could not be introduced at first, and after the current was turned on it went in easily.

Dr. W. P. Chunn referred to one of the cases mentioned in which Dr. Earle said there was a neoplasm in Douglass cul-de-sac.   This disappeared after treatment.   Did he think it was a growth removed by the electricity ?

Dr. Preston said he had not used electricity in this connection, but only in facial blemishes, etc.   He thought the idea was only to decompose tissue by a weak current, and not to cauterize it by a strong current as Dr. Earle seemed to do.   Some currents are too high.

Dr. Earle said, in reply to Dr. Chunn, that it was not a myoma, but simply an infiltration of tissue around the rectal walls.   In reply to Dr. Preston, he said his experience with both weak and strong currents in these cases was that the strong current was decidedly better.   These currents do not produce cauterization.

The next paper was read by Dr. S. K. Merrick on *"Some Observations on Fibroma of the Nose and Naso-Pharynx, with report of three cases.*   Before the debate Dr. Jno. N. Mackenzie spoke on the subject of *"Adenoid Growths as Obstructions in the Nasal Pharynx in Children."*   Drs. Goldsboro and Merrick further discussed the two subjects.

SOME OBSERVATIONS ON FIBROMA OF THE NOSE AND NASO-PHARYNX WITH REPORT OF THREE CASES.

This term is used to designate a neoplasm which is composed almost entirely of fibrous tissue.   According to the best authorities it springs when naso-pharyngeal almost exclusively from the basilar process of the occipital bone.   It grows rather slowly, filling up the naso-pharynx impinging upon contiguous parts, often sending prolongations into neighboring cavities.

It forces its way relentlessly in the direction of least resistance, often pushing bones and cartilages before it, resulting in the absorption of both.

The tumor may invade the pharynx, pushing the soft palate forward and in some instances so filling up the faucial space as to intefere with respiration.

Etiology.—It is hard to discover the cause of fibromata, as they spring from tissue, showing no evidence of morbid action and occur in individuals apparently in the enjoyment of perfect health.

More cases occur in males than in females, and generally about the age of puberty. "Nealaton, Dolbeau, Gosselin, and others of the earlier surgeons believed that they occurred exclusively among males."

Pluyette, however, made a special investigation of this point and found nine cases at least among females of undoubted fibromata.

Between the ages of 15 and 25 years is the period in which most cases are met with in the male, while in the female the age is probably somewhat greater.

It has been observed by Mackenzie that the frequency with which these cases are reported by the French surgeons might indicate their greater frequency in France than in England. Bosworth thinks the greater activity of both French and German surgeons would account for any difference found —the German reports corresponding to the French in point of numbers.

It is well-known that uterine fibroids among the negro race are exceedingly common, and it might naturally be inferred that a like frequency of fibromata of the upper air passages would be encountered. On the contrary it is doubtful if there is a well authenticated case of fibroma of the naso-pharynx, occurring in this race, on record. In a service of ten years in the Throat and Chest Department of the N. W. Dispensary, and five years in the Dispensary of the Baltimore Medical College—Nose, Throat and Chest Department—I have failed to find a single growth which resembled at all fibroma, among the hundreds of negroes examined and treated for various other affections of the nose and throat.

Symptomatology.—Fibromata of the naso-pharynx generally show early evidence of their presence by repeated attacks of epistaxis, which may be very severe. The source of this bleeding may be the mucous surfaces pressed upon by the growth, causing erosions, or the blood-vessels coursing over the tumor itself, which are often visible in the rhinoscopic mirror. Same cases will have only slight oozing, while others will bleed for hours and even days, under such circumstances, endangering the life of the patient. The liability to recurrence should be borne in mind. This bleeding may take place with or without an assignable cause. Violent exercise should be interdicted, as at all times dangerous. The tendency to hæmorrhage increases with the growth of the tumor.

Bosworth relates two cases occurring in his own practice where hæmorrhage manifested a tendency to appear during sleeping hours—while I have seen one case showing this disposition. As soon as nasal stenosis becomes at all pronounced, the "dead voice," as it is called, manifests itself. When the patient is made to pronounce the consonants M and N they simulate closely eb and ed. Interference with the proper reflection of the wave-sounds of the naso-pharynx is the cause of this vocal phenomenon. This is not peculiar, however, to fibromata—any tumor encroaching upon the lumen of the post nasal fossæ to any considerable degree will cause this peculiarity of the voice.

When naso-pharyngeal growths attain large proportions they give rise to a peculiar facial expression, which is caused partly by "an apparent broadening of the bridge of the nose and partly by the open-mouth, giving the idea of dullness of apprehension." The photograph which I here exhibit gives some idea of this facial expression. This is the photograph of a young school girl, 16 years old, upon whom I operated during the past summer for adenoma of the vault of the pharynx, where complete nasal stenosis was present before the operation. The mouth, you will observe, is open—so would it be with fibroma with nasal stenosis.

When prolongations from the fibroma are sent into the nasal cavity and sometimes even into the accessory passages, and the nasal bones are crowded forward, then results a conspicuous facial deformity, known as "frog face." These nasal prolongations have been known to traverse the entire nasal fossæ and make their appearance at the nostrils. The pressure towards the orbits may be so great as to cause exopthalmos. The presence of the growth causes excessive secretion, both in the nasal passages and naso-pharynx. They consist of tenacious mucus and muco-pus from the naso-pharynx, but are often serous or serum mixed with pus from the nose. Any of these secretions may be mixed with blood which, in most instances, comes from the superficial vessels of the neoplasm.

As the growth extends into the lower pharynx, it pushes the soft palate forward, and thus interferes with deglutition, preventing the complete closure of the upper pharynx during the act and permitting regurgetation of fluids into the nose. Dyspnœa may be caused by the further extension downwards of the growth, mechanically interfering with the entrance of air into the lungs.

Pathology.—The pathological characteristics of fibroma of both the nose and naso-pharynx differ in no essential particular from those of fibromata situated elsewhere and need not be enumerated here.

Diagnosis.—A fibroma may be recognized early in its development by means of the rhinoscope. A small irregularly rounded growth is seen attached to the upper portion of the cavity, giving the appearance as Bosworth says, of "a whitish mass seen through a pinkish veil." The density and mobility of the growth can be ascertained by the index finger introduced behind the soft palate, or by the nasal probe through the anterior nares. Denseness, hardness and slight mobility, together with the rhinoscopic appearances, make the diagnosis certain.

Digital exploration must be conducted with much care, however, as troublesome and even dangerous hæmorrhages have thus been induced. Osteoma and chondroma are the only growths of the upper air passages likely to be mistaken for fibromata. The rhinoscopic appearances of these differ, however, from those of fibroma, and when any doubt exists as to the nature of the growth the needle may be used to test its density. This can often be done through the anterior nares, the parts being previously well exsanguinated by the use of cocaine.

Prognosis.—Fibroma of the naso-pharynx is a very grave and often fatal disease. The fact that there is scarcely any limit to its growth, and that vital organs may be encroached upon, not to speak of the dangerous and even fatal hæmorrhages which may take place during its development and finally the serious nature of the operations, which have hitherto so often been resorted to for its removal, combine to make it a most formidable and serious affection. Nealaton reported one case in a boy, five years old, where the growth invaded the lower pharynx and caused death by asphyxia. Another, where the growth gained access to the cranium through the sphenoid cells, causing also the death of the patient. These cases are both cited by Bosworth, Treat. on the Dis. of Nose and Throat, 1889, Vol I.

Dr. Shrady reported a case in the N. Y. Med. Rec., Sept. 9th, 1882, where the growth sent a prolongation through the foramen lacerum medius. The patient died on the operating table, after resection of the Sup. Max. and the complication was discovered after death.

Fibroma of this region is a disease of youth, seldom occurring after puberty and retrogressive action may set in at this time and result in the complete disappearance of the growth. La Font, Grynfelt, Vimont and Berkett, each has reported a case of spontaneous cure—the two former by absorption—the two latter by sloughing. These cases are so rare that they cannot negative the proposition, that the disease is one of a grave character, as a large proportion of cases have a fatal issue. Bosworth says in the work cited :

"If we carefully examine statistics we find that death results from the operative procedures instituted in more cases than from the growth. These cases would, however, die if not operated upon, and in former times these radical measures, such as removal of the upper jaw, etc., were fully warranted, in that they afforded the only available means of reaching the tumor." "But," he continues, "with the improved methods of the present day by which all affections of the upper-air passages are rendered accessible to operative procedure, we may expect a great falling off in the mortality incident to such operations—we, therefore, must not base our prognosis on cases subjected to the radical operation of opening the face, but upon more recent statistics when the nicer surgical methods were employed." Lincoln reported in the Trans. of the American Laryngological Assoc., for 1883, fifty-eight cases collated, on whom seventy-four operations were done. Thirty-eight operations involved opening the face. Of these thirty-eight severe operations, but ten were cured—fourteen were operated on by gal. caut. Ecraseur and eleven were cured; in three, growths recurred. The milder operations were not done on selected cases. When the growths are large and serious complications have arisen (the reports would indicate) we are often warranted in giving a favorable prognosis if the milder operation is done.·

Treatment.—Hypprocrates, Albucasis, Fabricius, Celcus and other surgeons of ancient times recognized these tumors and used for their removal the ligature, forceps, the hook and other instruments, most of which have fallen into desuetude in the presence of the better instruments of the present day.

Syme and Mott, in 1832, each without the knowledge of the other, made a successful operation by cutting through the Sup. Max. Since that time about thirty different operations, bearing the names of as many surgeons, have been with varying success employed—all cutting operations through the face. The brillant investigation which these facts indicate, attest a universal desire among surgeons to attain better results.

Injections of chlor. zinc, evulsion, the curette, ligation and excission with the knife are all methods applicable to a very limited number of cases, but against all, valid objections may be made, except in *certain* cases.

The potential cautery, in the form of red-hot iron or Paquelins Caut., "gives rise to ill-smelling sloughs, is slow in its action and hence does not commend itself" in the presence of other measures to be mentioned presently.

Electrolysis, suggested by Nealaton in 1864, offers an attractive method of treatment and in view of the success claimed by its advocates, in the treatment of uterine fibroids, there would seem to be no good reason why it should not be as successfully employed in fibromata of the nose and naso-pharynx. There are some cases reported which were successfully treated, but it required from 25 to 100 sittings or more. The tediousness and length of time required for these sittings are serious drawbacks to its popularity. If, however, we could *often* expect a cure, even with the great number of applications of the electrode, it would deserve to be used, as it is usually devoid of danger. But Lincoln, Ingalls and Paquet found it only efficacious in reducing the size of the growth, so that a radial operation could be done ; while Gosselin failed even to get reduction of size. I have had no experience with this method, but removed a growth in one case, where electrolysis had apparently somewhat reduced the size of the tumor.

The chain ecraseur, wire snare or gal. caut. loop, all have their field of usefulness in removing nasal and naso-pharyn-geal growths, but the two last, viz : wire snare and gal. caut. loop, I feel sure are the best means we have at our command for this purpose, where the growth has not attained proportions which make an operation through the face necessary. Of course there will always be some cases where entrance to the growth and its complete extirpation are only possible by cutting through the face in some one of the thirty or more ways laid down by surgeons. In the Trans. of Medico-Chir. Fac. of Md., 1878, p. p. 180-187, will be found the report of a case operated on by Dr. Tiffany, of Baltimore, by the method known as the Cheever's Double Operation. This operation was brilliantly done for naso-pharyngeal fibroma, and was successful. It is to be hoped, however, that in the future (however brilliant the operations) they may become as infrequent as possible. The disfigurement and danger are insurmountable objections to them and only where the wire snare or cautery loop cannot be used should they, in my opinion, be resorted to.

Jarvis' wire snare or some one of its numerous modifications, I believe to be at least equal, if not superior to the gal. caut. loop for the removal of these growths. The great danger to be feared in any of these operations is from hæmorrhage. It is claimed for the caut. loop that this accident is prevented by the heated wire. Bosworth says, the " red-hot wire will not burn through these dense growths readily"—that it requires white heat. It is well known that white heat does not control hæmorrhage, whereas, red heat does.

If three or four hours are taken with the wire snare to sever the growth, hæmorrhage will rarely occur. Facility of adjustment is in favor of the wire-snare, while rapidity of removal (the loop once around the growth) is in favor of the caut. loop. The wire is liable to break in either instrument.

The wire snare should be larger than those kept in instrument stores. Dr. Jake Hartman, of Baltimore, has devised an improvement on Jarvis' snare, where strength and security of attachment of wires, with bar instead of milled nut to tighten loop around growth, make it a useful instrument, but it has one serious fault which was conspicuously brought out in one of the cases I shall report.

Little has been said in the foregoing pages about fibromata occurring within the nasal cavities and little need be added for much that has been said of fibromata of the naso-pharynx applies with equal appropriateness to nasal fibromata. It is worthy of note that they occur much less frequently in this region than in the naso-pharynx, but pursue generally the same relentless course, causing at an earlier stage of their development the facial distortion referred to as "frog-face."

These growths are sessile as a rule, and the great danger in
their removal is hæmorrhage. The best methods of operating generally are by means of the wire-snare or gal. caut.
loop, when a cutting operation through the face is not
required.

Cases one and two of the three cases which follow in the
reports were nasal growths.

Case 1. Mr. M., age 28, lawyer, came to consult me for
nasal catarrh, Jan. 17th, 1887. Inspection revealed a highly
congested pharynx and the rhinoscopic mirror showed the
naso-pharynx and nasal fossæ posteriorly to be in a similar
condition. The turbinates instead of presenting their normal
hue, gray or pinkish-gray, were very red and much engorged.
Anterior illumination and inspection revealed much redness
and tumefaction and there was an appearance of great
hypertrophy of the middle turbinated body on the right
side. For two years he had from time to time been under
the care of one of our most distinguished throat specialists
for his "catarrh" as he said. My patient said he had recently
caught cold and was somewhat hoarse then. I used locally
antiseptic and astringent sprays and gave quin. sulph. internally for a few days. As the acute symptoms seemed to
subside there was observed a muco-purulent discharge,
occasionally streaked with blood from the right nostril. This
he told me had existed for a long time. I noticed no dimu-
nition in the size of the right middle turbinate and probed it
a number of times. It appeared firm and immovable. The
treatment was continued and this muco-purulent secretion
continued, but the general turgessence of the parts became
markedly improved, when at the end of three weeks, in
probing at the middle turbinate again, I observed slight
movement. I at once made the diagnosis of fibroma and
told my patient of the discovery and asked him to come next
morning and have the growth removed. Next A. M. he presented himself at the office, and after cleansing the nasal fossæ with an antiseptic spray and applying a 4 per. ct. sol. of
cocaine I introduced Jarvis's snare, and in one hour completed the operation. The growth was sufficiently pediculated to admit of easy adjustment and retention of the loop

so that at least fifty minutes of the hour were occupied in severing the tumor. Getting the growth out of the nostril after it was separated from its attachment, caused more pain than the operation. The growth was symmetrically ovoidal and about the size of a large pigeon's egg. The growth, when washed, was whitish, dense and hard and undoubtedly composed almost entirely of fibrous tissue. My patient, by my advice, remained at the office half an hour. No bleeding occurred and I let him go. When he had walked eight or ten squares a copious hæmorrhage came on and he went into a drug store and a doctor across the street was called and after some trouble arrested it. Three hours should have been taken to remove the growth. He bled no more and no recurrence of the growth has taken place. I examined him not two weeks since.

The failure to recognize the tumor was due to the fact that the great congestion of the nasal fossæ had imprisoned the growth in a certain position over the middle turbinate and rendered it immovable by the probe, until the astringent sprays relieved this surrounding congestion.

Case No. 2. Mr. M., Hardy Co., Va., age 52, occupation distiller, was brought to me by Dr. G., of the same county, on September 17th, 1890. The man seemed to be suffering from an acute coriza. The voice was nasal, the eyes weeping and intolerant somewhat of light. The nasal passages, naso-pharynx and pharynx were all intensely red, and complete nasal stenosis existed on the right side. The rhinoscopic mirror revealed a white nodular tumor projecting from the middle meatus, right side, about one and a half inches from the post-nasal margins. Anterior illumination with inspection revealed little additional information, as the mucous membrane of the right nasal fossæ were greatly tumified and bathed in serum. Cocaine 10 per cent. sol. had no effect in exsanguinating the parts, and none in producing anæsthesia. The man also sneezed on slight provocation. Under these unfavorable conditions I determined to attempt the removal of the growth with the wire snare. After one hour's unsuccessful efforts to place the loop over the growth I desisted and sent my patient out for some fresh air. When the mirror was placed in position so as to reveal the growth—the snare being in the nasal-fossæ—the least movement of the wire to place it around the tumor induced sneezing. Failure under such circumstances was inevitable.

My patient returned to the office after an hour. In the meantime I had attended a number of cases, thinking all the time how I could relieve this man and send him back to his home in Virginia that night. I tried the forceps with negative results. I then bent a silver nasal probe in the shape of a hook, introduced it, and succeeded in fixing it into or around the growth. I made traction until the probe straightened and came away. I then took an ordinary copper cotton applicator which had not been annealed for a long time, and by means of a strong pair of forceps, fashioned it into a blunt hook. This was introduced and the tumor secured as on the former occasion. Traction and tortion were made until blood flowed freely from the man's mouth and nose. I desisted until the bleeding was arrested by plugging with cotton, when I introduced the hook, caught the tumor and kept up traction and tortion until the growth came away. The growth could be easily recognized as a fibro-mixoma.

I then learned from my patient that for many years one or more neighboring doctors had made many unsuccessful efforts by means of the forceps to remove this growth. The tumor proved this statement. Originally the growth had doubtless been a myxoma, by the numerous wounds it had received from the forceps left scar tissue behind, and each scar acted as a nidus for fibrous degeneration and nearly the entire mass was, at the time of removal, fibrous tissue. This growth was an irregular mass about the size of an English walnut. The custom among many physicians of using the forceps in the nose and attempting the removal of any and every growth is a bad one, and should not be resorted to until other less injurious methods fail.

Bosworth thinks nearly all fibro-myxomota are caused by injury done with instruments.

This case shows that the hook of the old surgeons may still on occasions do what cannot be done by the more fashionable instruments.

Case 3. Mr. F. C. M., of Dorchester County, Md., merchant, age 30, single, was brought to my office by his physician, Dr. J., November 11th, 1889. Patient from earliest recollection had always had one nostril closed, never breathing through both at once an hour at a time in his life. Uninterrupted obstruction of left nostril began about December 15th, 1887, and had continued ever since. The right had gradually become obstructed; but a small amount of air could be forced through it. Hearing of left ear had become impaired. On several occasions patient came near bleeding to death. The foregoing is the substance of the history as given by patient.

Rhinoscopic mirror revealed a symmetrical, ovoidal, sessile tumor, apparently attached to the bassilar process of the occipital bone—filling up the entire naso-pharynx—the apex of the growth reaching below the inferior margin of the posterior nares. Patient was compelled to breathe through his mouth. The color was nearly white, with a superficial pinkish hue. Digital exploration revealed a tumor apparently the size of a small hen egg, dense, but slightly elastic and nearly immovable. The diagnosis of fibroma was made and its removal advised. After the gravity of the affection as well as that of the operation was explained to the patient, he consented to the removal of the growth. The only methods of operating which I held under consideration were by the galvano-cautery loop and cold wire snare. The latter method was, I thought, better adapted to my case.

Jarvis' snare, as modified by Dr. Jake Hartman, of Baltimore, was the instrument used. I proceeded to apply the loop of No. 5 steel wire about the tumor, first spraying the parts with Dobell's sol., and then a 10 per cent. sol. of cocaine. After many unsuccessful efforts to force the loop into the naso-pharynx, first through one nasal fossæ and then the other, I replaced the straight nasal tube of the snare, with the one bent upon itself at right angles, and after some

minutes manipulation succeeded in placing the loop, with the
index finger of the left hand, introduced behind the soft
palate, the right holding the snare in situ, while an assistant,
(Dr. Jones,) by a few turns of the bar, tightened it about the
base of the growth.   About one revolution of the bar was
now made every four minutes for an hour and then half of a
revolution every four minutes for another hour, when the
wire broke.   It broke at its attachment to a steel post, which
is cut half way through, and the wire is bent over same at
right angles, and where a nut screws down upon it to keep it
from slipping.   The wire passes on the outside of the instrument, and when it breaks can often be secured again without
disturbing the loop.   If this accident happens with Jarvis'
snare the loop must be removed as a rule, and the often difficult manipulation of replacing it, repeated.

I had decided to occupy three hours at least in completing the removal of the growth.   After readjusting the
wire, where it broke, I proceeded in the same manner as
above, and at the end of another hour the wire again broke.
I again fastened it, and at the end of four hours from the beginning of the operation the wire again parted—always at the
same point. viz.: where it was bent at right angles over the
post.

The rhinoscopic mirror was now used, and the tumor was
almost black and seemed to be completely strangulated.
The wire was now too short to again fasten and the loop was
removed and the patient allowed to go to his hotel with his
physician and ordered to report at my office next morning,
an antiseptic wash being advised in the meantime.

I fully expected to find next morning a sloughing mass.
On the contrary, the rhinoscopic mirror showed the natural
color restored, somewhat heightened, with here and there
spots of gangrenous tissue.   The patient's condition was excellent, and he was anxious to have the operation completed.
I now took the largest wire that is kept in the instrument
stores, and, after some manipulation, got the loop in good
position, expecting to complete the operation in about three

hours. When this length of time is taken it is rare that hæmorrhage occurs.

After proceeding as before the wire parted in two hours. Twice more the wire broke during a five hours' sitting. The tumor was now black.' The patient was again allowed to go to his hotel in the company of his physician, and next morning when he appeared at my office by appointment, I saw at a glance he was a very sick man. His temp. was 104 and pulse 120. Rhinoscope revealed a sloughing mass, and the odor of decomposition was marked. I now insisted on my patient going to bed, as it was evident the growth was almost entirely necrotic and the man had septic fever. He declined, however, to be governed by my advice, and took the steamer that night (under the intelligent care of his physician), and arrived home next morning. I directed a mercuric chloride wash and quin. sulph. in suitable doses.

I received a telegram a day or two after, asking me to come across the bay to see him, but owing to circumstances, I was compelled to wire my regrets, and Dr. Goldsborough, of Cambridge, Md., was called, at my suggestion.

I subsequently received a letter from Dr. Jones, telling me what was thought to be septicæmia, he believed to have been rheumatism ; that patient was rapidly convalescing, and that the tumor must have nearly or quite sloughed, judging from the re-establishment of nasal breathing, and that our patient was much pleased with the result. I am of the opinion, however, that the fever was septic.

About two months since Mr. M. walked into my office, looking well and breathing quietly through his nose, presenting an appearance in marked contrast to that observed on his first visit.

I seated him at the laryngoscope and found on rhinoscopic examination a small atrophied growth, (the remains of the once formidable fibroma,) about the size of a pigeon's egg. I insisted on removing it, (with an improved snare,) but he declined, saying he was perfectly satisfied with the result.

The successful removal of the growth would have been accomplished at the first sitting I believe, if the instrument

I now show the Society had been available. Hartman's snare will not permit slipping of the wire at a critical juncture in the operation, as so often occurs with Jarvis', but the wire, when it is brought at right angles around the slotted post broke five times during my operation, and this fact is what suggested the improvement which I have made in the instrument.

The instrument which I exhibit is Hartman's, plus something to prevent the wire from breaking—that something being a steel post about ten times the diameter of that used in the Jarvis' snare, and placed in a steel plate, which projects three-quarters of an inch in front of the Hartman device for securing the wire. Around this post the wire may be wrapped once or twice, and the direct tension thus transferred from a sharp, cutting edge to a large curved surface, where the bend in the wire is so gradual that it is as little liable to break here as at any other point.

This is not a great change in the instrument, but one, which, in my judgment, will make all the difference between successful extirpation and failure, when a large dense fibroma is to be removed.

DISCUSSION.

Post-Nasal Obstruction in Children.

This is a subject of the utmost importance. It is wonderful that only in the past fifteen years it has been studied. Meyer, of Copenhagen, was the first to introduce it, in 1875. He called it adenoid growth of the naso-pharynx. The adono-adenoma of the vault of the pharynx is the most common cause. It is generally said that post-nasal obstruction is incompatible with viability of the foetus. It is most common in children from the fourth to the fifth month. Pliny spoke of it. It grows from the vault of the pharynx as a mass of adenoid tissue, called by the Germans the tissue Luschka, although discovered by Schneider. It begins by a proliferation, then small tumors appear, which may hang down in the pharynx like stalactites or bunches of grapes. The papillomatous form of pharyngeal growth is more frequently met with in this part of the country, while in patients from the West and Lake regions it presents the greatest varieties of growth. In Boston the stalactite variety preponderates. In England he found this very common. The diagnosis is sufficiently easy. It may be confused with a fibroma at the vault of the pharynx, but the treatment is the same. Those who do not make the diagnosis with the rhinoscopic mirror may use the finger. It is like touching an earthworm, and if blood is on the finger when withdrawn, those two facts will confirm the diagnosis. He uses the forceps which bear his name. When a child is brought to him with nasal obstruction or with symptoms of non-suppurative otitis media, he introduces these forceps without making a diagnosis and rarely failed to bring away the growth. These growths have a great effect on the child, who breathes through his nose ; his nose becomes flattened and he has a frog face. This facial expression is characteristic. Meyer, of Copenhagen, uses a "Ring-messer," or guillotine-knife, introduced through the nose. The best methods seem to be the forceps. As a rule he does not give anæsthetics. Occasionally the hæmorrhage is very severe.

Dr. B. W. Goldsborough, of Cambridge, in referring to Dr. Merrick's paper, said he had seen one of the patients and he was well.

Dr. Wilmer Brinton asked what was the smallest child operated on by Dr. Mackenzie.

Dr. Mackenzie said he did it to those in arms three or four months. In referring to Dr. Merrick's paper, he said the instrument was apt to break, as it had done once in his case. He said he did the operation every day, and at the Johns Hopkins Hospital in one month he did it 170 times.

Dr. S. K. Merrick said he used Mackenzie's forceps. In one case when he could not reach with the forceps, he used his fingers with success.

On motion, the Faculty adjourned at 1 P. M. to meet at 3 P. M.

AFTERNOON SESSION.

The Faculty was called to order at 3.15 P. M. Dr. Wilmer Brinton read a paper on the subject of "*Prolapse of the Funis*," it was discussed by Drs. W. P. Chunn and B. W. Goldsboro, and referred for publication.

PROLAPSED CORD, WITH REPORT OF A CASE COMPLICATING AN OTHERWISE NORMAL VERTEX PRESENTATION, TREATED BY INTERNAL PODALIC VERSION, FOLLOWED BY ALARMING HÆMORRHAGE FROM A LACERATED CERVIX.

In one thousand cases of obstetrics, I have seen four cases of "prolapsed cord," all complicating vertex presentation. Two of these cases were seen in consultation; auscultation, as well as examination per vaginam, proved the children to be already dead, therefore no operative procedures were instituted. The other two cases occurring in my private practice were under my control from the first. One of them came under my care on the morning of September 7th, of this year, and I mention it only briefly in connection with the case I shall report later on in this paper.

Mrs. F., a German woman, living on Chew street, summoned me at 2 A. M., September 7th, to attend her in her sixth confinement. I arrived at her house at 2.30 o'clock, and upon making a vaginal examination found the cervix dilated and dilatable, the "bag of waters" unruptured, child presenting vertex, and to the left of the child's head I found the pulsating cord presenting. Upon auscutating the mother's abdomen, I found the fœtal heart sounds distinct and clear to the mother's left. I therefore determined to institute no active measures, and waited. In less than thirty minutes I was informed that the "bag of waters" had ruptured, and upon making another vaginal examination I found the cord

prolapsed in front of the presenting part of the child. At
this time I was surprised at the small amount of cord prolapsed. The woman having no pain at this moment, and still
lying on her back, I found no difficulty in pushing up the
cord, then immediately fixing the child's head in the pelvis
by pressure from above, waited anxiously for a "pain,"
which finally came, and within ten minutes and by not more
than six expulsive contractions, a male child was delivered,
crying vigorously. I found the cord around the child's neck
three times, which explained why such a short portion had
prolapsed. This circumstance no doubt was also a factor in
saving the life of the child.

Before relating the case in which I performed podalic version in the interest of the child, I would like to call your attention to the definition, history, causation and treatment of
the complication in question.

Definition.—By "prolapsed cord" is meant that condition
where the cord is found in the vagina or beyond the vulva,
differing from the so-called presentation of the cord, in which
condition the cord is found above the external or internal os,
or still within the uterus, but in the majority a presenting
cord becomes a prolapsed cord. (Winckel.)

Frequency.—It varies seemingly in different localities, notably so in the lying-in hospitals of Europe, Collins having met
it once in 245 cases, while Crede has had it to occur as often
as once in 63 cases. Churchill, of Dublin, collected 98,512
cases of labor in which it occurred 401 times, or in the proportion of 1 to 243 cases. On the other hand, a Mr. Bland,
quoted by Lusk, has met with it only once in 1897 cases.

Causation.—This complication occurs only in cases in
which the presenting part does not completely occlude the
lower uterine segment. This condition is caused by very
different circumstances, and any defect which prevents the
lower segment of the uterus from having uniformly regular
contractions, may be a factor in causing a prolapsed cord.
Among the recognized causes are pelvic anomalies. Winckel
has proved by actual measurement in 55 cases of prolapsed
cord, that 40 per cent. occur in narrow pelves. Faulty state

of the uterus, especially faulty shape, faulty position and faulty contractions, favor prolapse of the funis. Myomata of the uterus, pendulous abdomen, faulty engagement and presentation of the fœtus, especially footling and transverse presentations; it is also favored by multiparity, multiple pregnancies, hydramnios, excessive length and other anomalies of the cord, anomalies of placenta previa.

Winckel, in analyzing a number of cases of prolapsus of the cord, says: "It will be easy to prove that it was not a single predisposing factor alone, but that, as a rule, several of them have co-operated, and this, too, in the most varied combination.

Diagnosis.—When a loop of the cord has slipped down and is found to present in the os uteri alongside of or in advance of the presenting part, a thorough examination will readily discover it, and it will be found to pulsate more or less vigorously when the child is living. Still, the absence of the pulsation does not always mean the death of the child, for Spiegelberg has demonstrated, to his own satisfaction at least, that in some cases the child's heart continues to beat for a few minutes after the circulation in the cord has ended. Then, one may be deceived by examining the patient during a pain, at which time no pulsation can be detected, yet the pulsation in the cord may return in the interval between the pains.

Prognosis.—So far as regards the children, it is extremely unfavorable, but it depends, to some extent, however, on the time at which the case is seen, and if proper assistance be given. Engelman found that of 365 cases of prolapsus of the cord, 171 children (or 48.7 per cent.) were saved, and therefore 52.3 per cent. succumbed, 71 per cent. being saved in footling presentations, 70 per cent. in breech and only 36.7 per cent. in vertex. In the four cases coming under my notice, two of the children were dead when the mothers were first examined. In the other two cases efforts were made to save the life of the children, resulting in saving one child and the delivery of the other, partially asphyxiated, and which, if proper efforts at resuscitation could have been continued, would have lived. The ,results have been, therefore, in the four cases which I have seen in practice, 75 per cent. mortality. Yet in the cases treated the mortality has been 50 per cent. The enormous fatality attending prolapse of the cord is caused by the pressure to which the cord is subjected during the passage of the child through the pelvis. Death of the child, according to Winckel, generally results from suffocation and apoplexy combined, according as the circulation is interrupted quickly or slowly, at a time when the heart still preserves its full energy.

Treatment.—The one indication for treating this comparatively rare complication of an otherwise normal labor, is to relieve the cord from pressure. All authorities agree that, as a rule, the best results are obtained by reposition of the cord, still Lusk has truly said "the conduct of the physician in each individual case will depend upon the presentation and the modifying circumstances."

If reposition fails, then version in the interest of the child should be performed. In the majority of cases reposition of the cord should be first attempted, being a mild procedure, but too much time should not be lost in fruitless efforts to replace the cord. The methods of reposition are those of Thomas— the knee and chest position, with the aid of the hand, and the various instruments that have been devised for the same purpose, and which are, as a rule, worse than useless, even if they be at hand in the emergency. Lusk, in his last book, in describing Gaillard Thomas' method, "Postural Treatment of Prolapsed Funis," says: "By this method the simple plan of reversing the direction of the uterine axis, all the conditions which had previously favored the descent of the cord are made to promote its return into the uterine cavity. Thus the intra-abdominal pressure is removed, the amniotic fluid is retained, the head is easily pushed to one side so as to permit the introduction of the hand, and the cord tends to glide by its own weight over the declivity furnished by the anterior wall to the fundus. The prolapsed loop should be seized in the hollow of the hand, and should be carefully sheltered from pressure. It should go beyond the greatest circumference of the head, and, when possible, to the back of the child's neck. As in all cases where the hand has to be passed through the cervix, the uterus should be sustained by pressure from without; with the advent of a pain all manipulations should cease, to be renewed, however, as relaxation follows. If the replacement prove successful, the hand should be withdrawn gradually, while the head becomes fixed in the lower segment: this latter result may frequently be expedited by judiciously directed external pressure. This method so thoroughly described meets with Lusk's approval, but can not always be carried out, and if in a given case the cervix is almost or quite fully dilated, the head still high up, and the pelvis not greatly narrowed, while the lessened pulsations of the cord indicate danger to the child, direct internal version with subsequent extraction is indicated. If the cervix admits but one or two fingers, the child being still movable, its head high up, and the pelvis little if any contracted, combined version according to Braxton Hicks, should be performed.

The case of "prolapsed cord" which I report in full occurred in June, 1889, and is as follows : Mrs. E. R. P., aged 24, engaged me to attend her in her fourth confinement which was expected to take place in the early part of June, 1889. I had attended Mrs. P., in her three previous confinements. Her first child was born previous to the completion of her seventeenth year ; after her labor a physical examination revealed a unilateral laceration of the cervix and an enlarged uterus. As her labor had been a perfectly normal one, this condition of affairs I believed to be due to lack of care during the *lying-in-period* on the part of the patient ; among other indiscreet things done during this period was to go to the opera with her husband before her child was three weeks old, walking there and back, the distance being over one mile. Declining any operative procedure she resumed her usual household duties. During the next four years she conceived twice and carried her children to full term, nothing worthy of note occurring, but profiting by previous experience she took better care of herself during her lying-in-period on both occasions. I was summoned at 4.30 P. M., June 7th, to attend Mrs. P., in her fourth confinement, found upon my arrival she was just beginning to have her labor pains. The os dilating and dilatable, child presenting vertex, and the fœtal heart sounds could be heard very distinctly to the mother's left. I remained in the room of my patient for a short time, and saw that labor was progressing, advised her during this stage to keep out of bed, and left, promising to return about 7 o'clock, requesting to be telephoned for if needed sooner. Having heard nothing from her and having been detained in my office, it was after 8 o'clock before I visited her again. Upon entering her room I found her in bed, and having decided expulsive pains, I was informed that the "bag of waters" had broken some twenty minutes previously, and since that time her pains had been more decided in character. Upon making a vaginal examination, I found, to my surprise, the head well in the pelvis and the cord prolapsed about six inches, as far as I could decide. I kept my fingers on the loop for a short time and found no pulsation during the pains and very feeble pulsations in the interval between the pains. I then immediately examined for the fœtal heart sound, and found it very indistinct in comparison with the examination made on my first visit. I then spent a minute or two (the woman being in the knee elbow position,) in efforts to replace the prolapsed cord, but seemingly my efforts to replace it increased the expulsive efforts of the uterus, and finding that I was not succeeding in my attempt at reposition, I determined at once to turn in the interest of the child. Having no time to send for an assistant, I gave the woman chloroform and proceeded to perform version. I at first brought down one foot, but found some difficulty in turning. I therefore brought down the second foot, and without much traction the breech and trunk of the child, but the head was detained by the cervix. After considerable pulling, I delivered a large male child, asphyxiated, but which gave some evidence of life after efforts on my part at resuscitation. I was unfortunately not able to continue these efforts, for my attention was drawn to the large amount of blood coming from the mother. She was having an alarming hæmorrhage, the source of which was not clear to me for a short time. I found the uterus well contracted, and the after-birth was at once delivered by Crede's method. Ergot was given by the mouth and hypodermically, the uterus still well contracted, but the hæmorrhage continued. At one time I thought the patient was dying, so great was the amount of blood lost. During this time I had explored the cavity of the uterus with my fingers, and finding no cause for hæmorrhage there, and that organ being most of the time well contracted, I determined the source of the hæmorrhage to be the cervix, which had been lacerated in my efforts to extract the head of the child. I immediately tamponed the vagina with towels, the only material I had at hand, with the effect of controlling the hæmorrhage. This permitted me to give some attention to the child, but no efforts at this time on my part could make it manifest any evidence of life.

I am thoroughly satisfied that if any competent assistant had continued efforts at resuscitating it from the time of birth, its life would have been saved. The mother, from the effects of chloroform, loss of blood, and shock of operative procedure, was in a very bad condition for twenty-four hours. Finally she rallied, and after a protracted lying-in period recovered. A recent examination confirms a previous examination that the patient, Mrs. P., has a bilateral laceration of the cervix, with a large subinvoluted uterus, but she declines with a persistency "worthy of a better cause" all operative procedures.

DISCUSSION.

Dr. W. P. Chunn, asked what the hæmorrhage was from in Dr. Brinton's cases.

Dr. B. W. Goldsborough, of Cambridge, said he had a case of this kind. He tried to stop the hæmorrhage in vain. Everything failed until he applied turpentine to the fundus of the uterus and all bleeding stopped.

Dr. Brinton said in the case reported, there was no doubt that the source of the hæmorrhage was from the lacerated cervix. In regard to the treatment of "prolapsed cord," he insisted upon prompt and decided treatment, and advised very short delay in attempts to replace the cord, and would advise version in the interest of the child in the vast majority of cases.

Dr. W. S. Gardner said such cases were very difficult to treat and needed prompt attention.

Dr. J. C. Clarke of Federalsburg, Md., produced a patient with obscure diagnosis simulating chronic anæmia. He was examined by Prof. Osler and others. Arsenic was recommended in large doses.

Dr. W. S. Gardner read a paper on "*The Relation of Albuminuria to Puerperal Eclampsia.*" The subject was discussed by Drs. Preston and Osler, and the paper ordered to be published.

THE RELATION OF ALBUMINURIA TO PUERPERAL ECLAMPSIA.

It has not been the object of the writer of this paper to speculate concerning the causes of either albuminuria or eclampsia, but to record a few observations that have some bearing upon the prognosis in cases of albuminuria during pregnancy, and also upon the possibility of the prediction of puerperal eclampsia. The observations include a report of the percentage of cases of albuminuria discovered in one hundred and eighty pregnant and parturient women taken consecutively, and an abstract of the records of the cases of eclampsia occurring within the selected period.

The patients whose urine was examined were confined at the Maternite Hospital, Baltimore, between April 1, 1889, and August 1, 1890. The examinations of urine were made by Drs. Todd and Allen, resident physicians. The heat-test and the nitric-acid test, being undoubtedly the best tests for practical purposes, were used. The figures represent the volume of coagulated albumin which settled to the bottom of a test-tube, after a test-tube full of urine had been acidified with acetic acid, boiled, allowed to cool, and left to stand twenty-four hours, as compared with the quantity of urine boiled. Where a "trace" is recorded, it means a quantity that could have been easily detected by anyone reasonably expert in urinary analysis.

The urine of each patient was examined soon after admission, and where albumin was once found, or where there were indications that it was likely to be found, the urine was examined repeatedly up to the time of labor. Patients who were admitted to the Hospital while in labor were necessarily exceptions to this rule. Urine from all patients was examined on the first and eighth days after labor.

Quantity of albumin found.

No.	Before labor.	1st day after labor.	8th day after labor.	No. of child.
1.	o	$\frac{1}{16}$	o	1st
2.	o	$\frac{1}{16}$	o	4th
3.	$\frac{1}{16}$	$\frac{1}{8}$		1st
4.	—	$\frac{1}{16}$	o	2d
5.	in labor $\frac{1}{4}$	$\frac{1}{16}$	o	3d
6.	—	$\frac{1}{16}$	trace	5th
7.	o	o	$\frac{1}{16}$	2d
8.	trace	o	o	1st
9.	—	o	trace	1st
10.	$\frac{1}{8}$	$\frac{1}{8}$	$\frac{1}{8}$	2d
11.	o	$\frac{1}{16}$	o	2d
12.	o	$\frac{1}{8}$	o	1st
13.		o	$\frac{1}{16}$	1st
14.		o	trace	1st
15.			$\frac{1}{8}$	2d
16.			trace	1st
17.	—		trace	1st
18.	trace	o	o	2d
19.	o	o	trace	1st
20.	$\frac{1}{4}$	$\frac{1}{4}$	$\frac{1}{4}$	3d
21.	o	$\frac{1}{4}$	o	1st
22.	o	trace	o	1st
23.	trace	o	o	2d
24.	o	o	$\frac{1}{8}$	3d
25.	o	$\frac{1}{4}$ in labor	—	1st
26.	o	$\frac{1}{16}$	o	1st
27.	$\frac{1}{16}$	$\frac{1}{4}$	—	1st
28.	o	o	trace	1st .
29.	—	trace	o	4th
30.		trace	o	2d
31.		$\frac{1}{3}$	trace	1st
32.		trace	trace	1st
33.		trace	o	1st
34.	o	o	trace	1st
35.	o	trace	$\frac{1}{16}$	1st
36.	$\frac{1}{8}$	trace	o	1st
	8	22	17	

34 of the 180 cases were in labor when admitted, so that it was not possible to examine their urine before labor. In the urine of the 146 cases examined, albumin was found eight times, or in about 5½ per cent. The urine from all cases was examined within twenty-four hours after labor, and albumin was found twenty-two times, or in about 12¼ per cent. The urine from 177 cases was examined on the eighth day, and albumin found seventeen times, or in about 9½ per cent. Taking the whole 180 cases, albumin was found one or more times in the urine of 36, or in 20 per cent. 96 of the patients were primipare ; of these albumin was found in the urine of 22, or in 23 per cent. 84 were multipare ; of these, 14, or 16⅔ per cent., had albumin in their urine one or more times.

Included in the 180 cases were 4 who had convulsions. This proportion is much greater than is ordinarily found ; the rate, as is well known, being usually about 1 case of convulsions in 500 pregnancies.

The following notes are abstracts of the records of the cases as kept by Dr. William J. Todd and Dr. Samuel H. Allen, resident physicians at the Maternite :

CASE No. 1487, aged twenty, primipara, was admitted to the hospital March, 28, 1889. Her urine was examined repeatedly before labor, and was always found to have a very low specific gravity, but perfectly free from albumin.

She was delivered at 4:40 A. M., May 25, 1889. Between 3:55 P. M. and 9 P. M. she had fourteen convulsions. From May 26th to May 30th inclusive, she had numerous convulsions and passed large quantities of urine involuntarily, which upon examination was found to contain no albumin. She died at 9:40 A. M., May 30th.

The autopsy was held next morning by Dr. N. G. Keirle. A small area of the lower lobe of each lung was in the first stage of pneumonia. The kidneys were small, flat, and lobulated. The other organs were found normal. Dr. Keirle gave the opinion that the cause of death was chronic interstitial nephritis.

CASE No. 1595, aged twenty-three, primipara, was admitted to the hospital, January 4, 1890. A specimen of her urine was examined January 11th, with the following result: specific gravity 1020; acid reaction to litmus; no albumin. Since she had no edema of the limbs, no headache nor other symptoms pointing to a possible derangement of the kidneys, her urine was not again examined.

At 12:30 A. M., January 25th, she had a convulsion, which was followed by twelve more before 2:15 A. M. Early in the forenoon labor came on spontaneously. There were no more convulsions until 7 P. M., when she had one which was followed by a second at 9 P. M. A few minutes after nine she was delivered by short forceps of a dead child weighing six pounds. At 7:45 the convulsions again returned. She died at 12:55 A. M., January 27th, forty-eight hours after the first convulsion.

After the first convulsions some urine was drawn from the bladder, and the examination gave the following result: specific gravity 1012; albumin ¼ volume. The next day at noon the urine was again examined; specific gravity 1020; albumin ⅝ volume.

The kidneys were examined post-mortem, and found to be very much congested, but the changes had not gone sufficiently far to say that they were inflamed.

CASE No. 1624, aged nineteen, primipara, was admitted to the hospital March 12, 1890. She gave a history of having had dropsy subsequent to scarlet fever when a child. The urine was examined March 14th; specific gravity 1020; acid reaction to litmus; no albumin.

One week afterward she complained of headache and sleeplessness, and her extremities were edematous. Analysis of her urine revealed a trace of albumin. Her bowels were kept moving with saline cathartics, and she drank potassium bitartrate lemonade during the daytime. Under this treatment her headache disappeared entirely, she slept well and was bright and cheerful. Her urine was examined March 21st, April 5th, 8th, 10th, and 19th. At each examination a small quantity, never more than 1-16 volume, of albumin was found.

Labor began about 9 A. M., April 25th. It progressed slowly, but there was nothing unusual until the next morning at 9:25, the labor then being in the second stage, when she had a convulsion. Chloroform was given and she was promptly delivered. After the effect of the chloroform passed off she was perfectly rational and said she felt much better.

After the convulsion her urine was examined and ¼ volume of albumin was found, or four times as much as the largest quantity present at any previous examination.

During the afternoon she had a number of convulsions. After 8 o'clock that evening there was complete suppression of urine. She died at 2:05 A. M., April 27th.

No post-mortem examination was allowed.

CASE No. 1658, aged thirty-eight, primipara, was admitted to the hospital June 9, 1890. Her feet were slightly swollen. Examination of her urine showed, specific gravity 1010; acid reaction to litmus ; no albumin.

She was given a saline cathartic and potassium bitartrate-lemonade.

Her labor began about 1 P. M., June 13th, and was completed at 2 A. M. of the 14th. After she was put into bed she said she felt well except a slight headache. At 5:15 A. M. she had a convulsion, followed by a second at 5:45 A. M. At half-past six four ounces of a dark-colored urine were drawn off and analyzed ; specific gravity 1028; acid reaction to litmus; ⅔ volume albumin. At 9 A. M. she had a third convulsion. She was kept under the influence of chloral and the convulsions did not return.

Her urine was examined subsequently with the following results :

Date.	Specific Gravity.	Reaction.	Albumin.
June 15	1026	Acid.	None.
" 16	1024	"	"
" 17	1026	"	Trace.
" 18	1032		None.
" 19	1030		"
" 20	1030		"
" 21	1028		

The following case, although it occurred at the Maternite, is not included in the list of 180, because she was not confined until after that list was completed; but I report it because of its bearing upon the subject.

CASE No. 1682, aged eighteen, primipara, was admitted to the hospital August 2, 1890. The result of the analysis of her urine before labor was: specific gravity 1028; acid reaction to litmus; a trace of albumin.

Her labor began about 9 P. M., August 19th, and progressed favorably until 11:40 P. M., when she became suddenly unconscious and was immediately seized with a convulsion lasting about one minute. This was quickly followed by two more convulsions—the patient being perfectly rational in the intervals. A catheter was passed at once and some urine was drawn. Analysis of this specimen showed: specific gravity 1010; acid reaction to litmus; and no albumin.

She was delivered of a living child at 1:16 A. M., August 20th. She had seven more convulsions within the sixteen hours immediately following delivery.

The following are the results of further examinations of her urine:

Date.	Specific Gravity.	Reaction.	Albumin.
August 20	1012	Acid.	Trace.
" 21	1022	"	None.
" 23	1024	"	"
25	1030		"
" 27	1024	"	Trace.

Briefly reviewing these cases we find that case No. 1487 was under observation almost two months, and though her urine was examined frequently a low specific gravity was always found, but never a trace of albumin. There was no headache, no edema, nothing but the low specific gravity to indicate that the patient was not in perfect health; yet, within less than twelve hours after labor, she began to have convulsions which continued until she died. These convulsions were not of the type usually observed, but resembled more closely the convulsions of hysteria—her body and limbs being thrown into the most grotesque contortions. Her urine was repeatedly examined, both before and after the convulsions set in, but no albumin was found at any time.

CASE No. 1595 was under observation three weeks before confinement. No albumin was found in her urine before the accession of the convulsions, and there were no symptoms that gave warning of impending danger. After the first convulsions her urine was examined and found to contain ¼ volume of albumin. The next day, there having been a number of convulsions in the interval, her urine was again examined, and found to contain ⅝ volume of albumin, or more than double the quantity of the previous day.

CASE No. 1624 gave a history that pointed to the probability that she had suffered from parenchymatous nephritis subsequent to scarlet fever. Under these circumstances her urine was examined with great care. The first examination showed a perfectly normal urine; a number of other examinations before labor each revealed a small quantity of albumin. During the second stage of labor she had a convulsion. Her urine was examined and found to contain ¼ volume of albumin. Later, there was complete suppression of urine.

CASE No. 1658 was under observation four days before labor. Analysis of her urine gave no trace of albumin. More than three hours after delivery she had a convulsion, which was followed in half an hour by a second. One hour and a quarter after the first convulsion, analysis of her urine showed ⅓ volume of albumin. Her urine was examined each day for one week after the convulsions, and a trace of albumin found only once.

Unfortunately, the urine from case No. 1682 was examined but once before labor, when a trace of albumin was found. As soon as the convulsions appeared a catheter was passed and some urine drawn off, which must have been secreted before the convulsions came on. It was examined and found to contain no albumin. Several hours afterward her urine was again examined, and the presence of a small quantity of albumin ascertained. Within the following week her urine was examined four times, and a trace of albumin found but once.

To make the statement general: In a series of 180 consecutive cases, 5½ per cent. were shown to have albumin in their urine before labor, and more than 12 per cent. of them the first day after labor. Included in this series were four patients who were attacked by convulsions. Of the four, in only one case was the presence of albumin detected before labor; in three cases there was a large quantity of albumin present soon after the convulsions; in one case there was never any albumin present, and in one there was no albumin present twenty-four hours after the convulsions.

Elliot reports, in his "Obstetric Clinic," ten cases of puerperal convulsions, the urine from each of which was examined before the convulsions came on. In these, albumin was discovered four times, and its absence was ascertained six times. In three cases there was no albumin in the urine either before or after the convulsions.

In connection with the above cases, are reported seven others of marked albuminuria, four of which died, but none of which had any convulsions.

Or, to put it in another way, he records eleven well-marked cases of albuminuria, only four of which had convulsions; and, on the other hand, there were six cases of convulsions where the urine was examined, but no albumin and no other signs of kidney lesions were discovered before the appearance of the convulsions.

If we add these to the ones already related we have a total of fifteen cases of puerperal convulsions. The urine from each case was analyzed before the convulsions .appeared. Albumin was found six times, and it was not found nine times.

The number of cases here presented is too small from which to draw any definite conclusions; but if we are allowed to consider these to be average cases we are warranted in drawing the following conclusions :

1. The presence of albumin in the urine of a pregnant woman is no sufficient cause upon which to base a prognosis of probable eclampsia.

2. The failure to find albumin in the urine of a pregnant woman is no evidence of the absence, or, at least, of the con-

tinuance of the absence of the condition that gives rise to puerperal convulsions.

3. Albumin is so frequently found in considerable quantities in the urine of patients immediately after the appearance of puerperal convulsions, that we are justified in making the statement that the convulsions are the probable cause of the albuminuria.

DISCUSSION.

Dr. Brinton was much pleased with this paper. He thought that if we could collect a large number of cases much more than presented in this paper, we should be warranted in drawing conclusions as he has done. We cannot always look to the kidney lesion as the cause of death.

Dr. G. J. Preston thought that some lesion of the central nervous system might cause the trouble.

Dr. Osler said that in Montreal he had made the autopsies for ten years, and that in not a single instance were the kidneys in such cases found normal, except one case, which showed an immense cranial hæmorrhage, the clot extending from the third to the fourth ventricle of the brain.

Dr. Gardner thinks this experience rather exceptional.

Dr. Preston asked if the women were systematically examined in each instance.

Dr. Gardner said that the urine was examined in a routine manner in each case, and was done with average care. The object of these urinary examinations was to see if the prognosis of eclampsia could be made before pregnancy.

Dr. Robt. W. Johnson read a paper on "*The Surgical Treatment of Non-pyæmic Abscess of the Liver.*" The paper was discussed by Dr. Randolph Winslow, Dr. Osler and Dr. G. J. Preston, and referred.

The Surgical Treatment of Non-pyæmic Abscess of the Liver, with Report of a Case.

Nothing impresses you more with the immense wealth of medical writing than the volumes that present themselves for recognition, when you map out the simplest subject for study or description. At first thought you might feel that abscess of the liver is not a very comprehensive subject, but I can assure you, you would have to write a book as large as Frerichs did on the whole liver to give a full detail of the etiology—symptomatology, relations of hepatic abscess to lesions of the intestinal tract as dysentery, or worms or its still more intricate relation to fractures of the skull, accidents, etc. Writers vie with each other in adding their mite to the general store, whether that mite bear on the causes or the cure of the disease. Have no fear however, I do not intend to rehearse to you the questions that have already been settled, or to ask your judgment on those still in doubt. I shall leave all but a very narrow selection to your careful study in your closet, and only ask your attention for a few moments to the very practical point of the surgical treatment of hepatic abscess; report a fatal case of my own, illustrating a late discovery in the microbic side of the subject which may or may not have escaped your notice, and which may or may not have practical relation to the future treatment.

The first element in surgical treatment is a correct diagnosis. This we obtain indirectly from the history of the case, a previous dysentery, residence in tropical or malarial climate, etc., chills perhaps, jaundice perhaps, though not a usual accompaniment, fluctuation, very deceptive and unreliable, at best not necessarily indicating the presence of pus, temperature chart, etc., all throwing a sort of twilight on the diagnosis, but not to be mentioned in comparison with the clinching story of the aspirator and the sight, not the feel—nor the suspicion of pus. What the sound striking the stone is to the lithotomist the aspirator is to the hepatotomist; without its tell-tale thrust we are uncertain, with it we have a safe (in all human probability, though Goodlee reports a fatal case in a bleeder) simple and conclusive guarantee that we are dealing with an abscess.

Suppose an abscess is found, can we afford to leave it to its own or nature's care? Not in most cases. A few may be absorbed, quite a number form adhesions and unless they break internally do so outside of the abdominal wall, but the risk is great and the history of abscess emptying into lung, pericardium, kidney, intestine, peritoneum, stomach or any neighboring organ show with the death rate of each that we should not trust to such blind luck, if our patient confides in us as scientific surgeons.

Between the abscess pointing through the abdominal wall with firm adhesions, which the merest tyro could open with a lancet, to the deep seated abscess threatening another organ, there is every grade of difficulty requiring every measure of scientific acumen in their treatment; and in these latter cases we need information from all sources. What does the exploring needle teach?

1, Presence of Pus. 2, Nature of Pus. 3, Direction. 4, Depth of abscess. 5, Thickness of wall and parieties. 6, Presence of adhesions by its mobility, during respiration; but diagnosis completed, the aspirator's function ceases, and should seldom be employed in treatment, for by its use the drainage is capricious, and not constant, and the presence of a metal tube of so small a calibre as an exploring trocar canula would be irritating and ineffective.

In cases where we may be sure adhesions exist, and the abscess shows a tendency toward pointing in the abdominal wall, the method recommended by Stephen Smith is good, who introduces a good sized drainage tube through the canula of the trocar and splitting the end of tube projecting, secures it with thread and sticking plaster, after he has withdrawn the trocar. This method would suit all cases except for the danger of pus innoculation in the peritoneum from the leakage along the side of the drainage tube which is necessarily smaller then the canula by which the opening into the liver is made.

In cases where there is no sign of adhesion between the abdominal wall and the liver, two principal methods for operation present, if we do not class such vain attempts as

blisters in the rational category.   The first or two stage operation where adhesions are artificially constructed rather
more rapidly than when nature is left to build her own barriers
alone, may be described as follows:—"This operation, based
on the readiness with which two peritoneal surfaces adhere is
a very satisfactory one, being free from risks of escape of
blood or other fluids into the peritoneal cavity.   An incision
four inches long was made through the abdominal wall
about two inches to the right of the median line, from just
below the ribs to the line of the umbilicus, and bleeding being
carefully stopped, the peritoneum was picked up and slit
open.   The liver recognizable by its characteristic color was
at once seen moving with respiration.   To make certain of
the position of the fluid a fine trocar was now thrust in, one
or two carbolized sponges being first inserted, any leakage
was stopped by sponge pressure, the parietal peritoneum was
stitched to the edges of the wound by a few points of
chromic gut suture, the sponges removed and dry gauze dressings firmly bandaged on with a good deal of pressure, so as
to keep the abdominal wall as far as possible in contact with
the liver.   On the third day the operation was completed by
incising the liver, now well adherent and inserting a large
drainage tube."   Surgical operations—Jacobson, p. 705.

The one stage method particularly championed by Tait,
whose opinion is a host in itself, may be described as follows :

" The parts being cleaned and the other preliminary steps
taken, the surgeon makes an incision about four inches long
on the most prominent part of the swelling, previously carefully percussed, down to the peritoneum ; all hæmorrhage is
next arrested and this layer carefully slit up.   The liver is
now recognized, and carbolized sponges or towels are carefully packed in on either side so as to prevent any escape of
fluid into the peritoneal cavity.   The needle of an aspirator
or a fine trocar is then thrust in, and the existence of fluid
beneath thus verified.   As the needle is withdrawn, the liver
is incised, and a finger quickly plugs and then enlarges to
1½ inches the opening made by the knife.   Hæmorrhage if
free is easily arrested thus by sponge pressure.   Escape of

fluids into the peritoneum is prevented by the use of the sponges already mentioned, by an assistant keeping the edges of the wound carefully adjusted to the liver, and lastly by the next step, which consists in hooking up the opening in the liver with the finger or forceps, and in stitching the edges of the wound in the liver to that of the abdomen with a continuous suture of carbolized silk. In inserting this, care must be taken to unite peritoneum to peritoneum, and to take up a sufficiency of tissue by inserting the needle well away from the edges of the wound. As the suture is inserted the sponges must be gradually withdrawn, and if the fluid escapes very freely, it may be well to turn the patient over on his side.

"Any escape of pus into the peritoneal cavity is prevented (1) by the careful sponge packing; (2) by the finger hooking up the liver against the wound; (3) by an assistant keeping steadily the parietes against the liver; (4) by seizing the edges of the liver with catch forceps, and so keeping them against the parietes. Hæmorrhage is prevented by the above forceps or sponge pressure. When the abscess is empty its opening is plugged with a sponge, and the liver and the parietes being still accurately together, the sponges first inserted are removed and the edges of the liver stitched with carbolized silk, passed with curved needles on a holder to the edges of the abdominal incision, care bring taken to keep peritoneal surfaces well in contact. If the pus is fetid, the abscess cavity should be well washed with a deluted aseptic solution. A considerable thickness of dry gauze dressings will be needed at first, easily renewed by means of a many tailed bandage." (loc. cit p. 707-709.) Comparing the two, the operation in two stages appears to be the safer. Nature's barriers protect the peritoneum, and though we speak of two stages, the final introduction of a drainage tube into the abscess after the liver has been exposed, is so simple a procedure that it does not rank with the primary incisions and stitching as an operation. The walls of the abscess tend to collapse after emptying and it seems to me it would require much greater care to prevent peritoneal infection in a wound when chinks might exist between stitches just put in, than in a wound whose chinks have all been closed by four days old lymph. If you can afford the four days wait, I would recommend the two stage operation. The drainage tube should remain until all discharge ceases, all medical means kept up to preserve the patient's strength, who at best will have a tough fight before him.

Permit me now to report a case of hepatic abscess, I have just had.

J. M., 40 years old.—White, married, born in England, been in America several years, was admitted to St. Joseph's Hospital, Baltimore, September 22nd, 1890, suffering from malarial or "bilious" dysentery, contracted while laboring in a malarial locality near the city. Prior to entrance he had been having chills, fever, and suffering with general malaise for three weeks.

His stools were painful, frequent, bloody and not copious nor otherwise abnormally colored, but very liquid. His temperature was not markedly high, varying from 101° to 103° F., with evening exacerbations until near the close of his illness. Two days before his death it ran up to 107° falling rapidly to 100°. Chills, at first with the characteristic regularity of malaria, in spite of the ten grains of quinia every three hours, became less frequent, and in the mid-period of his illness he was well enough to be about the ward and seemed on the way to recovery. Irregular chills set in with debilitating sweats about ten days prior to his death, which with pain in the right hypochondrium, not in shoulder, drew my attention to what I then considered a beginning hepatic abscess. All the while there was more or less irritation about the rectum which was best relieved by starch and laudanum injections after the bowel had been thoroughly washed out with a strong solution of boracic acid. On October 25th, he passed per rectum, while having a stool, about three pints of clotted blood, and hæmorrhage more or less profuse, kept up until the day of his death. On October 27th, I aspirated his liver which was enlarged and projected three inches below the margin of the ribs, but showed no tendency to point exter- nally and drew out six ounces of a creamy, gelatinous or syrup-like whitish pus, with no marked traces of blood in it, and had his condition warranted, I would have done hepatotomy in two stages as described above. He sank, becoming weaker and weaker, and died at 2 A. M., October 28th, having been in hospital thirty-six days. I considered, prior to the post mortom, his death due to protracted Hæmorrhage in a patient already debilitated by malarial dysentery, and the presence of abscess of the liver. I append the post-mortem report of Dr. Councilman, which shows a very important feature had been overlooked, namely the pneumonia. I confess I was surprised at the discovery, though I anticipated possible metastatic abscess in the lung. There were no symptoms during life which called my attention primarily to his chest, and I fancied he had enough trouble below his diaphragm to account for his illness and death. Dr. Councilman thinks that had he not had pneumonia he might have survived an operation.

Autopsy made on J. M. at St. Joseph's Hospital—Service of Dr. Johnson—Autopsy, Oct. 29, 12 M.

Diagnosis—Acute croupous pneumonia (grey hepatization) lower lobe left lung, acute pleurisy same place. *Abscess of liver following dysentery. Dysenteric ulceration of large intestine.* Fatty degeneration of heart and kidneys. *Erosion of small vein in transverse colon.*

Body, that of a tall, well built man, about 170 C. M. long—muscular, somewhat emaciated. Skin and mucous membranes pale. Post-surface of body slightly congested. Rigor mortis marked. On right side of the abdomen in line of nipple 1 C. M. below the margin of ribs is a small punctured wound (aspiration needle).

Subcutaneous fat slight in amount, muscles red.

Lungs—Right lung free from adhesions, anterior borders of both lungs in contact. The upper and middle lobe of right lung very emphysematous, lower lobe of same œdematous.

Upper lobe of left lung emphysematous. Almost the entire lower lobe consolidated—cut surface greyish white. A puriform fluid exudes on pressure. Nearly all this part of lung sinks in water.   Pleura over this lobe covered with a thin fibrinous exudation.

Heart in diastole.   Both sides contain fluid blood and soft partially decolorized clots, myocardium soft, flaccid, of pale brown color—coronary arteries normal.

Diaphragm on the right side at the lower border of 4th rib.   Liver in nipple line 8 C. M. below rib margin, in the median line 11 C. M. below the ensiform cartilage.   The liver is firmy adherent to the diaphragm over a space 9 C. M. in diameter commencing 1 C. M. above the ribs in nipple line.   Just below this adhesion there is a furrow 1 C. M. deep, extending downwards and backwards across the right lobe of liver.   There is a large abscess cavity in the right lobe of liver beneath the adhesions with the diaphragm.   At the adhesions there seems to be no liver tissue about the abscess. The abscess is 15 C. M. in diameter and contains a thin bloody fluid in the centre of the cavity.   This is surrounded by a mass of thick gelatinous looking pus containing masses of necrotic tissue.   The wall of the abscess of dark greyish necrotic tissue, not stained with bile.   In most places there is a sharp line of demarkation between the abscess and the surrounding liver tissue.   Here and there the abscess' wall extends down into the liver—liver elsewhere is very pale and soft.   The gall bladder contains a small amount of clear yellow bile.   The bile duct is open.   Portal vein and contents, normal.   Spleen of light brown color, softer than normal.

Pancreas and supra-renal capsules normal.

Kidneys large, very pale capsules easily stripped off.   In the cortex small yellowish diffuse foci.

Stomach and small intestines normal.   Mucous membrane of stomach softened from post mortem digestion.

The large intestine contracted.   Its mucous membrane contains numerous ulcers of various shapes and dimensions. In the beginning of the ascending colon they are most numerous ; these are, in some cases, round or elongated with the long axis transverse to the intestine.   The edges of all these ulcers deeply undermined and œdematous.   In the transverse colon the ulcers are largest.   The floor of the largest

of these ulcers (4 C. M. in diameter) is formed by the muscular coat.   In the floor of this ulcer there is an oval opening
2 M. M. in long diameter and from this a small blood clot protrudes.   A probe passed into this opening entered a small vein
about 1½ M. M. in diameter.   In the descending colon and
rectum there are similar ulcers.   In all these ulcers, beneath
the undermined mucous membrane there is a quantity of
greyish gelatinous pus.

Aorta smooth and normal.

Microscopic examination of the gelatinous pus from the
ulcers shows numerous amœbæ.   Most of these are round,
vacuolated, sharply refractive, and not motile.   A few amœbæ were found which were feebly motile.

In the liver abcess there are numerous motionless amœbæ.

Heart and kidneys show fatty degeneration.

Permit me to quote Dr. Osler's description of the amœba in
presenting, as far as I know, the third case reported in this
country :

"From the liver, the size ranged from 10 μ to 20 μ.,
which appears to be somewhat greater than indicated by
Katulis.   When at rest the outline was usually circular,
occasionally ovoid, but when in motion they presented, as
shown in the figures, the extreme irregular contour of moving amœboid bodies.   The protoplasm could be distinctly
differentiated into a translucent homogeneous ectosarc or
motile portion and granular endosarc containing the nucleus
vacuoles and granules.   The hyaline ectosarc was, as a rule,
very distinct, and in many examples the granular protoplasm of the interior was surrounded by a distinct rim.
Occasionally a form was seen in which this portion was much
less developed and the greater part of the organism seemed
composed of granular substance.   Within the endosarc the
vacuoles constituted the most striking feature ; sometimes
the interior substance appeared to be made up of a series of
closely set clearvesicles of pretty uniform size.   As a rule, one
or two larger vacuoles were present, the edges of which were
not unfrequently surrounded by fine, dark granules.   I never
saw a true contractile vesicle which displayed rhythmical

pulsation, but the larger vacuoles underwent, at times, changes in size. The nucleus was plain enough in some examples, in others very difficult or impossible to detect. It was usually pale, ovoid or rounded in outline and with a very delicate contour. No distinct nucleolus was seen, though there were sometimes coarser granules which possibly represented it. Their movements, however, constitute the most interesting and distinctive feature. From any portion of the surface a rounded hemispherical knob would project and with a somewhat rapid movement the process extended and the granules in the interior streamed toward it. It is impossible to speak with any certainty as to the relation of these organisms to the disease."

Finally I would call your attention to the conclusions arrived at by Rickman Godlee, whose experience, coupled with his association with Sir J. Fayrer, to use a familiar and in this case, entirely complimentary title, the great Indian Liver Doctor, to whom all flesh must come apparently after a sojourn in the tropic, I say Godlee's conclusions are worth noting and are as follows:

1. Pyæmic abscesses do not call for surgical interference or if in rare cases one should point it is only opened to relieve symptoms, but without hope of doing permanent good.

2. The same observations apply to abscesses resulting from suppurative phlebitis of the portal vein.

3. Multiple abscesses associated with dysentery or ulceration of the bowels are very unfavorable for surgical treatment. They must, however, be opened and treated on the same lines as the single or tropical abscess, because they cannot be certainly diagnosed.

4. Single abscess of the liver, whether tropical or not, must, if it approach the surface, be opened ; the following precautions being adopted :

A. If it present at the epigastrium, the presence of adhesions must be ascertained before incising the liver.

B. If through the chest wall, a spot must be chosen below the normal limit of the pleura; but if by chance either pleura or peritoneum be opened, the opening must be closed with a double row of stitches before incising the liver.

C. Strict aseptic precautions must be throughout adopted, either carbolic acid or some slightly soluble salt of mercury being employed in the dressing.

D. The tube must be of large size at first, and a tube of some sort must be kept in until the discharge is reduced to a very minute quantity.

If an abscess has busrt into the lung, pluera, pericardium, peritoneum or kidney and the position of the abscess can be clearly determined, it must be opened without delay. If the position of an abscess be only suspected, and the patient be losing ground, it is right to puncture the liver in the most likely situations, bearing in mind that though usually quite harmless, a slight amount of risk accompanies this very trivial operation. This rule applies to cases in which the abscess has ruptured into any of the cavities enumerated above.

If on the other hand, whether the abscess has ruptured or not, there are no means of diagnosing the whereabouts of the matter, and the patient be not losing or even gaining ground, the surgeon should hold his hand for a time.

5. Hydatids of the upper and back part of the liver are to be treated on the same lines ; but in cases of this sort, and in those of sub-diaphragmatic abscess, it must be remembered that the diaphragm may be pushed up to a great height, thus closely simulating intra-pleural suppuration.

6. Empyema, pericarditis and peritonitis, caused by rupture of an hepatic abscess or hydatid, must be promptly dealt with on general principles. (Brit. Med. Journal, Jan. 25, '90, p. 175).

Gentlemen, I have dealt largely in quotations, because the people quoted knew more of the subject than I did—but three points I hope I have made clear of my own accord. 1st. The aspirator is the best diagnostician, but a poor therapeutist. 2nd. The operation of incision is best done in two stages. 3rd. The presence of the amœba coli in dysenteric hepatic abscess, and last, but not least, instructive to you as it shall be to me, the fact that because we know sufficient cause, we must not flatter ourselves that we know the *whole* cause of a patient's illness or death, or relax our search for truth, while a single stone is left unturned.

DISCUSSION.

Dr. R. Winslow said that such cases were not so infrequent in this climate as many supposed. All cases he had seen were Germans. He does not agree with Dr. Johnson in the treatment with the aspirator. Small abscesses may be cured by the aspirator. An abscess of the liver should never be allowed to break. It may break inward and cause death.

Dr. Wm. Osler said he had seen more abscesses of the liver in the sixteen months that he had been in Baltimore than in five years in Philadelphia. Some abscesses will not get well by aspiration; often they are so low down in the liver that they cannot be found, except by incision. Very often this is due to a multiple pyelo-nephritis. He related a case in which the diagnosis was only made by a laparotomy.

Dr. Preston also related a case of hepatic abscess, occurring in his practice, and then Dr. Johnson closed the discussion.

On motion, the Faculty adjourned to meet at 10 A. M., Wednesday, November 12th, 1890.

Second Day.

CAMBRIDGE, Nov. 12th, 1890.

The Medical and Chirurgical Faculty met as per adjournment, at 10 A. M. this day. Dr. T. A. Ashby in the chair. The first paper was read by its author, Dr. Geo. J. Preston, on "*Differential Diagnosis and Treatment of Multiple Neuritis.*" The subject was discussed by Dr. Wm. Osler.

THE DIFFERENTIAL DIAGNOSIS AND TREATMENT OF MULTIPLE NEURITIS.

Multiple neuritis, poly-neuritis, peripheral neuritis are synonyms employed to denote an acute, inflammatory affection of the peripheral nerves. In looking over the older Medical Literature, one can find cases described, which were evidently of the nature of the affection under consideration, but no clear account of the disease with the post mortem appearances is to be met with prior to the case reported by Duchenne in 1864. He gave a full description of this case with a careful report of the autopsy, and a year or two later reported another case, announcing his belief that many cases of paralysis were due to affection of the peripheral nerves. Cases were afterwards reported by Eisenlohr, Eichhorst, Leyden, Joffroy and others. Not until recent years, however, through the labors of Grainger Stewart, Lancereau, Allen Starr, Buzzard, Ross and others, has the disease become generally known. The object of this paper is chiefly to show how difficult often, the diagnosis of multiple neuritis is, and how easily it may be confounded with certain other affections, especially when it is met with in its late stages after recovery has advanced to a certain point. It is necessary however, for the clear understanding of the disease to glance for a moment at the ætiology and pathology of this interesting affection. By far the most potent factor in the disease, and the most frequent and best known cause is alcohol.

The frequency with which habitual consumers of alcohol are attacked with peripheral paralysis, has long been recognized. It is remarkable how often motor and sensory disturbances can be observed in such cases if systematically looked for. I have recently made a number of interesting observations on chronic alcohol drinkers, testing the reflexes and sensation of all the cases met with, and in an overwhelming proportion of cases have found more or less indications of affection of the peripheral nerves. In the same category with the cases caused by alcohol may be placed, those due to poisoning by lead, the most frequent arsenic, illuminating gas and other agents. We find multiple neuritis following certain infections and other diseases as typhus and typhoid fever, small-pox, diphtheria and tuberculosis, especially the two latter. Perhaps syphilis may be added to the list. There are a large number of cases for which we can find no cause and are generally attributed to cold and dampness, overexertion are the causes generally, which seem to be provocative, to a certain extent, of acute cord lesions, as myelitis. Finally we must include that curious disease found in Japan, certain parts of Brazil and some of the Islands in the China Sea, known as Kake or Beriberi. This affection presents the symptoms of multiple neuritis, and many autopsies have confirmed the seat of the lesion to be the peripheral nerves. It is perhaps, due to a special micro-organism, and bears some resemblance to malarial affections.

A mere glance at these various ætilogical factors is enough to show us that very different causes may produce practically the same result, whether it be alcohol, lead, an infectious disease or a special mircro-organism, the pathological appearances are much the same, and the symptomatology sufficiently similar in the different varieties to warrant our including them all under the same head.

A word as to the pathology and pathological anatomy. There is perhaps no special difference between the degeneration of nerve fibres occurring in multiple neuritis, and that seen after other degenerative processes, or after nerve injury. There is first a disintegration of the myelin which breaks up and collects in drops, presenting a characteristic appearance under the microscope. As the degenerative process advances, the axis cylinder becomes involved, and finally destroyed. It would seem that this degenerative process includes two varieties, one in which the entire nerve structure is attacked by a general diffuse inflammation, the other in which the sheath of Schwann is first involved, and the consequent hyperplasia of connective tissue produces compression, and finally destruction of the other nerve elements. It is to be noted that the peripheral branches are the first to be affected, and show more marked changes than those parts of the nerve nearer the cord. The nerves of the extremities, as a rule, are alone affected, though occasionally the pneumo-gastric, phrenic, facial and hypoglossal suffer. It is true that occasional cases have been observed in which the degenerative process extended to the cord, and involved slightly its cellular elements. The muscles show simple degenerative atrophy.

The process of regeneration, a subject not very clearly understood, and concerning which there is some dispute, certainly takes place in a great majority of the cases of multiple neuritis.

The symptomatology of multiple neuritis, thanks to many carefully reported cases occurring in journal literature of late years, presents a fairly distinct picture. The disease is rather more common in males than in females, if we leave out the alcoholic cases, which curiously enough predominate in the latter.

The affection usually begins in an acute manner, with fever which may reach 103° or 104° F. Sensory symptoms appear almost at once; tingling "pins and needles," burning and often distressing pain. The pain follows the course of the nerves which are very sensitive to pressure, and the muscles become tender to the touch. Very soon anæsthesia shows itself, which may be moderate or profound. The pain is felt most severely in the extremities of the limbs. Muscular sense may be decidedly implicated. Motor paralysis comes on rapidly. It may begin in either upper or lower extremities, following the distribution of the nerves. Rarely the muscles of respiration are affected. Cases have been reported in which the pneumo-gastric, phrenic, hypoglossal and facial nerves have been involved. The paralyzed muscles soon begin to atrophy. Tendon reflexes are lost early, and the muscles respond not at all to the Faradic current, or only to a very strong current, and only to strong galvanic currents. There is usually double wrist and foot drop. Œdema is not infrequently observed. Bed sores and other trophic phenomena are rare.

The course of the disease is very irregular. After about a month, the symptoms become stationary. This stationary period may extend over several months, and then improvement set in. It usually takes some months, often more than a year before recovery is complete. A fatal result is not common from the disease itself, and when it does occur, is due, generally to involvement of the respiratory muscles or pneumo-gastric or phrenic nerves.

The differential diagnosis between multiple neuritis and affections which resemble it, is by no means always easy, and it is to this point that attention is specially directed in this paper. When the case is seen in its acute stage, or when the history is clearly given, the diagnosis is generally easy. On the other hand, when the case is not seen until all the acute symptoms have disappeared, or when improvement has begun, it is very easy to confound the affection under consideration with certain cord lesions. The disease with which it is perhaps oftenest confounded is polio-myelitis in the adult, (perhaps children.) This affection is very like the infantile affection, its pathology being the same, and its symptomatology very similar, so that it is doubtful whether we should separate them as is usually done. The following cases will show how closely the symptoms of multiple neuritis correspond to those of polio-myelitis.

Case 1. Female, aged 25. Has always been healthy. Family history good. Temperate. Thinks a fall that she had from a carriage had something to do with the subsequent disease, but this is improbable. In September, 1888, was taken suddenly ill with fever, and intense pains in limbs. Lost strength so rapidly that in 3 or 4 days she could hardly stand. Anæsthesia then began and was very general. Muscles soon began to waste. Patient came under my care at the Good Samaritan Hospital, March 1, 1889, or about six months after her illness began. Resembled a case of progressive muscular atrophy, in its last stages, so great was the wasting. Had weighed nearly 200 pounds, and was now not over 100 pounds weight, if that. Extremities wasted away to such an extent that the limbs appeared to consist of skin and bone. Muscles of the face were also atrophied. Double wrist and foot drop. Could not hold up her head. Was not able to turn in bed or feed herself. Some anæsthesia of the extremities remaining. No reaction to the strongest faradic, and but slight reaction to strongest galvanic current that could be borne.

From the history of the case, the pain following the course of the nerves, the anæsthesia, and the electric reaction, with absence of symptoms of cord lesion, a diagnosis of multiple neuritis was made. Patient was given strychnia in increasing doses, electricity and massage were regularly and systematically employed, and she made a rather slow, but perfect recovery. In about 10 months after treatment began she was perfectly well.

Case 2. Female, aged 26. Patient presented herself at the polyclinic with a history of having been ailing for several years. Was greatly emaciated. Double wrist and foot drop. Could not stand or walk without assistance. Reflexes were almost entirely abolished, as well as I can remember, for the notes of the case are very imperfect. No note as to sensation. Strong Faradic current applied to flexors, produced slight contraction; no response when the current is applied to extensors. Examination showed blue lines on the gums, and patient confessed to using white lead as cosmetic. Diagnosis; multiple neuritis due to lead poisoning, under appropriate treatment patient recovered perfectly.

Case 3. Male, aged 38. Good family and personal history, temperate in his habits, says he never recovered entirely from the "grippe" which he had in the winter. Last June was taken ill with pains in his limbs and gradual loss of strength, with atrophy of the muscles rapidly following. Came to City Hospital in September, presenting a typical picture of multiple neuritis. Extremities, particularly the lower, greatly wasted, unable to stand or walk, reflexes totally abolished, sensation very markedly impaired and over the distribution of some nerves entirely lost. Slight loss of muscular sense, pains in the limbs, over course of nerves and in the muscles. He was discharged last month entirely cured. Bearing in mind these fairly typical cases, the following are the points of differential diagnosis between the affection under consideration and polio-myelitis of the adult. In multiple neuritis the onset of the paralysis is more gradual and symmetrical, pain is generally a prominent symptom; both general muscular pains, and pain on pressure upon the affected nerves, and anæsthesia well marked as a rule. In polio-myelitis the paralysis is very sudden, and generally groups of muscles are affected at random, with no relation to their nerve supply, there is never any marked pain, never any tenderness along the course of the nerves, and no affection of sensation. In multiple neuritis if the case is severe, atrophy of the muscles begins rather sooner than in polio-myelitis, in which there is usually a decided period of stasis after the paralysis, before the atrophy commences. Contractions following the atrophy are much more common in polio-myelitis than in neuritis. There is a slight difference in the electrical reaction. In both diseases the faradic current gives no contraction, but in neuritis a very much stronger galvanic current is required to produce contraction of the muscles, than is necessary in polio-myelitis. Sometimes in this latter disease we find great susceptibility to the continuous current, in the early stages, with marked difference in the two poles, reversing the normal reaction.

Two other forms of muscular atrophy are to be borne in mind in making the differential diagnosis, namely chronic muscular atrophy and idiopathic muscular atrophy. The only danger is in confounding them with cases of neuritis that have gone on to great atrophy, and when these latter cases are seen very late in the course of the disease, and no clear history can be obtained.

If a good history can be gotten, mistakes in diagnosis are not apt to be made. The course of multiple neuritis is acute or sub-acute, while in the other named diseases, the onset and course is exceedingly chronic. In the latter diseases we have no pain or interference with sensation, and the gradual atrophy attacking certain groups of muscles, and then slowly extending to others is most characteristic. There are a few other rare forms of atrophy that need not be mentioned, as they are not at all apt to be confounded with neuritis.

There are certain cases of multiple neuritis that present a picture not unlike that of locomotor ataxia, and mistakes may occur in differentiating between the two. After a case of multiple neuritis has partly recovered, the diagnosis between it and locomotor ataxia is not always easy, unless we consider carefully the previous history of the two.

Case 4. Male, aged about 40. Presented himself at poly-clinic, and was first seen by my assistant, who made a diag-nosis of locomotor ataxia. Patient gave a rather indistinct history of pains and ataxia. Incoordination was not marked, knee-jerk totally abolished, slight loss of sensation, pupils sluggish and contracted. The fact there had been no inter-ference with vesical, rectal or sexual functions, that Argyl Robertson pupil was absent or not marked, that coordination was only slightly impaired, and that the history of the disease was not at all that of locomotor ataxia, led to the diagnosis of multiple neuritis which had practically recovered, a diag-nosis which was confirmed by learning that the man had been in hospital with a marked case of acute multiple neur-itis, some months previous to his visit to the polyclinic.

Case 5. Male, aged about 45. Was picked up on the street drunk, and sent to City Hospital. Had marked delu-sions of a characteristic kind, would give every morning a distinct account of a visit he had paid to some place in Ire-land the night before. Complained of pains in his legs.

Knee-jerk abolished. Pupils almost insensitive to light, and accommodated only slightly for distinct objects. Ataxia was so pronounced that for the first month he was in Hospital he could hardly walk or stand. Could not stand with eyes closed. Muscular sense was greatly impaired. Slight loss of strength and a little anæsthesia. He gradually recovered, though his mental condition was not by any means perfect, when he left the Hospital. This was a marked alcoholic case.

Case 6. Male, aged 38. Seen at City Hospital. Gave history of having had pains, ataxia, loss of knee-jerk, loss of sensation, loss of muscular strength with some atrophy about a year and a half ago. A diagnosis of locomotor ataxia had been made by a well-known physician. The man is now practically well, and able to attend to his business. Knee-jerk can be obtained only with difficulty, and there is still some slight loss of sensation. All the other symptoms have disappeared. The man had been very intemperate, and the history of his case, with its subsequent course, have no doubt about its having been multiple neuritis of alcoholic origin.

Case 7. Female, aged about 45. Has very marked ataxy, resembling closely that of a late stage of locomotor ataxia, absolute loss of knee-jerk, irregular anæsthesia, slight loss of power ànd Argyl Robertson pupil well marked. Opthal-moscopic examination showed a normal disc. The case would almost certainly be diagnosed tabes, but for the history which was that of an acute affection, rapid loss of strength, in a few days after the onset of the disease she was unable to walk, pain and anæsthesia confined to the lower extremities mainly, with some wasting, and no involvement of bladder or rectum. During the past three or four months she has improved greatly, and her improvement has been most marked while she has been in the City Hospital.

Of course when the case is seen early there is no likeli-hood of confounding neuritis and tabes, but the above cases show that there is a close resemblance between tabes and late cases of neuritis.

We must rely a good deal on the history of the case. In multiple neuritis we have the history of an acute or sub-acute affection, with paralysis coming on in a few days, anæsthesia which is often absolute, pain along the course of the nerves and muscular soreness, followed in a short time by the loss of electro contractility and muscular atrophy, with a strong tendency to recovery in a comparatively short time. All these symptoms are absent in locomotor ataxia. In this latter affection we have as distinguishing symptoms: girdle sensation, lightening pains, loss of sexual power, interference with bladder and rectum, and optic neuritis and atrophy, with Argyl Robertson pupil and the special trophic disturbances as perforating ulcer and Charcot's joint, and normal electric reaction. In case 7, the pupil phenomena were those of tabes, a fact that I have not seen mentioned in any reported cases of multiple neuritis.

Common to both affections are loss of knee-jerk, ataxia, numbness and tingling, general pains, and loss of sensation (marked in neuritis, slight in tabes).

Mistakes do undoubtedly occur in making the differential diagnosis between these two affections.

Diffuse myelitis, a rare affection, presents many symptoms in common with multiple neuritis. In the latter affection we have no tender spots over the spine and no affection of bladder and rectum, symptoms which are met with in the former. Occasionally we see cases which bear some resemblance to a transverse myelitis in the lumbar region.

Case 8. Female, aged 20. Gives history of difficult labor, with perhaps some pelvic cellulitis following and associated with hysterical attacks. Shortly after her confinement she was taken ill with great pain in limbs and gradual loss of strength. Had absolute anæsthesia, and muscles soon began to waste. When she came to City Hospital, was unable to bear any weight on legs, knee-jerk absent, some loss of sensation, double foot drop with contractions, and great wasting, involving mainly the leg muscles. She remained in Hospital a few months during which time she improved slowly. A favorable prognosis was given and she returned

to her home.   I received a letter from her a few days ago, or
about four months after she left the Hospital, in which she
says she has practically recovered.   Absence of girdle sensation and of tenderness over spine and bladder and rectal
involvement, with presence of tenderness of muscles and
pain along the course of the nerves are the distinguishing
points.   It is hardly necessary to mention, that very rare
disease, Landry's paralysis, which may be confounded with
multiple neuritis.   I reported recently a case of this curious
affection which resembled closely multiple neuritis, except
that there was preservation of the reflexes and normal electro
contractility.   Generally in Landry's paralysis sensation is
not affected, but it is occasionally involved, as in the case
referred to.   I have seen one case of multiple neuritis of
alcoholic origin in which the symptoms seem to have been
confined to the arms.

It must be that occasionally, as has been pointed out, the
inflammatory process may pass to the cord and involve its
cellular elements.   We may also have, as Starr has pointed
out, a multiple neuritis in the course of other affections,
notably myelitis and tabes.

From the above cases, which have been condensed in the
reporting, it may be seen that the diagnosis of multiple neuritis is by no means always easy, especially if the case be
seen late.   Yet careful attention to the history of the case,
and a minute scrutiny into the individual symptoms will generally clear up the doubtful cases.   It is important that a
correct diagnosis be made, for two reasons.   First, because
the affections with which multiple neuritis is liable to be confounded; offer an almost hopeless prognosis, while in multiple
neuritis, the prognosis is very favorable.   Second, multiple
neuritis is very greatly influenced by appropriate treatment.

The rules for treatment are simple.   In the acute stage,
the patient should be kept perfectly quiet in bed, on moderately light diet.   Morphia may be required to relieve the
pain.   I prefer to put the patient at once on a combination of
bromide and iodide of potash, in doses of gr. xx of former,
and gr. x of the latter, three times daily.   Starr recommends
the Salicin compounds in this stage.   The limbs may be

wrapped in flannel or oil silk, and very gentle friction or evaporating lotions employed ; a douche, sometimes hot, at others cold, according to the sensations of the patient is often beneficial. This treatment should be continued until the acute stage has passed. If the disease has been the result of poisoning by alcohol, lead, arsenic and the like, care should be taken that these substances no longer enter the system. In the case of alcohol this precaution is very necessary, for such patients are apt to continue its use unless they are placed under very close surveillance.

When the chronic stage has become established, that is to say the pains and anæsthesia passing off, and atrophy beginning, strychnine should be given in increasing doses, from gr. 1-40 to 1-20. A ferruginous tonic is often called for. Cold douches are found to be very valuable in this stage and systematic massage should be practiced. Electricity is of very great use in this stage of the disease. It should never be applied early, except very weak currents to test the reactions. The constant current of moderate strength 10 to 30 milliamperes should be passed through the diseased nerves. The sitting should last about half an hour daily. The patient should be encouraged to use the paralyzed limbs, and gentle exercise in the open air taken as soon as possible. The faradic current is not of much use in stimulating the nerves, but is of great value in exercising the muscles. Every muscle should be energetically faradised, and in this way much may be done to prevent atrophy and to restore the nutrition of those muscles which have already wasted. This very briefly is the outline of the treatment which of course varies somewhat with the individual cases. Space does not permit any elaboration of it, or any mention of the treatment of the cases resulting from alcohol, lead and arsenic.

My experience leads me to believe that multiple neuritis is a far more common disease than is generally supposed, and this with the fact that it is a comparatively recently recognized affection, and not perhaps very clearly understood by the general practitioner, makes one hope that these notes of cases may prove of some interest.

DISCUSSION.

Dr. Wm. Osler agreed with Dr. Preston in saying that peripheral neuritis was more common than usually supposed. There are often mistakes in the diagnosis, unfortunately. The gait is very characteristic. It is the "steppage" of the French, in which the foot is lifted high to get the toes raised off the ground. This is so characteristic that the diagnosis can be made from it alone. He had seen it after alcoholism, arsenical poisoning, and typhoid fever. It is so much like locomotor ataxia that an unfavorable prognosis is apt to be made. He referred to a case in his own practice in which neuritis was mistaken for ataxia.

The general order was suspended, and the following named gentlemen were elected to membership, having been at a previous session recommended by the Eastern Shore Examining Board:

A. C. Jones, M. D., Crapo, Md.; Enoch George, M. D., Denton, Md.; J. A. Stevens, M. D., Oxford, Md.; S. Chase deKrafft, M. D., Cambridge, Md.

The reading of papers was resumed, and Dr. Herbert Harlan read a paper on *"Pyoktanin in eye Diseases;"* before discussion of this paper, one of kindred bearing was called for, namely, *"The Injurious use of Remedies in Eye and Ear Diseases,"* by Dr. Hiram Woods. The papers were commented on by Dr. Harlan.

PYOKTANIN IN DISEASES OF THE EYE.

In the middle of August last my attention was called to an article on Pyoktanin in Merck's Bulletin for June.

The article was by the discoverer, Prof. J. Stilling, of Strassburg University, and gave a brief account of the origin and his laboratory and clinical experience with the new medical disinfectant which he named from "puon" *pus* and "kteino" *to kill.*

It is one of the coal-tar derivatives and can be obtained pure in the form of metallic green crystals, which dye a blue violet, and yellow crystals.

It is readily soluble and can be used in solution, in powder and in ointments, or in form of pencils, which are prepared of the two varieties, blue and yellow pyoktanin. Pyoktanin is claimed to be a *sure but harmless therapeutic agent*, i. e. an absolutely sure yet perfectly safe bactericide, adapted for permeation through animal tissues and fluids in the living body because it is

"1st, Devoid of any injurious effect on the human or animal economy or organization;

2d, Certainly and utterly destructive of all bacteria or other micro-organisms absorbing it;

3d, Rapidly and completely diffusible in and permeant of both healthy and diseased animal tissues or fluids and perfectly penetrant through the enveloping membranes and internal substance of all bacterial colonies harbored by them.

As reported by its discoverer, pyoktanin has so far completely cured pyoid corneal ulcers, hypopion keratitis, marginal eye ulcers *in one day;* parenchymatous keratitis in a week or two; serous iritis, panaritum, in two days; varicose ulcers in three days; burns, purulent sores and lacerations of various kinds in astonishingly brief periods."

Having read carefully the whole of the bulletin my thought was that the report was plainly that of an enthusiast, but that perhaps there was some good in the drug and as soon as possible I procured samples of both the yellow and blue varieties and began experiments on all suitable cases coming under my care, a few or which I here report—

A number of cases of

PURULENT OPHTHALMIA

were treated with the blue solution 1—1000 without benefit. The following is a fair sample:

CASE 1st, is that of a man of 32 having a purulent ophthalmia in the left eye. The case was a grave one of un-

doubted gonorrhœal origin as the patient admitted a clap at
the time. The usual blue solution was ordered to be used
three times a day, and after five days the condition of the eye was
unchanged and a microscopic examination of the pus at this
time showed great quantities of gonococci to be present. I
changed the treatment to the use of nitrate of silver and the
case went on to prompt and complete recovery.

Gonococci; although said to be easily destroyed by most
antiseptics, are clearly shown by this case not to be affected
by pyoktanin.

CASE 2d, is that of a very obstinate one of blepharitis mar-
ginalis in a man of 45 who had been under more or less constant observation for two or three years at the Eye Hospital.
He has a bad case of sycosis also, and I think the blepharitis
is caused by the same parasite. Under continual treatment
he has been benefited many times, only to turn up again
suffering from an aggravation of his symptoms and generally
on these occasions there are some corneal ulcers.

In September he made his appearance with his eyes in
worse condition than I ever remember to have seen them. I
used the blue solution of pyoktanin 1—1000 freely to the
corneal ulcer and the inflamed edges of the lids. The result
was most gratifying and the next day the eyes were in as
good condition as I had ever seen them.

The eyes were open, the ulcers healed, he faced a strong
light and expressed himself as better than for a long time.

I determined to try the pyoktanin on his sycosis and gave
him a prescription for a solution to be used at home. About
October 1st, he went to his work as a tinner for the first time
in two years. At the end of two weeks he again appeared
at the hospital with a small corneal ulcer. Unfortunately I
was out of the city that day and he fell into the hands of
another surgeon, who, seeing the ulcer and not knowing the
recent history of the case touched up the ulcer with the gal_
vano-cautery. October 31st, he again came to me saying
that he had had no rest except when under the influence of
morphia since the eye was burned. I instilled a drop of an
atropia solution and ordered pyoktanin. The following day,

November 1, he reported the eye comfortable and that he had slept well without morphia. November 6th, the eyes were in fair condition and the corneal ulcer quite healed, although the eyes were not in nearly as good condition as before the use of the galvano-cautery.

CASES OF INTRA-OCULAR INFLAMMATION.

CASE 3d, A. B., male, aged 42, an ironworker at Steelton, was struck in August last with a chip of steel, the particle penetrating the cornea, opening the capsule of the lens and injuring the iris. The history was clear that the particle did not remain in the eye. When seen there was a traumatic cataract and iritis. There was much ciliary congestion, the eye was always painful and much more so when exposed to light.

The indications were plain, to allay the iritis by the use of atropia and wait for results. A four-grain solution of atropia sulphate was given and he returned to his home, reporting for the next three weeks about twice a week. The irritation was lessened, but not subdued and, after three weeks treatment by atropia the eye was in much the same condition, *i. e.* fairly comfortable, but patient still suffered when exposed to light and was unable to work. The redness of the ciliary region still continued. Without much expectation of benefit, I instilled a few drops of pyoktanin solution 1—1000. The whole sclerotic was stained a deep blue and through the cornea it was seen that the coloring matter had penetrated to the iris. Without being directed to do so the patient came to town the following day and asked to have some more of the blue drops put in, saying that he had passed the first really comfortable night since the accident. I gave him a prescription for some of the same with directions to stop the atropia and use the blue drops three times a day. The patient was not seen again for two weeks when he gave as a reason for not returning that he had gone to work the day after his last visit, but had afterwards had an attack of chills from which he had just recovered. He had used the pyoktanin regularly, and the eye was in excellent condition. There was no redness and no evidence of pain. The lens was undergoing the process of absorption and he had already regained some vision.

On the other hand may be related the following:

CASE 4th, male, aged 37, appeared at the hospital with the left eye red and painful, having a large scar over the ciliary region extending across the cornea, the iris entangled in the wound and the whole eye plainly disorganized. There was a hesitating recognition of a strong light thrown upon the eye with an ophthalmoscope. It was evident that there could never be any useful vision in the eye. He had been advised some weeks previously at another dispensary to have the eye taken out but had declined. Having suffered two weeks he had come to ask to have the eye removed if I thought it advisable. I determined to try the effect of pyoktanin and had him admitted to the hospital. Blue pyoktanin was used for three days with only a little lessening of the pain and then the eye was enucleated. Had this case been treated earlier, the result might have been different, and the same may be said of the following case of that most unfortunate and intractable disease, sympathetic ophthalmia.

CASE 5th, in March last Mary McK., a child of 8, had the prong of a fork stuck into the left eye just at the inner sclero-corneal junction. When first seen there was a small piece of the iris which was clipped off under the influence of cocaine. The pupil was thus moved to the nasal side. The eye was bandaged and a simple collyrium ordered. The wound healed and the vision remained good, and the patient returned to school. A few weeks later she returned with a typical sympathetic ophthalmia affecting both eyes, but the injured one still retained fair vision. The iris was not dilatable with atropia, a film overspread the capsule of the lens and the vitreous was muddy. Under mercury internally and atropia locally there was some improvement for a time, with occa-sional outbreaks of inflammation. The case ran along with-out marked improvement until September 29th, when the vision with the right eye was 8-200, with the left eye she counted figures at one foot only. Having read Stilling's enthusiastic report of a case of sympathetic ophthalmia successfully treated with blue pyoktanin, 1-1000, I ordered a similar solution to be used twice daily. After two weeks use, on October 13, the vision was somewhat worse. In fact, my notes show it to have been on that date: R. 6-200; L. fingers at 8 inches.

At this season of the year in Baltimore there are many cases of what has been described as oyster-shuckers' corneitis. These are of the nature of corneal ulcers and are caused by small particles of shell or slime striking against the eye in the process of shucking oysters. The appearance of the eye and the cause of the disease in these cases is so peculiar that I have no doubt that they are due to some particular micro organism.

The cases do not yield readily to ordinary treatment. Although some years ago I reported successful results from use of a solution of eserine, I have lately treated about 20 cases with pyoktanin and in every case with marked benefit. The usual treatment was to drop in the eye a solution of cocaine and then after a moment rub the white spot or ulcer as the case might be with pencil of the yellow pyoktanin. This had the effect of staining the diseased spot a bright yellow, and in the milder cases a single application sufficed. The most severe case I had was one where the ulcer covered one-fourth of the corneal surface. This case was dismissed with a slight remaining opacity at the end of ten days.

In three cases of mucocele as an injection for washing out the lachrymal sac I have obtained good results from the blue solution, I think better than if I had used any other antiseptic or astringent solution.

In two cases of iritis when used alone pyoktanin was of no benefit. When used with atropia there was no reason to suppose that the latter was not the real curative agent, and I made no further experiments with that disease.

PEDICULI.

On the very day on which I obtained a supply of the drug under consideration and began my experiments to test its usefulness there happened to appear at the dispensary a boy of some fifteen years of age having the eye lashes of the right eye infested with crab lice (pediculi pubis.) Now these cases are interesting and not very common. The patient complains of an intense itching and irritation of the eyes. Close inspection as in this case shows a few lice which are seen moving about on the lashes and a great many eggs. These eggs are firmly glued to the lashes and it is very difficult to destroy them and prevent their further development. The usual and quite satisfactory treatment is the application of a red precipitate or a yellow oxide of mercury ointment. This readily destroys the living pediculi and if kept up a week or two effects a perfect cure by killing the lice as they are successively hatched out. The ointment, however, does not penetrate the glue-like covering of the eggs. As special stress is laid on the penetrating power of pyoktanin it occurred to me to try the effect of a solution of the same in this case. A 1-1000 of the blue solution was painted over the cilia and edge of the lid. The living lice were destroyed and all was stained a deep blue. By the following day the stain had worn off from the cilia and edge of the lid but the eggs had absorbed the pyoktanin so well that they were all with the exception of two or three of the characteristic blue color. These few had another application and after that the boy was kept under observation two weeks without one of the eggs developing. In other words two applications had destroyed all the lice and all the eggs.

In conclusion, my opinion is that pyoktanin is a harmless, yet satisfactory germicide for some micro-organism and while it is unreasonable to expect any drug to do what the enthusiastic discoverer claims for pyoktanin, still it ought not on that account to be condemned utterly. Only by continual and carefully conducted experiments can we learn the class of cases in which we can confidently expect positive benefit. It is equally important that we should know where it is of no value or of less value than other remedies.

To report practically from my own experience I think it useless in all cases of purulent ophthalmia. In fact, in all inflammations of the conjunctiva there are other well-known remedies much more efficient.

In many ulcers of the cornea it is very useful.

In intra-ocular inflammations probably due to pathogenic bacteria as sympathetic ophthalmia, and choroiditis disseminata, pyoktanin should be given a trial.

It will be a great gain if only a small percentage of these intractable cases are benefited.

The Injurious Effects of Remedies in Common use for Eye Diseases—Atropia, Yellow Oxide of Mercury, Nitrate of Silver.

The paper to which I ask your attention for a few minutes is founded upon observations made from time to time during the past 8 years in hospital and private practice. Although diseases of the eye and ear are generally recognized as calling for treatment at the hands of a specialist, few if any practitioners either care to resign all such patients to the oculist or aurist, or can do so, even if they desire. The diseases and remedies which I shall consider are those treated and employed by all physicians of considerable practice, and this brief study will not, I hope, be a waste of your time.

Even in my own brief experience there can be noted a marked change for the better in the diagnosis by physicians of eye and ear diseases and the general use of ocular and aural therapeutics. While such things are still occasionally seen, only rarely now are cases of glaucoma treated with atropia, simple conjunctival hyperæmia with blue-stone, iritis with nitrate of silver, the recognition of the dangers from ophthalmia neonatorum postponed until both corneæ are destroyed, the nasal douche used until acute otitis media develops from the entrance of fluids into the middle ear through the Eustachians, or ear-ache treated with Haarlem, carbolized or some other stimulating oil, irrespective of the etiology of the pain, until a severe otitis externa results.

But while these things are becoming matters of the past, other injurious effects of drugs upon the eye and ear are noted by those having access to large clinics in these two departments of medicine. In many instances these effects follow the proper and legitimate use of the remedy, and are entirely unforseeable. Sometimes they are transient, and, at the worst, only delay recovery, while again they may be more serious, and cause irreparable damage. It is to the possibility of these untoward results that one should be always on the alert.

Barring its use as a mydriatic in refraction work, the place of *atropia* in the treatment of eye diseases is generally appreciated. Broadly speaking, it is indicated in the following state of things :—a painful eye with cloudy cornea or muddy anterior chamber, a lustreless or dull looking iris, and most important of all, a small pupil, either stationary or responding feebly to light. The conjunctiva is always injected in iritis ; but usually a test of pupillary action will render clear the diagnosis between conjunctivitis and iritis, saving the patient, on the one hand, the useless annoyance from the use of atropia in the former disease, and, on the other hand, preventing the physican from making the serious blunder of not using it if the case be iritis. If one is still in doubt, a drop of a weak solution (gr. i-ʒvi) may be used for diagnostic purposes. Prompt and regular dilatation of the pupil follows in conjunctivitis while in iritis the pupil will either remain stationary or else dilate slowly and irregularly according to the firmness and number of adhesions between the iris and lens capsule. The general *contra*-indications for the use of atropia are *dilated* pupil and increased tension of the eyeball. There is a secondary effect of atropia when used for a long time which is given in most of the standard text-books but which is not always borne in mind. This is its irritating action upon the conjunctiva. Some men think its prolonged use may lead to trachoma or granular lids. This I have never seen, but cases like the following are not uncommon : Mrs. A., 48 years of age, was referred to me by my friend, Dr. T. A. Ashby, of Baltimore, in August, 1889. Dr. Ashby had treated her for kerato-iritis of the right eye. There was partial and irregular dilatation of the pupil, considerable photophobia, with marked catarrhal conjunctivitis of two weeks standing. The kerato-iritis had been treated for a month or so with atropia, which was still being used with a view of breaking up the remaining adhesions. In spite of the use of astringent washes the muco-purulent discharge from the conjunctiva persisted. For a week I continued the atropia and tried to cure the conjunctivitis with astringents. Getting no more pupillary dilatation from the atropia, it was evident that this remedy would not break up the remaining adhesions, so it was discontinued, as was also all astringent treatment. Within two or three days the discharge ceased and the eye cleared up. The atropia was clearly the cause of the conjunctival inflammation. I saw this lady a few weeks ago and the remaining adhesions have given no trouble at all. Should at any time a recurrent iritis develop, an iridectomy would be indicated. When the atropia conjunctivitis does not reach the point it did in this case, it will often produce persistent and annoying irritation. When, in the course of iritis, pain has ceased, and the eye becomes less congested, strong solutions of atropia are not, in my opinion, useful, even if a few adhesions remain. These are often so firm that atropia will not break them up. It is better to leave them alone if they are not causing pain, or else to perform an iridectomy to prevent subsequent recurrent attacks. Atropia will only irritate the eye.

While atropia is the standard remedy in corneal ulcerations, there are cases in which, it appears to me, it not only does no good, but really adds to the patient's suffering. This may be due to its irritating local effect, but more probably comes from the increased amount of light admitted into the eye by the dilatation of the pupil. Of course, if iritis be present with the ulcer, the atropia must be used, but when the ulcer is the only lesion, I have for some time used the sulphate of eserine (gr. i-ʒi) instead of atropia. I first obtained the suggestion of this from my hospital associate, Dr. Herbert Harlan, who published some time since an article upon it in the *N. Y. Medical Record*. The ulcer seems to me to heal more rapidly and comfortably, so to speak, than under the atropia treatment.

Passing to another very common eye disease, blepharitis, and its remedy, used everywhere, the yellow oxide of mercury ointment, we occasionally meet with annoying results not expected.   Blepharitis may be only a redness of the lids, coming on after prolonged use of the eyes, or it may manifest itself by more or less deep ulcerations along the margins of the lids, destroying the lashes.   In both cases, but especially in the former, an error of refraction may be found to be the cause of the trouble, and its correction cures the lid disease.   Again, the ulcerations may persist in spite of persistent treatment.   No remedy has yet been found, which in the majority of cases, equals the ointment of yellow oxid. hydrag. gr. ii, vasiline ʒi.   In a few cases, however, one will have his patient return in 24 hours, with his lids red and inflamed, while before the only evidence of disease was a few crusts on the margins of the lids, the conjunctiva hyperæmic, and possibly in the condition of catarrhal inflammation, while prior to the use of the ointment this membrane was healthy. Under these circumstances the ointment itself should be carefully examined.   Little crystals of the drug may be found in the vasiline, which act as irritants, and a more carefully prepared specimen will soon effect a cure.   The two samples of the ointment which are passed around show very well the difference between a well and badly made preparation.   Still, quite a number of persons cannot use the drug at all without having a more or less severe conjunctivitis.   They cannot endure the slightly stimulating effect of the mercury salt. Milder ointments of zinc oxide. bismuth, boracic acid or of acetate of lead (gr. i to lanoline or vasiline ʒi) will promptly effect a cure.   I believe that this form of conjunctivitis is much more common than is supposed.

Probably no topical remedy is more commonly used in eye diseases than nitrate of silver.   In its place it is invaluable.   Out of its place it can do a great deal of harm.   My object in speaking of it here is to record a fact, which I have repeatedly noticed, that it sometimes perpetuates the very condition it is used to cure.   The pathological conditions calling for nitrate of silver are tumefaction of the conjunctiva, with prominence of the papillæ, and the presence of a purulent or muco-purulent discharge.   These conditions are met with in gonorrhœal ophthalmia, and its kindred disease, ophthalmia neonatorum.   In the gonorrhœal conjunctivitis of adults, occurring simultaneously with the exciting disease, nitrate of silver must be used freely, at times even to cauterization with the solid stick. The bad effects of the drug, however, are more apt to be seen in the purulent conjunctivitis of babies—a disease so common and so destructive to sight as to cause about 33 per cent. of all the blindness, and yet a disease curable, if properly managed. It is not held that purulent ophthalmia in a baby always means gonorrhœal infection from the mother. This is the cause, is it true, in the *majority* of cases, and when the conjunctival pus contains the gonococcus of Neisser, the prognosis is always more grave than when this organism is not present. The dangers of the disease are generally recognized, and it is a well-known fact that of all drugs nitrate of silver is the most potent in effecting a cure. Nothing can be of any use without cleanliness ; but this being obtained, it is important to know when to use and when to stop a drug so powerful for good or evil. There are two uses of the remedy which are now in vogue, the prophylactic and curative. The former was introduced into the lying-in hospital of Leipsic by Crede, and consists of (1) washing the lids of the infant immediately after birth, and (2) instilling into the conjunctival sac one single drop (and no more) of a 2 per cent. solution (gr. x-℥i.) The effect of this was to reduce the cases of purulent conjunctivitis in this hospital from 7.5 per cent. to 0.5 per cent. The same method in the lying-in hospital at Halle brought the cases from 12 to 3 per cent. Special attention in this use of nitrate of silver is called to an irritation of the conjunctiva which may result from the caustic action of the remedy. This hyperæmia of the conjunctiva does not mean a commencing inflammation. No further medication is to be used until the progress of the disease—if it does develop—calls for it. The curative use of nitrate of silver in ophthalmia neonatorum is different. The disease usually sets in on the 4th or 5th day with redness of the lids, more or less swelling and hardness, increased heat, and possibly some watery discharge. If seen at this time much can be done by the use of cold (iced) applications. As a rule, however, the little patient is not seen till the second stage appears, when the

lids, while still swollen, are not so hard or stiff and there is a
purulent discharge.   The point of greatest danger to the eye
is the cornea, and the sources of danger are two : 1st, the
impeding of the conjunctival circulation and 2d, the presence
of the pus.   The cornea may slough in 24 hours.   It is in
this second stage that the remedy under consideration is so
beneficial.   If, after cleansing the lids, a 1 or 2 per cent.
solution (gr. v to x to $\tilde{3}$i) be applied a whitish flake will form
on the conjunctiva, due to the coagulation of the albuminous
discharge, the lids may become even hotter than they were
before, and for ½ to 1 hour after the application, there will
be a serous discharge from the conjunctiva.   Von Graefe
attributed the beneficial effects of the drug to its power to
contract the blood vessels and accelerate the circulation, and
thought that the serous infiltration of the conjunctiva was
relieved by the serous effusion which followed the cauterization.   To these influences must now be added the well established *antiseptic* property of nitrate of silver.   It is to this
that it owes its prophylactic power in Crede's method, and
it is by this that the pus is made innocuous in the established
disease.   Noyes, in his recent admirable work states that
the pus of purulent ophthalmia retains contagious properties when diluted to 1-1000, but is made innocuous by a ½
per cent. solution (gr. i½-$\tilde{3}$i) of nitrate of silver.

'The single drop from a small glass rod—Crede's method,
disinfects the conjunctival sac, and possibly lessens the absorbing power of the mucous membrane by its astringent
action.   Care must be taken to keep the solution away from
the cornea, and a second application is not to be made for
prophylaxis, lest the corneal epithelium be cauterized, and
this structure injured.   There is abundant clinical evidence
to show that the application of astringents and caustics to
mucous surfaces in the early stage of inflammation *i. e.* when
there is swelling and hyperæmia but no hypersecretion, is
followed by bad results. Before the pus appears in the
course of a purulent ophthalmia, the disinfecting properties
of the nitrate of silver, or certainly as much disinfection as is
necessary, can be gotten with remedies which are neither
caustic or more than slightly astringent.   Warm water, tan-

nic acid and weak solutions of corrosive chloride are examples. So strong a caustic and astringent as nitrate of silver, if applied to the conjunctiva, while the lids are swollen and hard, may increase the infiltration and make the disease more serious. Schmidt-Rimpler thinks it can produce diphtheritic conjunctivitis. These considerations preclude its use. before the stage of suppuration.

In reference to the time when it should be stopped there is more or less difference of opinion. The generally accepted doctrine is to continue its use once or twice daily till suppuration ceases; then to return to it if there is a relapse. While following this line of treatment in a number of cases last winter at the Presbyterian Eye and Ear Hospital, I was struck with the fact that some of them continued for several weeks without any improvement. The cornea was clear, the lids swollen but soft and succulent, the papillæ of the conjunctiva prominent, and the purulent discharge profuse. I could not make up my mind to apply the stick to the lids, for the *ocular* conjunctiva showed little or no congestion, and I did not think the eye was in enough danger to necessitate such severe methods. The treatment I was pursuing was the cleansing at home every two hours with a 1-8000 bichloride mercury solution, and the daily application at the Hospital of a 1 per cent. (gr. v-ʒi) nitrate of silver solution. In one baby whose case was between four and five weeks, I finally ordered a prescription of alum gr. viii, zinc. sulphat. gr. i, aq. ʒi, and stopped the nitrate of silver. The child got well altogether too quickly for alum and zinc to march off with the credit. Other cases were treated in the same way with like results.

Two cases have come under my care recently which well illustrate the point I wish to make. For the notes on them I am indebted to Dr. Hartwig, one of our hospital assistants.

Case 1. Emma O., three weeks old, white, was brought to the hospital Oct. 6th. The history showed eye trouble since the 3d day, a physician being called in on the 5th. The treatment then ordered, I have since learned from the physician, a careful and capable man, was the hourly clean-

ing with warm water, and the daily instillation of nitrate of
silver (gr. iii-ℨi.) The child's mother had gonorrhœa. It
was next to impossible to have the eyes thoroughly cleaned
more than once a day, when the physician did it himself.
(It is to be noted that the silver had been used 16 days before
we saw the child.) Examination showed swollen lids, and
on separating them, pus gushed out. The papillæ of the
conjunctiva were enlarged, and the entire membrane tumefied. The *right* cornea was sloughed, the left clear. Hourly
cleansing with a 1-4000 corrosive solution was ordered, and
a nitrate of silver (gr. v-ℨi) solution instilled once daily.
The child's nurse, an aunt, I think, was shown how to clean
the eye, and I am sure she did it well. This treatment was
continued 10 days with apparently no diminution of the charge.
On Oct. 16, I suggested to Dr. Hartwig the possibility of the
silver aggravating the disease. It was discontinued and an
alum solution (gr.x-ℨi) substituted. In 48 hours there was
a marked improvement, and in a week the eyes were well,
barring, of course, the sloughed right cornea.

CASE 2. October 19th, Nathan B., white, 1 week old.
Both eyes began to discharge on the 4th day. No treatment, save washing with warm water and milk, had been
used for the 3 days between the appearance of the discharge
and the visit to the hospital. Nothing definite could be
learned about the mother's condition. Examination revealed
the same state of things as recorded in Case 1, save that the
corneæ were both clear. The hourly cleansing at home
with a 1-4000 solution, and the daily instillation of the same
nitrate of silver solution were followed for two weeks without, apparently, any lessening in the discharge. The child's
sister, who cared for him seemed to do her work well. On
the 25th of October Dr. Hartwig stopped the silver solution
and substituted alum (gr.x-ℨi] every hour in the place of the
corrosive chloride. Improvement in the swelling of the lids,
and the amount of the discharge was at once apparent. In
3 days the eyes were open, and are now perfectly well.

Such cases as these are exceptional, and their occasional
occurrence is not to deter one from using nitrate of silver

when the indications call for it. From an observation of a large number of cases of ophthalmia neonatorum I have come to these conclusions upon the disease:

1. If a physician sees a case while the cornea is still un-affected, he ought to save the eye. The disease is thoroughly amenable to treatment. Cleanliness is the cardinal point in treatment.

2. If the case is seen within a day or two after the first appearance of the discharge, a 5 or 10 gr. solution of silver nitrate should be used at once. Often one or two applications will cure the disease.

3. If the case is 10 to 15 days old, the conjunctiva thick and its papillæ much enlarged, less is to be expected from nitrate of silver than in the more recent cases. Occasionally in these older cases the remedy aggravates the disease. Milder astringents will often effect a cure, while again the disease gradually dies out and is not much influenced by any treatment. To keep the pus from remaining in the eye is then the only necessary thing.

4. Cases in which the cornea survives several days of suppuration, and which do not readily yield to the silver solution, show, as a rule, very little involvement of the ocular conjunctiva, and are not apt to terminate badly.

Dr. W. P. Chunn read a paper on *"Vaginal Examinations."* The paper was discussed by Dr. Noble, of Philadelphia, Pa.

The next paper was read by Dr. W. B. Canfield on *"Immunity and Protection from Disease."* The paper was referred for publication.

IMMUNITY AND PROTECTION FROM DISEASE.

When a physician attempts to cure disease, he simply removes as far as possible the cause, clears the way to recovery and lets Nature do the rest. In many cases Nature does her work well, although not always getting due credit for warding off disease and protecting us from harm; in the other cases she succumbs to her stronger foe, disease. Those of us who live in crowded communities are surrounded by an invisible enemy, and with every breath are liable to draw in disease in some form, yet so many escape. We may open our windows and let in what we call "fresh air," and as the sunbeam slants across the room, what myriads of dusty atoms meet our eyes. If we inhaled at every breath this dust in a quiet room, what would we not breathe in in the streets of dusty cities, in mines and in mills. In the sanitary management of our cities the danger of flying dust with its many impurities is rarely considered, and the dust of city streets which should be properly sprinkled and carted away is simply stirred up by the indolent sweepers and much of it is probably taken away in the clothes and breathing apparatus of the unfortunate passer-by. Such dust when inhaled does harm both from the impurities it may contain, and from its mechanical action and irritation when present in appreciable quantity.

That germs float in the air in the most secluded spot the careless or unfortunate housewife knows to her sorrow when she leaves her jelly glasses uncovered for a short time and finds the surface covered with a most beautiful mould. Bacteriology has told us that the germs of some contagious diseases are found in the air and may be inhaled and produce disease. Thus diphtheria, glanders, measles, whooping cough, hay fever, pneumonia and consumption are all undoubtedly in part due to the inhalation of dust containing the germs of these diseases. If the disease is floating in the air in so many forms, it is strange indeed that so many escape, especially when we consider the crowded public and private rooms, cars, and other places where the sick and well meet together and breathe the same air. Fortunately for us Nature has erected a series of barriers against such an enemy as inspired dust and in exposing us to this danger, has given us certain means of protection which repel attacks unless made with unusual severity.

All inspired air in persons who breathe as they should passes first through the nostrils and in its passage through this channel is not only warmed up to the proper temperature for the throat and lungs, but the moist walls serve as a sieve by which the air thus inhaled is relieved as far as possible of dusty impurities. This shows at once the importance of breathing with closed mouth, especially in passing from a heated to a cooler atmosphere, and of always thus breathing in an atmosphere of visible dust. The moist walls of the lining membranes of the nasal cavities fills the inspired air with moisture making it more agreeable to the throat and lungs.

The nasal passage in almost every animal deviates from a straight channel, and this is according to the needs of the animal. In man who is upright and far from the ground the passage is only slightly curved and may almost be considered rudimentary in its development. In birds, which fly far above the earth the nasal passage is almost straight. In all quadrupeds and especially in those which graze or seek their food on the ground and in those exposed to sudden changes of temperature as in amphibious animals, the nasal passages are exceedingly tortuous and in a high state of development, and their extreme moisture, due to the active secretion of their lining mucous membranes, serves to catch and stop as far as possible the entrance of dust into the throat and lungs. This is familiar to us in the cold nose of the dog, cow, etc., and the constant sneezing of the horses.

Those individuals who breathe abnormally with open mouths are much more liable to diseases of the throat and lungs. In spite of the outward defence we have within the nose, dust and foreign substances do occasionally get into the throat and trachea, but the latter is so very sensitive to the slightest irritation that the presence of such foreign substance excites a cough and they are quickly expelled. The minute anatomical structure of the lining membrane of the trachea is much like the waving surface of a wheat field. The whole surface of the trochea and large lung tubes is covered with ciliated epithelium whose waving motion is from the lungs upwards to the throat and very minute particles of dust and foreign substances which find their way into this region are gradually removed by this motion. This membrane is also active during sleep as many throat sufferers and others may have noticed on rising as they go through their morning cough.

In spite of these defences which nature has raised against her enemies, disease germs and foreign substances find their way into the trachea and even to the ultimate ends of the finest lung tubules.   In this way disease germs, and especially the tubercle bacillus get into the lungs of persons and in those predisposed to this disease this organism easily thrives. From recent investigations in microscopical anatomy we now know that Nature does not give up even after these foreign substances and disease germs find a place in the body.   In the organism, and more particularly in the blood, there has long been known a cell or corpuscle called the white blood corpuscle, or leucocyte and in suppuration the same cell is recognized as the pus cell.   That this cell seems almost ubiquitous in the body and that it assumes different roles under different circumstances has also been the subject repeated investigation.

The most recent function now assigned to this cell is that of a "carrier cell," scavenger cell or phagocyte, because it has been discovered in parts of the body devouring or carrying off germs, bits of germs and foreign substances within its body.   This was noticed in those who worked in dusty atmospheres.   The dust was inhaled in such quantities that it got into the lungs, and as it could not be coughed up in sufficient quantity to ensure the proper amount of breathing space in the lungs, it worked its way into the lung substance where by its irritation it attracted these carrier cells or scavengers which promptly attacked as far as possible the bits of dust and carried them either to the nearest lymphatic gland where they could be quiet and harmless or the dust containing cells found their way into the lungs and were coughed up and out.

This has been repeatedly noticed in the case of coal miners in whose expectoration large numbers of these cells were found, and in these cells bits of coal dust could be easily recognized.   In some cases where the piece of dust was too large for one cell to devour, two or more would join together and close around it. These cells have certain movements called amœboid from their resemblance to the movements of the amœba, one of the lowest forms of life—the type of a cell found on the surface of fresh water ponds. These amœboid movements consist in a change of shape on the part of the cell by which it thrusts a part on one side and draws in another part and by thus changing its shape it surrounds the substance and assimilates it. That these cells endeavor to do their work as well as possible, is shown by the fact that years after miners have ceased to work in the coal mines, it has been noticed that the expectoration was dark and a microscopical examination showed these cells full of coal bit and pigment, thus proving that the carrier cells were still trying as far as possible to remove these foreign substances. Experimentally this has been demonstrated by introducing finely divided organic substances, such as powdered cinnabar into the tissues and lungs of an animal and after a short time examining microscopically the tissues and glands of this animal when these carrier cells are found loaded down with the red pigment, especially the glands. In all these cases the role of the foreign substance is undoubtedly passive while the cell is active.

Further study of these cells, especially by a Russian observer, showed that they acted antagonistically to bacteria, that between these cells and the bacteria there was a struggle for existence or supremacy and on the result of this struggle depended a condition of illness or health. These observations were made on a disease produced in a fresh water crustacean, the "water flea" a daphnia, by a fungus. The fungus swallowed by the crustacean produces spores which pierce the intestinal wall, enter into the tissue and are at once surrounded by these cells or phagocytes. Here a struggle took place which resulted in a victory for the cells, the latter closing around these fungus spores, devouring them and finally destroying by a process of "intracellular digestion." In this case the action is very simple, but in the case of other animals and man the process is not so simple.

A careful study, both biological and chemical of these bacteria, has fully proved that they exert their deleterious action not so much by their actual presence as by a poison or ptomaine which they secreted from their minute bodies and that each specific bacterium or bacillus has its own peculiar body product, which in the case of pathogenesis or disease-producing germs is a poison. This then complicates the struggle between bacteria and the body cells. There is then an actual life-and-death struggle between cells and bacteria. Inoculation of a frog with the bacillus anthracis showed this struggle very beautifully. A study of these cells of the frog revealed them with bacilli and part of the bacilli within the cell wall and these were in the process of digestion or disintegration.

Thus there is good reason to believe. that in the presence of a contagious or infectious disease, the germs floating about or in some way gaining access to the individual near by, find their way into the body and there a struggle takes place between them and these cells which are attached to the invaders. Now begins a struggle for supremacy. The cells close around the attacking host and endeavor to destroy them and carry them off, or at least to prevent the further ingress of the bacteria. If the cells are victorious they devour the germs, carry them away and thus the individual escapes the disease. But if the germs increase too rapidly and by the secretion of this poison or ptomaine from their bodies, cause the death of the cells, thus sickness results. In this case the accumulation of these carrier cells which are killed by the germs, results in suppuration for the cells of pus are but the white blood corpuscles, leucocytes or phagocytes when dead. As heat increases the motion of these carrier cells and also their protection activity, the rise of temperature which precedes and accompanies suppuration has been looked upon as an attempt on the part of Nature to assist these cells activity and destroy the winding bacteria.

Immunity from second attacks of certain diseases as well as the protection influence of certain inoculations and vaccinations has never been clearly understood, although various explanations have of late been offered.

In all probability, although this is but a theory sustained by analogy, after recovery from the contagious diseases usually occurring, but once, the bacteria are supposed to secrete some poison virus which hinders its own life, just as animals produce carbonic acid which is poisonous to them, or the yeast fermentation produces alcohol which stops the growth of the fungus. In the same way after these attacks the cells of the body are supposed to contain some substance which resists the second attack of these organisms. It may be that Koch's tubercle acts in this way. The strength and duration of this immunity differs in individuals. Of course the ability of these cells to struggle with bacteria is lessened in weakened conditions; hence, for example, it is very probable that the lowered vitality caused by being chilled below the recuperating point invites an attack of pneumonia or some other disease, not from the mere chilling alone, but from the weakening of the cells' strength. In hereditary diseases predisposition plays an important role.

Thus we have seen that before Nature succumbs or yields to what has been very wisely called an "attack" of a disease, she has many means of defence, and fortunately for us often comes off victorious.

On motion, the paper of Dr. Geo. H. Rohe on the *"Treatment of Fibroid Tumors of the Uterus,"* was, in the absence of that gentleman, read by title and ordered to be printed.

THE TREATMENT OF FIBROID TUMORS OF THE UTERUS.

The object of this paper is to advocate a rational discrimination in the treatment of fibroid tumors of the uterus.

Uterine fibroids differ greatly in size, situation, structure and character of the symptoms to which they give rise.

In structure, fibroid tumors are homologous with the tissue of the organ in which they are found. They are composed of muscular and fibrous tissue in varying proportions usually encapsulated by a connective-tissue capsule, in which large vessels ramify. In some cases the growth is made up principally of muscular tissue, in others almost exclusively of white fibrous tissue. In the majority of cases, however, the growths are composed of varying proportions of these two tissues, sometimes the muscular, at another the fibrous predominating.

Most fibroid tumors, especially if of moderate size, are firm and solid, but the larger growths frequently have cysts or cavities filled with a lymphoid fluid. . These fibro-cystic tumors often cause no little difficulty in diagnosis, being sometimes mistaken for ovarian cysts, at others confounded with pregnancy. It must not be forgotten that pregnancy and fibroid tumors may co-exist, although happily this combination is not very frequent.

Fibroid growths may occupy any portion of the uterus. Their site of predilection appears to be the fundus and posterior wall of the corpus uteri. Schroeder found 92 per cent. in the body of the uterus, and only 8 per cent. in the cervix.

With reference to their situation in the uterine walls, fibroids are usually classified into sub-mucous, sub-serous and interstitial.

The sub-mucous project into the uterine cavity, the sub-serous toward the cavity of the abdomen, and the interstitial occupy a more or less intermediate position between the inner and outer surfaces of the uterus. As a matter of fact, most large fibroid tumors begin as interstitial or intramural growths and become sub-mucous or sub-serous in consequence of the contractions they excite in the muscular walls which force them either inward or outward.

Fibroid tumors may undergo fatty degeneration and be absorbed; they may slough and be cast off through the genital canal; they may undergo calcareous change and become encysted and be thus carried through life, or may slough out in the form of concretions, which have received the name of uterine stones. Finally they may undergo sarcomatous degeneration and become malignant. All of these terminations are, however, exceptional. Generally the tumor continues growing until, or after, the menopause, and gives rise to symptoms more or less troublesome, and in many cases sufficiently serious to demand active measures of relief.

The most pronounced symptoms of fibroid tumors of the uterus are pain, hæmorrhage and interference with the functions of other organs by pressure. They may also produce great discomfort by their weight. Occasionally the submucous variety undergo sloughing, when they may cause the death of the patient by septicæmia.

The pain produced by uterine fibroids is sometimes so severe as to be alone a sufficient reason for medical or surgical interference. It usually manifests itself at the menstrual periods as dysmenorrhœa, but may be constantly present as severe backache, bearing down simulating labor pains, especially in the sub-mucous variety, or neuralgia of the sciatic nerves. Sometimes there is persistent pain in the uterus itself, or, more probably, in its peritoneal covering, which is subjected to irritation or inflammation.

Comparatively small fibroids, situated low down in the uterine walls or in the cervix, may cause severe irritation of the bladder by pressure. There is often vesical tenesmus with frequent micturition, causing the most intense suffering.

The pressure upon the rectum may also give rise to constipation and great pain on going to stool. Hemorrhoids and œdema of the lower extremities are not infrequent complications, due to interference with the venous circulation. During the menstrual periods these pressure symptoms are generally increased in severity. Intra-pelvic or intra-abdominal pressure may also cause ascites, and in some cases localized peritonitic processes.

Hæmorrhage is, in most cases, the symptom that urgently demands remedy. It is most frequent and gravest in the sub-mucous tumors, but may be an accompaniment of any variety. It may be alarming in cases where the tumors are so small as to be detected with difficulty on bimanual palpation. The bleeding usually occurs at the menstrual periods, which are prolonged and more profuse than normal. The menstrual interval may be normal in duration, but in many cases is shortened, so that the bleeding recurs in two or three weeks. The blood is frequently discharged in large clots. Indeed the discharge of clots at the menstrual period is an absolute indication of something abnormal, and should always invite attention to the condition of the uterus. In a very large proportion of cases it will be found to be an outward sign of fibroid growths.

A definite relation exists between uterine fibroids and sterility. Whether the sterility is a cause or a consequence of the morbid growths is not positively determined. Statistical compilations show that about 75 per cent. of the women having fibroid tumors have never borne children. This may be regarded as fortunate, for in cases of labor complicated with uterine fibroids over half of the mothers and nearly two-thirds of the children die.

The treatment of fibroid tumors of the uterus is pre-eminently surgical. Even the administration of ergot and savine may be looked upon as a surgical method of treatment, for the effect striven after in the use of these remedies is the extrusion, or partial extrusion of the growths, whose removal s completed by surgical means. While the deaths directly due to the use of ergot are probably few, most writers discountenance the treatment for these reasons : the ergot treatment is tedious, painful, often ineffective and even at times dangerous. When the tumor is forced into the uterine cavity, or through the cervix by the contractions induced by the medicine, the practitioner must be ready to interfere surgically, otherwise sloughing and sepsis are imminent.

The ideal operation for a fibromatous tumor is the removal of the tumor, leaving the uterus intact. Unfortunately in many cases this result cannot be attained. Nevertheless this should be striven for whenever possible. The marvelous success of Schroeder and Martin in enucleating fibroids and thus preserving the uterus should encourage us to an imitation of their work. The enucleation of fibroids whether by the genital canal, or by laparotomy is in the true line of conservative surgery.

When a sub-mucous tumor projects into the uterine cavity or the vagina, its attachment is usually by a pedicle of greater or less thickness. When the pedicle is thin the tumor may be twisted off. The torsion seems to arrest all hæmorrhage at the same time from the highly vascular mucous membrane covering the pedicle. When the latter is thick, the attachment may be severed with scissors, ecraseur, or galvano-caustic wire. I prefer the latter method as less dangerous, cleaner, more rapid and thoroughly aseptic.

When the tumor is attached by a sessile base, the mucous membrane and capsule over it may be split with a knife after carefully dilating the cervix under aseptic precautions and then enucleating the tumor from its base. To arrest hæmorrhage a tampon of iodoform or creolin gauze may be packed against the bleeding surface. Great care is requisite, however, not to allow the tampon to remain too long, as the secretions may be backed up through the tubes and cause salpingitis or other inflammatory disturbances in the pelvic cavity. I am sure I produced a pelvic peritonitis in one case by the improper use of a tampon to arrest hæmorrhage after amputation of the cervix.*

Sloughing of a sub-mucous fibroid is not necessarily fatal, as careful disinfection of the genital canal before and after operation will often avert sepsis.

Vaginal enucleation of sub-serous tumors of the cervix may sometimes be practised. The operation was first done by Czerny. An incision is made through the vaginal fornix, avoiding the large vessels on the sides of the cervix, and the tumor enucleated from the tissue of the cervix and the pelvic connective tissues.

Tumors of considerable size may be delivered by intra-uterine and vaginal enucleation. If the growth is too large to remove entire it may be diminished in size by subdividing it with scissors, saws specially devised for the purpose, or the galvano-caustic wire. The operation should always be completed at one sitting, for to allow part of the tumor to remain is an invitation to septic absorption. Judgment and experience are required, however, to decide when

---

*In reference to this point, Sir Spencer Wells says : " I have occasionally put on 1 or 2 pairs of pressure forceps to a pedicle, either before cutting away the polypus, or when bleeding occurred after the cutting away, and have left the forceps hanging out of the vagina for several hours ; and I prefer this method to the more common one of applying perchloride of iron and plugging the vagina."

the growth has reached a size that does not permit its safe removal by way of the vagina.

The enucleation of fibroids through an incision in the abdominal wall,—laparo-myomectomy—is indicated in certain cases where the tumor cannot be removed by the vagina. It is at once a graver operation than the latter, and accompanied by a considerable mortality. If the tumor is subserous and attached by a thin pedicle, its removal after section of the abdominal walls is not difficult. The pedicle may be transfixed by a double ligature and tied tightly, the tumor cut off above the ligature, the peritoneum stitched over the end of the stump, and the external wound closed. Unfortunately the tissues of the pedicle often shrink after the tumor is removed, and hæmorrhage may take place from the stump. To avert this accident various measures have been adopted by different operators. Some remove a wedge-shaped plug from the face of the stump and sew the opposing raw surfaces firmly together by deep and shallow sutures, lastly bringing the peritoneum together over all. This is usually efficient, but consumes valuable time. Other operators clamp the stump in a wire-snare (Kœberle's serre-nœud) or a constrictor of parallel steel bars (Keith's clamp) and bring it outside of the abdominal wound, where the constricted portion of the stump mummifies or sloughs off. The peritoneal covering of the sides of the stump is stitched to the parietal peritoneum and so closes the peritoneal cavity against any discharges from the end of the stump, This method gives better results than the intra-peritoneal method, but leaves much to be desired in the way of surgical neatness and rapidity of healing. It is also at times attended by other inconveniences and dangers, especially if the pedicle and uterus are much put upon the stretch.

When the growth of the tumor is sessile and directly under the peritoneum or covered by a very thin layer of uterine tissue, it may be enucleated by making a bold incision over the tumor, and shelling it out of its base.

To guard against excessive bleeding an elastic ligature—a piece of rubber tubing—may be tied around the cervix, including within the ligature the arteries supplying the uterus

and appendages. Even large growths may be removed in
this way. If the cavity left in the uterine tissue is too large
to get good coaptation between its walls, it may be packed
with iodoform gauze as practised by Fritsch and the edges
stitched to the abdominal incision, in order to secure free
drainage and make the cavity accessible to external treatment.

Deep intra-mural, or even submucous tumors may be
treated by this method, but the results are less and less
favorable the more the uterine cavity is opened.

Sometimes the uterine walls are so occupied by the new
growths that their total removal can only be accomplished
by the excision of the uterus, or at least that portion above
the cervix. This operation is one of the gravest in surgery
and gives, in the hands of nearly all operators a high mortality. The total extirpation of the uterus including the
cervix, by way of abdominal section has not been very often
done, but with present methods should give more favorable
results than supra-vaginal hysterectomy.

In the latter operation the stump very often gives trouble
either from hæmorrhage or sepsis.

Complete removal of the uterus at the vaginal junction,
approaches the conditions of vaginal hysterectomy and should
give very little higher mortality than the latter. However,
at best, the complete or partial extirpation of the uterus is
an operation of great gravity and should only be resorted to
when all other means promising success have been tried.*

Tait has called especial attention to the soft œdematous
myofibroma, which often gives the impression on examination, of containing cysts. This tumor frequently fluctuates
in size, being now larger, now smaller, without any apparent
cause. These, as well as fibro-cystic growths of the uterus
are particularly suitable for complete extirpation by abdominal section. No other operation or method of treatment

---

*Several American surgeons have done complete extirpation of the uterus success-
fully, and A. Martin reports eleven recoveries out of sixteen operations, a pretty high
mortality.

Fritsch's mortality in all cases of hystero-myomectomy, including enucleations is 25
per cent. Bantock's 22 per cent.

seems to control their growth or arrest the hæmorrhage which is a frequent accompaniment.

In 1872 Lawson Tait, of Birmingham, and Alfred Hegar, of Freiburg, almost simultaneously devised the operation of removal of the uterine appendages—ovaries and Fallopian tubes—with the view of artificially inducing the menopause and thus arresting the growth of fibroid tumors by cutting off the principal source of blood supply to the growth. This operation has now probably been done over one thousand times with very satisfactory results. Tait's[*] own results, as shown in a statement recently furnished by him, are extremely favorable. In 426 cases, 16 died, a mortality of 3.75 per cent. Tait also declares that 95 per cent. of the cases of fibroid operated by removal of the uterine appendages are cured—that is to say, the bleeding is arrested and a large proportion of the tumors diminish in size, some disappearing altogether. These effects have been established by many observers, especially when the cases have been properly selected. As above pointed out, in the soft œdematous growths the arrest of the bleeding does not seem to follow so regularly as in the hard, nodular fibroids.

The cause of the arrest of the hæmorrhages after removal of the appendages is probably due, as suggested by Mr. Knowsley Thornton,[†] to cutting off the blood supply by ligature of the large vessels in the broad ligaments, and not merely to removal of the ovaries and Fallopian tubes. As a matter of fact, the mere extirpation of the ovaries alone often fails in producing the expected results.

The high mortality of the abdominal hystero-myomectomy, and the opposition on many sides to the removal of the ovaries, which it is claimed by many, unsexed the woman,[‡] led Dr. George Apostoli, of Paris, about 1882, to experiment with the galvanic current in the treatment of uterine fibroids. It is true Cutter, Kimball, and perhaps others, had used gal-

---

[*]MacNaughton Jones, Diseases of Women, 4th Ed., p. 340.

[†]Am. Gynecol. Trans. 1882.

[‡]This objection is not tenable as the "unsexing" consists, merely in anticipating the menopause, which is one of the natural characteristics of the human female.

NOTE :—Trenholme, of Montreal, deserves the credit of having first removed the ovaries to establish a premature menopause.

vanism successfully for this purpose before, but Apostoli developed a method by which the application of electricity is reduced to scientific exactness. The improvements in the instruments for generating, measuring and applying electricity now permit the physician to administer this remedy with as much exactness in dosing, as any other therapeutic agent at his command. It would take too much time here to describe the apparatus or the methods in use. For a full description I refer to pages 327-350 of "Practical Electricity in Medicine and Surgery," by Liebig and Rohé, and to Dr. G. Betton Massey's excellent little book on "Electricity in Diseases of Women," both published by F. A. Davis, Philadelphia.

In 1887 Dr. Apostoli reported 278 cases treated by this method with a successful result (arrest of hæmorrhage, diminution in size, disappearance of pain and pressure symptoms) in 95 per cent. The average number of applications was fifteen in each case. In August, 1889, Dr. Thomas Keith* and his son, Dr. Skene Keith, published a detailed record, without commentary, of 106 cases treated according to the method of Apostoli. The average number of applications in the cases treated to a termination was twenty-eight. Three of the cases died during or shortly after the discontinuance of the treatment, but in neither case was the fatal result attributable to the applications. Admitting, however, for the sake of argument, that the electricity was the cause of death, a mortality as low as 3 per cent. cannot yet be claimed by any operator in hysterectomy, and even in the comparatively safe operation of removal of the appendages, very few operators can show as favorable results as Keith has obtained with electricity.

I have carefully gone over the record of the cases reported by Keith and have been surprised at the almost uniform improvement noted. Diminution in size of the tumor, arrest of hæmorrhage, relief of pain and general improvement in the nutrition and spirit of the patient are recorded in nearly every case.

*The Treatment of Uterine Tumors by Electricity, Edinburg, 1890.

August Martin,[*] the greatest living gynecological surgeon of Germany, has very recently referred to ten cases treated by him in the following words: "The results in these ten cases show that hæmorrhage, the most troublesome and dangerous symptom of myomata, may usually indeed be controlled, in fact, in those large multiple tumors, which apparently were situated intramurally, and included the fundus, hæmorrhage ceased nearly entirely. Several small tumors were not influenced in the same manner, and the hæmorrhages continued unchanged·in spite of very frequent sittings, so that here·the result must be regarded as a very doubtful one. One patient, who had a myoma of the size of an ostrich egg, had such violent pains after seven sittings that she insisted upon being operated. The operation was performed, and the patient recovered. A second symptom, often so frequently complained of, is the phenomenon of pressure. These disappeared in all of nine cases, so that in this regard the result is very satisfactory. An essential decrease in size has, up to now, not been obtained in any case."

This is not very enthusiastic, but Dr. Martin admits that the symptoms for the relief of which hysterectomy is at all justifiable, were relieved in his cases. He states that he shall continue "making experiments with the procedure."

Numerous other competent observers in France, Germany, England and in this country have had successful experience with this method, and although there is a good deal of sneering at the method as being useless, and withal dangerous, and those who use and advocate it are denounced as quacks and "low-down, no-account sort o' pussons" generally, electricity in the treatment of fibroid tumors of the uterus has come to stay, and demands investigation.

Ridicule and denunciation are no answers to plain records of facts submitted by Apostoli, Zweifel, Martin, Keith and many others, less eminent, perhaps, but still of some account in the world.

Some of those who use the electrolytic method, apply it in office or dispensary practice, allowing the patients to walk

---

[*]Introduction to Am. Translation of Martin on Diseases of Women, Boston, 1890, P. 29.

or ride considerable distances after the application. This, I regard as imprudent, and likely to cause trouble. All the cases in which serious symptoms or a fatal result followed after the use of electricity were such as had imprudently exposed themselves. I regard it as important that several hours at least of perfect rest should follow each application. To allow this course to be pursued it is requisite that the patient should be treated at her own home, or in a properly fitted institution.

It goes without saying that careful asepsis of the genital canal should be maintained during the electrical treatment as well as in the gravest and most delicate surgical operation.

Laparo-hysterectomy puts the woman in jeopardy of her life and keeps her a helpless invalid for at least one month. The electrolytic treatment keeps her under moderate restraint for a period of two or three months, does not endanger her life, and leaves her generally in such a condition of comfort and health that she is satisfied to live her allotted days, even though she is obliged to carry her tumor with her to the grave.

I would not advocate the exclusive use of electrolysis in the treatment of uterine fibroids. As stated in the beginning of this paper, a rational discrimination is demanded of those who treat this condition. Many cases are readily relieved by vaginal or intra-uterine division of the pedicle by scissors, ecraseur, or galvano-cautery wire; others are best treated by vaginal, intra-uterine or abdominal enucleation. Large œdematous tumors or fibro-cysts should be treated by laparo-hysterectomy; bleeding fibroids of not too great size are proper cases for the removal of the appendages, and most large chronic, immovable tumors, choking up the pelvis, causing pain, pressure symptoms and hæmorrhage, yield to the proper patient employment of the galvanic current, after the method of Apostoli.

No more papers having been presented, miscellaneous business was taken up, and the Secretary read a notice of Amendment to Article 5 of Constitution, offered by Dr. J. C. Hemmeter, relating to the appointment of Chairmen of Sections, and also ordering the *titles* of papers to be read to be sent in *one week before* the date of the Conventions; also effecting the appointment of members to open discussion.

On motion of Dr. Jno. N. Mackenzie, the thanks of the Faculty were voted to the county members for their hearty reception of the city members, and the semi-annual meeting of 1890 adjourned *sine die*.

G. LANE TANEYHILL, M. D.,
Recording Secretary.

MINUTES.
Annual Meeting.

HALL OF THE FACULTY,
N. W. Cor. St. Paul and Saratoga Sts.
BALTIMORE, MD., April 28, 1891.

The Faculty was called to order by the President, Dr. T. A. Ashby, this day at 12 M., it was the *93rd Annual Session.* About 200 physicians were present.

The proceedings were opened by prayer by Rev. Frank Ellis, D. D.

On motion the calling of the roll and reading of the minutes were dispensed with. Preliminary announcements were made by the Recording Secretary, in which he called attention to the extensive programme of proceedings as prepared by him, the first the Society has published, in the knowledge of the present generation.

The President read his address on "*The Relation of the Medical and Chirurgical Faculty to Professional Organization in Maryland.*"

On motion the thanks of the Faculty were voted the President, and a copy of his address requested for publication.

Dr. Joseph T. Smith, the Corresponding Secretary, read his report, which was accepted.

Dr. W. Fred A. Kemp, the Treasurer, read his report, which, on motion of Dr. Brune, was received and referred to the Executive Committee for audit; and he was instructed to so revise the same, so that to the liabilities be added the sum due the Library Committee, from dues collected and not yet paid to it, and, that this sum be paid to it from the first available funds.

The report of the Executive Committee was read by the Chairman, Dr. P. C. Williams, which on motion was accepted and referred to the Publication Committee.

Dr. Chas. H. Jones, the Chairman, read the report of the Examining Board in which they recommended the following members of the medical profession to membership in this Faculty :

Philip Brisco, Theo. Cooke, Jr., Julius Friedenwald, J. H. Kennedy, Alex. S. Porter, J. H. Robinson, Edw. M. Schaeffer, J. B. Schwatka, E. G. Welch.

Dr. T. Barton Brune, the Chairman of the Library Board, read his report, which was accepted and referred.

Dr. G. Lane Taneyhill, Chairman of the Publication Committee, read the report of the Committee, which, on motion, was accepted.

Dr. E. F. Cordell, Chairman, read the report of the Memoir Committee, which on motion was accepted and referred to the Publication Committee, with authority to condense, but not that part referring to Dr. Quinan.

Dr. C. H. Jones, Chairman of the Ethics Committee, read his report, which was accepted.

The Curator had nothing to report.

The Special Committee on Increasing the Membership, reported through the Chairman, Dr. Ashby, that a large number of applications would be presented during these sessions.

The SECTIONS being called, Dr. Tiffany, Chairman of *Section on Surgery* was allowed to read his paper by title, the same action was taken on the paper of Dr. Chambers. Dr. R. Winslow from *Section on Surgery*, read his paper, which was on motion accepted.

On motion a committee in regard to the "Telephone Question," consisting of Drs. Grove, Browne and Cathell, was appointed, with instructions to report at a future meeting.

The Faculty adjourned to meet at 8 P. M., April 28, 1891.

G. LANE TANEYHILL,
Secretary.

HALL OF FACULTY,
TUESDAY, April 28, 1891.

The Faculty was called to order at 8.15 P. M., by the President, a good attendance characterized this, the first " *night session*," of the Faculty which has taken place for many years. The minutes were read by the Recording Secretary, and adopted.

The *Section on Surgery* continued its report,—Dr. Jno. D. Blake, reading his paper from said section; the paper was debated by Dr. Michael, and on motion was accepted and referred for publication.

Dr. Jos. T. Smith, a member of the *Section on Practice*, read a paper, which was discussed by Drs. Bond, Sellman, Brinton and others, after which it was accepted and referred for publication.

On motion the reading of the paper of Dr. Osler, was at the request of that gentleman, postponed until a later hour.

Dr. J. E. Michael, Chairman of the *Section on Obstetrics and Gynæcology*, read a very interesting paper; it was debated by Drs. Rohe, Craighill, Blake, Wiltshire, Friedenwald, Bond and Gardner, after which the paper was accepted and referred for publication.

On motion the Faculty adjourned to meet at 11 A. M., Wednesday, 29th inst.

G. LANE TANEYHILL,
Secretary.

HALL OF FACULTY.

APRIL 29, 1891.

The Faculty was called at 11.15 A. M., this day.

The President, Dr. T. A. Ashby, in the chair.

The minutes of last night's session were read and approved.

The following candidates were elected to membership :

Theo. Cooke, Jr., Julius Friedenwald, J. H. Kennedy, Alex. S. Porter, J. H. Robinson, Edw. M. Schaeffer, J. B. Schwatka, E. G. Welch.

Dr. Michael, a member of, and for the Examining Board, recommended the following named candidates for membership, to be voted for Thursday, April 30, 1890.

Philip Brisco, J. A. Bonnett, J. T. Crouch, F. E. Fooks, Harry G. Harryman, W. T. Hall, S. B. Hammett, J. F. Martenett, J. H. Mittrick, Pedro de S. Moran, Frank D. Sanger, W. H. Schwatka, J. F. Somers, W. G. Townsend.

Dr. Wm. S. Gardner, of the *Obstetrical and Gynæcological Section*, read a paper which was discussed by Dr. Michael and others,—accepted and referred for publication.

Dr. J. W. Humrichouse, from the *Section on Laryngology*, read a paper which was accepted and referred for publication.

At this juncture, as per announcement, the regular order was suspended, and the Orator of the convention, Prof. Wm. H. Welch, of the Johns Hopkins University delivered an edifying address on "*The Causation and Treatment of Diphtheria.*"

On motion of Dr. W. T. Howard, the thanks of the Faculty were heartily voted to Prof. Welch for his masterly oration, and on motion of Dr. P. C. Williams, the author was requested to present a copy for publication.

Dr. H. Newell Martin, Chairman of the *Section on Anatomy Physiology and Pathology*, reported from his section; he was, on motion of Dr. Blake, requested to reduce his remarks to writing and transmit the same to the Publication Committee.

Dr. J. C. Hemmeter, of the same section, read a paper, which was accepted and referred for publication.

Dr. H. Newell Martin, of same section, made remarks on "*The Vaso Motor Nerves of the Heart.*" He was requested to reduce the same to writing and transmit the paper to the Publication Committee.

Dr. P. C. Williams, the Chairman of Executive Committee, announced other volunteer papers, which will be read under that heading.

On motion the Faculty adjourned to meet Wednesday night in "Executive Session."

G. LANE TANEYHILL,
Secretary·

HALL OF THE FACULTY,
APRIL 29, 1891.

The meeting was called to order at 8.30 P. M., the President, Dr. T. A. Ashby, in the chair. The Assistant Recording Secretary at the table.

The Telephone Committee reported through its Chairman, Dr. B. B. Browne. The report was accepted, and the President appointed Drs. B. B. Browne, W. F. A. Kemp and B. F. Grove, as the permanent committee.

The Recording Secretary read the minutes of this morning's meeting, which were adopted.

Dr. Jas. T. Smith announced that as there were very few members present from out of town, there will be no Banquet Thursday night, and that money in his hands would be refunded.

The Secretary then reported from the Committee on Increasing the Membership, and reported progress; the committee was continued.

Under Unfinished Business, the Library Committee through its Chairman, Dr. T. B. Brune gave notice of an Amendment to Constitution, Art. No. X. They also offered the following resolution, which was adopted after considerable debate :

Resolved, That the sum appropriated by the Faculty to the use of the Library, be disbursed to the Chairman of the

Library Committee in equal payments, the first to be made on or before May 15th, the second, on or before August 15th; the third on or before January 15th, and the fourth on or before April 15th, of each year.

Amendments to the Constitution, Art. 5, were brought up by Dr. Hemmeter and they were voted on seriatim.

1st, Art. 5, Constitution, effecting the appointment as far as possible by the chair and the Executive Committee of a member to open the discussion on every report and paper read by the various sections, (and possibly volunteer papers.)

2d, The *titles* of all reports and papers must be sent to the Recording Secretary at least one week before the opening of the meeting at which it is desired to read the paper.

3d, Members of Sections shall hereafter be appointed by the Executive Committee and the chair, instead of by the chair alone; this appointing Board must obtain personal assurance from every member appointed on Sections that he will contribute to the proceedings of the annual or semi-annual meeting by reading a paper; printed blanks to this effect are to be signed by the members.

After considerable discussion, the first amendment was laid on the table; the second was *adopted* as offered. To the third, the following substitute was offered, by Dr. G. Lane Taneyhill, namely:

The President shall secure in writing, *personal assurance* from *each Chairman of a Section* previous to appointment, that he will read a (his) paper at the annual meeting; he should, also, secure if possible an assurance from all appointees on the several sections, that they will write papers for the annual or semi-annual meeting. The number of papers from each section, shall be limited to *five,* and if by any uncontrollable circumstance a section member be unable to prepare a paper, the Chairman may, after notification to the President, invite a member in good standing in the Faculty to write a paper for the same section.

Both substitute and the third amendment, were on motion laid on the table.

By permission at this time the Examining Board for Western Shore recommended the following named physicians for membership in the Faculty:

I. R. Trimble, M. D., William Gambel, M. D., L. C. Horn, M. D., H. A. Kelly, M. D., Z. K. Wiley, M. D., J. C. Wunder, M. D., J. T. M. Finney, M. D., and J. L. McCormick, M. D.

Dr. Hiram Woods gave formal notice of intention to present at a future meeting the following *amendment* to the Constitution.

The Chairman of each section shall select some member of the Faculty to open the discussion upon one of the papers to be read by his section: he shall send to the Recording Secretary the name of the one selected when he sends the titles of papers to be presented by his section.

Dr. E. F. Cordell offered the following resolution, which was adopted:

Resolved, That the Committee on Publication be directed to publish in the Transactions of the Faculty for this year, the amendments to the Constitution and also all resolutions affecting the same—which have been adopted since the last publication of the Constitution and By-laws.

Resignations from the following named members were accepted: W. C. Sandrock, Isabella K. Godfrey, W. C. Kloman, W. Dulaney Thomas and J. J. Pennington.

The election of officers resulted as follows:

President.—Dr. Wm. H. Welch.

Vice-Presidents.—Drs. J. W. Humrichouse and David Streett.

Recording Secretary.—Dr. G. Lane Taneyhill.

Assistant Secretary.—Dr. Robt. T. Wilson.

Corresponding Secretary.—Dr. Joseph T. Smith.

Reporting Secretary.—Dr. Wm. B. Canfield.

Treasurer.—Dr. W. F. A Kemp.

Executive Committee.—Drs. T. A. Ashby, J. E. Michael, G. H. Rohe, P. C. Williams, Wilmer Brinton.

Examining Board of Western Shore.—Drs. J. W. Chambers, L. McLane Tiffany, E. F. Cordell, Hiram Woods, D. W. Cathell, W. H. Norris, B. B. Browne.

Examining Board of Eastern Shore.—Drs. B. W. Goldsborough, G. T. Atkinson, A. H. Bayley, J. K. H. Jacobs, W. F. Hines.

On motion the Faculty adjourned to meet at 11 a. m., Thursday, April 30th.

G. LANE TANEYHILL,
Recording Secretary.

HALL OF THE FACULTY,

APRIL 30, 1891.

The meeting was called to order by the President, Dr. T. A. Ashby. Present 115. The minutes of the previous meeting were read by the Assistant Recording Secretary and adopted.

Dr. Wm. Osler, Chairman of *Section on Practice*, read his paper—"*The Healing of Pulmonary Tubercolosis.*" It was discussed by Dr. Welch and Dr. J. T. Smith and referred for publication.

Dr. W. T. Councilman, Chairman of *Section on Microscopy and Micro-Chemistry*, read a paper on "*The Form of Dysentery produced by the Amœba Coli.*" It was discussed by Dr. Osler, Dr. Neff, Dr. A. Friedenwald, Dr. Hemmeter, Dr. Councilman and Dr. Harris, and on motion referred for publication.

Dr. Welch introduced Dr. N. A. Powell, of Toronto, Canada, an accredited representative of the "Ontario

Medical Association" to this Faculty; he was, on motion, invited to a seat in the Convention.

Dr. H. Woods, Chairman of *Section on Ophthalmology, Otology and Laryngology*, read a paper on *"Blindness in the United States."* It was discussed by Dr. A. Friedenwald, Dr. Rohe, Dr. R. L. Randolph, Dr. Brinton and Dr. Harris. It was accepted and referred for publication.

On motion, a special committee of four was appointed, as suggested by the paper of Dr. Woods; the committee consists of the following: Drs. H. Woods, Harry Friedenwald, J. E. Michael and G. H. Rohe.

Dr. Wm. T. Cathell read his paper from the same Section; it was accepted and referred for publication.

Under *Volunteer Papers*, Dr. E. M. Schaeffer read a paper, which was accepted and referred for publication, after being discussed by Dr. Norris and others.

The following candidates were elected to membership:

J. A. Bonnett, Philip Brisco, J. F. Crouch, F. E. Fooks, J. T. M. Finney, William Gombel, W. F. Hall, S. B. Hammett, Harry G. Harryman, L. C. Horn, Howard A. Kelly, J. F. Martinet, J. H. Mittnick, Pedro De S. Moran, I. L. McCormick, R. C. Rasin, Frank D. Sanger, W. H. Schwatka, J. F. Somers, W. G. Townsend, H. B. Thomas, I. R. Trimble, Z. K. Wiley, J. C. Wunder.

On motion the Faculty adjourned to meet at 8 P. M., this Thursday, April 30th.

G. LANE TANEYHILL,

Secretary.

HALL OF THE FACULTY,

THURSDAY, April 30, 1891. Night Session.

The meeting was called to order at 8.30 P. M., by the President, Dr. T. A. Ashby. The minutes of the morning session were read by the Secretary and approved. On account of the enforced absence of the Secretary, on motion of that officer, Dr. J. F. Martinett was authorized to act during the evening.

Dr. Samuel J. Fort's paper on "*The Physical Training of the Feeble Minded*," was on account of the absence of that gentleman, read by title and referred.

Dr. Geo. H. Rohe read a report of One Hundred Cases of Labor at the Maryland Maternite, it was discussed by Drs. Michael and Chisolm and referred.

Dr. Geo. J. Preston's paper was read by title and referred for publication.

Dr. John C. Hemmeter read his paper on "*Acute Miliary Tubercolosis*" treated by Koch's Tuberculin, it was discussed by Dr. J. W. Chambers and referred.

Dr. J. J. Chisolm read his paper on "*Intra-Uterine Diseases of the Eye*." It was, on motion, referred for publication.

Dr. Wilmer Brinton read his paper on "*Two Cases of Obstetrics*," it was referred for publication.

Dr. James Brown read a paper on "*Cancer of the Bladder*," and exhibited an interesting pathological specimen. His paper was referred for publication.

Dr. Thos. Opie read a paper on "*Supra-Vaginal Hysterectomy*." It was referred for publication.

On motion, on account of the absence of Dr.
Howard A. Kelly and Dr. N. G. Keirle, the papers
of those gentlemen were read by title and they were
requested to transmit copies to the Publishing Committee.

On motion of Dr. John Morris it was ordered that
Dr. Henry M. Hurd prepare a suitable memorial in
regard to the death of Dr. Richard Gundry and
transmit the same to the incoming Memorial Committee.

The President read the following as his list of appointments of Committees, Sections and Delegates
for the ensuing year :

STANDING COMMITTEES.

Library.—T. Barton Brune, G. Lane Taneyhill, B. B.
Browne, Wm. Osler, S. T. Earle.

Publication.—G. Lane Taneyhill, W. F. A. Kemp, J. E.
Michael, H. M. Wilson, C. H. Riley.

Memoir.—E. F. Cordell, J. McP. Scott, G. T. Atkinson, C.
F. Bevan, Alice T. Hall.

Ethics.—L. McLane Tiffany, P. C. Williams, E. G. Waters,
Caleb Winslow, Alan P. Smith.

Increasing the Membership.—T. A. Ashby, B. W. Goldsborough, G. Lane Taneyhill, W. F. Hines, S. T. Earle.

Curator.—L. F. Ankrim.

SECTIONS.

Surgery.—Drs. R. W. Johnson, John G. Jay, E. R.
Walker, A. S. Mason, H. H. Biedler.

Practice.—Drs. S. C. Chew, F. C. Bressler, David Streett,
B. W. Goldsborough, H. M. Salzer.

Obstetrics and Gynæcology.—Drs. L. E. Neale, J. Whitridge
Williams, Hunter Robb, R. T. Wilson, Arthur Williams.

Materia Medica and Chemistry.—T. B. Brune, J. W. Humrichouse, I. E. Atkinson, J. T. Smith, A. K. Bond.

Sanitary Science.—E. F. Cordell, G. H. Rohe, W. B. Platt, E. M. Schaeffer, A. H. Bayly.

Anatomy, Physiology and Pathology.—J. W. Chambers, C. O. Miller, Randolph Winslow, J. C. Hemmeter, J. D. Blake.

Psychology and Medical Jurisprudence.—H. M. Hurd, C. G. Hill, H. J. Berkley, S. J. Fort, E. M. Reid.

Microscopy, &c.—C. Hampson Jones, W. D. Booker, J. W. Funck, N. G. Keirle, Wm. Osler.

Ophthalmology, Otology and Laryngology.—S. K. Merrick, J. N. Mackenzie, R. L. Randolph, G. W. Thomas, Harry Friedenwald.

DELEGATES.

American Medical Association at Washington, D. C.—Jos. Brown, J. W. Branham, Wilmer Brinton, W. B. Canfield, E. M. Chamberlaine, J. J. Chisolm, W. P. Chunn, Jno. Dickson, F. Donaldson, S. T. Earle, R. H. P. Ellis, T. B. Evans, A. Friedenwald, N. R. Gorter, H. Harlan, H. F. Hill, B. M. Hopkinson, C. Johnston, T. S. Latimer, R. B. Morison, W. B. Platt, Wm. Osler, G. J. Preston, J. McP. Scott, Alan P. Smith, David Streett, E. M. Schaeffer, W. A. B. Sellman, G. Lane Taneyhill, S. Theobald, W. C. VanBibber, Arthur Williams, Wm. H. Welch.

DELEGATES TO STATE MEDICAL SOCIETIES.

West Virginia.—B. B. Browne, W. A. R. F. Carr, Thomas Opie, J. M. Craighill, J. G. Wiltshire.

Virginia.—J. E. Michael, J. S. Conrad, A. C. Pole, I. R. Page, H. P. C. Wilson.

North Carolina.—C. G. Hill, W. T. Howard, Hiram Woods, I. E. Atkinson, R. T. Wilson.

On motion of Dr. Michael the thanks of the Faculty were voted to the retiring President, Dr. T.

A. Ashby for the commendable manner in which he had executed the duties of his office ; this action was supplemented by a general vote of thanks to all the retiring officers, and the President declared the 93rd Annual Convention of the Medical and Chirurgical Faculty of the State of Maryland adjourned *sine die*.

G. LANE TANEYHILL, M. D.,

Recording Secretary.

REPORTS.

REPORT OF CORRESPONDING SECRETARY.

BALTIMORE, MD., April 28, 1891.

The Medical and Chirurgical Faculty of Maryland:

GENTLEMEN :—Your Corresponding Secretary has the honor to report that he has carried on the correspondence of the Faculty during the year. As the programs of the meeting at this time were sent to the profession throughout the State, it did not seem necessary to notice the meeting in the county papers.

This is respectfully submitted,

JOSEPH T. SMITH,
Corresponding Secretary.

REPORT OF TREASURER.

Mr. President and Members:—The report of your Treasurer at this 93rd Annual Convention of our time honored Faculty should receive the careful study of our membership. The last year has witnessed our attempt at an annual dues per member of $5, and a continuation of the Semi-Annual Meetings. It will be observed that the large increase in membership acquired at our last meeting, has made our income reach nearly that of our preceding year, whilst on the other side it has added corresponding expenses which have exceeded those of last year—our increased expenses are mainly from larger issue of Transactions—from expenses of Reporting Secretary and the larger incidental account—a comparison of which I take liberty to present at this time.

Transactions, print'g, mail'g and directing, 1889, $355.51.   1890, $435.31
Reporting Secretary,...................... 1889,   15.00.   1890,   35.48
Sundries,................................ 1889,   38.15.   1890, 162.16

     These items total,...................... $408.66 $632.95
or an extra expenditure of $224.29.

Some of this increase is only incurred once, whilst that which is credited to Transactions must abide and increase in a ratio with acquisitions in membership. The incidentals must ever remain uncertain, as in every well ordered house that which is necessary for comfort must depend largely upon contingencies.—The Semi-Annual Meetings are too much of an experiment to justify positive predictions concerning them. We cannot compare aroused interest with the hard figures of paid in and paid out. I will therefore only compare the in and out. You will be told Semi-Annual Meeting cost $40 for hall rent and announcements ; for bill allowed Reporting Secretary $11.50, making $51.50, at which meeting the Secretary reports there were 4 new members elected.

One more item it is well for you to remember, is that our income from rent of local societies cannot in the coming year exceed $175 ; whilst this year we received $212.50. Again, when our telephone was introduced into our hall, this Faculty was expected to pay one-quarter of the cost, now that some local societies have removed to other quarters, we have the privilige of paying one-half. It is but due you, gentlemen, that you devote more than a passing thought to our Faculty, and its necessities. On April 1st, as per resolution of our body, I mailed 78 bills to members who had as yet not paid their dues; from that number 23 responded, you can easily make the calculation, and find that at this writing 50 odd of our membership so ardently love this Faculty, that they are unable or unwilling to pay the debt due. These brethren I'm sure would resent any imputation upon our fair name, and yet fairness to us, attention to the Treasurer's appeals, or the collector's call would relieve our debt due, and would go far toward making us a thing of beauty and a joy forever.

Our greatest attraction in the Faculty undoubtedly is the Library, and we ought to do honor to ourselves in increasing its efficiency. This first year of our new departure has had its effect upon its operations, of this the Library Board will make mention in their report; they should report their actions in detail. They will mention that they received from sales and fines $8.39, from dues $448, making a total of $456.39, being $115.12 less than they received last year.

Our accessions this year have been by the election of the following ninety-two members at Annual Meeting, April, 1890.

L. F. Ankrim, Thos. H. Buckler, Bobert Bond, S. B. Bond, J. B. Baxley, Jr., Joseph Blum, W. S. Blaisdell, F. C. Bressler, C. Bernie, J. E. Bromwell, J. W. Branham, C. L. Buddenbohn, Wm. M. Barnes, H. J. Coffroth, Frank M. Chisolm, J. H. Christian, W. P. Chunn, J. M. Craighill, M. A. R. F. Carr, G. H. Chabbot, Wm. D. Corse, R. G. Davis, G. E. Dickinson, E. Dorsey Ellis, J. W. Funck, Geo. A. Flemming, Jno. S. Fulton, Harry Friedenwald, A. B. Giles, Isabel K. Godfrey, N. R. Gorter, E. C. Gibbs, H. H. Goodman, H. B. Gwynn, W. S. Gardner, Henry F. Hill, J. M. Hundley, J. W. Humrickhouse, H. S. Herman, W. F. Hines, H. L. Hilgartner, E. M. Hartwell, Alice T. Hall, Wm. N. Hill, Henry F. Hurd, C. Hampson Jones, C. C. Jacobs, Edwin E. Jones, J. T. King, N. G. Keirle, S. A. Keene, W. F. Lockwood, Thos. M. Lumpkin, A. S. Mason, A. H. Mann, Jr., C. O. Miller, S. K. Merrick, Russell Murdock, W. E. Mosely, Arthur Mansfield, Wm. H. Norris, Winton M. Nihiser, H. C. Ohle, Wm. Osler, J. J. Pennington, J. E. Prichard, J. Randolph Page, Hunter Robb, O. H. W. Ragan, M. Rowe, R. L. Randolph, M. Laura E. Redding, John H. Rehberger, J. B. Saunders, J. M. Spear, Norman B. Scott, John McP. Scott, Alan P. Smith, Jno. T. Spicknall, W. C. Sandrock, W. R. Shaw, W. D. Thomas, W. J. Todd, J. G. Van Marter, Jr., W. W. Virdin, Hiram Woods, Jr., Mactier Warfield, E. R. Walker, R. B. Warfield, E. J. Williams, J. Jones Wilson, Charles B. Ziegler, and the election of A. C. Jones, Enoch George, J. A. Stevens and S. Chase DeKraff at the Semi-Annual Meeting in Cambridge, November 12, 1891.

Our losses have been by resignation, Dr. Jos. F. Perkins; by death, Richard Gundry, A. M. Drought, R. W. Eareckson, Jno. R. Quinan; by non-payment of dues, A. M. Chilton.

RECEIPTS.

Initiation Fees,	$	460 00
Rent of Hall		212 50
Rent of Telephone,		36 00
Pharmaceutical Exhibit,		145 00
Advertisements,		65 00
Dues of members,		814 00
Sales and Fines at Library,		8 39
	$	1,740 89

DISBURSEMENTS.

Annual Orator,	$	5 50
Advertising Annual Meeting,		47 00
Janitor,		70 00
Chairs for Annual Meeting,		22 50
Gas,		13 50
Library Board Sales and Fines,		8 39
" " Dues of Members,		448 00
Rent of Hall,		600 00
Rent of Telephone,		72 00
Transactions, Printing,		400 51
" Stamps,		24 80
" Directing,		10 00
Corresponding Secretary,		16 94
Reporting Secretary,		35 48
Semi-Annual Meeting,		40 00
Commissions for Collecting dues,		15 20
Treasurer's Expenses, including Stamps, &c.,		35 00
Incidental Sundries,		162 16
Making a total of	$	2,026 98
To which add deficiency reported last year of,		231 97
Making total,	$	2,258 95

Our Assets—

Amount to Credit Building Fund,	$	192 00
Library and Fixtures estimated,		7,500 00
Dues from Members in Arrears,		350 00

Our Liabilities—

Deficit of 1889		$231 97
Deficit of 1890		286 09
		$518 06

And by resolution adopted April 29, page 144, of this year's transactions, as due Library Board   47 10

Making total of $565 16

Gentlemen you have heard the report as presented. It becomes you to so arrange and adjust our affairs, that the Faculty may make a showing that will reflect honor upon ourselves. Our deficiency of last year $231.97, has been increased by our expenses over income of this year, which is $286.09, to $518.06.

Your Treasurer frankly acknowledges that it has been with no little trouble to himself to meet the calls for money necessary to pay our indebtedness, and he takes this public occasion to personally thank those who have loaned him moneys to dispense for our relief. I would appeal to the honor of our delinquent membership, that they respond to their duties more promptly. Our dues are collectible in advance, and only by prompt payment on the part of our membership can we establish and confirm in the community the name we deserve, the name in which we delight to honor, and the name we would imperishably stamp upon the future. I would in concluding again call attention to the facts afore-stated, and urge upon you an increased desire and action to add to our ranks those who will honor and assist us, and enjoy the advantages, we, by our Journal Library, are offering to all. Speculate upon our possibilities, if all would pay their just dues, and think upon our halting gait which is necessitated by our delinquent list; this is a burning shame. It has been a source of perplexity to this officer of your association. Finally whatsoever things are true think on these things. Let not to-days' sun go down to cover thy delinquency and have it reappear on the morrow, as the canker that mars our possibilities, that hampers our progress, that makes us unsightly, but let every one give of that which he hath, that the Faculty may arise in her strength and that as she approaches her Century of existence she may grow stronger, spreading wider her influences, gathering into her fold those embued with the spirit of her purpose, and desirious to have her unsurpassed in all that is good and excellent.

All of which is hoped for by your reporter and respectfully submitted.

W. F. A. KEMP,
Treasurer.

REPORT OF EXECUTIVE COMMITTEE.

The Executive Committee begs leave to report that during the past year its duties have been unusually light, very few subjects of importance having been brought before it.

At its first meeting a letter was received from Prof. I. E. Atkinson in which he resigned the Chairmanship of the Library Board, but expressing his willingness to remain a member of the Committee. The resignation was accepted and Dr. T. Barton Brune was appointed Chairman. He at once entered upon the discharge of his duties, which he has performed with zeal and fidelity.

Your Committee appropriated money to pay for necessary repairs of the room occupied by the "Directory for Nurses." It also authorized the Treasurer to pay the Reporting Secretary for extra duty at Semi-Annual meeting.

The Committee also appropriated $50.00 for the use of the "Committee for the increase of the Membership of the Faculty."

Your Committee has the great pleasure of announcing that Prof. William H. Welch, of the Johns Hopkins University has accepted its invitation to deliver the Annual Oration. His subject will be the "Causation of Diphtheria." His oration will be delivered to-morrow (Wednesday) at 12 o'clock.

P. C. WILLIAMS, *Chairman.*
J. W. CHAMBERS,
S. T. EARLE,
A. FRIEDENWALD,
R. WINSLOW.

ROB'T T. WILSON,
    Sec'y to Ex. Committee.

REPORT OF THE BOARD OF EXAMINERS.
WESTERN SHORE.

Mr. President and Members:—The Board of Examiners for Western Shore have considered the applications of the following named, eight, members of the medical profession, and recommend their election. The names have, as ordered been placed on the bulletin board. Theodore Cook, Jr., Julius Friedenwald, J. H. Kennedy, Alex. S. Porter, J. H. Robinson, Edwd. M. Schaeffer, J. B. Schwatka and E. G. Welch.

Your Committee has assurance from the energetic *Committee on Increasing the Membership* that this list is only one-fourth of the names that will be presented during the sessions of this Convention.

All of which is respectfully submitted,

CHARLES H. JONES, M. D.

Chairman.

REPORT OF LIBRARY COMMITTEE.

Mr. President and Gentlemen:—In behalf of the Library Committee I have the honor to report that the Committee duly organized under the chairmanship of Dr. I. E. Atkinson, Dr. Brune being elected Secretary.

After a few months of service Dr. Atkinson found himself obliged to resign the chairmanship, tho' not his membership in the Committee, and Dr. Brune was appointed Chairman in his place, Dr. Taneyhill being elected to the Secretaryship thus made vacant.

Dr. A. K. Bond was elected Librarian and Registrar of the Nurses' Directory for the year ensuing from June 1, 1890.

Dr. W. Guy Townsend was elected Assistant Librarian for the same period.

Immediately upon its organization the Committee was confronted with the grave problem of a great diminution in its already small income.

No doubt you will recall the fact that at the last Annual Session a majority of members present and voting, decided to reduce the annual dues from $8.00 to $5.00 for city members, and from $3.00 to $2.00 for county members, the Library to retain its former proportion.

This has resulted in a net loss to the Library of about one-ourth of its income.

As we all know, the membership of the Faculty increased unprecedently this past year—thanks to the exertions of the Committee on New Members—and a large sum was received by the Treasury of the Faculty on account of the initiation fees of the new members, but, as new members pay no annual dues the first year and as the Library has no share in initiation fees, it derived no pecuniary benefit from the increased membership. It simply suffered a net loss of revenue from the reduction of the dues.

Moreover, your Committee has been seriously hampered by delay in receiving from the Treasurer even the pittance appropriated to it. This delay is attributed by him to the remissness of members in settling their accounts.

In consequence of this combination of untoward circumstances the Committee has been much embarrassed and the smooth working of the Library impaired. Not for years has its revenue been so small and so hard to obtain. Indeed had it not been for the use of individual credit and the increased earnings of the Directory for Nurses, it would have been impossible to conduct its affairs.

So strapped have we been that we have not been able to bind a journal, rebind an old volume or purchase a new book, to say nothing of our inability to provide the new shelving imperatively demanded by a growing Library.

Such a state of things is certainly deplorable, if not disgraceful.

On the other hand your Committee is glad to report that it has not given up a Journal subscribed for last year and has kept the Library open the same number of hours daily as when its income was largest. Moreover, it has incurred no indebtedness.

The Library has grown through the generous contributions of certain gentlemen to the extent of 307 volumes, making the number of volumes now upon our shelves 7,027, exclusive of 840 duplicate volumes.

We are indebted to Dr. B. B. Browne for 16 volumes ; Dr. Jas. A. Steuart, 166 volumes ; Dr. A. K. Bond, 16 volumes; Dr. W. B. Canfield, 10 volumes ; Dr. F. Donaldson, 4 volumes; Dr. C. C. Shippen, 2 volumes; and Dr. Baldwin, 19 volumes of the North American Review.

Drs. A. K. Bond, B. B. Browne, T. B. Brune, H. Harlan and Jas. A. Steuart have contributed collections of pamphlets and journals.

Eighty-two journals are regularly received and placed upon our tables.

We have received as exchanges from the University of Erlangen, 186 Theses; University of Goettingen, 26 Theses; University of Heidelberg, 22 Theses; University of Strasbourg, 63 Theses; University of Tuebingen, 22 Theses; University of Leyden, 11 Theses.

The Health Reports of Baltimore City have been regularly received.

The increased demand for Nurses from the Directory made by physicians and the public has been gratifying.

The percentage of hospital-trained nurses on its roll has markedly increased and the standard of nursing is being decidedly raised.

An especially desirable class of nurses is being added to our list from the training schools here and elsewhere.

Physicians, however, are not yet fully alive to the advantages of the Directory, and even those who are accustomed to use the Directory would save the Registrar and their patients much annoyance by reminding the latter that the valuable information furnished them by the Directory cost $1.00 or $2.00.

There are upon the roll of the Directory 56 nurses. Of these 6 are male and 50 female. Four (one male and three females) devote themselves to massage.

Of the 15 nurses added to the roll during the present year 13 have been trained in hospital; 4 having graduated at the Maternite in this city, 5 in the Philadelphia training schools, and 3 in the training schools of Ireland.

The Directory has 34 hospital trained nurses as against 24 last year, and its work so far as known, has been very satisfactory to both physicians and the public. The large amount of business done by it this year has enabled it, after paying all of its own expenses, including the salary of the Registrar, to turn over to the Library a cash balance of $92.80.

The Receipts and Expenses of the *Library* for the year have been:

RECEIPTS.

From old Committee,	-	$ 4 05
" Fines and Sales,		8 39
" Treasurer,	-	448 00
" Nurses' Directory,	-	92 80
Total,	- -	$553 24

EXPENSES.

Salaries, Librarian and Assistant,	$240 00	
Journals, - - -	297 01	
Sundries,	-	6 37	
Total,	$543 38	
Cash Surplus,	- - - ˗ -	$9 86
Due from Treasurer on dues collected,		. . . .
Total receipts of *Nurses' Directory*,	$182 00	
Total expenses of Nurses' Directory,		89 20
Cash Surplus,		92 80

In conclusion your Committee would earnestly recommend for your adoption the following suggestions which will be offered as resolutions at the proper time:

1.   That the sums due the Library from the Treasurer be paid in equal quarterly instalments on May 15, August 15, January 15 and April 15 of each year.

2.   That *one-half of all initiation fees and annual dues be paid to the Library*, instead of ⅝ of dues from city and ⅔ of dues from county members, as at present.

Respectfully submitted,

T. BARTON BRUNE, *Chairman.*

B. BERNARD BROWNE,

G. LANE TANEYHILL,

WILLIAM H. WELCH,

I. E. ATKINSON,

Committee.

REPORT OF PUBLICATION COMMITTEE.

Mr. President and Members:—Your publication Committee went to work early in the year :—they elected Dr. George J. Preston their Secretary, and as there had been a large increase in the family, they contracted for 700 instead of 500 copies of the Transactions. Griffin, Curley & Co., were the successful bidders for the printing, and the first-class typographical execution of the contract demonstrates their ability to meet the exacting demands of your committee. The volume in printing and contents has been universally commended.

A copy was promptly mailed to each member, to all State Medical Associations, to many Libraries and Medical Journals throughout the world, for which we have received many valuable exchanges.

The new feature of publishing the papers read at the Semi-Annual meetings has increased the volume in size, and we believe, in merit.

It is the opinion of your committee that authors should be compelled to deliver to the Recording Secretary within 15 days after adjournment of the conventions, either the original manuscript or a perfect copy, in order that the committee might not be subjected to those vexatious delays which have too often in the past tried the patience of this hard worked committee, and, that they may at an earlier date issue the Transactions.

Your committee has adopted the regulation as endorsed by all other State Medical Associations, of devolving the expense of photographs, wood-cuts, electrotypes, etc., on the authors of papers.

All of which is respectfully submitted,

G. LANE TANEYHILL, *Chairman.*
WM. FREDERICK KEMP,
GEORGE J. PRESTON,
RANDOLPH WINSLOW.

REPORT OF MEMOIR COMMITTEE.

MEMOIR OF ALBERT MATHEWS DROUGHT.

Dr. Drought was born in Baltimore, May 17th, 1866. He was a grandson of the late Captain Francis Drought, of the English army, and a nephew of Colonel Drought, of Drought-ville, Ireland, and of the Rev. Adolphus Drought, of the same place. His maternal grandfather was Thos. Mathews, Esq., a member of an aristocratic Irish family. At the age of fourteen he entered the drug store of the late Philip Rogers, No. 6 West North Avenue, and when only seventeen became the proprietor of a similar establishment on the corner of Presstman and Stricker Streets, which he successfully managed for five years. At the age of eighteen he graduated from the Maryland College of Pharmacy, and during the succeeding year studied chemistry under the direction of Professor Simon. At the age of nineteen he began the study of medicine at the University of Maryland, and graduated, after attending three sessions, in 1888. Entering then upon practice in the northern part of the city, by his intelligence and assiduity he soon acquired the confidence and patronage of a number of excellent families, and his prospects were very bright when his career was cut short by a shocking and unusual accident. Whilst diving at Tolchester Beach on the 16th of July, 1890, he sustained a fracture of the fifth cernial vertebra. He was brought to the city and treated at the City Hospital, but no relief could be afforded him and he died on the day following the accident. Dr. Drought was a young physician of genial and courteous manners, and endeared himself to all who knew him.

At a meeting of this Faculty, held November 15th, 1890, to record our sentiments upon the loss of Dr. Drought, Drs. Sandrock, Giles, Norris, Baldwin and Cordell were appointed a committee to prepare resolutions, who brought in the following :

WHEREAS, It has pleased an allwise Providence to take from our midst our esteemed young friend and associate, Dr. Albert M. Drought, at an age when his future seemed so bright, and under circumstances so sad to his bereaved friends and family,

Resolved, That we place upon record our appreciation of his excellent qualities of mind and heart, and offer his example and success for the emulation of those who are just. entering upon their professional career.

Resolved, That a copy of these resolutions be sent to his family.

<hr>

MEMOIR OF JOHN RUSSELL QUINAN, M. D.

By Wm. Stump Forwood, M. D., of Darlington, Md.

<hr>

The lives of the dead are committed to the memory of the living.—CICERO.

Man is but the sum of his ancestors.—EMERSON.

<hr>

Mr. President and Members of the Medical and Chirurgical Faculty of Maryland:—As a member of the Committee on Memoirs, and as a warm personal friend of the deceased, it becomes my painful duty to make the formal announcement to you of the death of *Dr. John Russell Quinan*, one of the most able, and valued members of this Faculty, which occurred, suddenly, on the 11th of November, 1890, in the 69th year of his age.

As the last hours, or moments, as in this case, of our friends, always possess a peculiar interest for their survivors, I will begin by narrating the sad incidents of the final scene, which have been kindly furnished me by the son of the deceased, Mr. Allen B. Quinan, who was present, and witnessed what he states. In answer to my request for information in regard to the shockingly sudden death of my friend, Mr. Quinan wrote me as follows, under date of November 17th—six days after the sad event :

" I feel stunned, and can scarcely realize that I shall never again, in this life, see his face. For some weeks past he had been working very hard on the Medical Dictionary (the great Dictionary being published by the Appletons, and of which Dr. Q. had been assigned the preparation of a part,) and at times I observed in him more or less dyspnœa after walking; but, with this exception he was apparently in as good health as I have ever seen him.

"On the afternoon of the 11th instant, after dining, he was called out hurriedly to attend a child suffering with convulsions. He had to hold the child, which was about six years of age, while the mother, who was half distracted, went for hot water. The child struggled violently, and befouled my father's clothing. He came home, took a cold sponge bath, changed his clothes, and returned to finish his attendance. On his second return home he showed no signs of excitement, nor of exhaustion, but appeared to be in his usual good spirits. Within ten minutes after resuming the writing, upon which he was engaged (the Dictionary), he complained to me of a very disagreeable sensation of nausea; remarking that the room, in which he had been with the child, was so filled with disagreeable odor that he felt sick at his stomach, he thought, in consequence.

"He went into the dining room, and asked my mother for some soda and water, which she gave him, and which he drank, and then lay down on the sofa. My mother had not been out of the room more than a few moments when she heard him groan. She ran to him, and found that he had reversed his position on the sofa, and seemed to have fainted. I hurried into the room and found him half lying on the sofa, his head hanging toward the floor. I raised his head, and while mother bathed his feet in hot water I ran for a physician. I suppose that it was fifteen or twenty minutes before I could get one; and when we reached the house, the doctor pronounced him to be dead.

"The death certificate said: 'Apoplexy and heart disease.' I cannot believe that it was *Apoplexy*. (Neither can I. W. S. F.) My father's habit and condition preclude the idea of brain disease. There was no foaming at the mouth, no stertorous breathing nor flushed face. He had never shown any confusion of intellect. * * * It would appear to me that he died from heart-failure, or heart disease of some kind, as a result of the over exertion and excitement, to which he had just been subjected."'

Within a few months of Dr. Quinan's death, as though he felt a premonition of the approach of that event, he prepared "for the use of his children," as he expressly stated, a full genealogical record of his family—occupying more than 70 type-written pages, and showing an intimate relationship with some of the most honorable and patriotic families of Ireland—the land of his ancestors.

As it is " appointed for man but once to die," such a man as Dr. Quinan, whose life and daily walk was an ornament to our profession, is entitled at our hands, to at least one memorial sketch—such as he would have given the present writer had he survived. I propose to enter very briefly upon a notice of his ancestry, and upon the history of his life, conforming to the proper limits of the present occasion.

The following facts I copy from the record just referred to as having been prepared by the deceased himself.

John Russell Quinan, son of Rev. Thomas Henry Quinan and Eliza (Hamilton) Quinan, was born at Lancaster, Pa., August 7th, 1822. He was educated classically at home and at Woodward High School (now College), Cincinnati, Ohio, and also at Marietta College, Ohio.

He studied medicine under the preceptorship of the late Dr. John K. Mitchell, Professor of Practice at the Jefferson Medical College, Philadelphia ; at which college he was graduated M. D. on March 20, 1844. He married Elizabeth Lydia Billingsley, of Calvert County, Md., on August 31, 1845, and had ten (10) children ; only five of whom, together with his wife, survive him.

The father of the subject of our sketch, (Rev.) Thomas Henry Quinan, was born in Balbriggan, Lienster County, Dublin, Ireland, on February 12th, 1795. He married Eliza (Hamilton) Quinan, who was born at Enhiskillen, Ulster County, Fermanah, Ireland, August 18th, 1799; the marriage taking place March 18, 1817, at St. Peter's Church, Dublin— soon after which event they moved to the United States, and had six children.

We learn from the genealogical record, already referred to, that William Henry Hamilton was his maternal grand-father; he being a son of Johnstone Hamilton, a solicitor of Enniskillen.

His grand-father became deeply infected with the Revolutionary mania of that day—occupying a somewhat similar position we are led to believe, under different circumstances, toward English authority, as that occupied at the present day by Parnell and his followers. And just as he was about to receive a commission in the army through the friendly offices of the Earl of Enniskillen, he delivered a speech of such an inflammatory tendency as to place, forever, a bar to any further patronage from his Lordship.

He afterwards married a sister of Thomas Russell, and embarked with that celebrated Irish patriot in all of his Revolutionary schemes.

His ancestor, Thomas Russell, was such a conspicuous and formidable enemy to the government—in intimate association with O'Connor, T. A. Emmet and McNeven—that, as a consequence, he frequently suffered imprisonment, which, instead of teaching prudence, appeared to increase and aggravate his disloyalty; until finally he was tried for high treason October 20, 1803, and was beheaded on the following day—defiant and reckless to the last, like his compatriot Robert Emmet, who suffered in like manner for similar offences, about the same time.

As before stated, Dr. Quinan had prepared a very full and complete genealogical record, for which his tastes and education peculiarly fitted him, of his own and of his wife's ancestors; which, on the title page is "Affectionately dedicated to my children and grand-children." This record chiefly relates to the "Quinans, Hamiltons, Russells, Barbers and Billingsleys," with the incidental mention of minor connections; with the following sentiment as a motto upon the title page, in the antique spelling of the author:

> "I, upon my later age,
> To sett an end to all my werke,
> Do make this testament of Love."
> —*Gower.*

As an evidence of his appreciation of the value of such memorials, he quotes the following lines:

> "To neglect the memory of one's ancestry
> Is to court oblivion for ourselves."

I here simply refer to the existence of the full records of Dr. Quinan's ancestors, which it has been my privilege to read, and which show that he had descended on both sides from the most honorable lineage. I will now give a brief sketch of the man himself. Having been an honorary member of the *Historical Society of Harford County, Maryland*, he prepared a short sketch of his life, in accordance with the Society's rules, for preservation in its archives upon his election; and having that sketch before me, I find that Dr. Quinan was born in Lancaster, Pa., as already stated; and after moving with his father to different cities in the West, he was finally graduated in medicine; and then embarked upon his honorable career of medical practice in Calvert County, Maryland, in the year of 1844. Here he labored assiduously, with the unquestioned title of being *the leading physician* in the county—achieving more honor than profit, as is the rule with our profession—especially in "country practice" for a period of twenty-five years—the best years of life for physical labor; at the end of that period, in the year 1869, feeling that his health and strength were failing under the strain of increasing and of largely unremunerative labors, to which had been added the non-paying office of "Superintendent, Examiner and President of the Board of School Commissioners, of Calvert County," he removed to the City of Baltimore, and there pursued the practice of his profession until the very hour of his death.

He, being a man possessed of uncommonly fine sympathies, of quick perception, and skilful diagnosis, I learn that his patients were most warmly attached to him; feeling that in him they had a friend, as well as a physician. His presence in the sick room was ever welcome, and carried with it the light of hope and comfort in support of the ebbing vitality of the sick, and happy cheer to the anxious sufferings of watching friends.

My personal acquaintance with Dr. Quinan has dated back only about ten years; and was brought about on seeing his Memoir of *John Archer*, *M. B.*, late of Harford County, Md. and who was the first of the great multitude, which has since passed, full-fledged, from the portals of Medical Colleges to take a medical degree in America (1768.) The memoir referred to was prepared for and read before this Faculty.

I wrote to Dr. Quinan for a copy of this paper, which he immediately sent, accompanied by a brief letter. Thus, unconsciously, as it were, the strong *historical* bearings of our natures brought us together, and bound us more closely, day by day until the hour of his death.

That it may be understood upon what grounds my estimate is made of the character and abilities of Dr. Quinan, I will state that we were in close correspondence during the last eight years of his life,—his last letter being received by me only three days before his death—and that our letters were frequent; and his were always of a cheerful and charming character. His letters were full of interest, and suggestive of much learning. He was ever ready to aid with his knowledge—especially in consulting the City Libraries for information of every kind that might be desired by his friends. Upon entering a Library, he possessed the rare faculty of being able to lay his hands upon any class of authorities desired without a moments' loss of time; and then would run through a book and make full notes of the passages of interest to his correspondents; and generally all completed within the brief space of an hour or two—in less time indeed, than would be required by many of us to hunt the shelves, and find the book. I am free to say that his faculty for making rapid and thorough search of Libraries as was developed in Dr. Quinan, was truly wonderful; and by thorough training it became a work of comparative ease; and instead of feeling annoyed, as many of us would, by frequent demands upon his time, in making such researches for his friends, in the various Libraries of the City, it really appeared to afford him pleasure to thus be able to aid kindred spirits in historical, and in other work. No sentiment of *self* entered into the elements of his mental constitution. His knowledge, which was extensive and exact, he freely shared with his friends—only being too happy upon finding those who were interested in similar lines of thought.

Dr. Quinan was, *par excellence*, the *medical historian of Maryland*; not that he had written such a formal history, but by his extensive researches, and various publications, he has shown a familiarity with the subject far in advance of any other medical writer whatever. And if we were left to consider only this one phase of his character, in it alone the "Faculty" has sustained an irreparable loss. He was familiar with everything connected with its history from the date of its organization to the present day ; and always stood in a position to correct errors regarding its past, and to assert the truth when occasion required.

It was a sore disappointment to him when the "Faculty" refused to claim and maintain its *Chartered Rights*, under the law, as set forth, and exemplified in his *Presidential Address*, 1886.

It was a well-deserved honor that he should have been elected the President of the "Faculty," 1885–1886. It may not be known to all of you, but such was the fact, that his extreme modesty and keen sensibilities, on account of his defective hearing, had almost determined him to decline the acceptance of the office of President of the Faculty. I flatter myself that it was chiefly through my influence, and arguments, brought to bear upon his sense of justice, that he finally consented to submit to the wishes of the "Faculty." And it is a comforting and happy reflection now, after our friend has departed this life, to know that his name has been enrolled with those of his distinguished predecessors who have occupied the honorable position of *President* of the venerable MEDICAL AND CHIRURGICAL FACULTY OF MARYLAND.

Dr. Quinan held membership in the following named Societies : *Medical and Chirurgical Faculty of Maryland*, its vice-President in 1884, and its President in 1885–86. Member of *Baltimore Medical Association* ; of the *Clinical Society of Maryland* ; of the *Microscopical Society of Baltimore*, and of the *Historical and Political Science Association* of the Johns Hopkins University, etc. He was also an honorary member of the *Historical Society of Harford County, Maryland* ; and a mutual friend in the membership of this Society, Dr. Geo. W. Archer has paid his memory a warm, and well-deserved tribute, as a man and as a historian, at the meeting of the Society, held January 24th, 1891.

The list of the published writings of Dr. Quinan are thus recorded by himself in his autobiographical sketch, which was filed with the *Historical Society of Harford County*, April

1888, soon after his election to honorary membership. He then said :

"My literary contributions have been: 1. '*A Report of the History and Condition of the Public Schools of Calvert County, Maryland*,' in the report of the State Superintendent of Schools of Maryland, 1866, p. 87. 2. '*Non-Identity of Croup and Diphtheria*,' read before the *Baltimore Medical Association*; published in the *Maryland Medical Journal*, August, Vol. viii, pp 211-239, 1878. 3. '*The Uræmic Theory*,' read before the *Clinical Society of Maryland*, published, *ibid*, Vol. vii, pp. 198, 217-224. 4. '*An Historical Study of the Invention and Publication of the English Midwifery Forceps*,' *ibid*, Vol. viii, pp. 293, 296, 1881. 5. '*The Introduction of Inoculation and Vaccination into Maryland, Historically Considered*,' read before the *Baltimore Medical Association*, May 14, 1883; published in the *Maryland Medical Journal*, June 23-30, 1883. 6. '*Illustrations of Medicine in Maryland in Ye old time*;' *Inquests and Autopsies*,' *ibid*, May 26, 1883 and September 1, 1883. 7. '*Juries of Matrons*,' *ibid*, July 21, 1883. 8. '*Medical Fees*.' *ibid*, Sept. 22, 1883. 9. '*Drs. Alexander Hamilton and Upton Scott and the Tuesday Club*,' *ibid*, Aug. 4, 1883. 10. *Comments on Dr. Gee's Address on the Literature of Children's Diseases*,' *ibid*, Dec. 1, 1883. 11. And another paper (and perhaps others), published since this list was made, was a very excellent contribution on the value of early '*Bleeding in Pneumonia*,' published in the Philadelphia *Medical and Surgical Reporter*, on (if I remember right,) August 2, 1890.

"The last work mentioned on the list, and by far the most important, is 12. '*The Medical Annals of Baltimore from 1608 to 1880, including Events, Men and Literature; to which is added a Subject Index and Record of Public Services, Baltimore: Friedenwald, 1884, 8vo. pp. 274.*'"

This is but a brief and imperfect record of the voluminous writings of Dr. Quinan. His modesty forbade his mentioning many minor medical articles, and numerous sketches from his prolific pen, published through many years, in the various newspapers of the day—especially *historical data*, in the form of notes and queries, which the editors frequently called upon him to furnish.

His fame as an author, however, will rest with his *Medical Annals of Baltimore*. This work will endure as a finger-board to the historical student perhaps for centuries; and will be quoted by all future historians as their guide in the early Medical History of Baltimore. It is a monument to his pains-taking and patient labor—a labor of love.

That inaccuracies, as to dates, ages, etc., should exist in a work of this character, is not surprising, when we consider the varied and uncertain sources from which his information was obtained. I have heard the author say in many instances he had written repeatedly to the families of deceased physicians for the necessary information, without receiving in return any reply whatever; thus compelling him to rely upon data from less reliable sources. For this reason, and for others inherent in such a work, many minor errors exist, but in comparison with the grandeur of the work itself—extending over a period of two hundred and seventy-two years, they are but the comparatively invisible spots upon the sun, which but slightly obscure the brilliant rays of that great orb.

It may be added that Dr. Quinan contemplated the preparation of a much enlarged work, comprising the Medical Annals of the entire State (Md.). Knowing the limited demand for such books, however accurate they may be ; and knowing too that he, like the majority of our poorly paid profession, could ill afford pecuniary loss from such an undertaking, I used my influence to dissuade him from the weighty and fruitless labor. I believe however that, notwithstanding my advice, he would have proceeded with the work, had not Dr. Foster, of New York, the editor of the most extensive *Medical Dictionary*, already referred to, ever attempted, succeeded in enlisting his invaluable services in aid of that great work. This work, besides the research for definitions, requires a knowledge of the various languages, dead and living, to supply the full list of synonyms ; in all these particulars Dr. Quinan was quite equal to the demands made upon him, and all of his spare time (if such a man ever has any " spare time,") was devoted, during the last year or two of his life, and up to the day of his death, to work upon this Dictionary.

CONCLUSION.

I now approach the end of my memorial remarks, which some may hastily consider as already too long; but my friends, such a man as JOHN RUSSELL QUINAN rarely demands a memoir at our hands; and therefore do not let us grudge his memory the few pages in history to which it is so justly entitled.

I may properly conclude by giving the personal language penned by himself for the before mentioned archives of the *Historical Society of Harford County*, which brings us in closer association with the inner feelings of the man than any language or reference that I could give. His concluding remarks in that autobiography are as follows:

"On attaining manhood, I hesitated about a profession. The fact that many of my paternal ancestors had been physicians, had, perhaps, its influence in determining my choice. Be that as it may, I cannot be too thankful that I was finally led to decide on medicine—the noblest calling that man can pursue. Nor have I ever regretted it. It does not yield the readiest route to fortunes' favor; yet to be able to spend one's life in the study of the wonderful exhibition of God's handiwork in man, with his complicated structure, and mysterious union of soul and body—to be able, as I hope I have been, with my sympathy, at least, if not my skill, to relieve the pangs and pains of human suffering; to soothe the anguished brow; to moisten the fevered lips, and whisper words of consolation in the ear of the bereaved, or of the dying—what can be a better lot than this?

"I do not mean that I have always accomplished what my heart desired, or done all the good I might have done; O, no! Looking back to-day over a long life, I see enough of time lost, of opportunities neglected, and feel but too keenly how small the sum of all the little knowledge I have gained; yet, even *scire ut nihil sciam*, to know one knows nothing, in comparison with the unexplored region before him, is better than presumptious ignorance, and affords a fitter start for entering on the never-ending, ever-widening study of God's wisdom and omnipotence, which I hope to begin in Eternity.

Yes :

> " Let the thick curtain fall ;
> I know better than all,
> How little I have gained,
> How vast the unattained !

"If sometimes, through man's ingratitude, or my own weakness, life has seemed a burden, and the way dark, I have never blamed Providence, or destiny ; and though my barque may have drifted from its true course, the anchor of belief in a just and merciful Ruler of the storm, still held.

But my life nears its close, and 'what is writ, is writ; would it were worthier !'

" But whether for good or evil, let not my foes strike the balance.

> " O, living friends who love me,
> O, dear ones gone above me,
> Careless of other fame,
> I leave to *you* my name." '

Thus closed the solemn adjuration of our *living* friend— *now* speaking to us from the tomb. I for one, believing that as close a friendship existed between us as is possible to exist between men, have here assumed to mark and guard his fame, in simply stating some of the chief elements of his character that distinguished his public life. Socially he was a delightful companion—full of happy sallies of wit and jocular rejoinders, with a hearty, honest laugh. When not engaged in conversation, his countenance indicated that he soon fell into serious meditation ; showing that the serious part of his nature, when left to his own thoughts, largely predominated. I can sincerely say that I respected and loved Dr. Quinan more than any other man outside of my immediate family. In my eyes he possessed every virtue necessary for man's perfection. His loss falls as a great darkening shadow upon my own declining days. In his death much of my own sunshine has been extinguished. The good physician, in the best sense of the term ; the wise historian of his profession in our beloved State ; the perfect gentlemen, and the true, warm-hearted friend, has departed from our midst forever, and in accordance with his firm belief, has joined his honored and noble ancestors.

In conclusion, Mr. President and gentlemen, we must all realize that this Faculty has lost a most valuable member; one who contributed to its advancement; one who loved its history, and who revered the memories of its founders, and of the good men who followed them ; and I have lost a dear, dear friend, whose like I shall ne'er see again.

In accordance with a resolution adopted at a meeting of the Medical and Chirurgical Faculty of Maryland, held Nov. 15th, 1890, we have the honor to report as follows :

WHEREAS, Death has removed from our midst our colleague and former President, *Dr. John Russell Quinan*,

Resolved, That we now place upon record the sense of our great bereavement at his loss and our high appreciation of his many virtues and accomplishments. As a physician, assiduous, sympathetic, courteous and enlightened, as a man unselfish, pure, honorable and high-minded—it is not often that Nature vouchsafes to the profession and to the world an instance of so high a model. In the field of letters, especially, his work among us was unique and few men even of independent means and ample leisure would have devoted themselves to the indefatigable research to which he gave his time, talent and money. This Faculty but honored itself in honoring him with the highest office within its gift. His efforts, while President, to restore the lost privileges and authority of this Association, although they failed of success, will ever remain a monument to his zeal and public spirit. We cannot but regard his loss as a personal one to each of us and trust that others may rise to fill the place he so worthily occupied.

Resolved, That we extend to his family in their bereavement our deepest sympathy and condolence.

Resolved, That the Secretary be directed to send a copy of these resolutions to the family of the deceased.

MEMOIR OF RODERICK W. EARECKSON.

Dr. Eareckson was born on Kent Island on February 12, 1825, was office student of Prof. Samuel Chew, and graduated in medicine at the University of Maryland, in 1848. He practised medicine until just before the war when he formed a company of volunteers and was commissioned as captain by the State. When the war broke out the company was broken up by the Federal troops, and some of the members imprisoned. After the war the doctor took to peach growing and attained great success in that industry. Mrs. Eareckson's health failing in 1873, he came to Baltimore and opened an office on Lafayette Avenue. In 1875 he bought out the practice of the late Dr. Henry, at Elk Ridge, and since that time held a large and lucrative practice in that village and vicinity. Dr. Eareckson was a man of large experience and great clinical skill, and added to his strictly professional ability such personal charms as endeared him to all who knew him. He was kind and gentle to a fault, and seemed to pursue his professional labors more with a view to ameliorate the sufferings of his patients than in the interest of his own emolument. His health had been failing for some months, several slight apoplectic attacks having occurred, when on the evening of March 13th, after returning from a visit to a patient in whose case he took great interest, and who in fact died within 24 hours, a severe attack occurred from which he never rallied. He died at 2.10 a. m., March 14th, 1891. Thus, his last conscious act, was one of charity and kindness.

WHEREAS, Death has removed from our midst Dr. Roderick W. Eareckson, a member of this Faculty,

Resolved, That in his death the profession of the State has suffered a great loss,

Resolved, That in his personal character, in his professional acquirements and in his well earned success, Dr. Eareckson has illustrated the highest type of the physician and has left with us a most honorable record.

Resolved, That a copy of these resolutions be sent to his family.

Memoir of Richard Gundry, M. D.
By Henry M. Hurd, M. D

Richard Gundry, M. D., was born in Hampstead, a little village in the vicinity of London, England, October 14, 1830. His father, Rev. Jonathan Gundry, was a Baptist clergyman, who early imbued his son with a love of learning and was able to send him to a private school in the neighborhood, where he gained his first knowledge of the classics. At the age of 15, he came with his parents to Simcoe, Canada, where after a brief period of study in a Latin School he was thrown largely upon his own resources. He obtained the means for pursuing his professional education by writing in the office of an attorney. He began the study of medicine under Dr. Coverton, Toronto, and graduated in 1851 at Harvard Medical School. At Harvard he had the advantage of instruction from, and personal contact with such men as Oliver Wendell Holmes, Jacob Bigelow, John Ward and James B. Jackson. He took an excellent stand in his class, and graduated with honor. He settled in Rochester, N. Y., but before he had' been long engaged in practice, was able by a fortunate legacy, to realize his desire to travel abroad. Returning in 1853, he settled at Rochester, N. Y. again, but during the year, in company with Dr. E. M. Moore, an eminent surgeon of Western New York, removed to Columbus, Ohio, where soon after he was appointed Demonstrator of Anatomy in Starling Medical College. In 1855, he received a provisional appointment as Second Assistant Physician in the Central Insane Asylum at Columbus, one of the earliest institutions established in Ohio for the treatment of the insane, to fill a temporary vacancy caused by the absence of one of the Physicians who had gone to the Crimea. His fitness for the work was so apparent the temporary appointment soon became a permanent one. From 1855-1857, he was one of the associate editors of the Ohio Medical and Surgical Journal. In 1857 he was transferred to the Southern Ohio Asylum at Dayton, as Assistant Physician, of which Asylum he became Medical Superintendent in 1861. This position he filled with signal ability until 1872, when he was transferred to the South-Eastern Asylum, at Athens, Ohio, then in process of erection, to complete and prepare the buildings for occupation. Subsequently on the completion of the Asylum in 1874, he was appointed its first Medical Superintendent, and retained the position until 1877, when he was transferred to Columbus, Ohio, to complete and make ready for occupation, the very extensive buildings of that Asylum. This position he held until May, 1878, when the exigencies of practical politics forced his resignation. The Asylum was "reorganized" in consequence of a vicious custom which still exists in Ohio, to the end that its medical officers may be of the same political faith as the dominant party in the State.

After twenty-three years of most faithful, devoted and self-sacrificing service to the insane of Ohio, in three of the asylums, he was forced to resign because his political affinities did not correspond with those of the newly-elected Governor. To a sensitive, high-minded physician like Dr. Gundry, the blow was a severe one, and he felt the injustice of this treatment to the day of his death. He was immediately appointed Medical Superintendent of the Maryland Hospital for the insane, at Catonsville, and held the position until he died. In the opinion of his friends, his change of residence to Maryland was most fortunate. He was thrown at once into a circle of high-minded, cultured and appreciative men, with whom his relations were most pleasant, and under the genial influences of whose companionship his mind was stimulated to new and fruitful effort. In 1880 he received the appointment of Professor of Mental and Nervous Diseases in the College of Physicians and Surgeons, of Baltimore, and in the following year, upon the sudden death of Prof. Howard, was appointed Professor of Materia Medica, in the the same College, and there lectured with great acceptance during the remainder of his life. In January, 1890, he suffered severely from influenza, and for a time was very seriously ill; but he subsequently rallied, and apparently regained his usual health. It was however, evident, that his vigor had been seriously impaired by this illness; and during the last year of his life he seemed to have lost the buoyancy and elasticity which had previously characterized him. Although he lectured as usual, his duties cost him much effort. In March, of the present year, the Trustees of the Maryland

Hospital perceiving his condition, voted to give him a long leave of absence with the hope that his health would be restored. He went to Atlantic City, and for a time, seemed to improve. Subsequently, however, symptoms of Bright's disease developed, and it was evident that his days were numbered. In accordance with his earnest desire, he was brought home, where, four days later, he passed away, surrounded by his family and devoted friends.

Dr. Gundry's career as the chief medical officer of an institution for the insane, was most successful. He possessed a rare executive ability, and the happy faculty of judging of men and their fitness for the proper discharge of duty. It is interesting to note, that many able men grew up about him in the various Asylums and Hospitals with which he was connected, who, under the stimulus of his presence, developed a great degree of efficiency and usefulness. He was eminently helpful to young men; was ready to recognize their talents, and took great pleasure in their advancement. He wholly discarded the use of mechanical restraint in the treatment of the insane while at Athens, and during his whole after life was the consistent and fearless advocate of greater personal freedom for the unfortunate victims of mental disease. He had an intuitive appreciation of the mental processes of those who suffered from insanity, and was fertile in expedients for relieving their distress or for adding to their comfort. The literature of alienism was familiar to him, and his speeches and writings upon all matters touching insanity, showed an intimate knowledge of the work which others had done. He was also an expert in asylum construction, and the asylums at Dayton, Athens and Columbus, were in turn built by him. He took much interest also in landscape-gardening, and was never so happy as when directing the planting of trees, or the decoration of a lawn. It was a pleasure to visit the wards of his hospital with him. His genial presence and ready flow of wit, his quick sympathy with his patients, his ability to impress the most irritable or wayward with a conviction of his genuine interest in them— all tended to make his daily round of duty, a delightful one.

He was an omnivorous reader—a ready writer—a clear and pleasing speaker, with rare gifts of expression and vast stores of knowledge at instant command. His memory of names, dates, facts, incidents, and of verbal quotations, was phenomenal.

Some of Dr. Gundry's feats of memory were remarkable. The writer has known him to repeat from memory the names and dates of birth and death of the Lord Chancellors of England; also, the names and dates of birth and death of the signers of the Declaration of Independence.

He had great intellectual grasp, and in debate could marshal his forces most effectually. The writer often heard him in public discussions, where he measured swords with the keenest and brightest of his associates in scientific or philanthropic work, and never without the conviction that few men were able to wield so many weapons in their own defense, or had such wealth of ammunition. He also wrote with equal facility, and the list of titles of his articles and addresses is a long one. It is to be regretted that no full record of them seems attainable. Among the number were "Observations Upon Puerperal Insanity," 1860; "The Psychical Manifestations of Disease," 1881; "The Care of the Insane," 1881; "Separate Institutions for Certain Classes of the Insane," 1881; "The Regulations of the Powers of the State to the Rights of the Individual in Matters Concerning Public Health," 1883; "Valedictory Address to the Graduating Class, College of Physicians and Surgeons," 1883; "Some Problems of Mental Action," 1888; "The Care of the Insane," 1890.

Dr. Gundry was married in 1858 to Miss Martha M. Fitzharris, of Dayton, Ohio, who, with eight children—four sons and four daughters—survives him. His domestic life was eminently happy. Kind, affectionate, interested in his children and proud of their development, he watched over them with more than a father's care, and was rewarded in turn by a love and devotion on their part rarely seen. His children were his companions in travel, in study and in recreation.

His attitude of mind towards religious matters was a reverent one. He was a Unitarian in his religious belief and affiliations. He was full of charity toward all, and was sin-

gularly tolerant of the rights and feelings of those with whom
he differed.

In private life he was seen at his best. His rich stores of
knowledge were poured forth freely in conversation, and he
was equally at home in all fields. Without neglecting his
scientific work, he was a devoted student of history and of
English literature. Pure in life, an enthusiast in his chosen
work, an able physician, a profound scholar, an affectionate
husband, a devoted father, a steadfast friend—such was his
character.

WHEREAS, This Faculty has learned with deep sorrow of
the death of our late colleague, Professor Richard Gundry,
of Spring Grove Asylum,

Resolved, That whilst we bow in submission to the Divine
decree of Him who doeth all things well, we lament our own
irreparable loss.

Resolved, That in our deceased colleague, who has departed from us at an age when his experience was ripe, his
wisdom most matured, and his usefulness most manifest, we
recognize the highest example of the good citizen, the learned
and skilful physician, and the wise and successful teacher.
Possessing a scholarship and acquirements of the highest
order, with strong literary tastes, perfect self-command, a
dignified and impressive bearing, an acute and observing intellect, a robust constitution and the best opportunities for
clinical observation, he has left his impress not only upon
ourselves and upon this community, among whom he resided,
but upon our literature and the American profession. More
especially in the specialty to which he devoted himself, he
was in the advance. Keeping pace with the rapid progress
of psychology, he was able with his subtle intellect to master
all its details, and thus he became an authority among his
co-workers. In the management of a large institution for
the insane, he evinced the highest executive abilities, and in
the treatment of the unfortunates committed to his care, by
abolishing those restraints and rigors to which a supposed
necessity had previously condemned them, he strove, and we
may believe, successfully, "to minister to minds diseased,"

and thus to mitigate somewhat the wretchedness and hopelessness of their lives.

Resolved, That our warmest sympathy is extended to the family and friends of the deceased, and that a copy of these resolutions be forwarded to them.

All of which is respectfully submitted,

EUGENE F. CORDELL, M. D.,
D. W. CATHELL, M. D.,
W. STUMP FORWOOD, M. D.,
THOMAS B. EVANS, M. D.,
Committee.

PRESIDENT'S ADDRESS.

THE RELATION OF THE MEDICAL AND CHIRURGICAL FACULTY OF MARYLAND TO PROFESSIONAL ORGANIZATION IN MARYLAND.

By T. A. Ashby, M. D., of Baltimore.

MEMBERS OF THE FACULTY:

We meet again in Annual Session, under auspicious circumstances. The year which has passed since the last annual meeting of the Faculty has been singularly exempt from disturbing influences and favored with many indications of an encouraging progress in work and methods which tend to advance the usefulness and prosperity of this organization. The roll call of members has been greatly enlarged by the addition of many useful and active men, from whom we may confidently expect earnest work and co-operation. Our ranks have been depleted by but few deaths and resignations, thus making a large gain in material strength and in numbers.

The Faculty is, however, called upon to deplore the loss, by death, of our honored ex-President and faithful historian of its "Annals," in the person of the late Dr. John R. Quinan, whose genial nature, stern integrity, eminent virtues and ripe scholarship endeared him to us all. The name and fame of Dr. Quinan are the property of this Faculty. I need not dwell upon his labors and services in the cause of medical work and culture, and in behalf of this Faculty.

He was an ornament to his profession and his memory will ever be preserved among our archives as an honored and distinguished member.

It likewise becomes my sad duty to announce the death of Prof. Richard Gundry, whose professional eminence and personal worth were recognized in every section of our country, and whose earnestness and interest in the work of this Faculty have been conspicuous since he became a resident of this State. Removed from this life in the midst of a most useful and honored career, we may pause here to consider the personal loss this Faculty has sustained, and to express our earnest sympathy with his bereaved family and friends in their sudden and unexpected grief. Only a few weeks ago we had hoped to have his presence with us upon this occasion. He has passed away, leaving with us the pleasant memory of a pure character and genial nature, and, above all, the legacy of an honored place in his profession.

The reports of officers and committees to be presented at this meeting exhibit an encouraging condition. These reports will indicate the routine work which has been discharged, and will present such practical suggestions as will enable the members of the Faculty to appreciate the important duties which devolve upon these officials, and the relations which the various departments bear to the general prosperity and usefulness of the entire body.

Whilst recognizing the faithful discharge of duties by every official of this Faculty, I feel called upon to mention by name the work of the different committees.

The Library Committee has been greatly embarrassed by want of money in the conduct of its work, yet, despite this fact, the library has not materially suffered. The actual gain in books, pamphlets and periodicals, though small, is encouraging. The library has been kept open for the convenience of the members on an average of six hours each day during the year, excepting Sundays and holidays. The service has been prompt and efficient.

The Nurses' Directory has become, under the management of the Faculty, a source of revenue and a bureau of practical information of decided value to the profession and to the citizens of this State. This department is worthy of every care and attention, as it bids fair to assume a position of im-

portance not to be disregarded among the influences which
this Faculty presents as a claim upon the profession of
Maryland.

The Publication Committee has presented a volume of
transactions which for the size and practical value of its contents has not been surpassed for a number of years. We
have in this volume a report of the Semi-Annual Meeting,
held in Hagerstown, in November, 1889, showing the practical work accomplished by that meeting.

During the month of November last the second of the
Semi-Annual Meetings was held in Cambridge, under circumstances of extreme interest and profit. The results of
this meeting, as of the previous meeting held in Hagerstown,
were of sufficient value to convince all who were in attendance that a continuation of this work upon the part of the
Faculty will ultimately bring about a complete and successful reorganization of the profession in Maryland by bringing
to the support of the Faculty a large addition of useful and
loyal men.

The Faculty should take pride and interest in this work,
and not relax in the undertaking which these semi-annual
meetings impose. This work is, without doubt, in the line of
progress and of professional advantage. The meetings held
have brought the city and county members into closer and
more cordial relations, agreeable friendships and acquaintances have been promoted, a more generous interest in
medical work has been stimulated, and the needs and interests
of the profession, as such, have been discussed and considered in a way which no other system of work can more successfully foster. As a further outcome of this work we may
confidently anticipate the growth of a spirit of organization
and of co-operation which should be the aim and duty of
this Faculty to advance in the most earnest manner.

The founders of this Faculty were men who were thoroughly
imbued with the spirit of professional organization and of
co-operation. When the Faculty came into existence, ninety-
two years ago, the State of Maryland had but recently
emerged from the struggles and triumphs of an imposing

and eventful historic contèst. Many of its founders and members had served in one capacity or another in the War of the Revolution and in those civil contests which made Colonial Maryland a commonwealth, Baltimore Town a municipality, and which had moulded the American Colonies into a federation of States under a republican form of government. The forces and influences around these men were assertive of those broad principles of co-operation and of fraternity, which were at the very foundation of our National progress under a representative form of government. Liberty, equality and justice were the bulwarks of individual rights, whilst truth, learning and ethics were the cardinal principles which gave support to a social and political scheme which proclaimed the doctrine of human brotherhood in associated work and advancement.

These principles gave shape and character to the organization of this Faculty which, in the very beginning of its existence, gave consideration to those methods of work which promised the largest development in membership and the largest influence which could be made to flow from co-operative work. The scheme of organization contemplated that every assistance should be given to the growth of science, learning and ethics in their relation to professional work and that from this authoritative source should flow those influences of organized effort which would develop individual strength and encourage associated labor. The strength and usefulness of the Faculty were made to depend on the aid and influence of each individual member. Its plan assigned to each member in proper rotation a part in its system of work, and sought to stimulate each one to contribute his proportionate share to the growth and efficiency of the entire body. Hence we observe that its scientific work was divided into sections, that its members were assigned to these sections, so that each might contribute in some way or another to the improvement of the whole.

But apart from the encouragement which was in this manner given to individual effort, in the scientific work of the Faculty, its founders had larger views before them. They recognized the various agencies which could be made to contribute to the cultivation and advancement of the individual in other channels of thought and labor. Public addresses, prize essays and lectures, which offer a scope for the presentation of original work and for literary and historical statements, were established under its supervision and authority.

Later on in the progress of its work the education and cultivation of the member were further provided for by the establishment of a hall, library and museum where facilities were presented for research and study in medical literature, and history. Access was in this manner made easy to those volumes of professional learning not within the reach of the individual. Opportunities and aids to self-improvement were made available by the joint contribution of the entire membership. Such a stimulus as this to work and to self-culture was as wide reaching as it was beneficent. Another principle of far reaching import was recognized by our predecessors in the establishment of a system of legal supervision over the status of the medical profession in this State. A charter was obtained from the Legislature of Maryland in 1798, which made the Faculty virtually responsible for the character and qualification of every practitioner within the borders of the State. Every practitioner of medicine was by the laws of the State forced to enter upon professional work through this doorway.

His habits, character and educational fitness were called in question and passed upon by his professional brethren before he was deemed worthy of their association and fellowship. None can dispute the wisdom of this system. It gave a guarantee to the medical fraternity and to the citizens of Maryland that incompetency and incapacity were discountenanced and that the legal right to engage in a most responsible work implied the moral assurance of fitness and reliability.

Under the exercise of the privileges conferred by the charter granted to this Faculty, its affairs and the interest of legitimate medicine were conducted with moderation and success.

At no time in the history of the profession in Maryland were the influence of quackery and irregular methods so slightly experienced. The records of the Faculty show that the profession throughout the entire State gave a zealous support to the organization, that so long as the charter was enforced the pride and dignity of the professional body were maintained. The encouragement given to the medical profession of the State, by the laws of the State was most salutary.

In an address delivered before the Faculty in 1815, by Dr. Richard Wilmot Hall, in defense of this law, the following language is used: "Since its provisions have been acted upon, medicine has gained a general accession of respectability and public confidence throughout the State.†

"They who were desirous of building up characters as physicians have been encouraged to press on with increased ardor to the attainment of that knowledge which held out the promise of future usefulness, honor and competence. Talents of the first order now enter on the medical career, which, without the provisions of this law, would have remained torpid and useless. The desire of holding an elevated rank among their brethren of the Faculty is shown; of submitting to the decision and approbation of this corporation and its officers, such qualifications and such claims as shall be, not bravely and coolly admitted, but warmly applauded; such claims as are not founded on mere sufficiency or mediocrity of knowledge, but on pre-eminence of talents and science; such claims as their friends and an enlightened public may with more than justice admire and admit.

"But the ordeal which this corporation presents to the ignorant is truly appalling. They shrink back from the disgrace which must be the consequence of attempting to secure its sanction, while on the other hand they know that without the credentials derived from this body, public confidence will be withheld from them and they must sink in public estimation in proportion as the expediency, the justice and the humanity of the law shall become more apparent. Hence the number of empirics is comparatively small in our State and is daily diminishing."

---

†This is confirmed by the report of a committee at a former meeting of the Faculty and recorded in their minutes.

We have in these earnest words of Dr. Hall a clear and forcible presentation of the status of the profession in Maryland at the time of which he writes, when the profession and the citizens of Maryland were protected in their respective interests by wise and careful legislation. We may picture the satisfaction and pleasure of professional work under such conditions and appreciate the force of Dr. Hall's remarks, when he says, "There is no longer a necessity to resort to those *little* expedients which disfigure the dignified character and noble simplicity of science, a less ostentatious and more rational conduct amongst physicians now meets with applause and confidence."

The law of 1798, which conferred such benefits upon the medical profession and upon the citizens of Maryland, was enforced by the Medical and Chirurgical Faculty, with a few slight modifications, for a number of years. The justice and necessity of its provisions were often assailed. Its legality was contested and denied, while its sanctity was often violated. Its vindication and defense became necessary from time to time as its enemies increased and multiplied in the State. In the eloquent defense of the law by Dr. Hall, from which I have quoted, we obtain an insight of those influences which were combining against it. Its enemies began to cry out against the injustice of a law which deprived the individual of the power of confiding his health to whatever hands he might choose. The law, they claimed, was an infringement of the rights of the citizen. This argument found advocates in the persons of demagogues, irregulars and pretenders. As the population of the State increased this class of men grew stronger and more aggressive. The arrival of a class of medical practitioners designating themselves Eclectics, Thompsonians and Homœopaths, men deficient in educational and professional attainments but possessed largely of the spirit of assurance and avariciousness, found in the provisions of the law effectual barriers to position and progress. Through these various agencies, which secured the aid and sympathy of an ignorant and indiscriminating class of citizens, the law was vigorously assailed, and from year to year its provisions were openly violated until it finally became a dead letter upon our statute-books.

The records of the Faculty fail to disclose the various steps by which this position was reached. As late as 1822 the law was in successful operation. It is probable that its final overthrow was not accomplished until some 10 or 15 years subsequent to this time.

The prejudice and aversion of the members of the Faculty, composed entirely of reputable physicians of the regular school of medicine, toward this class of irregulars were so decided and pronounced that we must assume, in the absence of authentic evidence, that the Faculty virtually assented to a relinquishment of its chartered privileges in preference to a legal recognition of irregular practitioners.

The law of 1798 has never been repealed and remains to-day upon the statute-books in the same form as when originally granted by the Legislature, with the exception of the amendments of 1801, 1816, 1818 and 1821, which were unessential modifications and in no respect derogatory to the character and influence of the original charter. The only legislation of a medical character which could in any way infringe upon the charter of 1798 was an act passed by the Legislature of 1838, authorizing Thompsonians or Botanic physicians "to charge or receive compensation for their services and medicines."

Whether the passage of this latter act of Legislation was construed by the Faculty a t that day as an abridgement of its authority we are unable to determine, but it is quite evident that the influence of irregular practitioners, yearly growing stronger in this State, had a most damaging effect upon the Faculty in weakening its authority as a licensing body. This authority virtually ceased about this time, and the Faculty either voluntarily, or without marked resistance yielded to the influences waged against it. At this late day we are in no position to criticise or to condemn the action of our predecessors for surrendering the chartered rights of the Faculty. We have no way of estimating the nature and force of the conditions which surrounded them and we must assume that the motives which governed them were pure and patriotic, since we find that whilst the Faculty was being robbed of its legal authority as a licensing body it continued to exercise a most beneficial and elevating influence in behalf of its membership in other channels of labor and fellowship.

The unexampled prosperity of the Faculty cannot be said to have been overthrown by the violation of its charter. It continued to be to the physicians of this State the doorway through which all should pass who wished to rise to honorable professional position and usefulness in medical work. To those who sought an entrance to medical work through any other route eminent position and cordial fraternal relations were long denied them. Membership in the Faculty was now sought as a mark of honor and as a professional privilege accorded only to those deemed worthy.

The loss to the Faculty in shrinkage of membership came gradually from year to year, resulting in diminution of its revenue and in impaired usefulness to the profession throughout the State. Through these influences the Faculty began to assume the characteristics of a local as distinguished from a State organization. Its membership in Baltimore held fast whilst that from the Counties was reduced yearly by death and withdrawal.

But in compensation for these unfavorable conditions which prevailed, a spirit of loyalty and devotion to the traditions and work of the Faculty continued to inspire many of its members with a zeal and faith in its perpetuity and purposes. Reduced in numbers, but not discouraged, these members set in motion those enterprises and influences which come down to us to-day as noble emblems of a spirit of liberality and of devotion to the cause of medical science and culture. The need of co-operation and of fraternal helpfulness was only intensified by the influences of quackery, ignorance and selfishness which assailed them. Unable longer to control and to influence the status of the profession in Maryland by the processes of law, the Faculty, as it were, resolved to exercise an intellectual and moral force upon professional and public opinion. It sought to surround its membership with the motive and stimulus of culture, refinement and honorable endeavor.

As far back as 1832 the Faculty established the nucleus of the Library, which to-day is its most honored and valued possession. Here was inaugurated a force and influence of wide-reaching importance and significance. Here it put in operation an aid and stimulus to professional ambition and culture which the present and succeeding generations must recognize as a most valued and noble inheritance. To the library in its very earliest organization the Faculty gave a liberal and earnest support. In further recognition of the value of this influence we find that as early as 1839 a movement looking to the purchase of a hall as a repository for its library and museum, and as a place for holding its meetings, was successfully inaugurated. In later years this purpose was happily consummated.

In 1840 the Faculty attempted the publication of a medical journal, under its auspices, which it was forced to relinquish after a brief period of unprofitable journalistic enterprise. This effort was none the less commendable, for it gives evidence of the spirit of progress and of enterprise which animated its membership at that time.

Time will not permit me to enumerate the various steps in enlightened progress and in useful work which the Faculty continued to make from year to year until the beginning of the civil war in 1861.

Up to this period it had changed its character in only one essential respect. It had ceased to be a licensing body and the only doorway to professional recognition in Maryland. It had come to be an organization of commanding influence and respectability not only in Maryland but throughout the entire country and wherever known abroad. It gave encouragement to and fostered all of those agencies which were promotive of the highest aims and results of professional work.

The golden area of the Faculty's usefulness was reached in the year 1858. At the annual meeting held in the month of June in that year, it assembled for the first time in the hall which had become but recently the property of the Faculty. In the annual oration delivered upon this occasion by an honored and distinguished member, the late Professor Sam'l Chew, this event is commemorated in the following happy and encouraging words: "The present annual meeting of our Society is an occasion of more than ordinary interest. The building in which we assemble to-day for the first time is one which has recently become the property of this Association. We have heretofore had no fixed and regular place of convocation. To-day we inaugurate a wiser and better arrangement of our polity. From to-day we are prepared as a body to experience the happiness ascribed by the wondering hero of the Roman Epic to those who possess a local habitation, '*Fortunati quorum jam mœnia surgunt.*' The hall in which we are now gathered together will probably be the usual, or perhaps the constant, place of all our future meetings. May its use be auspicious to the best interests of our fraternity. Happy for us all if its name be henceforth associated in our minds with recollections of the knowledge, the good sense, the urbanity of deportment and the friendly and cordial feelings which should subsist among the members of a scientific, liberal and honorable profession."

The occasion so felicitously celebrated, contrasts most happily with subsequent events. The Faculty was scarcely housed in its own hall and secure in the possession of those means which could be made to contribute to its usefulness and renown when disturbances began to arise in the political and social affairs of the country, which brought temporary disaster upon the work so successfully inaugurated.

In 1859 a decline in the work of the Faculty was already apparent. From 1860 to 1870 the interests of the Faculty were so completely overlooked in those disturbances which were going on in the State during this decade that no record remains of any work having been done during that period. Its membership was scattered and disorganized, its work was suspended, its revenues were cut off, and but for the watchful care and loyalty of a few members living in this city its library would have been totally destroyed and its property sacrificed.

Fortunately for this and coming generations this work of our predecessors escaped the ravages and ruin of war and remains with us to-day safely shelved in the building we now occupy. The finances of the Faculty suffered much during this decade, and the crippled condition of our treasury to-day may be largely traced to the period of which I now speak. The building erected by the liberality and perseverance of our predecessors was swept away by accumulated debt. We have only the example and noble self-sacrifice of these members to stimulate our pride and liberality in the new work of rebuilding a library hall which both duty and expediency demand of our hands.

The war over, wisely enough no attempt was made to resume the annual meetings of the Faculty until sufficient time had elapsed to bury out of sight the memories of a struggle in which its membership had been arrayed in hostile relations toward each other.

In 1870 the scattered and depleted ranks of the Faculty were again assembled, under the presidency of that venerable and honored member, the late Professor N. R. Smith. The traditions and memories which had gathered around the sixty odd years of work prior to the war were now recalled, its high aims and purposes and its honorable record of usefulness in the work of professional organization were remembered and a movement was set on foot looking to a revival and renewal of its interests and objects. The machinery was in proper working order. All that was required was the stimulus of its membership to set it in motion. We of the present generation know how successfully this was done, and we are here to-day to bear testimony to the fact that this work established by our forefathers in medicine is a vigorous, earnest and healthy organization as fully devoted to the welfare of the medical profession as in the past.

The work of this Faculty from 1870 to the present is familiar to all. It has been a continued and onward movement from year to year, from achievement to achievement, until we stand to-day in a position to push forward this work upon such terms of advantage as this Faculty has never before enjoyed.

I have attempted to show that the founders of this Faculty had before them a large and intelligent plan of usefulness for the Faculty as a State medical organization. The plan, under its charter, conferred upon the Faculty full powers as a licensing body. The authority which it exercised whilst its charter was in force was eminently advantageous to the interests of the medical profession and to the public welfare. The influences which led to the overthrow of this authority have been referred to. We have seen that this result changed the characteristics of the Faculty to a very marked extent, and led to the inauguration of other features of its work which have exercised a most beneficial influence upon its membership.

It is not my purpose to discuss the questions which have been raised in regard to the legal rights conferred by the charter of this Faculty. I assume that any attempt to revive the legal authority conferred by the charter is as impracticable, as it is ill-advised. The Faculty is not now, in my humble opinion, in a position to inaugurate any movement looking to a renewal of its functions as a licensing body. There are other features appertaining to its work which claim more earnest consideration and demand more serious attention at this time. When these interests have been furthered, the Faculty can then, if it sees proper, advance a step forward and assert its influence in matters of medical legislation to far more eminent advantage. In my judgment, the most important work now before the Faculty is the work of general organization of the medical profession in Maryland. This work implies that every effort should be made upon the part of the Faculty to enlist in its ranks and place on its roll-call the name of every worthy member of the regular school of medicine in Maryland. When this has been done it will bring to its aid and purposes a material and moral force which will elevate the profession of this State to a position of usefulness and of respectability such as it has never before enjoyed. Other influences will at once flow from this result. Local medical societies in the counties and cities throughout the State will organize, professional pride and ambition will be stimulated, an interest in medical work and progress from a scientific standpoint and as a means of public advantage will increase, and, not least, the exercise of those courtesies and civilities which come from closer professional intercourse and association will be promoted. A large and intelligent class of men bound by such fraternal relations as this Faculty can and should present cannot fail to have the strongest influence over that class of men who repudiate its principles of work and ethics. The moral force and authority of thorough organization would reach beyond the limits of its own body. Mere strength in numbers should never be the aim of the Faculty, but the bringing in of men, strong and true, and raising them up to a standard of usefulness as professional workers, which the scheme of this Faculty contemplates, is quite within its scope and capability. It seems to me that the principles of this organization contemplate the greatest good to the greatest number. It was never designed that this Faculty should become so select and so eminent as to exclude from its ranks the great body of professional workers in Maryland. In the early years of its organization its membership embraced the entire body of medical practitioners in the State. It was during this period that the standard of the profession throughout the State was raised to its highest plane of usefulness and activity. The influence of the Faculty upon the ethics and culture of the profession was then most marked. In one sense this influence has never been lost, but it has been narrowed and localized just in proportion as it lost the support of the profession in the counties and gained in membership in this city.

The circumstances and conditions which led to this result have ceased to exist. The time has arrived when this Faculty can earnestly and patriotically claim and demand the support of the profession over the entire State. Nor can the profession of Maryland, without injury to its pride, prosperity and high character, and disregard for those higher interests of professional work, neglect the claims which the Faculty makes upon their loyalty and co-operation. This work of organization has commenced and it must go forward or the medical profession of Maryland will continue to lag behind the profession of our sister States in enterprise, pride and earnest work in all undertakings looking to professional and public advantage.

As an outcome of a larger growth in the membership of the Faculty we may confidently look for marked progress in other matters of importance to professional interests in Maryland. Virchow has made the remark that "the object of medical associations should be to unite the world in a struggle against disease and death, not to get shorter hours and more pay, but to increase our ability for research and to diminish the dangers which surround humanity." These words seem to express the highest aim of associated work coming within the scope of all organized medical bodies. To increase our abilities for research and to diminish the dangers which surround humanity, we must look largely to the philanthropy and beneficence of endowed institutions and societies. But it seems clear that an organization, such as this, should assume an important and responsible relation in furtherance of such sentiments and considerations. It comes within the scope of our work to give a helpful stimulus to research, both in the field of science and in the mines of knowledge and learning. And if this be true, how much higher is the duty to give aid and attention to those conditions of our environment which diminish the dangers which surround the citizens of the communities in which we reside.

The means of accomplishing these highest aims of an organized body, such as this, lead to practical results by indirect methods. This Faculty can only make progress in general philanthropy along such routes as run parallel with its plan of organization and methods of work. Its influence upon scientific work and upon medical culture must be felt from a literary as distinguished from an experimental and investigative standpoint. It is not within its scope to provide the facilities and appliances for original research, but it can offer the stimulus both in word and in action. It can express its sympathy with the work of research by extending encouragement to the investigator. Through prize essays, public addresses and honorary testimonials it can aid and uphold the hands of men who constantly tell us in the language of Bruno, "when science is made traffic, wisdom and justice shall perish from the earth."

The agencies which represent an educational and moral influence upon medical ethics and culture were clearly recognized by the early members of this Faculty. These agencies have been handed down to us in such shape as to suggest the importance of a more careful consideration of their claims upon our pride and liberality.

I need hardly present an argument in behalf of the claims which the library of the Faculty makes upon the profession of this State and city. Every intelligent and thoughtful physician must feel the need of literary assistance in his medical work, and yet how few of us are there who fully appreciate the value of such a repository of medical literature as a properly conducted library can and should present. This single agency, the property of this Faculty, apart from every other consideration, should entitle the Faculty to the respect, support and liberality of the entire profession of Maryland. It is a common centre, an imposing obligation, around which we should unite as a means of the highest advantage to an educated class of men. We have not sufficiently appreciated the value and usefulness of this single educational and refining influence upon the professional body, in consequence, I venture to suggest, of the fact that we have not fully made a personal application of its advantages. To the individual it has probably represented too little, but if we consider the opportunities which it offers to the profession as an entirety, its importance at once grows upon our attention. Libraries, whether technical or general in their scope and characteristics, are as essential to large communities as the purity of the atmosphere which surrounds them. They create intellectual wants, stimulate ambition, promote culture and refinement to a degree not within the reach of any other single educational influence. These facts have long since been recognized, yet be it said to our discredit, that within a city and State of the size, intelligence and wealth of our own, we have permitted this influence to remain undeveloped and dwarfed. In this respect we are far behind some of our sister cities of less population and wealth and surrounded with inferior advantages. I can not but believe that this neglect is remediable and that we are now in a position to take hold of this work and place it upon a higher plane of usefulness and importance. The plant is here and the machinery is in motion, but we must awake to a realization of the importance of greater liberality and progressiveness on our part in relation to this interest. The profession of this State, much less of this city, can not, in duty to its intelligence and out of respect for its prestige, remain passive and indifferent to the claims of the library owned by this Faculty. A work which our predecessors, numbering less than one-third our present numerical strength, set in operation and by liberal contributions housed in a building of their own purchase, we find to-day stored on shelving and under a roof owned by another corporation. Is not this a reflection upon our liberality and professional pride? Is it not an indication that we are lacking in enterprise and in interest toward the higher obligations of medical achievement and progress? Whatever may have been the cause of our present position in respect to so important an interest the time has come for a new movement and for larger activity. I cannot but believe that among the members of this Faculty there are many who will liberally contribute to an endowment fund to be used for the purchase of a hall or building in this city to be dedicated to the purposes of a medical library and to the uses of permanently organized medical bodies. Is not such an enterprise worthy of our encouragement and undertaking? Are we here in Maryland wanting in those generous and elevating sentiments which have enabled the medical profession of New York, Philadelphia and Boston to become the exclusive owners of noble and beautiful temples, erected to the uses of science and literature, and as places for the assembling of medical bodies.

I, therefore, confidently appeal to the pride and liberality of the medical profession of Maryland to recognize the importance and utility of such an undertaking. I cannot make this appeal in words of sufficient earnestness, for I feel that the circumstances and the situation are alike binding upon us.

If Baltimore is to be the great centre of medical education and research of the future, as we have just reason to anticipate, we must not only encourage and foster endowed institutions and great educational bodies but we must provide every possible facility for the education and cultivation of medical practitioners who have but a limited contact with these larger organized influences. It is proper that this Faculty should assume some such relation as to this great body of medical workers throughout this State. It is to the wisdom and liberality, to the influence and leadership of such an organization as this that the profession of Maryland should look for larger growth, influence and prosperity.

Organization is the great lever of the human will and intelligence, it is that principle which coördinates the functions and movements of society into harmonious and efficient action, and directs the mental and physical energies of men in work of the highest aim and advantage. The medical profession of Maryland cannot and should not remain indifferent to such important considerations and interests as are involved in this work of professional organization. The highest interests and aims of professional service are connected with and dependent upon the good fellowship, the urbanity of deportment, the correctness of conduct, the purity of motive and action, and the integrity of purpose which characterize the relations between physician and physician and between physician and patient. These relations cannot be strengthened and developed apart from the influence and aid of organized effort, nor can the moral standard, the legal status, and the educational qualifications of the profession as such, be advanced to their highest plane of usefulness through any other human agency or instrumentality. I, therefore appeal to the membership of this Faculty and to the great body of intelligent practitioners of medicine throughout the State to realize the dangers and duties of the hour which alike confront them, and to arouse to the responsibilities of labor and fellowship which devolve upon them.

ANNUAL ADDRESS.

THE CAUSATION OF DIPHTHERIA.

BY WILLIAM H. WELCH, M. D.,

Professor of Pathology, Johns Hopkins University.

The subject which I have selected for this address is so largely a topic of the day, and fills at present so much space in medical journals, that the main facts which will be here presented must appear familiar to those who have followed recent medical literature. Nevertheless, many of these facts are so new and so important, and the disease to which they relate is one of such great interest, that no apology is needed for bringing before you a brief summary of recent investigations concerning the causation of diphtheria, and the light which these discoveries have shed upon our knowledge of the pathology, prophylaxis and treatment of a disease more dreaded, and justly so, than any other infectious disease always present among us. Although these new discoveries are mainly the results of bacteriological work, it will be my purpose to dwell not so much upon minute bacteriological descriptions, more suitable to the laboratory and to special articles than to a general address of this kind, but rather upon those points which illustrate the application of these discoveries to a fuller and more correct knowledge of the nature, etiology, pathology, diagnosis, prevention and treatment of diphtheria.

The history of our knowledge of diphtheria illustrates the difficulties which we encounter in endeavoring to reach a full understanding of a disease upon the basis of its symptomatology and pathological anatomy alone. Consider for a moment what are some of the uncertain and still much disputed questions concerning this disease.

Is diphtheria primarily local or constitutional in its origin? Are all pseudo-membranous inflammations of the throat, not directly referable to caustic irritants, diphtheria? Is there a purely local, non-contagious pseudo-membranous laryngitis called croup distinguishable from diphtheria? Are the pseudo-membranous anginas secondary to scarlatina, and less frequently to measles and some other infectious diseases identical with diphtheria? Is there any relation between follicular tonsillitis and diphtheria? May diphtheria occur in a mild form as a simple catarrhal inflammation of the throat? Are pneumonia, acute nephritis, suppuration of the glands in the neck, etc., referable to the direct action of the diphtheric virus; in other words, what lesions belong to the disease and what are complications? Shall reliance be placed chiefly upon local or upon general treatment?

These are some of the questions which the most careful study of the clinical history and of the anatomy of diphtheria has not been able to answer clearly and unmistakably. Nor are these matters only of theoretical importance. Referring to the two doctrines of the local and of the constitutional nature of diphtheria, Dr. J. Lewis Smith, one of the most painstaking and profound investigators of this subject in this country, says: "It is a matter of great importance—an importance transcending that of almost any other subject relating to the pathology of this dreadful scourge—that we should ascertain certainly and clearly which of the two prevailing theories is true, since the theory influences practice."

I hope to be able to show in the course of this address that this question, as well as others mentioned, have now been answered "clearly and certainly," and that we are in a position to solve other of the problems still remaining in doubt. All of this gratifying widening and deepening of our knowledge has come from the discovery of the microscopic germ which is the specific cause of diphtheria, and from the study of the singular and interesting properties of this germ. There is, perhaps, no other disease, with the exception of tuberculosis, upon which greater light has been shed by the discovery of its specific cause than upon diphtheria.

Permit me to present to you, in the first place, the evidence that the so-called Klebs-Löffler bacillus is really the specific agent of infection in diphtheria; and then to describe the most important properties of this microörganism, so far as they bear upon the subject of this address.

There are three things especially which have rendered difficult the convincing demonstration that a given micro-örganism is the specific cause of diphtheria.

The first is the uncertainty as to what shall be called diph-theria, and the possibility that included under this name are various affections which may be due to different causes. Hence it might happen that one investigator studying one class of cases—for instance, the pseudo-membranous anginas associated with scarlet fever, measles, etc.—might obtain results different from another who observed another class of cases. In view of this uncertainty, it is clear that conclusions as to the causation of primary diphtheria should be derived from the investigation of cases which all are agreed in regard-ing as genuine primary diphtheria. When the etiology of this undoubted class of cases has been determined, we are in a position to examine whether the secondary and other doubtful forms of diphtheria have a different causation or not.

A second difficulty has been not in the demonstration of microörganisms in diphtheria, but rather in the abundance of bacteria present in diphtheritic membranes. Of the various species of bacteria found in the false membranes of diphtheria we must determine which are constantly present and which are inconstant. If we find one species always present in large number and absent in other conditions, the presumption is that this is the specific cause of the disease, and this pre-sumption becomes a certainty if we are able to reproduce experimentally, by inoculation with pure cultures of this germ, a disease in all respects identical with human diphtheria.

Just here we meet the third difficulty, which consists in bringing positive evidence that our experimental disease is in reality identical with human diphtheria. We are accustomed to regard the fibrinous pseudo-membrane on the mucous membrane of the tonsils, pharynx, and air-passages as the most certain anatomical criterion of diphtheria, but we have long known that it is possible to produce experimentally in animals, by a variety of agencies which have nothing to do with diphtheria, false membranes histologically identical with the diphtheritic membrane. Hence the mere produc- tion of a false membrane by the inoculation of a germ suspected to be the cause of diphtheria, although it constitutes weighty evidence, cannot be considered absolutely conclu- sive that such germ is really the cause of diphtheria. But are there not other anatomical changes in the body character- istic of diphtheria besides the diphtheritic membrane? We owe especially to Oertel the demonstration of the fact that the diphtheric virus is a most peculiar poison to the cells of the human body, and that it produces areas of cell death not only on the surface of mucous membranes, but also in deeper parts, in various lymphatic glands at a distance from the local lesion and in the spleen. These changes can be demonstrated by histological examination. Now, if we find that our suspected germ, besides causing pseudo-membra- nous inflammations, produces identical foci of cell death ; if we find that it injures the kidneys, as we have long known it does in human beings ; and if we find that it causes late muscular paralyses resembling the post-diphtheric paralyses which the clinician regards as of such diagnostic value in doubtful cases of sore-throat, then we shall have evidence strong indeed that this germ is the real specific cause of diphtheria.

It is not surprising that all these difficulties were not over- come in the first important publications of Klebs in 1883, and of Löffler in 1884. We owe to Löffler the first bacteriological study of diphtheria by the modern culture methods. Although his work was most valuable and accurate, he was compelled to express himself reservedly as to the significance of the bacillus which we now believe to be the cause of diphtheria. No such complete chain of proof was brought forward as Koch presented in his first memorable publication upon the tubercle bacillus two years previously. Hence it came about that the Klebs-Löffler bacillus from the first assumed a doubtful status, and that even to-day it is often referred to in writings on diphtheria as only one among many claimants to be regarded as the cause of diphtheria.

I shall not weary you by following the historical path in which obstacle after obstacle has been removed which stood in the way of the full recognition of the Löffler bacillus as the infectious agent of diphtheria, but I shall simply direct you to the goal which has been reached.

It is now established that this bacillus is constantly present in large number in the pseudo-membranes of all cases of primary diphtheria, and that no other species of bacteria is constantly to be found in this situation. The expectation expressed a year ago by Löffler that the results on this point would not be found to be different in this country from those in Europe has been fulfilled by the bacteriological examination by Dr. Abbott and myself of a series of cases of primary diphtheria occurring in Baltimore, in all of which we found the Löffler bacillus, as the only constant organism, as well as by the latest publication of Dr. Prudden. The occurrence of a bacillus, with all the properties of the virulent diphtheric bacillus, in persons not affected with diphtheria is so extremely exceptional that Löffler, notwithstanding years of searching, has been able to find it only once under such circumstances.

The Löffler bacillus can be readily obtained in pure cultivation on artificial media and its properties studied outside of the body. The sum of these properties suffices for its positive and ready identification.

Inoculation of pure cultures of this bacillus is found to be pathogenic for guinea-pigs, cats, pigeons, rabbits, and some other animals. By such inoculation a disease can be reproduced identical in all essential features with human diphtheria, and there is no other species of microörganism known capable of reproducing all of these features. In suitable animals we can cause by inoculating them with the diphtheric bacillus pseudo-membranous inflammations of mucous membranes indistinguishable from those of natural diphtheria, swelling of adjacent lymphatic glands, multiple ecchymoses, serous transudations, fatty degenerations and other lesions in the kidney and liver, late muscular paralyses, and foci of cell death resembling those in human diphtheria. Upon this last point the investigations in full have not yet been published, but researches have for some time been directed, in the pathological laboratory of the Johns Hopkins University, to the detection of areas of cell-death in the internal organs of the animals inoculated with diphtheria, and I may say here that we have been able to confirm and extend in animals Oertel's researches on this subject in human beings.

By the labors, therefore, of many investigators since Löffler's first publication in 1884, including those of Löffler himself, all of the conditions have been fulfilled for diphtheria which are necessary to the most rigid proof of the dependence of an infectious disease upon a given microörganism, viz : the constant presence of this organism in the lesions of the disease, the isolation of the organism in pure culture, the reproduction of the disease by inoculation of pure cultures, and similar distribution of the organism in the experimental and in the natural disease. We are then justified in calling the Klebs-Löffler bacillus, the bacillus diphtheriæ.

Let us now turn our attention to the most important properties of this bacillus. However great may be the scientific interest of the discovery of the specific germ of an infectious disease, this discovery by itself is after all only the realization of the faith of enlightened physicians that the infectious diseases are all caused by specific living organisms. The practitioner is fully justified in inquiring how this discovery helps him to a better understanding of the disease, to a more certain diagnosis, to a more accurate interpretation of symptoms, to more effective measures of prevention and of treatment. Although these expectations have been met only in part, enough has been accomplished already to show that great practical value has come and is likely to come in still larger measure from the discovery of the bacillus diphtheriæ.

The specific germ of diphtheria is a bacillus, devoid of independent motility, averaging in length about that of the tubercle

bacillus, but thicker than this.   It presents itself both in diphtheritic membranes and in cultures often in such bizarre forms
that these belong to its most characteristic morphological
properties.   It grows upon our ordinary culture media, best
upon Löffler's blood-serum and bouillon mixture, but it will
grow even upon steamed potato.   As bearing upon a possible
source of infection it is important to note that the bacillus
will multiply readily in milk, without altering the appearance
of the milk.   It does not multiply or it does so only very
sluggishly at a temperature below 18° C. (about 64° F.).   It
is killed by exposure for ten minutes to a temperature of 58°
C. (136.4° F.).   It is not necessary to describe here in detail
the peculiarities of its growth upon the various culture
media, although to the bacteriologist these are the guides for
the isolation of the bacillus in pure culture.   The series of
cultures which I here exhibit to you illustrates the characteristic appearances.   It suffices here to draw the conclusion
that, unlike the tubercle bacillus, the bacillus of diphtheria
may readily find conditions outside of the body suitable for
its multiplication.

But, as is well known, it is not necessary that an infectious
organism should actually propagate itself outside of the
body in order to produce ectogenic infection.   Such infection may occur if the organism simply preserves its vitality.
On this point we know that the diphtheric bacillus, although
it forms no spores, is among the more resistant bacilli of the
non-spore-forming class, withstanding for a long time drying
and other influences injurious to the less resistant forms.
The specific bacilli have been obtained in cultures made
from diphtheric membranes preserved dry in a piece of linen
cloth for five months. This prosperity is in harmony with the
experience that rooms, clothing, and other objects may retain
for months the diphtheric virus in an active state. As the
bacilli diphtheriæ may live for a still longer period in the
moist state, and as moist, damp dwellings have long been
held to be particularly favorable for the development of
diphtheria, it is probable that statements as to the preservation of the diphtheric virus in such situations for a year or
more are not without foundation.

Of capital importance is the establishment of the fact that the bacillus diphtheriæ develops only locally at the site of infection, and does not invade the tissues or the circulation. It is found only in the diphtheritic pseudo-membrane, and not even in the subjacent mucous membrane. Indeed, it is only the superficial parts of the false membranes which contain the bacilli. The determination of this fact gives at once a clear and decisive answer to the long-mooted question as to the primarily local or constitutional nature of diphtheria. Diphtheria is, without a doubt, local in its origin. The germ which causes this disease not only makes its first appearance and multiplies where the pseudo-membrane is formed, but it does not subsequently invade the blood and organs. As we shall see later, the constitutional symptoms are due to the reception of a chemical substance or substances of remarkable toxic properties, produced by the local development of the diphtheric bacillus.

This settlement of the controversy as to the local or the constitutional origin of diphtheria is one of the most important outcomes of the bacteriological study of this affection, for the question pertains to a fundamental point in our conception of the disease. Nevertheless, from the point of view from which this controversy has usually been waged, the triumph is, in my opinion, only a partial one for the localists, for, as will be shown later, I believe that there are reasons as strong as ever for the employment of constitutional measures of treatment in combination with the local ones.

From what has already been said we are prepared to consider for a moment in what ways a person affected with diphtheria becomes a source of danger to those around him, and to the locality.

The bacilli diphtheriæ are conveyed from the body in particles of diphtheritic exudation, saliva, and other secretions discharged through the mouth and nose. (It is not necessary to consider the comparatively exceptional localizations of the disease.) In this way the infectious substance may readily become attached to the person and clothing of the patient, and of those around him, as well as to the bedding, furniture, floor and walls of the room, dishes, and other objects.

Notwithstanding the statements current in nearly all text-books, there is no evidence that the breath of the patient contains the diphtheric germ, except as bits of false membrane or secretion may be mechanically expelled in the act of coughing, hawking, or sneezing. It has been proven experimentally that the expired air is incapable, during ordinary respiration, of detaching bacteria from the moist mucous surfaces over which it passes.

The specific germs are not so readily conveyed by air currents from a diphtheric patient to those near him, as they are, for instance, from a patient with scarlet fever, in which the germs are in all probability thrown off from the surface of the body on light epidermal scales.

Nor are the chances of infection of the sources of supply of drinking-water with the diphtheric bacillus so great as is the case with such diseases as cholera and typhoid fever, in which the stools contain in large number the specific bacteria, and are likely to be disposed of in such a way that under bad sanitary conditions these bacteria may find their way into wells and streams. While there are some accounts intended to show the conveyance of the virus of diphtheria through the drinking water, we do not hear much of this as a source of infection, and it is not likely that it plays an important role, although it is probable that the diphtheric bacillus may sometimes be discharged by the stools.

Diphtheria is one of the infectious diseases the germs of which may be taken into the body by the inspired air. Inasmuch as bacteria cannot, under ordinary conditions, occur as floating matter in the atmosphere until they have been completely dried down so that air currents can detach as dust the little particles to which they adhere, it is evident that only those infectious germs are likely to be conveyed by the air which are not destroyed by complete drying. As has already been mentioned, the diphtheric bacillus withstands for months desiccation which is so injurious to the cholera vibrio and to many other species of bacteria. While, therefore, we must admit that air-infection with the bacillus of diphtheria is a real and conspicuous danger, it is well to bear in mind that modern bacteriology has taught us the great lesson that the most frequent and important mode of infection is by contact with infected substances. When we consider the manifold ways in which the diphtheric bacilli may be widely distributed, and when we consider the habit of young children—who are the most numerous victims of the disease—of handling everything and of putting everything into their mouths, we are led to appreciate that infection by contact must play the leading part in the transmission of diphtheria.

I will now ask your attention to a brief consideration of the most deadly of all the properties of the bacillus diphtheriæ, namely, the power of producing extraordinarily poisonous chemical substances. That the grave constitutional symptoms of diphtheria are referable to such substances has long been surmised, and as soon as it was found that the bacilli causing diphtheria develop only locally it became certain that toxic substances must be formed. The results of the investigations as to the nature and properties of these substances are not only most important for the etiology of diphtheria, but are among the most significant acquisitions of bacteriology in recent years. We owe these results chiefly to the researches of Roux and Yersin and of Brieger and Fränkel.

If bouillon cultures, four or five weeks old, of the diphtheric bacillus—preferably containing some blood-serum—be sterilized by heating them at temperatures of about 55° C., or if they be deprived of bacteria by filtration through a Chamberland porcelain filter, it is found that the sterilized culture fluid possesses highly poisonous properties when injected, even in small quantity, into animals. The toxic substance is not of a crystallizable, alkaloidal nature of the kind known as a ptomaine or a toxine, for no such substance can be detected in these cultures. The poisonous material, although it has not been separated in a condition of absolute purity, has been shown to be probably of a proteid nature. It is precipitated by alcohol and by saturation with ammonium sulphate and sodium phosphate. It is mechanically dragged down by fine precipitates, such as those of calcium phosphate. It is soluble in water. Obtained in a state approaching purity it appears as a white, amorphous mass of light specific gravity. In the moist state it loses, in great part or entirely, its poisonous properties when subjected to heat above 60° C., but when dry it stands temperatures of 70° C. It is not volatile, and can be preserved for months at least in the dry state, without loss of its characteristic properties.

Some idea of the extraordinarily poisonous nature of this substance can be obtained from the statement of Roux and Yersin, that four-tenths of a milligramme of the substance (after deducting the weight of the ashes and of the non-poisonous part insoluble in alcohol) obtained by evaporating to dryness the active culture fluid, is sufficient to kill at least eight guinea-pigs, weighing each four hundred grammes, or two rabbits, weighing each three kilogrammes. As the major part of these four-tenths of a milligramme is represented by other substances than the diphtheric poison, it is apparent that the poison must be of appalling potency.

If this poison, or the sterilized culture fluid containing it, be injected into a guinea pig or rabbit or other susceptible animal, it is found to be capable of producing all of the changes in the body which follow the inoculation of pure cultures of the diphtheric bacilli, with the exception of the pseudo-membrane. For the production of this membrane the bacilli are necessary, but the other lesions, such as the local œdema after subcutaneous injections, the ecchymoses, the serous transudations, the changes in the kidney, liver, and other parts, are observed after the injection of the toxic albumin, as the diphtheric poison is sometimes called, as well as after inoculation with the bacilli. If the animals live sufficiently long, muscular paralyses may develop.

The most remarkable property of this toxic albuminoid substance, or these substances (for we do not know positively that there is only one such substance), is that when injected in a single sufficiently small, but fatal dose, it may produce no apparent disturbance for days, and the death of the animal may occur many days or even weeks, or months after the injection. This is a quality which we have not been accustomed to attribute to chemical poisons, and it is evidently one of the greatest practical significance. If it is true that the bacilli of diphtheria are capable of producing at the site of their local development poisonous substances which, when at first received into the system, may cause no manifest harm, but which may destroy life perhaps after days, then it is clear that even if we succeed in killing the bacilli in the pseudo-membrane, the individual may still die of toxæmia.

That the bacilli of diphtheria may produce apparently identical toxic proteids in the animal body has been demonstrated. The poisonous proteids are probably allied in their constitution to the poisonous substances found by Weir Mitchell and Reichert in the venom of rattlesnakes and of other serpents, and belong to a group of interesting chemical products now known to be produced by various pathogenic bacteria and other organisms, and which have been and are still being carefully studied, among others, with especial success by Sidney Martin and by Hankin in England. While there is reason to believe that the diphtheric poison is a proteid this view cannot be regarded as established until the poison has been isolated in a state of purity. As we know that the poison can be mechanically dragged down by fine precipitates, it is possible that it is intimately united to the precipitates of albumose without being itself an albumose. Interesting as it might be to tarry longer at this point, we cannot complete this outline sketch of the properties of the diphtheric bacilli without the consideration of certain other important characteristics which they possess, and time admonishes us to hasten on.

It is well known that the character of the symptoms, and especially their gravity, vary in a marked degree not only in different cases of diphtheria, but also in different epidemics. There are epidemics of a mild character, and there are epidemics, such as some of those of recent years in the north-western part of this country, which sweep away nearly all the children of a neighborhood or a town. In estimating the value of different methods of treatment, this is a point not always kept sufficiently in view. The question suggests itself whether there is anything known concerning the attributes of the bacillus diphtheriæ which will explain these differences.

As to this point, it is to be said that this bacillus, as obtained in pure culture from different cases of diphtheria, varies in its virulence, as tested upon animals, to a greater degree than any known pathogenic organism. Diphtheric bacilli isolated from different cases of diphtheria, will sometimes kill guinea-pigs by subcutaneous inoculation in twenty-four hours ; in other cases they require two, three, four, even nine days to accomplish this result. From two cases of diphtheria of slight severity recently examined at the Johns Hopkins Hospital, Dr. Abbott obtained in pure culture a bacillus identical in its morphology and its behavior on culture media with the diphtheric bacillus, but incapable of killing guinea-pigs by subcutaneous inoculation. In this respect it resembles the so-called pseudo-diphtheric bacillus, but it differs from this organism in having been present in the diphtheritic exudate in large number.

While observations are as yet insufficient to justify a positive statement, there seems to be a general correspondence between the virulence of the bacilli and the gravity of the case in which they are found, but there are exceptions to this. It is interesting to note that as a case progresses toward recovery a tendency has sometimes been observed toward a diminution in the virulence of the bacilli. It has been demonstrated that the less virulent the bacillus, the smaller is the amount of the toxic proteid which it is capable of producing in cultures, this substance being replaced, according to Fränkel and Brieger, by another albuminoid product devoid of toxic properties. While other factors may be, and doubtless are, concerned in determining the severity of a case of diphtheria, it is evident that the demonstrated variability in virulence of the diphtheric bacillus affords an explanation of many of the differences observed in the onset and decline of an outbreak of diphtheria and in different epidemics of this disease. The existence of an attenuated variety of the bacillus diphtheriæ, which may, under circumstances which we do not now understand, acquire virulence, is unquestionably of great significance in the epidemiology of diphtheria.

Roux and Yersin have brought forward a number of reasons for regarding the so-called pseudo-diphtheric bacillus (that is a bacillus resembling, if not absolutely identical with the diphtheric bacillus, in its morphology and its behavior on culture media, but incapable of killing animals) as an attenuated form of the bacillus diphtheriæ. In the two cases of apparent diphtheria referred to, in which a bacillus, which we could not distinguish from the ordinary diphtheric bacillus, save by absence of pathogenic properties when inoculated into guinea-pigs, there was a thin, grayish pseudo-membranous deposit on the tonsils, and the symptoms were of a mild character. The bacilli were present in large number and were mingled in each case with a large number of the golden pyogenic staphylococci. It would be interesting to determine whether the virulence of the diphtheric bacilli may be modified by the presence of other bacteria. Whether or not we are justified in regarding the two cases of pseudo-membranous angina referred to as genuine diphtheria cannot be decided until the status of the pseudo-diphtheric bacillus is settled.

I wish now to say a few words concerning the diagnostic value of the bacillus of diphtheria, and this will afford a convenient opportunity of touching also upon the existence of very mild cases of diphtheria and upon pseudo-membranous anginas, which are not due to the diphtheric bacillus.

While typical cases of diphtheria, especially when occurring during an epidemic, offer no especial difficulties in diagnosis, every practitioner of experience will admit that cases occur often enough which he does not know whether to call diphtheria or not. If the case is a mild one, with whitish patches on the tonsils or pharynx, which soon disappear, and constitutional symptoms are slight, he does not generally venture to make a diagnosis of diphtheria. Still the diagnosis in just this class of cases is of great importance, for such a case may be a dangerous source of infection to others.

Now we possess in the detection of the Klebs-Löffler bacillus a positive means of diagnosis of diphtheria, and it is to be considered how far this means is available to the general practitioner. The bacteriological method of diagnosis involves, first, the microscopical examination, with an oil-immersion objective, of properly stained cover-glass specimens of the suspected inflammatory exudation; second, the preparation and study of cultures from this exudation made upon suitable media, preferably Löffler's blood-serum and bouillon mixture; and third, in some cases the inoculation of a guinea-pig with the pure culture. In some cases the mere microscopical examination of cover-slip preparations from the exudation may suffice, but the diphtheric bacillus cannot be identified in this way so positively as the tubercle bacillus, for instance; and in just the class of cases where doubt as to the diagnosis is likely to exist, this procedure is most apt to prove insufficient. The examination of the cultures can be made the day following their preparation, and in nearly all cases this will afford a positive answer. The preparation of the cultures requires some training in bacteriological methods, and also a modest outfit of bacteriological apparatus. To a person thus equipped the examination offers no especial difficulties. Now, although Roux and Yersin have attempted to popularize the method, and have urged its general adoption by medical practitioners, I do not think that under existing circumstances it is likely to be widely applied in general practice. The method can be readily employed in hospitals and children's asylums, where it is calculated to be of great service, and in most large cities probably some one will be found who can be called upon to conduct such examinations. As the importance of practical training in bacteriology becomes more widely recognized in medical teaching, a larger number will enter upon the practice of their profession prepared to employ bacteriological methods of diagnosis.

The bacillus diphtheriæ has been found in a number of cases of inflammation of the tonsils and pharynx in which the exudation and the symptoms were not sufficiently characteristic to permit a positive diagnosis in any other way than by the recognition of the specific bacillus. We do not possess sufficient information to be able to say how frequent these cases, which are generally of a very mild character, are, or how they can be diagnosticated by a merely clinical or anatomical examination. That they are not infrequent during the epidemic prevalence of diphtheria seems probable from clinical experience.

The view which has been widely advocated, that most cases of so-called follicular tonsillitis, which, as is well known, may prevail as an epidemic and may present marked but usually not dangerous constitutional symptoms, is a form of diphtheria is not supported by bacteriological examination. In these cases the diphtheric bacillus is usually absent, but under the rather vague name of follicular tonsillitis are doubtless included some cases of genuine diphtheria, generally mild, but occasionally developing into unmistakable diphtheria.

Not all pseudo-membranous inflammations of the throat are caused by the specific bacillus of diphtheria. It has been demonstrated by Wurtz and Bourges that this bacillus is absent, and that a streptococcus is present in nearly all cases of pseudo-membranous angina developing in the early stages of scarlatina, so that most cases of so-called scarlatinal diphtheria are not diphtheria at all, if we limit, as seems best, the term diphtheria to the affection caused by the Löffler bacillus. The Löffler bacillus is, however, present in the diphtheria appearing in the late stages of scarlatina and during convalescence, and it seems that scarlet fever is a predisposing cause of the development of genuine diphtheria.

In a series of cases, numbering 24, of pseudo-membranous inflammations of the tonsils, pharynx and larynx, designated at the time as diphtheria, Dr. Prudden found in all but two a steptococcus, and in none the Löffler bacillus. These cases were, for the most part, either secondary to scarlatina, measles, whooping-cough, or erysipelas, or developed under the same epidemic influence as these diseases, so that these cases probably should not be regarded as genuine diphtheria. This is the view now held by Dr. Prudden himself in his latest publication, according to which renewed observations in cases of primary diphtheria have convinced him of the causative significance of the Löffler bacillus. Roux and Yersin, whose work has contributed largely to the present recognition of the Löffler bacillus as the cause of diphtheria, have also examined with negative result, so far as this bacillus is concerned, a few cases with pseudo-membranous deposits on the tonsils and pharynx of such a character that the clinician had no doubt of the existence of diphtheria. We must admit, therefore, that pseudo-membranous inflammations of the throat resembling diphtheria occur, both secondary to infectious diseases and apparently primary, in which the Löffler bacillus is not found. The further etiological study of these cases and their more precise characterization as to clinical history and pathological anatomy constitute a promising field of investigation. Until certain points have been cleared up by such investigation, there may be a certain amount of confusion as to the conception of diphtheria, but this affection seems to me even now sufficiently well characterized as to its symptomatology, pathological anatomy, and etiology to constitute a definite and independent disease which need not be confounded with other diseases.

A few words may be appropriately introduced here as regards the use of the terms diphtheria and diphtheritis. The term diphtheritis or diphtheritic inflammation is used in an anatomical sense to designate a certain kind of pseudo-membranous inflammation of a mucous membrane which may be produced by a variety of causes. The designation of certain other varieties of pseudo-membranous inflammations of mucous membranes as croupous and as pseudo-diphtheritic still further complicates the terminology. It is now generally recognized that it is best to limit the use of the word diphtheria to a definite disease and not to an anatomical process, thus making a distinction in the employment of the terms diphtheria and diphtheritis, the former being applied only to the disease due to a specific cause and the latter to an anatomical condition due to a variety of causes, of which the specific cause of diphtheria is only one among many. The adjective derived from diphtheria would be diphtheric, and that from diphtheritis diphtheritic. The disease diphtheria may appear in the form of each or all of the varieties of pseudo-membranous inflammation mentioned. It has for some time been clear that the boundaries of the disease which should be called diphtheria cannot be sharply drawn save on etiological grounds. So long as these grounds were lacking the boundaries were uncertain, vague, and fluctuating. We now possess definite criteria for the recognition of the disease, and it seems to me that instead of saying that diphtheria may be caused by a variety of microörganisms, a statement which is undoubtedly true if we understand by diphtheria all pseudo-membranous inflammations of the throat, it conduces to clearness and definiteness to confine the term diphtheria to the disease caused by the Klebs-Löffler bacillus. This will not necessitate material deviation from ordinary usage. The etiological basis of classification of disease is the surest and best, and in this case it will doubtless be found to correspond to a symptomatic and anatomical entity.

The data at present at hand are insufficient to settle the burning question as to the existence, independent of diphtheria, of a disease called membranous croup, supposed to be of a purely local, non-contagious character. Not a few cases of pseudo-membranous laryngitis without membranes on the tonsils or pharynx have been examined with the result of finding the Löffler bacillus. One such case, diagnosticated by the physician as croup, will be found in the series reported by Dr. Abbott and myself. In this we detected in large numbers the diphtheric bacilli on the mucous membrane of the pharynx, although no membranous deposit was visible, and similar results have been recorded by others, so that there is no doubt that diphtheria may occur with membranous inflammation limited to the larynx. In Dr. Prudden's first series of cases there were some instances of pseudo-membranous inflammation confined to the larynx and trachea in which steptococci, but no Löffler bacilli were found, so that it is probable that pseudo-membranous laryngitis, without involvement of the tonsils or pharynx may be produced by the streptococcus. But whether or not membranous croup may occur in the sense advocated as a purely local, non-contagious affection cannot be said to have been settled by bacteriological investigations.

An account of the results of the bacteriological study of diphtheria would be incomplete without some reference to pathogenic bacteria, which are frequently, although not constantly found associated with the Löffler bacillus in diphtheric exudations. These associated bacteria may be the cause of grave complications. Diphtheria is no exception to the rule that all necrotic and ulcerative processes on mucous surfaces where bacteria normally occur open the way to the invasion of pathogenic bacteria, especially to the widely distributed pyogenic streptococci and staphylococci. Mention has already been made of the probable causation of certain secondary pseudo-membranous anginas by a streptococcus. The same or apparently the same streptococcus is very commonly present in diphtheria. It is usually held to be identical with the streptococcus pyogenes. This organism, unlike the Löffler bacillus, is capable of invading the blood and tissues. The most frequent and important complication produced by this streptococcus in diphtheria is broncho-pneumonia, which develops as an aspiration pneumonia, as has been shown by the investigations of Prudden and Northrup. The common pus-producing bacterium, the staphylococcus pyogenes aureus is, next to the streptococcus, the most common pathogenic bacterium complicating diphtheria. It is to the invasion of these secondary bacteria that such complications of diphtheria as acute ulcerative endocarditis, suppuration of lymphatic glands, inflammations of serous membranes, and erysipelas are referable.

A matter which, although not new, has attracted much attention in recent years, may prove to be of such importance in the etiology of diphtheria that I will direct your attention to it for a few moments. Evidence has been brought forward intended to show that diphtheria may be communicated to human beings by domestic animals afflicted with this disease. The animals chiefly concerned are cattle, cats and fowls. There have been reported in England during the last decade epidemics of diphtheria in which the evidence is strong that the diphtheric germ was conveyed in milk. There are two theories as to these milk epidemics. One is that the diphtheric virus got into the milk from persons affected with diphtheria, the other is that the cows yielding the milk were affected with diphtheria. This second daring hypothesis Klein has attempted to support by experiment. He claims that by the inoculation of two cows subcutaneously on the shoulder with a broth culture of the bacillus diphtheriæ he has succeeded in producing genuine infection with the appearance of vesicles and pustules on the udders and the elimination of the specific bacilli by the milk. These experiments should be received with great caution, as they are in opposition to all that we know concerning the exclusively local development of the bacilli at the point of inoculation. We possess no satisfactory evidence that cattle are ever affected with a natural disease identical etiologically with human diphtheria, although it is known that an affection sometimes called diphtheria may appear in calves.

That cats may acquire diphtheria and may be a means of transmitting the disease to human beings is a widely-spread belief. Medical literature contains many instances in which on the one hand, cats appear to have contracted a disease by eating substances contaminated with the discharges from diphtheric persons; and, on the other hand, children seem to have become infected with diphtheria by handling sick cats. Noah Webster, in his curious book on *Epidemic and Pestilential Diseases*, published at the end of the last century, noted the coincidence of cat distempers with malignant angina. In the recently published *Annual Report of the Local Government Board of England*, Klein has brought together the evidence to be found on this point. Inasmuch as cats are among the animals most susceptible to inoculation with cultures of the Löffler bacillus, acquiring a disease resembling human diphtheria, there is no *a priori* reason why they may not be the subjects of a natural disease etiologically identical with diphtheria. But the possibility of the experimental production of a disease in an animal is no proof of the natural occurrence of such disease; and thus far there is not satisfactory evidence that diphtheria occurs as a natural disease in cats. What is necessary to settle this question is to make careful bacteriological studies in cases of suspected diphtheria in cats. The matter is of sufficient interest and importance to merit careful study, and we should be glad of the opportunity of making examinations in suitable cases which may come to the notice of physicians in this vicinity.

Pigeons also are susceptible to inoculation with the Löffler bacillus, and it is well-known that a membranous inflammation of the mouth, fauces, and trachea occurs as a destructive epidemic in chickens, turkeys, pigeons and other birds. This so-called diphtheria of fowls has not, however, been found to be caused by the same microörganism which causes human diphtheria, so that notwithstanding some rather striking observations according to which human beings have appeared to contract diphtheria from fowls, there is no positive proof of the dissemination of genuine diphtheria in this way. It may be that human beings may become infected by the germs producing the so-called diphtheria in domestic animals, but if so, there is no proof that the disease produced is etiologically identical with the disease caused by the Löffler bacillus.

We have now passed over, gentlemen, in rapid survey, some of the leading factors concerned in the causation of diphtheria. The limits of an address do not permit an exhaustive consideration of the subject even from the bacteriological point of view. Many circumstances of great importance in the etiology of diphtheria, such as the influence of unsanitary surroundings, particularly those of a domestic character, and the often dominant *role* of school attendance upon the dissemination of the disease could not be considered. These, however, are etiological factors which can be more profitably discussed from an epidemiological than a bacteriological point of view.

I have already made such demands upon your patience that I have not left myself sufficient time for any adequate consideration of the prophylaxis and treatment of diphtheria —subjects, indeed, which would furnish ample material for a separate discourse. I am glad to see that the subject of the treatment of diphtheria is to be presented in a special paper before this meeting. I cannot refrain, however, from directing your attention to a few of the general principles controlling methods of prevention and of treatment of diphtheria, and from pointing out the directions in which our increased knowledge of the causation of diphtheria leads us in our search for more effective measures to these ends.

The very fact that we are no longer groping in the dark, but that we know the enemy, his strength and his weakness, should inspire our courage and hope, should make us forge new weapons and sharpen our old ones, and should point out where to ward off attack and where to force the battle.

The possibility of making an early diagnosis of diphtheria by the aid of bacteriological examinations enhances the chances of success in coping with this disease, both in prevention and in treatment, and, as already intimated, provision should be made in hospitals and children's asylums for making such examinations.

Inasmuch as the diphtheric bacilli are present only in the false membranes and other local products of the disease at the site of infection, and are distributed outside of the body primarily through these, it is apparent that the patient should be strictly isolated; that unnecessary fabrics and other objects, especially such as cannot be readily disinfected, should be first removed from the room where the patient is placed; that care should be taken to prevent, as far as possible, the soiling of the person and clothing of the patient, of the attendants, and of the physician, as well as that of other objects in the room, with the discharges of the patient; that opportunity should not be afforded for the desiccation of these discharges, which then may contaminate the air, and that efficient measures of disinfection of the room and of all objects which by any possibility can become infected should be employed. That the enforcement of the measures indicated is capable of restraining the spread of the disease, even in crowded infants' asylums and hospitals, has already been demonstrated by actual experience. They require for their accomplishment education on the part of the community, of physicians, and of sanitary authorities in the principles of disinfection, and an intelligent appreciation of the dangers to be guarded against. I seize this occasion, as I have others, to urge the importance in cities of public disinfecting establishments, constructed according to improved modern principles, and of a corps of men in the employment of boards of public health, trained in proper methods of disinfection.

The length of time that the patient should be quarantined depends evidently upon the duration of the period in which active diphtheric bacilli remain on the mucous surfaces attacked. As to this point we possess some definite information, which shows that the period varies within wide limits. In some cases the bacilli can no longer be found after the false membranes have completely disappeared. In many cases they vanish within three or four days after the local inflammation has subsided, but they have been found as long as fourteen days after the inflammation has gone, and when the mucous membrane appeared healthy. In a case reported by Löffler, the bacilli were found three weeks after the return of the temperature to the normal, and were present for a month altogether in a state capable of carrying infection. It is evidently not possible to set a precise limit for the period of isolation of the patient. Löffler suggests that the patient should not be permitted to mingle with others or to return to school for at least eight days after the disappearance of all local manifestations, and he reckons four weeks from the beginning of the disease as the period for keeping the children out of school. Where it is possible to do so, the length of this period can be controlled by bacteriological examinations of the mucous membrane of the throat.

We have thus far considered the patient as the immediate source of infection. The evidence already mentioned in favor of the occasional dissemination of the diphtheric virus through the milk suggests at once the importance of controlling, not only the condition of the milk as received for distribution, but also of inspecting the sources of milk supply. Evidently milk should not be permitted to be sold from dairies attached to households where there are cases of diphtheria.

It does not seem to me permissible to throw out altogether the possibility of the conveyance of diphtheria by domestic animals, especially by cats, which are likely to be fondled by children even more when the animals are sick than when they are well.

In considering what can be done to render children less vulnerable to diphtheria, and to ward off an attack after exposure to the disease, the question arises, what conditions of the individual we may regard as predisposing causes. Clinical experience, as well as experiments upon animals, indicate that morbid states of the mucous membrane of the throat, such as ordinary catarrhal inflammations, swollen tonsils, sensitiveness to "catching cold," the existence of measles and scarlatina, are predisposing factors. At all times, but especially during the epidemic prevalence of diphtheria, it is important to hold in check these morbid states as far as possible. Experiments upon animals would seem to indicate that some lesion of the mucous membrane is essential for the lodgment and multiplication of the diphtheric bacilli, but it would be entireiy unjustifiable to transfer directly to human beings the results of these experiments without warrant from clinical experience, and while this experience shows the importance of such lesion, it also shows that perfectly healthy children may be attacked by diphtheria, so that we have no right to assert that in human beings infection with the diphtheric bacilli cannot occur without pre-existing alteration of the mucous membrane. The frequency and readiness with which the tonsils become the seat of the diphtheric process may be explained by the peculiar anatomical structure of these parts, as has been shown by the researches especially of Stöhr and of Hodenpyl. The rarefaction of the covering epithelium and the emigration of leucocytes to the surface found as a normal condition, seem to render the tonsils particularly vulnerable to the lodgment of the diphtheric bacilli ; and the lymphatic structures, here normally laid almost bare, are favorable for the absorption of the toxic products of the bacilli, as has been pointed out in the recent interesting paper of Hodenpyl, "On the Anatomy and Physiology of the Faucial Tonsils."

The prophylactic value, in persons liable to exposure to diphtheria, of cleanliness of the teeth and mouth and of the frequent use of weak antiseptic mouth-washes, nasal douches, and gargles, is worthy of the attention of physicians. For this purpose Löffler recommends aromatic waters, weak sublimate solutions [1 : 10000 to 1 : 15000], or, perhaps better, solutions of mercuric cyanide [1 : 8000 to 1 :10000] also, chloroform water, chlorine water [1 : 1100] thymol, [1 : 500 parts of 20 per cent. alcohol]. The use of some of these solutions evidently involves danger of poisoning in children unless special precautions are taken.

The suggestion recently made by Dr. Jacobi, that, in addition to caring for those sick with diphtheria, places of refuge should be provided for the temporary stay of children sent from home to escape infection, seems practical and calculated to meet the circumstances of many families.

The dominant role often played by schools in the spread of diphtheria throughout a community renders especially urgent the introduction of a system of daily medical inspection of the schools.

The importance of letting air and sunlight into dark, damp dwellings, and of attending in general to matters of domestic sanitation, is a lesson plainly to be drawn from the history of such places as nests of diphtheria.

If the researches relating to the etiology of diphtheria which have been so fruitful in recent years have not added to the list of agents—whose name is legion—employed in the treatment of this disease, they have given precision to the indications for treatment. From what has been said concerning the localization of the diphtheric bacilli, and the peculiar characters of the toxic substances produced by them, it is apparent that the strongest indications exist, on the one hand, for the earliest possible local treatment by germicides, and, on the other, for the destruction of the poison in the system, and, in the absence of any antidote, for supporting measures of treatment which shall enable the body to withstand the effects of the poison.

The superficial situation of the specific bacilli in diphtheria seems to render this disease especially favorable for effective local antiseptic treatment, but the difficulties encountered in actually destroying the germs in the diphtheric deposits, even when these are accessible to local applications, emphasize the fact that the obstacles to thorough disinfection within the human body are exceedingly great. Many of our most powerful antiseptics, when they come into contact with the tissues and fluids of the body form precipitates which render them largely inert, and for this and other reasons they penetrate but slowly or not at all beyond a very superficial extent. But above all we are hampered by the fact that nearly all disinfectants are many times more poisonous to the cells of the human body than they are to bacteria.

But notwithstanding the difficulties mentioned, and still others suggest themselves, it has been shown both by bacteriological examinations and by clinical experience that local disinfectant applications in diphtheria are useful and may cause the specific bacilli to disappear. An important experimental study of the action upon the diphtheric bacilli of many germicides and agents used in treating diphtheria has been recently published by Löffler, who endeavored to imitate as far as possible in test-tube experiments the conditions present in the mucous membrane when affected with diphtheria. I can only refer you to Löffler's work and his recomdations. Any attempt to consider here therapeutic agents would lead us far beyond the limits of our subject as well as of our time.

Even if it were within the power of the physician to bring about the complete destruction of the bacilli diphtheriæ after the disease has taken a firm hold, he would nevertheless in many cases be called upon to combat the effects of the toxæmia resulting from the absorption of the toxic albumen already produced by the bacilli. In this respect there is an analogy between diphtheria and tetanus. In both of these diseases the specific bacteria develop only locally at the site of infection, where they produce substances of extraordinary poison-

ous power which enter the circulation.   In the case of tetanus
we are familiar with the fact that even the complete removal
of the infected part will not prevent a fatal issue after a certain amount of poison has been produced and has entered
the system.   Experiments already mentioned have shown
that animals may be killed by the injection of an amount
so small of the toxic albumen produced by the diphtheric
bacilli that for several days no symptoms are manifested.   The
physician certainy cannot neglect the dangers of intoxication
by such a substance as this.

The interesting experiments of Behring and Kitasato upon
the production of immunity against tetanus and diphtheria
encourage us to hope that we may in time come into the
possession of direct antidotes to the chemical poisons of
these diseases.   These experiments have shown that the
blood and the blood serum of animals naturally or rendered
artificially immune against diphtheria, possess the remarkable
property of neutralizing or destroying the toxic substances
produced by bacilli diphtheriæ, and that immunity depends upon this property.   The same is true of tetanus.
Whether or not any therapeutic application in human beings
can be successfully made of this property of the blood of
immune animals, has not yet appeared.

Failing any such antidote, it should be the aim of the
physician to assist nature to withstand the poison by supporting the strength of the patient in every way possible by remedies and food.

I have attempted, gentlemen, in this address to show,
although necessarily in an imperfect and fragmentary manner,
that the discovery of the bacillus diphtheriæ and the study
of its properties have rendered our knowledge of diphtheria
in many ways more accurate and fuller, have settled many
questions of controversy, and have dissipated some errors.
The new light has not yet penetrated into all of the dark
corners, but when we consider what has been gained in less
than a decade, we are justified in expecting that here also
obscurity will disappear, and that diphtheria will become in
all respects one of the best understood, and, we may hope,
one of the most successfully combated of the grave infectious
diseases.

Report of the Section on Surgery.

SOME CONDITIONS OF THE URETHRA REQUIR-
ING PERINEAL SECTION.

By J. D. Blake, M. D.

As the title of my paper indicates, I propose to consider at this time, only a few of the conditions of the urethra, which may necessitate perineal section for their relief, indeed, only three, and they may be stated as follows :

First. Tight organic stricture of the deep and otherwise healthy urethra.

Second. Urinary Fistulæ.

Third. Infiltration of urine, the result of unrelieved retention due to stricture.

The history of this method of relieving urethral obstructions, dates back to the time of Wiseman, who (in 1652) was the first to perform external perineal urethrotomy for the relief of stricture. A few years after this Solingen, at Livourne, resorted to the same method for relieving similar conditions. From this time to the time of Petit and Le Dran (1740) external incisions for the relief of internal conditions, was carried to the uttermost extent. Think of a patient in his wretched condition suffering the tortures of the damned, coming in the day of Solingen to a surgeon for relief from an over full and bursting bladder, only to be tied hand and foot, fastened to an operating table, and his urethra laid open from meatus to the prostrate, as was the practice of that day, or in the time of Desault, Boyd and Coffinere, who practiced what was called forced catheterism which consisted in forcing a sharp or blunt-pointed poorly made and poorly curved instrument through the obstruction and healthy tissue alike, into the bladder, allowing the instrument to remain in situ for days only to be followed in most cases by infiltration and death.

Petit in the line of advance introduced his button hole operation, which he describes as follows : for tight strictures of the urethra, a sound or catheter is passed down to the obstruction and held in position by an assistant, the scrotum is raised by the left hand of the operator, while with his right he makes a large button-like incision in the perineal wall opposite to the conducting instrument, which is to be withdrawn a short distance, the surgeon then attempts to find the urethra at the bottom of the wound, at this time he would instruct the patient to make an effort to pass his water. During the effort on the part of the patient to pass his water, the surgeon makes an effort to pass an instrument into the urethra ; this accomplished, the opening in the urethra is increased and a cathuter is passed into the bladder where it is permanently kept until the wound has healed by cicatrization, or the death of the patient. Without the use of an anæsthetic I imagine this was a very difficult, tedious and painful operation.

It remained, however, for John Hunter, in 1783, to first perform what is now known as Perineal Section, but it was rarely employed as suggested by Hunter until advocated by Mr. Grainger, of Birmingham, in 1815—and afterward by Mr. Arnott ; the cases for which any of these operations were recommended, was, of course, where no instrument in their possession could be passed. But in 1844 Mr. Syme advocated external division of the stricture in cases where, although a catheter can be passed, no other treatment has afforded sufficient or permanent relief.

As to the first of the conditions stated, viz: Tight organic stricture of the deep urethra, I would say, that they are so frequent and the accidents which they occasion are so serious, that the ingenuity of surgeons everywhere has been constantly occupied in seeking a remedy for their relief, during which time the most painful, and at the same time the most dangerous methods have been employed.

In my judgment there is no operation that may be more necessary, or become more urgent, than those necessitated by tight urethral stricture, and I do not remember any surgical affection that is calculated to give more pain, or cause more mental anxiety on the part of the patient, or more patient and persevering effort on the part of the surgeon, than tight organic urethral stricture ; this is even so in this day and generation, with all the modern appliances known, at our disposal, with chloroform and ether, by which the patient can be brought absolutely under our control, with the aspirator with which without pain or suffering, the patient can be relieved of his more urgent and painful symptoms, with the filiform bougie and all the other scientifically made instruments by which an entrance into the bladder can be effected ; what must the difficulties and obstacles in the way of the surgeon have been, in the dark and gloomy days of the sixteenth, seventeenth and eighteenth centuries.

Notwithstanding the large number of cases of tight urethral strictures that come under the observation of the surgeon, I am convinced that under proper treatment comparatively few will be found to be persistently impassable, and fewer still will require perineal section for their relief, in order, however, to accomplish this desirable result, the patience and dexterity of the surgeon, may be taxed to their utmost extent. Again it is to be noticed that the environments of one suffering from tight stricture will have considerable to do with whether or not perineal section will be required, it will also depend to some extent into the hands of what surgeon he may chance to fall, for we find Holmes requesting that he may not be considered ignorant, when he states that he is skeptical as to the real value of the aspirator and prefers to puncture the bladder through the rectum with a trocar, while we find so great an authority as Keys claiming that electrolysis like caustics, must be condemned.

That great good can come from the use of either the aspirator or electrolysis, in the treatment of tight stricture and its consequence, singly, or combined, I have not the slightest shadow of doubt.

The aspirator is a temporizing agent whereby perineal section can not only be postponed, but often averted; in my hands it has been an invaluable aid. I have time and again by the use of the aspirator 2 to 3 times daily, from 2 to 4 consecutive days, where not a drop of water would pass the stricture, been able, after the lapse of from 1 to 4 days to pass a filiform, and eventually relieve the obstruction by electrolysis, the condition of the bladder and urethra always serving me as a guide for perineal section. If I find the bladder does not become irritable or painful from frequent use of the aspirator I continue to use it until such reasonable time as I may hope with the use of the bougie, and electrolysis to relieve the obstruction.

The following typical case will illustrate my method. In June, 1889, I was asked to see a case with a medical friend who requested me to come at once and prepared to perform perineal section, as he was convinced that no other method was left by which the patient could be relieved, he having ineffectually tried to effect an entrance into the bladder. Upon arriving at the bedside of the patient I found an enormously distended bladder with absolute retention, not even a drop of urine had passed for 22 hours; he was 34 years old, single, and had suffered from stricture for five years, it having followed his first gonorrhœa, he was a rather fast young man, indulging at times to excess in stimulants but had not taken a drink for over two months previous to this attack. Believing that nothing could be gained by further efforts to overcome the urethral obstruction, I aspirated the bladder, passing the needle in the middle line about a $\frac{1}{4}$ of an inch above the pubis, relieving him of over 3 pints of urine; he was now put to bed and given 5 grains quinine and $\frac{1}{4}$ gr. morphine; this was about 9.30 a. m. He fell asleep and slept for 4 hours, when he aroused, took a soft boiled egg and cup of milk. I saw him again at 6 p. m. when he said that he felt all right. I now made an effort for the first time to pass a sound; failing in this, I tried a filiform bougie and failed. He was now put under chloroform when every effort was made, only to fail, to pass the obstruction. I aspirated again, drawing this time about a pint of urine.

Another 5 grs. of quinine and ¼ gr. morphine was given. The next morning at 10 a. m. patient had a good night, but no water had passed, bladder not distended but full. No bougie would pass. I aspirated again, and at 12 o'clock same day used electrolysis with a No. 11 insulated electrode, using 12 milamp. for 20 minutes, but could not effect an entrance. 7 p. m. could not pass bougie, aspirated again drawing about a pint. Next morning (3rd day) 10 a. m. no water has passed yet, bougie will not enter, aspirated again (the punctures ranging from a ¼ to ½ inch from pubis). Same day 3 p. m. This time I had returned to the bedside of the patient determined to get into his bladder either by way of the urethra or through the perineum under chloroform. I used the bougie and failed. I then resorted to electricity, increasing the strength of the current to 18 M. A. when to my satisfaction No. 11, which is the smallest electrode, under the current for 13 minutes passed through the obstruction, after withdrawing the electrode I attempted to pass a steel sound, No. 5, same size of electrode, but failed, the best I could do was to pass a No. 1 flexible bougie which I tied in the urethra, keeping it there until next day (4th day). At 9 a. m. when I found that the urine was dribbling from the bladder alongside of the instrument, the No. 1 bougie was at this time withdrawn and a No. 3 flexible bougie passed with some difficulty. From this time on by the use of electricity, I succeeded in completely relieving the patient who now, after the lapse of nearly two years remains well. This is only one of many somewhat similar cases that have come under my observation during the past year, and all successfully treated as above described. The advantage of this method of treating tight stricture over perineal section without a guide, must be manifest, as that is not only an operation extremely difficult to perform but which is attended with considerable danger. Besides this, the time required of the patient during the healing process, providing that goes on uninterruptedly, to say nothing of the danger from the shock of the operation, and the risk of a fistulous opening as the result, which would require possibly a secondary operation. Therefore, many of the cases which are laid down in the books as being eminently suited for perineal section, in my judgment, can and should be relieved by other and safer means. I am of the opinion then that only those cases of deep urethral stricture with extensive cartilaginous induration involving the greater part of the bulbo membranous or membranous portion of the urethra, also involving the surrounding tissues in the induration, require perineal section for their relief.

Fistulæ.—In those cases where we find fistulæ complicating stricture, I have obtained good results from free perineal incisions carried down through the cartilaginous induration (which is almost always found implicating the surrounding tissue) to the spongy tissue, immediately beneath the urethra, having thus relieved the urethra from extra pressure which such induration is bound to exert, and making a ready exit for urine escaping from the urethra through the fistulous openings during efforts at micturation. At the same time I make an effort to relieve the tight stricture which, as a rule is not impassable to a filiform, in the same way and manner as if I had only simple stricture to deal with, that is to say, I use bougies, followed by electrolysis and in this way save the patient from the sometimes fatal effect of cutting into the urethra, for there does seem to me to be a much more severe shock imparted to some patients by cutting even a diseased urethra open than is imparted by almost any other method of instrumentation. There is also vast difference between the effect produced on the patients by perineal section and that of perineal incision, with stricture treated in the way stated. Therefore it is only in those cases that after the incision is made the urethra is found to be extensively strictured and the bladder and urethra very much diseased and that I find perineal section absolutely required. When this is done the bladder should be washed out with some antiseptic solution aud a drainage tube inserted, in order that absolute drainage of the bladder may take place, the after treatment to consist of passing, in the course of 24 to 30 hours a large size sound through the urethra into the bladder, which operation should be repeated in 48 hours from the first, and continued at intervals of 2 to 4 days, gradually lengthening the time for the passage of the sound until the wound has healed. Great care should be exercised in the passage of the sound during the healing process, which generally takes from 4 to 6 weeks; during the later part of such period the patient need not be confined to his bed, and when finally discharged should either be taught to use a full size conical sound upon himself and instructed to pass it at least once a week for some time, or kept under observation and have it passed by the surgeon, or else in many cases retraction will surely take place.

Infiltration of Urine.—Notwithstanding all that has been said of the innocuous character of urine injected into the tissues, and its ready and rapid absorption without deleterious effect upon the system, I am convinced from experience that whenever a comparatively sudden swelling occurs outside of the triangular ligament, when it can be detected by the finger, manifesting itself in a somewhat hard circumscribed swelling of the perineum, attending with burning and a sense of distention upon attempting to pass water, whether it be small and painful, or not, it should be cut down upon and a free opening made in the perineum in order that the urine, which is incapsulated as it were, may find free exit, and thereby save many patients from the danger of having a rapid and general infiltration; the incision will also facilitate the passage of a sound through the strictured urethra by relieving the pressure which the swelling of the tissues exerts upon the urethra, the incision should not be carried into the urethra, but simply through the indurated tissue surrounding the cavity, or into the little pocket of urine, after which the stricture is to be gradually dilated to the full extent of the urethra, during which time the little fistulæ, opening into the urethra behind the stricture will heal as dilatation goes on. If there should be sudden infiltration as sometimes occurs, perineal section should be done at once, and a drainage tube passed through the perineal cut into the urethra in order to prevent further damage by infiltrated urine to the tissues. As the class of patients in which we find these conditions existing have generally suffered for a long time, their health is usually very much impaired. We should therefore not overlook or underestimate the value of constitutional treatment.

DISCUSSION.

Dr. J. E. Michael, said : I agree in some points with Dr. Blake and disagree with him in others. As to aspiration, when it is used as a temporizing means, it is good practice. When the instrument is used with proper antiseptic precautions there is little danger. I have used it as often as a dozen times in a given case with good results. I am sceptical with regard to the use of electricity. I have tried it, and found it to disappoint me. I have struggled with filiform bougies for a half hour and then passed a larger instrument over them. As to the danger of perineal section, this is a proper subject for discussion. I reported nine cases of deep perineal section to this society a few years ago, and all of them were successful. In one of these cases that had an impassable structure, every time I tried the passing of an instrument with sweet oil and perseverence, he would have a chill and be so shocked that every attempt was attended with danger. I did a perineal section without a guide and he stood the operation better than he did the attempt to pass the instrument. I am sceptical as to the greater danger attending perineal section than in attempting the passing of instruments. I believe that a free incision is attended with less shock than an attempt to pass bougies.

Dr. J. D. Blake said : As regards the use of electricity, Dr. Michael confesses that he has had little experience with it. I have found that in tight strictures an instrument will pass with a current easier than without it. A patient presented himself at my clinic with a tight stricture at the external meatus, which was the result of a chancroid ; he came in to have a circumcision performed, and having all the paraphernalia in order, I attempted to pass an instrument with a current 14 millamperemetres for a few minutes, which was very painful, as it was impossible to prevent the instrument from coming in contact with some of the healthy tissues. He came back in three days and showed that about one-half of the indurated tissue had disappeared. I applied the instrument again and in 4 days he returned and he could retract the prepuce over the glans penis without any difficulty whatever,

INJURIES TO THE KIDNEYS.

By Randolph Winslow, M. D.

On the evening of Oct. 17, 1890, a gentleman aged about 33, and weighing 170 pounds, whilst driving with a friend in a light buggy, was thrown out, through colliding with another wagon. The horses were going very fast, and the wagons collided with great force, pitching this man out violently. He must have fallen upon his abdomen, though there were no marks upon the surface. After recovering from the stunning, he was able with assistance to walk to a neighboring house, where he was put to bed. He was shocked and nervous, and some stimulants were administered. When I arrived, some three-quarters of an hour later, he was still in a condition of shock, cold, clammy, pale ; his pulse was, however, good. He complained of severe pain between the right ribs and ilium on the lateral aspect of the abdomen, pressure was not very painful, the abdomen was soft and there was no percussion dullness. He vomited freely after the accident. With great difficulty he was able to walk to a carriage about three hours after the collision, and was brought home, a hypodermic injection of morphia was administered and he was put to bed. There were no bladder symptoms present. The next morning the urine was heavily loaded with blood, so that it appeared to be almost pure blood. The bowels at no time contained blood, the pain in his right side continued, and severe sticking pain over the liver was complained of, and there was nausea and vomiting. The bloody urine gradually diminished, but did not disappear entirely for a week or more. Fever was early developed, reaching 102°, with a pulse 115 on the second day. The belly remained soft and at no time could any collection of fluid or exudation in the right lumbar region be detected. At times the urine would clear up entirely, and after an interval considerable quantities of blood would reappear.

There was complete anorexia, and insomnia except when an anodyne was administered. As the renal symptoms abated a new series of phenomena appeared on the opposite side. The left scrotum and cord were attacked with severe pain, radiating down the left thigh, and extending upwards along the cord. A deep-seated swelling could be detected, which was elongated and appeared to be the cord itself. This swelling was tender and painful. The left leg began to swell, and a phlebitis occurred, causing marked œdema and great aching in the limb. The right sided symptoms subsided in about two weeks, but the left sided symptoms lasted many weeks and only gradually disappeared.

This case, whilst it is not remarkable in any way, presented symptoms which were both rather uncommon and quite alarming, and I thought it might serve as a text to discuss a subject which, as far as I am aware, has never been brought to the notice of this Faculty.

A man who falls from a greater or less distance or in some way receives a severe degree of violence, and is stunned and suffers pain referred more or less to the region of the kidney, with or without external marks of violence, presents no symptoms of a diagnostic character. With the appearance of bloody urine, a sign of positive diagnostic value is presented, but one which is by no means pathognomonic of any particular lesion.

Injuries to the kidney may be divided into those which are associated with a wound of the integuments and those which are not. Of these the subparietal injuries are much the more common. According to Henry Morris, out of 2,610 inspections of persons dying of all kinds of injuries, there were 13 of injured kidney, and of these, twelve were subparietal, and one a penetrating wound. The renal injury may vary of from a slight contusion, to a complete rupture into two or more parts. Of the twelve cases mentioned above there were seven lacerations, extending through not more than one-half the thickness of the organ. In two the kidney was ruptured completely into two portions, in one the kidney was crushed to pieces, whilst in two there was no rupture of the organ, but an extravasation of blood, under the capsule and in the ureter respectively. In most cases there is an extravasation of blood into the perinephric connective tissue. The rent ·in the kidney may extend in any direction and may involve any portion of the organ. The right kidney is more frequently involved than the left, and the liver is also frequently ruptured. In the case narrated above, there was persistent pain in the region of the liver. Amongst the symptoms of injury to the kidney, hæmaturia holds the most important place, though it should be remembered that bloody urine does not necessarily indicate a renal injury, nor does its absence absolutely prove that no lesion of this viscus has been sustained. The degree of injury cannot be determined from the hæmaturia, but the persistent presence of blood in the urine in large quantities would afford a strong probability of some serious lesion. The blood may be voided in the form of casts of the ureter, or in small clots. Sometimes a collection of blood may form around the kidney, giving rise to a swelling in this region. Pain is a marked and early symptom, being situated usually in the renal regions, but it may shoot down the spermatic cord into the testicle, causing a retraction of this organ. There may or may not be external marks of injury. Micturition may be increased in frequency and painful, or in some cases there may be total suppression of urine from plugging of the ureters with clots. Shock is usually marked, and is followed by decided reaction, quick pulse, fever, nausea and vomiting, and persistent pain, which is increased on inspiration, producing a stabbing sensation.

One of the complications to be feared is peritonitis, with its concomitant symptoms of pain, tenderness and tympanitis. The hæmorrhage may be so severe as to produce death rapidly, or more slowly by exhaustion. Sometimes suppuration occurs from the irritation of the perinephric tissues with blood and urine, and requires to be evacuated by surgical means. Amongst remote complications are hydro and pyonephrosis from distension of the kidney, due to an obstructed ureter, and traumatic nephritis is always a serious danger. The prognosis of an injury to the kidney must always have in it a large element of uncertainty ; taken as a rule, all renal injuries are serious and may be followed by death, whilst recovery may follow even complete rupture of the organ. Cicatrization of renal wounds has been frequently observed in cases in which death has been due to intercurrent affections.

Treatment.—Rest is all-important in the treatment of suspected or recognized injuries to the kidney. The patient should not be allowed to raise up, all sources of excitement should be sedulously avoided, the food should be liquid and unirritating, pain should be controlled with morphia. If the hæmaturia is moderate in quantity, fluid extract of ergot, or ergotin, should be administered every two or three hours, or gallic acid or turpentine. The bowels should be moved by enema if-constipation exists, but this ought not to be done more frequently than is absolutely necessary, as the passage of feces along the colon is liable to cause increased bleeding or to start it afresh if it has ceased. Strapping the injured side with adhesive plaster tends by its immobilizing and compressing action to relieve pain and check hæmorrhage. Vomiting and retching are liable to detach clots from thrombosed vessels and cause renewed or increased bleeding, hence should be controlled or prevented by attention to the diet, etc.; if the stomach is excessively irritable, rectal feeding should be employed. When there is cause to suspect that hæmorrhage is going on, as from the presence of large quantities of blood in the urine or bladder, or swelling in the loin, indicating extravation around the kidney or within the kidney itself, or from the increasing collapse, ice bags or Leiter's coils with a stream of ice water running through them should be placed over the affected region. Still more urgent symptoms of hæmorrhage demand an exploratory incision into the loin, and if the bleeding cannot be arrested by pressure or ligature, the kidney should be extirpated. A patient should not be allowed to bleed to death without a nephrotomy or nephrectomy being performed. When the bladder becomes filled with clots, cystitis and possibly pyelonephritis and pyæmia may result, unless a cystotomy is performed through the perineum, which will allow the decomposing clots to be removed and the bladder to be kept at rest. Small clots will pass from the bladder naturally or may be removed through a large-eyed catheter or by the lithotrity aspirator. Sometimes a swelling occurs in the lumbar region, which is due to the escape of urine into the connective tissue around the kidney, caused by rupture of the pelvis or calices of the kidney, as rupture of the kidney tissue is not followed by the escape of urine. This is liable to set up suppurative inflammation and a perinephric abscess, which must be relieved by incision. A circumscribed fluctuating or elastic swelling in the loin may be a pyo or hydro-nephrosis, which will require nephrotomy and possibly nephrectomy.

Report of the Section on Practice of Medicine.

TREATMENT OF DIPHTHERIA.

BY JOSEPH T. SMITH, M. D.

It is with much hesitation that we venture to call the attention of the Faculty to the subject of the treatment of diphtheria, but in view of the increased interest in the disease, especially its causation, we thought it might not be amiss for some member of the Section on Practice to bring forward the subject of treatment in order that those so disposed might discuss the many vexed questions which still wait for an answer. It is then our purpose rather to furnish food for discussion than to present any new and untried means of cure, rather to more fully emphasize what we know than to call off the attention to fields unexplored and speculative ; we desire rather to more fully use the knowledge we have and from that, endeavor in the future, to build up a rational mode of treatment, which shall be more efficient than that employed at the present day. We need to have our knowledge affirmed and reaffirmed, if we would be kept from the domain of speculative and irrational forms of medication.

The knowledge we will gain from the orator at this session, on "The Cause of Diphtheria," will doubtless set many to thinking anew of the treatment, and he will doubtless give us food for thought that will keep us in the path of rational medication. Before the knowledge that germs caused disease, how meagre were the results of all forms of speculative treatment in preventing the suppuration of wounds and its attendant consequences, in keeping woman from the many forms of disease attending her lying in, and in preventing diseases which have now become so rare that they have almost passed out of our vocabulary. All this has been brought about by those engaged in the active duties of professional life following the lead of those who have enabled us to throw aside speculation and trust to knowledge.

We have learned that certain diseases are produced by microörganisms. Kill these minute bodies or keep them away and the diseases ought to cease or be altogether prevented. We act upon such knowledge in regard to some of the diseases and the result has very far surpassed our most sanguine expectations. May not what is true of other diseases be true of diphtheria? Can we not say it is true? Shall not this disease, like pyæmia, septicæmia and many others, yield to rational means of prevention and cure and it too become a thing of the past? We have every reason to believe that if rational means were in every case fully carried out the disease could be prevented. If we exercised as much care in regard to antiseptics in diphtheria as the surgeon does in his cases of abdominal section who can doubt but that we would be amply rewarded.

But many will and do say, that we need not trouble ourselves so about rational medication, that much that is of inestimable value has been the result of accident, as even to this day we cannot explain the action of quinine nor the preventive influence of vaccination. To such we can only answer, let us take all such discoveries and use them for our benefit, but as we know nothing of them we cannot control their coming; we must not, therefore, sit with folded hands waiting for something to turn up. Again, with how much more confidence and satisfaction we use the means that are the result of knowledge than we do those of accident or speculation.

That these apparently trite remarks need to be often brought to our attention is evidenced by the many and varied remedies which are brought to bear upon this disease, so that often times in sheer despair at the apparent hopelessness of many cases which come under our care, we are sorely tempted to abandon the knowledge we have and to launch out into the great field of speculative medicine, which will lead us we know not where. The temptation in this disease is peculiarly great, owing to the many and varied conditions which arise in the course of its development, the results of which even the most experienced cannot with any certainty foreshadow. When we look at the subject it seems in such a chaotic state that we are tempted to say that we know nothing about it. Indeed, we often hear it said, not only by those outside, but by many in the profession, there is no need to do much, the disease will take care of itself. It is the object of this paper to bring anew to our attention the fact that we have much valuable knowledge in regard to this disease and the importance of holding all else subsidiary to this knowledge. If we go over the field we are bewildered by the varied forms of medication.

Note a few of them :   Lime water and ice bags come to us with loud praise from Königsberg ; tripsin, papoid and lactic acid have been highly lauded as solvents of the membrane ; great praise is bestowed upon pine-apple juice as used among the negroes in Louisiana ; Burghart calls attention to the great benefits derived from insufflations of quinine and sulphur ; Nelson brings to our notice the great good obtained from applications of pure salicylic acid ; Dr. Manchester lauds the vapor of bromine ; Dr. Hall uses sodii hyper sulph. and tannin with marked benefit ; Dr. Roese gives spts. terebinth, $\mathfrak{z}$ i with spts. nit. ether three times daily ; Dr. Boyd puts verat virid in the front rank for its controlling influence upon the heart ; Dr. Mulhall advises the thorough washing out of the pharynx with a household syringe ; Dr. Braddon praises in no unmeasured terms the oil of peppermint ; Dr. Corbin refers in terms of praise to mercurial fumigations ; Dr. Jacobi claims great good from the bichloride of mercury gr. ¼ in divided doses during the day in infants four months old ; Dr. Hoyer uses acid gallic and glycerine ; Cholema is fond of using plugs of cotton for the nares wet with a 20 per cent. sol. of menthol in oil ; Parker speaks highly of a strong solution of hydrochloric acid one to three of water or glycerine or carbolic acid of the same strength. From all of this, and the list can be made much longer, one must bring order if he is to have any firm ground to stand upon. We know three things of diphtheria :

1. It is due to the presence of a poison produced by a microörganism which itself does not invade the blood.

2. This poison exerts a depressing influence upon the heart's action and interferes with the functional activities of the red-blood corpuscles.

We know of nothing as yet which will destroy the organisms when once they have found a lodgment upon the tonsil, so must content ourselves with meeting the results of their growth and development. We trust some day to be able to destroy the bacilli, but that knowledge is most likely to come from those specially trained to work in the laboratories of the world. .

The conditions presented by the nares, pharynx and larynx first demand our attention. That we have not yet found a solvent for the membrane is amply proven by the many articles tried and abandoned because they failed of universal acceptation, and the fact that no one thing is used by any large number of the profession to-day for that purpose. That we have found no one antiseptic that meets all of the requirements is proven in the same way. Failing thus to freely dissolve the membrane and not being able to use well known antiseptics in sufficient strength to fulfill a good purpose, as such, it seems clear that in dealing with irritable, sensitive, easily frightened children, as we do in most cases, it is best that we should confine ourselves to such applications as will afford the child the least annoyance, and at no time be tempted from them. The applications should also be made in the way most agreeable to the patient. Lime water and carbolic acid as a spray, seem to meet these indications best. The quiet, ease and comfort of our patients must be our first thought, and we should be jealous of any remedy which will disturb them.

Should the disease invade the larynx a surgeon must be called in early, that he may seize the proper time in his judgment for interference.

Any form of treatment for the throat should embody simplicity and ease of application ; the remedy the patient takes to most kindly is the one for our use, as we know of nothing which will offset the harm done by resistance.

We know of no antidote to the poison and so must rest content with combating its effects. That the symptoms produced are due to a poison is stated clearly and positively by Dr. Prudden in his recent article on the "Etiology of Diphtheria." He says: "That the poison locally produced by the Löffler bacillus can, and usually does, cause the characteristic systemic effects in primary diphtheria is well established." The one effect of the poison which gives us most concern is the failure of the heart to do its duty. This we know, and this knowledge is to be a constant stimulus to keep us from doing anything which will add a feather's weight to the work of the heart ; not only so, but that work must be made as light as possible ; the patient must keep the prone position from the outset, the rule to be relaxed under no conditions, even for one, though better,.for two weeks after convalescence has been established ; the patient should be kept rigidly on the back. Alcohol is the ally called in by universal consent to aid us in overcoming this tendency of the poison.. In view of this condition of the heart any applications to the throat or forms of medication which call out any resistance on the part of the patient or the exercise of his bodily powers must be looked upon with suspicion, for it is best that we should hold to the knowledge we have, that any increase in the work of the heart will aid the poison in its work of death. Calomel may ordinarily do no harm, but if it cause an increase in the number of stools, the exertion caused by the more frequent use of the bed-pan may result in much harm. The stomach is also to·be guarded, in that it receives only nourishing food, easy of digestion ; · thus the heart muscle shall have plenty to feed upon and a full stomach, even after convalescence shall have been some time established, shall not be allowed to diminish the space needed for the full action of the heart. Milk is the diet upon which we rely and which will usually meet the indications.

We know, in the second place, that the red blood corpuscles fail to fully perform their functions. They do not carry oxygen as they should, the pale, often profoundly anæmic condition of the patient proving this to the most careless observer. As we looked to alcohol to meet the indications in regard to the heart, so we look to iron to meet the indications in regard to the blood, and experience confirms our trust. The iron must be quickly and readily absorbed, and the muriated tincture with glycerine seems to be one of the best forms of administration. This, at the present day, seems to be the extent of our knowledge ; and if we push on further we must enter the field of speculation ; as witness the use of the bichloride of mercury. We do not rally about this as we do about alcohol and iron ; its use is speculative, and if what we have heard of the habits of the bacillus of diphtheria be true, as from the evidence it must be, it is difficult to see how a germicide given by the mouth can kill microörganisms which do not get into the blood, and this seems confirmed by the fact that there is no consensus of opinion as to its utility.

Another point upon which we possess valuable knowledge is, that by destroying the bacilli by means well known and easily applied, the spread of the disease can be prevented. This disease is thus made to rank with typhoid fever, phthisis and others in which, if the discharges from the parts affected be thoroughly and at once destroyed the disease can be confined to the person affected. The difficulty here is not that we are deficient in knowledge, but for many reasons we do not put it to a practical use. A writer has said, with much truth, that municipal prophylaxis in diphtheria is as useless as in puerperal fever ; that is, we are forced to the personal equation, take care of the thorough disinfection of the patient and his surroundings and the spread of the disease will be stopped. Dr. Prudden, in the article noted above, says: "It should be clearly held in mind by those eager to draw from experimental studies on the etiology of this disease such practical lessons as shall be of value in treatment, that whether one or more causative agents are at work in setting up those acute infectious diseases which are associated with the formation of a pseudo-membrane, it seems to be fully established that in all cases the seat of infection and the origin of the mischief is a local one. All these experiments point to the paramount importance of efficient local germicidal treatment, and this is equally important whether the bacillus of Löffler

or the streptococcus or both together be the infecting agent."
The evidence thus seems clear that we know the following
in regard to the treatment of diphtheria, and whatever else
we do should assume a secondary place.

1st.   The effect of isolation and thorough disinfection in
preventing the spread of the disease.

2nd.   The need of alcohol and iron to influence for good
the heart and blood ; the value of milk as the chief article of
diet.

3rd.   The need of quiet and rest in bed and the importance
of looking upon these as governing our choice of applications to the throat and other forms of medication.

4th.   The necessity of calling early upon the surgeon when
the disease invades the larynx.

5th.   The value of as great cleanliness of the pharynx and
nares as the condition of the patient will permit.

Three vexed questions still wait for answers :

1st.   How shall the membrane be dissolved ?

2nd.   How shall the bacilli be destroyed at the seat of invasion ?

3rd.   What is the antidote to the poison ?

We are patiently waiting for an answer to one or all of
these questions, and as the ablest men are putting forth all
their energies in the search for answers, we look confidently
for the day when diphtheria shall be as rare as pyæmia or
small-pox.

DISCUSSION.

Dr. A. K. Bond.—I believe papers like Dr. Smith's are
quite as valuable to the general practitioner as more scientific dissertations are.   I think it well in this age of scientific
experimentation, we should stop to sum up what we do
know, as he says "to review at times what is actually known
from a practical stand point."   Sometimes we have to leave
our cases alone and do nothing that will interfere with the
comfort of the child.   The blowing of some of the powders
will frighten some children into convulsions.   Among the

remedies that seem both good and yet are mild and agree, are alum water, lemon juice and hydrogen peroxide, which latter can be given freely diluted with water as a drink to rebellious patients. There is probably some value in repeated small doses of mercurials, as some of the older practi-.tioners have gotten excellent results from their use. By the use of the steam spray we may fill the air of the room with carbolic acid and other vapors. An interesting point has of late been made by writers, namely, that swelling of deeper lymphatics of the neck is associated with disease of the nasal cavities and should attract especial attention to those three cavities.

Dr. W. A. B. Sellman.—I am glad to hear Dr. Bond speak as he did. I have lost but one case in eighteen and that was one where there were very enlarged tonsils and on my first visit I gave a grave prognosis. When I am called to a case of diphtheria, I provide my patient with three sprays, a nasal spray, a post-nasal spray, a post-nasal syringe and a spray for the throat. I use Marchants peroxide of hydrogen (1 to 3) I spray the interior nares, then use the post-nasal syringe and then the spray for the throat. As to constitutional treatment I use iron and quinine. Equal parts of iodoform and sulphur to be blown into the nostrils and fauces I find is also good local treatment. I do not think that we should use stimulants in the early stages, but when they are to be used, I use carbonate of ammonium and whisky, whisky and milk punches, etc., a diet of beef extract and milk. In answer to inquiries he said : I spray the patients throat myself and do not trust it to the nurse, even if I have to go six times a day, I prefer to use it myself unless I cannot get to the case early enough and have an intelligent nurse, then I intrust it to her.

Dr. A. K. Bond asked what was the fatality of the epidemic?

Dr. W. A. B. Sellman said there was a large number of fatal cases. The fatality in his cases was one in 18. Some of these cases were slow in convalescence, some extending over a period of several months. In answer to Dr. W. Brinton, he said the average duration was from 4 to 12 weeks.

Dr. A. K. Bond said : I saw in my reading somewhere that a diluted solution of the tincture of the chloride of iron was put at the bedside of the patient and he was allowed to to drink it freely and he took as much as an ounce of th tincture in this way, in some cases and the condition of th patient was rapidly improved. He had not had any expe rience in this method but thought it a valuable suggestion.

Report of the Section on Obstetrics and Gynæcology.

OBSTETRICAL ANTISEPSIS.

By J. Edwin Michael, M. D., *Chairman.*

The too indulgent courtesy of our former president has laid upon me a task for which I feel that I am little fitted, but since the appointment signalizes the new departure I have taken in professional work, I cannot but express my gratitude for it, and the hope that what I have to lay before you may at least be worthy of your attention. Following the custom which has grown up in the Faculty since the increase of current medical literature made it unnecessary to give an epitome of progress in the whole subject under the control of a section, I have carefully scanned the field of obstetrics and selected that which seems to me to be of most importance to the general practitioner, as the subject of my remarks. The matter is somewhat old and has been much written upon, but it still occupies the first place, and there are still certain points about which there are differences of opinion both as to theory and practice which are well worth consideration. Obstetrical antisepsis like surgical antisepsis, has had its periods of development. The neglect of pre-antiseptic times gave place to the complicated and dangerous technique which the first burst of enthusiasm is responsible for, and careful study at the bedside has had the effect of eliminating dangerous procedures and simplifying methods, until, while we are not yet justified in saying that the method has reached its ideal perfection, it has undergone very marked development and reached a stage of wonderful utility. The able paper read by Prof. T. G. Thomas, on December 6th, 1883, before the New York Academy of Medicine, and in which advanced ground was taken in support of antiseptic precautions in all obstetrical cases, attracted widespread attention in this country and abroad, and while it did much good in making the profession aware of the importance of the subject, was not without evil effect in that, following the natural bent of humanity, to go to extremes, many physicians gave intrauterine douches without stint on the smallest provocation, and in many cases did much, even fatal mischief thereby. Two cases present themselves in this connection. The wife of a physician was confined, and I was called to see her on the fourth or fifth day in consultation. I found her in *articulo mortis*. Inquiry revealed the fact that after delivery, her uterus had been washed out, and that without any very definite indication, and that the washing had been done through a catheter which had previously been used for another purpose. In the fall of the same year, I was called to see a beautiful young woman who complained of certain well known symptoms. She had been married several months, and, not to mince matters, was in the family way. Less than a year afterwards I saw the husband with a black band on his hat. Upon inquiry he told me that his wife had been confined normally and she had so far recovered on the tenth day that she was sitting up. Her physician was called away and she was placed in the care of a brother practitioner. Upon paying his first visit the new doctor inquired if her womb had been washed out. Upon a negative answer being given he insisted that this should be done and did it. On the third day thereafter there was a decided chill followed by high fever and in four or five days the woman was a corpse. These cases, it is true, show more to the discredit of the physicians in charge than of the theory of antisepsis, but they are but types of what occurred in many instances during what might be called the meddlesome stage in the development of obstetrical antisepsis. Such experiences made a well nigh indelible impression on the minds of many practitioners, and created a prejudice against obstetrical antisepsis which in many cases still endures. My own observation in conversation and consultation with my professional acquaintances shows me that the subject has not been followed and studied as it deserves to be, and convinced as I am of the immense importance of it, I feel myself constrained to bring it before the Faculty. It would profit us little to go over the various theories which have been advanced to explain the nature of puerperal fever, and the many facts which have sufficed to overturn them. It is sufficient for our purposes to note that the recognition of the true nature of the malady as a septicemia, is the basis upon which has been founded all the work which has resulted in almost eliminating it from the practice of well conducted lying-in hospitals, and making it possible to so eliminate it from private practice. We have, but to glance at some of the results achieved by the adoption of the antiseptic method in order to convince ourselves that it is based on a true understanding of the nature of puerperal fever.

The crude antisepsis of Semmelweiss in Vienna, reduced the septic mortality in the lying-in wards from 12 to 1.27 per cent. In 1857 the septic mortality in the Paris maternity was 10 per cent.

In 1884 Tarnier was enabled to say : "Thanks to antisepsis, among 1000 women entered at the maternity, we have had but one death, the poor woman of whom we have spoken who entered with rupture of the neck of the uterus and the neck of the bladder. But for this case we should have had 1000 cases without a single death." What an experience this is for Tarnier, who had seen seven women die of puerperal fever in a few hours ! Such changes in the mortality statistics could well justify the enthusiastic proposition of Pajot " Messieurs, nous pouvons ecrire sur le fronton de cette clinique : Ici on nait mais on ne meurt pas." The closing of the London General Lying-in Hospital on account of the terrible death rate from puerperal fever, and its subsequent successful reopening under rules laid down by Lister is too well known to require more particular description. The figures given by Garrigues showing the changed death rate after the introduction of antiseptic methods in the New York Maternity, a reduction of septic mortality from 4.17 per cent. to .27 per cent. are interesting as illustrative of the benefits of antiseptic practice.

Dr. Rohé reports 377 deliveries without a single septic death in the Maryland Maternité.

Dr. Neale reports 308 deliveries without a septic death in the Free Lying-in Hospital.

The report of the first 1000 cases in the Sloan Maternity in New York, shows one septic death, and that one in the person of a woman who entered the hospital in a septic state. The literature of the subject is so full, and the result of antiseptic practice as compared to the older methods so brilliant that it would be impossible in the short space allotted to us to give even an epitome of the work of the last ten years. Moreover, the general subject is too well known to justify any attempt at a full consideration of it. Antiseptic midwifery has won its fight in a general way. All lying-in hospitals, so far as I am informed, are conducted, as far as their circumstances will allow, upon the antiseptic basis, and all obstetrical teachers are as one as to the advantages of preventing puerperal fever over attempts at curing it. Nevertheless, the general practitioner resists the teaching of the hospitals in but too many cases, and the septic results in private practice justify the statement of Leopold; that women delivered in lying-in hospitals are much safer than those attended at home, thus reversing the state of affairs which existed not very many years ago. The practice of antiseptic midwifery is the attempt to prevent certain pathological processes which are generally grouped together under the name of puerperal fever, and which depend for their origin upon the activity of pathogenic organisms either found in contact with the generative tract of the woman, or brought into contact with it during delivery or lying-in. The study of the method therefore involves, first, the question of auto-infection and hetero-infection, second, the principles involved in prophylaxis together with a consideration of the clinical results achieved, and third, the practical application of the results of the foregoing, to hospital and private practice.

The experience of Semmelweiss showed him conclusively that by far the largest proportion of cases of child-bed fever, was due to direct infection from the attendants and he had no hesitation in declaring this view. When for example the women were divided into two classes, among one of which the students practised, and the other was reserved exclusively for the midwives, and it was found that the mortality in the former class was far in excess of that of the latter it was perfectly clear that the students brought the infection. The students attended post mortem examinations, and contagious diseases, while the midwives did not, and hence the explanation of the difference was clear. Nevertheless, Semmelweiss believed that there were certain cases which were not due to infection, but were due to an intrinsic poison developed in the discharges of the patient. "In rare cases," says he, "will the decomposed organic material, the absorption of which causes child-bed fever, be produced within the affected organism, and these are cases of auto-infection." This view is not sustained by modern investigation and has no adherents at the present time, so far as I know. In the masterly discussion of the whole subject which took place at the meeting of the Congress of German Gynecologists at Freiburg, in 1889, not a single participant embraced this view. The question of auto and hetero-infection, as now understood, is quite different, and there is much to be said on both sides of it of great importance as bearing on the practical question of treatment. The views of the majority of obstetricians are expressed by Miltenberger in his admirable paper published in the fall of 1889, when he says: "So far then—and I have stated but received facts—we must conclude that the so called puerperal fever, including sapræmia, septicemia and pyæmia, is unquestionably a disease of bacterial origin, and that in all cases we must acknowledge in its history only exosepsis or hetero infection, and that its cause is always heterogenetic." The presence of the well known pathogenic organisms, staphylococcus aureus, s. albus and streptococcus is so constantly associated with puerperal fever in its various forms that there is no doubt that these organisms are justly regarded as the causative factors in the disease. These organisms, are, however, found in the vagina in normal cases as well as in the cervix uteri, and the question arises as to whether these resident germs are to be regarded as pathogenic and dangerous, and capable of producing puerperal fever or whether the disease is always due to some contagion brought in from the outside. This question is of the utmost importance, since upon its solution must depend certain points of prophylaxis about which there is considerable discussion. It cannot be denied that clinical experience has done much to eliminate the question as a practical one, for it is the universal result in all cases where large amounts of clinical material have been subjected to rigid precautions. Whether the prophylactic douche was used or not, the number of septic cases has notably diminished and the possibilities of auto-infection been largely reduced. The results of Leopold's investigations are very instructive in this connection. The immense material of the Dresden clinic has been used for the elucidation of this question with the following results: From September, 1883, to Easter, 1884, carbolic acid was used as the antiseptic, and afterwards sublimate came into vogue. Both objective and subjective disinfection, including the vaginal douche before and after delivery, were used, and the consequence was that successive series of 1300 and 1600 cases were recorded without a septic death. The discovery of germs of the kind usually considered dangerous in the vagina in otherwise normal cases seemed to show the necessity of a more thorough cleansing of the vagina before delivery, and the plan of thoroughly scouring out that organ was adopted. The results were by no means so favorable. There were more septic cases, and besides this the natural pliability of the vagina was so interfered with that there were many more lacerations to deal with, and the labors were in general less satisfactory. The plan was then adopted of using objective disinfection alone, with the addition of thoroughly scouring the external parts and using no injections whatever, nor allowing any internal examination whatever to be made. This plan was naturally restricted to the normal cases, i. e., cases which required no obstetrical aid, and excellent results were to be expected The results were indeed brilliant. In 510 cases so treated there were nine in which there was a moderate elevation of temperature, as follows: .

In No. 1 hæmatoma vulvæ, three days fever. No. 2 macerated child, four days fever. No. 3 syphilis, chill and high fever for ten days. No. 4, macerated fœtus, mammary inflammation, four days fever. No. 5, entered with membranes ruptured and a foul discharge, four days fever. No. 6, macerated fœtus, four days fever. No. 7, atonic hæmorrhage, pulse 140, three days fever. No. 8, moderate parametritis of the right side, (in this case it was not clearly proved that the patient had not been examined before entering the hospital.) No. 9, unsutured vaginal rupture with œdema of the vulva. Leopold thinks that this series of cases justifies the conclusions : 1. The word "auto-infection" is only allowable when every other possible source of infection has been most diligently sought for and there is no other possibility. 2. Sources of infection, especially in institutions used for instruction, are often concealed, but present and removable. 3. In cases of auto-infection other sources of infection can generally be easily demonstrated. 4. The word auto-infection is hence a dangerous one. It leads to false conceptions and, in practice, to improper procedures and doubtful excuses. Those women have the best lyings in who are not internally examined. 6. Especial stress should be laid on external examination. It nearly always gives satisfactory information in regard to the progress of the labor. If internal examination becomes necessary the greatest care should be exercised in cleansing the examiner and the external genitalia of the patient. 8. It is only in pathological labors that an antiseptic cleansing of the internal generative organs is necessary. This experience of Leopold is especially interesting from the practical point of view as showing what may be done by avoiding causes of hetero-infection, and while it does not by any means prove the point announced by Miltenberger, as I shall show later, it does prove beyond question that the possibilities of auto-infection even in the modern sense are very limited. I must again call attention to the fact that the cases upon which this experiment was tried were selected cases in that they were cases in which the process of parturition was normal and no obstetrical aid was needed. Let us consider for a moment what is the significance of this. Admitting as in the face of the demonstated facts, we must admit that there are in the many otherwise normal cases germs of the kind which are usually considered capable of producing fever in the vagina, let us follow the course of labor as seen in a normal, and compare it with the same process under abnormal circumstances. As was pointed out by Kaltenbach, the normal progress of labor is well calculated to cleanse the parturient canal, is in fact nature's aseptic method. We have the increasing discharge from the vagina as the labor progresses, the flow carrying along with it all loose germs in the vagina. Finally the bag of waters ruptures and the vagina is flushed out with the aseptic amniotic fluid. The second stage then begins in earnest, the head descends, there is a close fit, the vagina is brushed out by the head, and then follows another copious flow of amniotic fluid, the placenta passes and the birth canal is pretty well cleaned out. If not meddled·with there will probably be no trouble. On the other hand, what happens with premature rupture of membranes, bad presentation, inefficient pains and the like. The amniotic fluid trickles away, the process lasts much longer, there is more pressure and hence more wounding and bruising of the parts, many examinations are made, in short we have all the conditions which favor the activity of pathogenic organisms, if such are present, and experience shows that the longer the labor and the greater the necessity for interference the more probable is fever as a sequel to the labor. Germs are demonstrated to be present in a large proportion of cases.

But germs must be placed under favorable conditions before they become dangerous. Halstead has recently found staphylococcus in organizing blood clots, Gönner made inoculations with germs found in normal vaginæ and failed to produce pathological processes, and hence declared the germs so found non-pathogenic. Döderlein found germs (and even streptococcus in one case), in ten per cent of feverless cases in the vaginal discharges. Rosving's interesting experiments bear upon this point. He injected pure cultures into the bladder and so long as the outlet was free they simply passsd out with the urine and did no harm. But when the urethra was tied and favorable conditions for their development otherwise produced, they underwent their normal development and produced characteristic disease processes. We are indebted to Steffeck, of Wurzburg, for the most elaborate and practical combination of clinical and bacteriological work on this subject, a labor apparently stimulated by the discussion at the Freiburg Congress, and one which seems to set at rest many points of interest. The whole question of auto-infection rests on the determination of the powers of the germs found in the vagina in normal cases. Gönner's experiments, referred to above, proved negative since he failed to produce characteristic processes by the injection of vaginal secretion containing what seemed to be disease germs, and Leopold's clinical experience seemed to point the way to the denial of the possibility of auto-infection. Steffeck experimented with the vaginal secretion of women, most of whom had not been examined at all, and who were regarded as normal, healthy women. His method was to secure the secretion under the most careful antiseptic precautions, to inoculate a culture tube and a guinea-pig at the same time. If abscess or general infection ensued he compared the organisms found in the tube and in the pathological product. When they agreed he injected a pure culture and noted the result. In 29 cases there were 12 positive results; 7 abscesses and 5 general infections, followed by the death of the animal. In all the positive cases the staphylococcus auyeus or albus or the streptococcus was found, and in not one of the negative cases were these organisms discoverable. As he says, in commenting on the work, "the most important result of the experiments is that in every case from the organs containing abscesses and from the heart blood of the animals the same cocci which had been found in the secretions, and none other, could be cultivated." Steffeck feels himself justified by these experiments in the conclusion that "the micro-organisms, staphylococcus aureus, staphylococcus albus and streptococcus found in the genital canal of healthy women who have not been examined are pathogenic." The practical outcome of the laboratory work is that in order to reach the ideal perfection of antiseptic obstetrics these pathogenic germs should be removed from the vagina prior to the birth of the child, and hence the material at the Wurzburg clinic is subjected to a preliminary douche as well as protected by the usual objective disinfection. The results thus far are 439 births with 7.5 per cent. morbidity, these cases showing mere transient rise of temperature, no serious case, much less a death, having occurred. This among cases, all of which are examined by both students and midwives, is claimed by Steffeck to be superior to the results of Leopold. It appears to me that we must admit the possibility of auto-infection in the modern sense ; that is, that the germs found so often in the genital canal of healthy women can produce puerperal fever under circumstances which favor their development, and the unexamined cases of Leopold show this as conclusively as the bacteriological experiments of Steffeck. Ideal results are then only to be expected in cases where the resident germs are removed or rendered harmless as a preliminary measure, and all the points of both objective and subjective disinfection attended to as well. The practical question, however, is this : Can we disinfect thoroughly by a process which does no harm? This question seems to have been answered in the negative by the results of Leopold's clinical researches, and in the affirmative by the work of Steffeck. And there are many other obstetricians of large experience and excellent judgment who attach themselves to one or the other of these views. By far a majority, so far as I have been able to learn, prefer the preliminary douche, and especially in cases belonging to a clinic in which instruction is given and where examinations are made by students and widwives. For example, in the Baudeloque clinic under Pinard, a douche of 1 to 4000 biniodide of mercury is given. At the Paris Maternite, under Gueniot, 1 to 4000 sublimate. At the Lariboisiere, under Porak, 1 to 2000 sublimate. At the General Lying-In Hospital of London, 1 to 4000 sublimate. At the Sloane Maternite, in New York, 1 to 5000 sublimate. The Germans generally use sublimate of moderate strength, but Leopold, Fehling and a few others depend exclusively on objective disinfection, and use no douche at all, except in the presence of a positive indication. The opponents of the theory of auto-infection claim that the view is a very dangerous one, and that its acceptance is apt to cause undervaluation of the means used to prevent hetero infection. This is an important point in practice, for while we, I think, must admit the possibility of auto-infection in the sense explained, we must at the same time be mindful of the fact that the horrible ravages which in former times were made by puerperal fever were due, in the immense majority of cases, to hetero-infection ; in plain English, contagion. This was made clear by Oliver Wendell Holmes years before the present discussion arose. The present state of the question admits of discussion only with reference to the preliminary vaginal cleansing and the details of the technique by which objective and subjective disinfection can be carried out.

It is unfortunate that we are prone to substitute a name for a fact and to suppose or claim that we have adopted a certain method when we have only gone through certain of the motions, so to speak, appertaining to the method. If one watches the preparations and the progress of the work in an ordinary so-called antiseptic operation, one will ordinarily be able to discover more sins of omission and commission than the operator is aware of. Nevertheless the conduct of an antiseptic operation is but child's play as compared to the conduct of an antiseptic labor. In the surgical case we have all our things together, we make all our preparations, we perform our operation, dress our wound, and are done. In the midwifery case, on the contrary, we must wait several hours, perhaps several days, the possibility of infection being present all the time, and even after the case is over we cannot occlude the wound as in a surgical case, on account of the necessity of a free escape for the lochia, and so our disinfection is a much more difficult task, and as a consequence is much less thoroughly done. In fact, the general practitioner, as a rule, makes no regular attempt at disinfection, and beyond ordinary cleanliness, conducts his cases about as he used to years ago. The result justifies the statement of Leopold, that women confined in lying-in hospitals are safer than those confined at home. There is no difference of opinion as to the propriety of the most thorough disinfection of all persons and things which are to come into contact with the patient, and the first movement in this disinfection, which is a thorough scouring with soap and water, with the aid of a nail brush.

This cleansing should be most thorough. Not a mere ordinary rub, but an aggressive and persistent scouring, with plenty of good clean soap and water, as hot as can be borne with comfort. This treatment should be applied to nurse and doctor as well as to everything else washable. The patient should be given a full bath, with plenty of soap, and the genitals and all the parts adjacent, with particular reference to the anal region, should receive special attention, an enema having been previously given. All linen, for sheets, pads, etc., should at least have been boiled, and, preferably, treated with sublimate. I speak of this simple cleansing first and alone because it is within the reach of all, and is, indeed, the most essential part of the antiseptic treatment. There can be no practical antisepsis which is not preceded by careful use of soap and water. So far as chemical disinfection is concerned, there is some difference of opinion as to the best and safest drug to use, but there is such a large preponderance in favor of the bichloride of mercury that the other candidates for favor need not be considered. I do not mean by this that carbolic acid, biniodide of mercury, creolin and other drugs used are not useful. They are undoubtedly good, but not so good as the sublimate. Indeed, I was told that all the great change which has been wrought in the confinement results at Blockley was attained by the use of creolin alone. It would take my paper far beyond reasonable limits to discuss the merits of the various disinfectants recommended. For disinfection of hands, cloths, the external generative organs, etc., the strength of 1 to 1000 is usually preferred, while for vaginal and intra-uterine douching 1 to 4000 is generally used. Galabin, it is true, claims that 1 to 4000 is not sufficiently strong, but most obstetricians are afraid to use a stronger solution for fear of mercurial poisoning. The disinfection of the hands of the obstetrician and nurse is the most important process; and should not be slighted. We do not want a mere dip of the fingers into the solution, but the whole hand and forearm should be allowed so remain in the solution at least five minutes. Moreover, the solution should be as hot as can be well borne. Cases used for instruction should undoubtedly be douched with the 1 to 4000 solution both before and after examination and labor, and all cases in which the labor is unusually long or difficult, or in which any operation has to be done, the same treatment should be adopted. The intra-uterine douche should be reserved for cases in which the uterus has been subjected to the danger of infection. This cleansing and disinfection, which appears such an easy matter, upon description is not so, in fact, in ordinary hands. It is a matter of routine, and one must be somewhat trained in it or else something will be forgotten, some essential point neglected. Mermann, who uses no douche, had, as a result of his earlier efforts, 21 per cent. of fever cases. In his late cases in the same institute, and with theoretically the same method, the fever rate is reduced to about 6 per cent., a result which, as he says, is in no degree due to accident, but attributable solely to the training of the hospital staff. The only way in which satisfactory disinfection can be accom-plished is by rigid adherence to a given plan. This is espe-cially important in the hospitals whose material is used clini-cally, but not to be neglected in private practice. The ques-tion of the douche is one which each individual must answer for himself. If one is assisted by a nurse who has been well trained in antiseptic midwifery, I believe the habitual use of the douche will yield the best results, but if one has to trust to the ordinary midwife the douche is dangerous. Between the two evils—*i. e.*, neglect of the douche and the danger of letting an ignorant nurse give it—I would unhesitatingly choose the lesser and let the douche go. As was said by Stadfeld, of Copenhagen, at the Berlin Congress, we shall probably have to wait until the present generation of nurses passes away before we have such midwives as we desire. As expressing my ideas as to the proper conduct of a labor so far as antisepsis are concerned, I will mention the method pursued at the Free Lying-in Hospital. The following rules for personal disinfection are rigidly carried out under the direct supervision of the resident physician, and apply equally to all persons who approach the case :

1. Remove coat and roll up shirt sleeves above the elbow; pare and clean nails, scrub arms, wrists and hands with nail brush, soap and warm water.

2. Put on disinfected gown.

3. Rinse hands and wrists in alcohol.

4. Immerse hands and wrists in a 1 to 1000 bichloride of mercury solution for at least three minutes.

5. The hands are not to be dried on a towel, but may be wiped on front of gown.

6. Students who are engaged in dissecting, or who have witnessed a postmortem examination, or attended a case of infectious disease within a week, must not enter the lying-in hospital.

The woman is given a full bath and enema and the external genitals are disinfected with the 1 to 1000 sublimate solution. The douche of 1 to 4000 is used before and after labor in normal cases, and in delayed and operative cases repeated several times. Intra-uterine douches are only given in cases where the uterus has been exposed to infection, and then by the doctor.

Under these rules our results have been satisfactory, but not brilliant. Our house is not well adapted to the purposes of a hospital. We are much crowded at times, and not supplied with the advantages of well appointed maternities. Nevertheless, in 94 cases delivered since this time last year, in 51 the temperature did not exceed 100°, of the 43 above 100°, in 13 the rise was for one day only; in 17 the rise was between 100 and 101; in 12 cases only did it go above 101, and of these one died—a miscarriage case, who was brought into the house with a temperature of 104.8, and a pulse of 140. It was probably a criminal case. There was 1 case of grippe, 2 of malaria. In one case milk-leg developed on the 13th day, the temperature not having previously gone above 100. There was one case of salpingitis, the only definite septic case, except the fatal case, unless the milk-leg be counted. The other elevations of temperature were slight and transient, and largely associated with congested breasts in cases where the babies were sent away. We have had no case of breast abscess. This question of antisepsis is too big a one to be discussed in a single paper, and I must be satisfied to leave it where it is for the present, that is, as applied only to the delivery and the preparation for the same. The important matters of treatment during the puerperium, treatment of puerperal fevers, training of nurses with special tendency to antiseptic doctrines, the use of external rather than internal examinations, the prophylaxis in regard to the infants' eyes, mercurial poisoning and breast inflammation, must be left to a future occasion. I regret that I must leave the subject without a fuller consideration of these important matters, but I have already made an excessive draft on your patience, and must defer them to another time. For the present I think the following conclusions justifiable :

1. Antiseptic midwifery, by reducing septic mortality in lying-in hospitals from 10.19 per cent. to less than .50 per cent., has saved myriads of lives and made the clinical teaching of obstetrics safe and humane.

2. The neglect of antisepsis by the general practitioner makes his obstetric results, obtained under the most favorable circumstances, worse than those obtained in lying-in hospitals.

3. Antiseptic prophylaxis consists, to a large extent, in cleanliness, but is made more efficient by the use of chemical disinfectants, especially corrosive sublimate, used in a judicious and conservative manner.

4. The vaginal douche is requisite in operative and pathological cases, and desirable in all, where it can be properly administered, but had better be omitted in normal cases not under the care of a well trained nurse.

DISCUSSION.

Dr. Geo. H. Rohé—I heartily endorse the conclusions of Dr. Michael. The results brought to my attention in an official capacity and many of the results of private practice, confirm me in the belief that hospital practice is less fatal than private practice. I am sorry Dr. Michael discussed the question of auto-infection. Just as soon as this question is brought forward, it sets someone to thinking. I may cause some comment in what I am about to say, but I do believe that the thinking obstetrician is a dangerous obstetrician. When antisepsis is properly carried out I do not think it makes any difference how often the case is examined, but when a man thoroughly disinfects his hands and makes an examination, and has to wait for an hour or so, he sits about and puts his hands in his pockets, and after while he makes an examination after simply anointing his hands, he then makes an examination with infected hands. To be thoroughly antiseptic, he should prepare his hands in the same way every time he makes an examination. As to the preliminary vaginal douching, I think it of much importance, and I think in the Maryland Maternité, the only cases of sepsis we had were where the case came in too late for the preliminary vaginal douching to be carried out. I also deem the care of the infants' eyes important. I believe that if these antiseptic and aseptic precautions were more frequently used in private practice there would be as great an advance in the reduction of the percentage of mortality as there has been in hospital practice in the past few years.

Dr. J. M. Craighill said one point in Dr. Michael's paper that has not been noted, and that is, should a doctor attend an obstetrical case when he has a case of the milder infectious diseases on hand—scarlet fever, for instance. This is an important question, especially to the young doctor. I must confess if I were to have a case of puerperal fever develop while I was attending a case of scarlatina, I should feel as though I was the cause of the infection.

Dr. J. D. Blake said I cannot see for the life of me why we should use an ante-labor vaginal douche except in cases where there is a condition of the vagina that may infect the eyes. In a natural, healthy case nature, as Dr. Michael says, always provides for a clean canal by washing the channel by the bursting of the water. In addition to this, the secretion forced out in the canal for lubricating purposes is recognized to have some antiseptic properties. Now, by giving a bichloride of mercury douche, the bichloride coagulates the albumen of the secretion and adds to the difficulty a body has to encounter in traversing the canal by destroying the lubricating properties of this secretion. When we examine the records between hospital and private practice Dr. Michael says that an attendant is not allowed to enter the house within a given time after being in contact with any septic material, of course, where you can control all the actions, you ought to have a good record, but in private practice, you do not always have the selection of the nurse, nor can you quarantine your patient from the visits, free advice and misdirected efforts of her friends.

Dr. J. G. Wiltshire said he had always used the antiseptic and aseptic precautions, and had the usual good results, but one of the professors at the Hopkins announces that after he had scrubbed his fingers with a nail brush for ten minutes, he found the pus germs by cultivation, etc.; that the bichloride of mercury encapsulates the germ, and when brought under favorable condition it can be cultivated. They now prefer to disinfect their hands with a solution of permanganate of potash; the discoloration it makes can be removed by oxalic acid.

Dr. A. Friedenwald said one source of infection in child birth seems not to have been touched upon and that is the bowels. Sometimes the patient will have a passage and soil the linen and time is not allowed to clean the source of infection before the obstetrician is engrossed in the delivery of the child. Particular attention should be paid to the condition of the patient's bowels, and then avoid this possible source of infection.

Dr. Bond said my experience shows that it takes a great deal of septic dirt to kill a woman. If, in private practice, I even get my patient washed I think I am doing well. If I ever get the nurse to wash her hands, I am fortunate, and if I can get the nurse to wash her hands with a bichloride solution I am perfectly happy. I think that healthy tissue can throw off a great deal of bacteria. In a case where a woman was delivered by a clean doctor, a clean nurse, that

I know to have been clean, in four or five days there was a rise of temperature. Now, what was the source of infection there?

Dr. W. S. Gardner said the only case in which there was trouble that I was connected with was when the preliminary douche was neglected, when labor came on immediately after the patient came into the hospital. Another point is the cleanliness of the external genitals. This is a region that is difficult to keep clean, and if we get reasonable cleanliness there it can only be by considerable effort. As to the intra-uterine douche *after* labor, I think it is of no use, but may be a positive harm unless there is some special indication for it; for by it we may introduce septic material, as there is a possibility that everything which is introduced into the uterus at this time may become the vehicle of contagion.

Dr. Michael said, as to the necessity of the ante-partum douche, if the choice lay in giving it by an ignorant nurse, and letting it alone, I would leave it alone. What was said about having trained nurses in private practice is perfectly true. Now, any old woman who fails in everything else goes to nursing women in childbirth, where two lives are involved. Now, if it came to giving a douche by such a nurse and leaving it alone, I would leave it alone. Nothing can be clearer than the fact that women do not die in the hospitals now, as some say, "people are born here but never die here." The point that Dr. Friedenwald makes is of interest. There is probably no one point that gives rise to more discussion than the matter of attention to the bowels, and when this precaution is neglected a fruitful source of infection is left open. This point was touched upon in my paper. As to pus germs being found under the nails after washing and disinfecting the hands as thoroughly as possible, this has been known for some time. A streptococcus that will not be brushed off with a nail brush will not be apt to drop off in a vagina that is being examined. One staphylococcus will not kill a woman. Dr. Bond says it takes a great deal to kill a woman. This we all know. Sometimes a dirty woman will get well in spite of the dirt, and these are accidental cases.

MILK FEVER.

By William S. Gardner, M. D.

For about twenty-four hours after delivery the breasts of the puerperal woman remain apparently in about the same condition that they were before labor. At the end of this period the blood flow to them is increased, the secretion which had been present for a large portion of the period of gestation flows more freely, and at the end of forty-eight hours from delivery the milk flow is established. It is commonly stated that the milk comes in on the third day, but this apparent error is due to the custom of counting the day of delivery as the first day of the puerperal period. I have investigated this point and find that it is rare in normal cases for the flow to be delayed more than a very few hours beyond the normal average of forty-eight.

The older authors attributed almost every disorder of the puerperal period to some perversion of the milk flow. If a woman had phegneasia alba dolens it was due to a metastasis of the milk to the leg; if she had a peritonitis the coagulated caesin was found on the intestines ; if she had any disorder it was always due to the milk, which, by metastasis was charged with affecting first one organ and then another until everything from the vertex to the great toe was included. Happily the light of scientific investigation has revealed at least partially the true causes of a considerable number of the diseases formerly attributed to a determination of the milk to parts beyond the region the mammary gland, and in this way relieved the much maligned milk from many unjust charges. But even at the present time it is asserted that the milk secretion, especially at the beginning, causes an increase of the pulse rate and a rise of temperature of one or two degrees. It is a common thing to hear it spoken of, and our text books still cling to the statement.

Lusk says: "A temperature of 100.5° belongs within physiological limits. Schroder attributes the increased heat production to the combustion of organic substances which attends the involution of the uterus. To this are to be added, as provoking causes, the reaction of small wounds in the course of the genital canal, *and disturbances attendant upon lactation.*"

Playfair says: " For a few days there is often a slight increase of temperature, especially toward evening, which is probably caused by the rapid oxidation of tissue in connection with the involution of the uterus. In about forty-eight hours there is a rise of temperature connected with the establishment of lactation amounting to one or two degrees over the normal level, but this again subsides as soon as the milk is freely secreted."

Latterly through the medical journals these statements have been denied, but little or no evidence has been produced to substantiate the denials. Since we attach so much importance to the condition of the pulse and temperature during the puerperal period it is highly important that we should be familiar with the normal pulse and temperature for that time. To learn this it is necessary to study the temperature and pulse of the whole lying-in period, and especially that portion of the period in which is beginning lactation. Some three years ago, when revising the record blanks for use at the Maternité I inserted spaces for noting the time at which the milk flow began, a special record of the temperature and pulse, taken at the time which was nearest this beginning flow, and also for the temperature and pulse at the observation just twenty-four hours previous to the flow.

To get at the average pulse and temperature for the whole lying-in period I have taken fifty normal cases, and averaged them with the following results :

DAY.	MORNING.		EVENING.	
	Pulse.	Temp.	Pulse.	Temp.
	71	98.75	73.1	98.96
2	70.7	98.26	71.2	98.88
3	74	98.48	72.5	98.73
4	76.6	98.5	71.8	98.66
5	76.4	98.51	72	98.68
6	77.3	98.63	72	98.67
7	75.3	98.63	69.7	· 98.66
8	77.6	98.68	75.2	98.66
9	79.7	98.65		

In reviewing this table one of the most striking points is the fact that we do not find the marked depression in the pulse rate that is spoken of by almost all the text books. The lowest morning pulse is on the morning of the second day, and then it is almost 71. This certainly cannot be counted as being far from the normal. The highest morning pulse, nearly 80, is on the ninth day; and this slight acceleration was, no doubt, partially caused by the anticipation of getting out of bed that day. The lowest evening pulse, nearly 70, is found on the seventh day; the highest 75, on the eighth. A glance at the chart will show that the pulse is almost invariably slower in the evening than in the morning of the same day. The only exception being the second day and then the evening pulse averages only one-half a beat more than the morning pulse.

From the statements that have been made in regard to the effect of beginning lactation upon the pulse we would expect to find an acceleration of the pulse on the third day, but the table shows that there is no such acceleration either morning or evening.

It is well known that the pulse is increased in frequency during labor, and I am inclined to think that the fallacy upon which the statement is based that a slow pulse is usually found during the puerperal period is due to the fact, that after labor the pulse does decrease in frequency; but this decrease is from a rate much above the normal down to or about the normal rate, and not a decrease from the normal rate to below the normal.

If 75 pulse beats per minute be considered normal for women, the table shows that on the average during the uncomplicated puerperal period there is no marked variation of the
pulse from the standard of perfect health.

In reviewing the temperatures of this table it is seen that
none of the morning temperatures, after the first day, was
more than 0.15° above normal.   The highest average morning temperature being that of the ninth day ; the lowest that
of the morning of the second day.   The highest temperature
of the table is that for the evening of the first day.   But
twenty-one of the fifty patients were confined less than ten
hours before the observations were made,—a time too short
for the elevation of temperature caused by the labor to subside, and at a time of the day when temperatures fall with
least readiness.

After the rise of temperature, caused by the labor, has
passed off there is, as a rule, a slight daily fluctuation ; the
evening temperature being usually slightly higher than the
morning temperature.   But when the puerperal period is uncomplicated these fluctuations should not be greater than that
of the usual temperature variations in health.   When the
temperature exceeds this limit, even for a short time, some
local exciting cause should be looked for and can generally
be found.   It will be noticed that the temperature for the
evening of the third day is lower than that of the second day,
and is less than one-quarter of one degree above 98.5°.

To get as accurately as possible what the pulse and
temperature are just when lactation begins, and to show
whether there is any rise of either or both with the beginning
milk flow, I have taken the observations of the pulse and
temperature of one hundred cases recorded at the nearest
practicable time to the beginning milk flow, and also the observations recorded for the time just twenty-four hours previously and averaged them.

Fifty of these cases were taken from the records of the year
just ended, and fifty from the records of the previous year.
The cases were taken as nearly consecutively as possible; the
cases dropped being those which presented evidence of some

influence not in the breasts that affected the pulse and temperature. A large portion, but not all of these observations correspond to the observations for the evenings of the second and third day after labor.

The average pulse and temperature for these one hundred cases for the period just twenty-four hours before the milk flow was: pulse 73.7, temperature 98.91° ; for the time corresponding to the beginning milk flow the pulse was 74.6, the temperature 98.79°.

These averages show that while the pulse is increased a fraction of one beat per minute the temperature is actually on an average one-eighth of a degree less on the day the milk comes in than it is on the previous day ; and that the temperatures correspond very nearly with the temperatures for the evenings of the second and third days ; and that the flow of milk does not interfere with the gradual reduction of the average evening temperature from the first day when it is highest to the fourth day when it is as low as it ever goes.

The conclusions to be drawn from more than two thousand recorded observations of pulse and temperature during the normal puerperal period may be stated in a very few words :

1st. The average pulse for the whole normal puerperal period does not vary more than a few beats from 75 per minute.

2nd. The average temperature for the whole normal puerperal period does not vary at any time as much as one-half of one degree from 98.5°.

3rd. The beginning of lactation does not influence to an appreciable extent, either the pulse or the temperature.

DISCUSSION.

Dr. J. W. Williams congratulated Dr. Gardner on the able way he has presented the subject. His own experience was about the same. The normal puerperium is feverless and the results of Dr. Gardner do away with this milk fever theory. These statistics are of great value. Milk fever should be a thing of the past. In the German hospital reports, milk fever is never mentioned, and all above 99° are regarded as septic processes.

Dr. J. E. Michael was also of the same opinion. He thought the records very valuable, but thought the observations of the pulse if taken in another way would show different results. Dr. Gardner took them at 9 A. M. and 7 P. M. If a case were delivered at 10 A. M., for example, the pulse would not be taken until 7 P. M. The pulse should also be taken the first hour after delivery.

Dr. Gardner said the point he wished to prove was that while books say the pulse goes down and stays down below normal for three or four days after delivery, it was not so at all. It might do so exceptionally, but the exceptional case proves nothing. He always takes the pulse after delivery.

Report of the Section on Anatomy, Physiology and Pathology.

RECENT DISCOVERIES IN THE PHYSIOLOGY OF GANGLION CELLS.

By H. Newell Martin, M. A., M. D., D. Sc., F. R. S., *Chairman.*

It has been the custom for the chairman of the section which I have the honor to represent to-day to search recent physiological literature for some topic which may be of special interest to medical men. The literature of physiology is now so voluminous, and one has to seek it in so many journals, that even the physiologist himself cannot keep abreast of it, much less the busy practitioner. On making such a search it occurred to me that some work done during the last three years on the structure of ganglion cells and the changes undergone by ganglion cells when they were irritated would have interest for you, especially as it seems to open up quite new branches of research in the pathology of the nervous system.

Thanks to the work of Heidenhain and Langley, we have known for several years that the cells of a gland at work differ in their microscopic appearance, and differ in their staining qualities, from the cells of a gland at rest ; and it occurred to Mr. Hodge—then at the Johns Hopkins, now at the Clark University—it occurred to him to see if he could not discover whether histological changes take place in ganglion cells when they are stimulated.

I may use a moment in recalling to your memory the structure of the typical spinal ganglion cell, the cell marked A in the diagram. There you see the capsule, with its many nuclei, surrounding the cell, generally supposed not to be nervous but of connective tissue nature. Within the capsule we have the general granular cell substance, containing in the typical cell a rounded well defined nucleus, sharply marked off from the general protoplasm of the cell and with a single nucleolus in it. When prepared as this specimen was, by the aid of osmic acid, the nucleus shows a few darkly stained points around the nucleolus, but most of it remains clear and unstained and is a conspicuous whitish object in the general darkly stained mass of the osmic acid specimen.

It will hardly be necessary for me to go into details as to Dr. Hodge's earlier work, because, like most work of the kind, one has to begin tentatively and find out the best methods and the way to get the best results. In general I may say that his hardening was done by alcohol, and his subsequent staining either by osmic acid or by what is known as the Gaule method, which those of you who are histologists will remember. His work does not constitute the first set of observations made on histological changes produced in ganglion cells by various conditions. Some researches had been made on nerve cells at rest compared with ganglion cells in pathological conditions, with the result that the most marked changes in the cell were found in the nucleus; and some ten or eleven months after Dr. Hodge published his preliminary communication in the American Journal of Psychology, there appeared a paper in which observations were made by stimulating one sciatic nerve in a frog while leaving the other at rest, and subsequently comparing sections of the two sides of the spinal cord to see if the cells differed in appearance; it was found that the nuclei of the cells on the two sides were a little different in their relation to staining fluids. It had also been noticed that in starved animals the nuclei of the nerve cells seemed shrunken and the protoplasm less dense, more or vacuolated than normal; but Dr. Hodge was the pioneer in the discovery that stimulation of normal ganglion cells caused changes in them, which could be recognized with the aid of the microscope.

His work has been continued at Clark University with the greatest care. In order to get comparative results it was necessary to know the strength of the electrical stimulation, (that he used electrical stimulation I need hardly say). That was done by aid of galvanometer and rheochord, and every device was used to keep the strength of the stimulating current uniform. Then apparatus was devised to secure that the number of stimulations given in a second to the nerve was always the same : so each animal so far as one can assume that one young cat is like another young cat was brought under practically the same conditions.

His first idea was to etherize or curarize the animal in order to keep it quiet ; but observations on animals who had been given curare or ether showed that those drugs brought about changes in the nerve cells apart from all extrinsic nerve stimulation ; so it was necessary to eliminate their use. That was done by a method devised by Ludwig some years ago, in which a small hole is trephined in the skull of the animal, then a thin blunt glass rod introduced and passed through the brain until it reaches the crura cerebri. Both crura are destroyed by moving the rod to and fro, and thus all motor and sensory paths from the cerebral hemispheres to the lower parts of the body are cut off. After the operation the animal immediately goes into a state of apparently sound quiet sleep, and under those conditions it is experimented upon. Dr. Hodge used kittens, and each animal was carefully packed in cotton batting after destruction of the crura and its temperature observed from time to time and kept as constant as possible. So far as I can see every precaution to ensure reliable results was taken.

Next, the brachial plexus was exposed on the right side of the body and placed between electrodes and, by clockwork during the continuance of the excitation, the nerve was stimulated for fifteen seconds out of every minute, and rested the remaining forty-five ; and so on, minute after minute ; thus in five hours stimulation the nerve would have had on the whole an hour and fifteen minutes of stimulation, and during the remainder of the time would have been at rest. The lower part of the nerves going from the brachial plexus to the muscles of the forelimb was not divided, and the test that the sensory fibres were probably active was that the muscles always moved when the stimulus was applied. Since the muscles responded to the stimulus, showing the motor fibres were irritable, it was assumed that the sensory fibres going to the spinal ganglion were also irritable.

Working in this way Dr. Hodge found on staining the ganglion cells remarkable changes; those changes are of three kinds, and come on in different order. In the first place, the nucleus of the stimulated cell loses its well defined contour, and takes more of the appearance of the nucleus of the figure marked B in the diagram. In the second place, the body of the cell loses its general dark granular appearance and becomes vacuolated, filled apparently with little spaces containing liquid, instead of the ordinary granules which normally fill the interstices of the meshwork of fibrils which constitute the essential part of a ganglion cell. Third, and most remarkable, though Dr. Hodge only refers to it and does not attempt to explain it, the nuclei of the capsule which surrounds the ganglion cell and are not part of it at all, undergo changes. They shrink and become spherical rather than oval. It may be that the waste products secreted by the stimulated nerve cell affect these nuclei of its capsule.

Dr. Hodge takes up next the question whether these changes are physiological and not pathological; whether they are due to this gross method of electrical stimulation; which must be more crude than the normal afferent nerve impulse: if normal, the changes ought to be progressive with increase of the time of stimulation. This he tested by having the nuclei measured by persons who did not know what had been done to the cells, who did not know anything about the object of the research, but simply sat down to measure nuclei in their diameter: the concurrent testimony of these observers shows that the diminution of the diameter of the nuclei increases as the time of stimulation increases. If you stimulate one hour you will get perhaps an average diminution in volume of the nuclei as calculated from their diameters of about fifteen per cent. If you stimulate two hours, the diminution is not much more marked. If you stimulate four hours, the average diminution in volume of the nuclei of the stimulated side is thirty-five per cent., and after prolonged stimulation of eight hours, sometimes the diminution in volume was as much as sixty per cent.

One point that is important I omitted to mention in its proper place. As soon as the stimulation is finished the kitten is killed as quickly as possible, the eighth cervical ganglion on each side excised and the two put together in the same hardening fluid, they are fixed together on the same slide, stained in the same vessel, mounted side by side in the same paraffine, and cut with the same stroke of the knife, so that as far as any action of any reagent on the ganglion of the right side which had been stimulated, and on the ganglion of the left side which was left at rest, there is no possibility of the reagents producing any of the differences observed.

Next came the thought, if this change in the ganglion cells be really a result of their physiological activity, if they lose matter and alter their structure during functional activity, then they ought to recover with rest, and the recovery ought to be proportionate to the time of rest; and in a paper which has just appeared in the last number of the Journal of Psychology Dr. Hodge discusses that question.

Taking a number of kittens, from six to eight weeks old, they were well fed and then experimented upon; after experiment they were given no food until they were killed. Each animal was used for five hours, each minute of each hour indicating fifteen seconds of stimulation and forty-five seconds of rest. Then one kitten was killed at once, another was kept an hour before it was killed, a third two hours, and so on. The general result was this: In the kitten killed immediately, there was very great histological difference between the ganglion of the stimulated and un-stimulated side. In the kitten killed an hour later the difference was less, the nucleus had begun to enlarge again, and did not stain quite so deeply with osmic acid; and so it went on hour after hour, but even at the end of eighteen hours the nucleus on the stimulated side was smaller than the nucleus on the rested side. At the end of twenty-four hours, however, most of the nuclei of the right ganglion (the stimulated one), had returned to the histological condition of the normal resting ganglion cell.

I have received within the last few days a note from Dr. Hodge, in which he says he is now applying this method to the normal alternations of rest and work in animal life. He first tried it with kittens and cats, but it is very difficult to get animals of that kind to sleep any definite nnmber of hours. It occurred to him that birds had more regular habits as to sleeping and waking hours than any other animals. He tells me, though not ready for detailed publication, that he finds very distinctly in English sparrows the same difference in ganglion cells at the end of a day, as compared with the ganglion cells of a sparrow killed early in the morning, that he finds between the rested and stimulated ganglion cells in the kitten.

It seems to me that this method of research which proves that one can discover by histological methods what special nerve centre has been active, combined with the recent discovery of Langley that we can by local application of nicotine throw certain ganglia out of functional activity for a time, puts us on a whole new course of investigation, or two new courses of investigation in regard to the physiology and pathology of the nervous system. Ultimately I think these methods will come to be used largely in the localization of nerve function instead of the more gross surgical methods we have now at our disposal. With this future prospect it seemed to me that it might interest you to hear about them : and that is my excuse for intruding upon your time to-day.

ON THE EFFECTS OF CERTAIN DRUGS ON THE VELOCITY OF THE BLOOD-CURRENT.*

By John C. Hemmeter, M. D., Phil. D.

The velocity of the blood-current in an artery is determined by the ratio of the quantity of blood that flows through it in a given time to the sectional area. In other words, the figures representing the volume of blood that passes through an artery in a given time, say in one second, divided by the figures designating the sectional area of that artery, will give as the quotient the mean velocities of the current in the various areas of the arterial system. As these sectional areas differ in various vessels, and in various parts of the same vessel, so must the velocity differ. The velocities are in fact inversely proportional to the sectional area.

As the total sectional area of the arterial system continually increases from the heart toward the periphery, the velocity of the current naturally decreases from the heart toward the periphery.

The velocity and the tension of the blood current at beginning of the arterial system is dependent upon two factors : 1, The energy of the activity of the heart; 2, and the sum total of the resistances of the vascular paths. Both of these factors —the energy of the heart activity and the sum of peripheral resistances—are variable.

The heart's action continually varies in the normal animal in the rate of its rhythm, the force of contraction, the tonicity, and probably conduction, and the sum of the peripheral resistances varies mainly through vaso-motor influences exerted upon the small arteries. To gain a better conception of the influences that govern the rate of the current it is most expedient to consider the possible variations to which these two main factors of heart activity and peripheral resistance are subject.

*Experiments made in the Biological Laboratory of the Johns Hopkins University.

I.   The energy of the heart contractions remains the same
and the resistance (*a*) increases, then blood-pressure increases and velocity decreases.   (*b*) Resistance decreases,
then blood pressure decreases and the velocity increases.

II.   The energy of the heart activity increases and (*a*) the
resistances are the same, then blood-pressure and velocity increase.   (*b*) The resistances increase, then blood-pressure
increases and velocity remains the same.   (*c*) The resistances
diminish, then blood-pressure remains the same and velocity
increases.

III.   The energy of the heart activity decreases and at the
same time (*a*) the resistances are the same, then blood pressure and velocity are reduced.   (*b*) The resistances are correspondingly greater, then blood-pressure remains the same
and velocity decreases.   (*c*) The resistances are correspondingly smaller, then blood-pressure sinks and velocity is the
same.

There is no constant relation between the sizes and volumes
of the various branches that develop from the aorta.   Experience has shown that variations of resistance occur in
circumscribed areas of the peripheral arterial system, while
heart-action and blood-pressure remain unaltered.   This is
possible only if the restriction of the discharge, *i. e.*, the
diminution of the current volume in one branch, is counter-
balanced by compensatory increase in the current volume in
other branches ; therefore the velocity in different arteries
varies at the same time in an alternating equalizing manner ;
from this it follows that in investigations of the velocity of
the current in one and the same vessel one finds great variations in the velocity in consecutive periods of time which
bear no constant relation at all to frequency of the pulse or
to blood-pressure.

To form an approximately correct idea of the rate of the
current in any artery one cannot judge from one measurement taken in one single period of time, nor even from two
or three such measurements.   From experience one learns
that the mean of the results of at least six measurements
must be calculated, taken in six consecutive periods of time.

In the experiments to be detailed the results are based upon the average of six measurements taken once every two minutes. There are, of course, measurements taken oftener than once in two minutes, but they are for brevity's sake excluded, and only the measurement at the end of every second minute taken, during twelve consecutive minutes, to make up the average.

We have studied the effect of ergot, digitalis, and alcohol on the rate of the blood-current in the carotid artery. The animals used were dogs and cats. The drugs were allowed to run into the jugular vein, diluted with defibrinated blood from another animal of the same kind. For this purpose, and also to be able accurately to determine the amount which entered the circulation, a cannula in the jugular vein was connected with a eudiometer. In case of ergot we employed a solution of the officinal fluid extract, 1 c.c. to 9 c.c. of defibrinated blood, and also a solution of ergotole (S. & D.), 1 c.c. to 29 c.c. of defibrinated blood. In case of digitalis a ten per cent. solution of the tincture and a twenty-five per cent. solution of the infusion, in defibrinated blood, were made use of. A solution of digitalin was also experimented with, in form of a solution in defibrinated blood, .005 gm. digitalin to 100 c.c. blood. In case of alcohol, solutions of varying strengths of Squibb's absolute ethylic alcohol in defibrinated blood were used. Defibrinated blood injected into the jugular vein as such had no appreciable effect on the rate of the current in the carotid, as far as could be determined by the instrument which was used for that purpose, and which will presently be described. The drugs were in every case mixed with 50 c.c. of normal salt solution, and this again added to 50 c.c. of defibrinated blood.

A number of instruments have been devised to measure the velocity of the arterial current—Volkmann's hæmodromometer, Vierordt's hæmotachometer, Chauveau's hæmodrometer, and the hæmodromographs of Lortet and Marey— all have been shown to possess objections. The best instrument which has thus far been invented for this purpose is the so-called stromuhr of Ludwig (stromuhr, current-clock);

even this instrument has not entirely surmounted the difficulties, still it is the most accurate we have.

The stromuhr consists of two ovoidal glass cylinders or globes, the capacity of which is accurately known and is equal in both. These two globes are continued upward in a tubular manner, and connect with each other by a U-shaped curvature. On the convex side of this curve there is a short exit tube which can be hermetically closed. The lower ends of the globes are held in two metal tubes (*m*, *m*,) the other ends of which communicate with two cannulæ, *h* and *k*, that are inserted in the ends of a divided artery. The course of these tubes is at one place interrupted by two metalic disks, which are accurately fitted upon each other. The two upper ends of the tubes coming from the ovoidal globes are fitted into the upper disk so that its perforation exactly strikes the lumen of the lower tubes in the lower disk. The part of the instrument resting upon the upper disk can be rotated in a

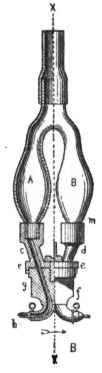

circle of 180°. By this rotation the globes of the current-clock can be alternately brought into communication with the two cannulæ.

In the experiment the globe nearest the cardiac end of the artery is filled with pure olive oil (this oil should be previously shaken with distilled water to free it from all oleic acid and mucin), while the globe nearest the distal end is filled with defibrinated blood. The globes each will hold 5 c.c. When a measurement is taken the blood enters from the artery into the first globe, displacing the oil, which is pushed over into the second globe, while the defibrinated blood is forced into the peripheral part of the artery.

As soon as all of the oil is forced from globe A to B, by the inrushing blood, the stromuhr is turned through 180°, by which the oil is again placed nearest to the cardiac end of the artery. In every new rotation after this the oil is displaced by blood, the blood in the second globe by oil, the main point of observation being to note the exact time it takes for the blood to displace 5 c.c. of oil. The velocity is measured by the ratio of the quantity to the sectional area.

Suppose the sectional area of a dog's carotid to be 3 1-5 mm., and the oil had been displaced ten times in 100 seconds, the space occupied ten times by the blood in replacing the oil being 10 + 5 ; hence 50 c.c. of blood have been delivered in 100 seconds, then

$$\frac{50.00 \text{ quantity,}}{3.2 \text{ sect. area,}} = 150 \text{ mm. of blood per second, the}$$

velocity.

The following are tables giving the results of one of the experiments each, that were made with ethylic alcohol, digitalis, and ergot :

Experiment No. 1, with Ethylic Alcohol, Ten per cent. Solution —Diameter of Carotid Cannula, 1.61 Mm.

A. NORMALLY.

Volume of Stream in 1 Second in Cubic Centimetres.	Mean Velocity in 1 Second in Mm.
0.33	190
0.25	142
0.28	142
0.33	190
0.23	143
0.19	140

Average of six measurements under normal conditions .... 158.0 mm.

B. UNDER ETHYLIC ALCOHOL.

1.6	338
1.3	339
2.0	410
2.3	432
2.5	460
2.0	416

Average of six measurements under ethylic alcohol............................ ...... 399.1 mm.

Increase of rate of current under alcohol .... , ... 241.1

Experiment No. 2, with Digitalis—Diameter of Carotid Cannula 1.61 Mm.

A. UNDER NORMAL CONDITIONS.

Volume of Stream in 1 Second in Cubic Centimetres.	Mean Velocity in 1 Second in Mm.
0.33	188
0.22	125
0.28	161
0.33	188
0.25	141
0.33	188

Average of six measurements under normal conditions .... 165.16 mm.

B. UNDER DIGITALIS.

0.20	120
0.14	84
0.10	72
0.20	120
0.20	116
0.12	80

Average of six measurements under digitalis .... 98.60 mm.

Difference between rate of current normally and under digitalis................ ...... 66.56

Experiment No. 3, with Ergot—Diameter of Carotid Cannula, 1.61 Mm.

A. UNDER NORMAL CONDITIONS.

Volume of Stream in 1 Second in Cubic Centimetres.	Mean Velocity in 1 Second in Mm.
2.0	340
1.7	312
1.69	314
0.72	392
0.72	390
1.7	318

Average of six measurements under normal conditions.............................. .... 344.3 mm.

B. UNDER ERGOT.

1.0	198
1.7	206
1.3	210
0.6	204
0.6	114
1.6	200

Average of six measurements under er-
got. .... 188.6 mm.

Difference between rate of flow under
normal conditions and under ergot...... 155.7

In the experiment we have recorded concerning ergot it is clear that the rate of the flow was diminished by 155.7 mm. Under digitalis the stromuhr showed a reduction of the rate of the current of 66.56 mm. Under ethylic alcohol, however, the rate of the current was increased by 241 mm. per second. These main conclusions are supported by the remaining experiments (four with each drug) and the figures are based upon the averages of six measurements.

A number of experiments have been rejected because in one way or other they were failures. It will probably be a safe method to use the stromuhr in the current of the femoral instead of the carotid artery, because of the easier manipulation of the instrument in this region; in the neck, the trachea, jugular vein, and vagus add to complicate the operation.

The result of every experiment showing, with very slight variations, that ergot and digitalis reduce the rate of the current while alcohol increases it, the question raises, "Are there any facts known concerning the physiological action of these drugs which could explain these observations?"

It is established beyond a doubt that ergot diminishes the frequency and force of the systolic contractions and that it constricts the arterioles. For the literature bearing on this we will refer to the writer's recent contributions to the subject (J. C. Hemmeter, "An Experimental and Clinical Study of Ergot," *Medical News*, January 31, February 7, March 7, and March 14, 1891). As ergot, therefore, diminishes the energy of the heart activity, and at the same time increases peripheral resistance, its effects must be classified under heading No. III., section *b*, on page 287 these influence being sufficient to explain the power of ergot to reduce the velocity of the blood-current.

Concerning digitalis it may be stated that it has been determined by many observers that this drug (1) decreases the work of the normal heart (see Jörg, *Archives de Medecine*, 1 er. ser., i. xxvii., p. 107; also Saunders, "On Foxglove;" Hutchinson, quoted by Homolle and Quevenne, *Arch. de Physiol. de Therap.*, etc., No. 1, 1854; and H. H. Donaldson and Mactier Warfield, "Studies for the Biol. Laboratory," Johns Hopkins Univ., vol. ii., p. 335). (2) That it produces contraction of the arterioles (see Fothergill-Schmidt's *Jahrb.*, vol., cliv., 1872; also *British Medical Journal*, July and August, 1871; Gourvat, *Gazette Medical de Paris*, 1871; Brieseman-Schmidt's *Jahrbucher*, vol. cliii., p. 29; Boldt, Inaug. Dissert., Schmidt's *Jahrbucher*, March, 1872; Ackermann, *Deutsch. Archiv. f. klin. Med.*, vol. xi., p. 125; Donaldson and Stevens, *Medical News*, Phila., xli., p. 697).

For fuller references to literature on the effects of digitalis in reducing the work of the heart, and in constricting the arterioles and capillaries, we would direct attention to the work of Donaldson and Warfield, and Donaldson and Stevens, above quoted, also to the works on therapeutics of H. C. Wood, Lauder Brunton, Ringer, Köhler and Binz.

The physiological actions of ergot and digitalis in reducing the rate of the blood-current are very closely allied, and might be arranged in the same category before stated, namely, No. III., section *b*.

The cause of the increase of the rate of the blood-current observed under alcohol will have to be exclusively sought in its property to cause dilatation of the arterioles and capillaries, thus diminishing peripheral resistance to the bloodstream, for Professor H. N. Martin has shown that there is no increase in the rate of the heart-beat, and therefore, probably, no increase in the work done by the heart in the normal animal (H. Newell Martin and L. T. Stevens, "Studies for the Biological Laboratory," vol. ii., p. 477). Professor Martin has also shown that the work of the isolated mammalian heart is actually diminished under alcohol, the character of the heart-beat being so altered through swelling of the myocardium that the ventricular cavity is not obliterated at the end of the systole. These observations have been confirmed by the author. It must be remembered in the clinical application of alcohol that the action of this substance is different in the organism that is pathologically altered from what it is in the normal one. Thus it is most probable that in fevers and acute inflammatory diseases the pulse-rate is reduced by alcohol. It was formerly held by some investigators that this reduction of the pulse-rate in fevers, etc., under the use of wine, whiskey, etc., was possibly the effect of some of the other constituents of these liquids, not to the alcohol contained in them. The author, however, has convinced himself, in a case of typhoid fever, and also in one of pulmonary tuberculosis, that 20 c.c. of absolute alcohol in 80 c.c. of water, will, within twenty minutes, reduce the rate of the pulse, in case of the enteric fever, from 112 to 96, this reduction was noticed three times in the same case of typhoid fever. Under the same dose a fall from 128 to 98 was noted in this patient on another occasion. However, the opinions concerning the action of alcohol in the work done by the heart may vary concerning pathological conditions. The most reliable observations, those already quoted, seem to point conclusively to the fact that the work of the normal heart is not increased at any rate; if, therefore, the velocity of the blood-current is increased under alcohol, this can be due only to its diminishing peripheral resistance to the blood-stream by dilating arterioles and capillaries; that alcohol has this effect was shown by Parkes, Bouvier, Marvaud, Zimmermann, Richardson, and the author. For fuller references on the literature of this subject we would refer to the work of Professor H. N. Martin, already quoted, and that of the author (J. C. Hemmeter, "Recent Experiments on the Physiological Action of Ethylic Alcohol," "Transactions of the Medical and Chirurgical Faculty of Maryland," 1889, p.

229; also, J. C. Hemmeter, "On the Comparative Physio-logical Effects of Certain Members of the Ethylic Alcohol Series on the Isolated Mammalian Heart," "Studies from the Biological Laboratory, Johns Hopkins University," vol. iv., No. 5).

The therapeutic significance, if any, of the results obtained we are not prepared to discuss, but we may point out that ex-periment confirms clinical experience, in case of ergot and digitalis, as applied to hæmorrhage, for if the quantity of blood that flows through an artery in a given time is reduced by these agents, their application to processes of transuda-tion and hæmorrhage becomes rational. And again the dila-tation of the blood-vessels and the increased velocity of the blood-current under alcohol may explain in part many of its clinical applications, for every physician knows how effec-tively the freer and fuller current of blood through the nobler organs acts, as a resuscitating stimulus in many diseases.

VASO-MOTOR NERVES OF THE HEART.

By H. Newell Martin, M. D., M. A., D. Sc., F. R. S.

There has come about in physiology within the last ten years the use of two new words, *anabolic* and *katabolic*. The justification for the employment of these words is mainly to be found in recent experiments made on the heart which show that certain nerves tend to help the nourishment of the heart and are in the old sense of the word, true *trophic* nerves, while certain other nerves, when active, tend to exhaust the heart and to prevent or hinder its nutrition. Experiments first made on the heart by Gaskell have since been extended to muscles and to other organs, so that the physiology of to-day is largely a question of an anabolic and katabolic phenomena. Investigation of the extrinsic cardiac nerves, with their ganglia, shows that although stimulation of the pneumogastric slows the pulse, or strong excitation entirely stops the heart beat, yet on the whole the nerve is a help to the heart ; that if in an animal you take a feebly beating heart stimulation of the pneumogastric will, after a time, strengthen the heart. If you take the dying heart of a frog, in which the auricles are still beating, but the beat fails to pass over to the ventricle, by stimulating the pneumogastric you can often get the heart back to its normal rhythm. Often one gets the phenomenon that the auricle in a dying heart makes two beats for the ventricle's one, and finds that on stimulating the pneumogastric one gets the normal beat, one stroke of the auricle corresponding to one stroke of the ventricle ; we can therefore on experimental grounds assert that the pneumogastric is essentially a trophic nerve for the heart.

The same observer (Gaskell) had also shown some few years before that, mingled with the motor fibres of an ordinary motor nerve were vaso-dilator fibres, fibres which ·

dilated the arteries of the muscle at the same time that the muscle fibres contracted.   One can paralyze the motor fibres proper by curare, and then, on stimulating the nerve trunk, get the vascular dilatation without the muscular contraction ; but normally the two things go together.   Whenever a muscle contracts, be the impulse that excites the contraction voluntary or reflex, the contraction is accompanied by an impulse which acts upon the blood vessels of the muscle and for a time paralyzes their muscular coats, so that its arteries allow more blood to flow through the muscle.

It occurred to me that it would be interesting to investigate this question in connection with the nerves of the heart. We there find the vagus of which I have just spoken ; and in addition the accelerator nerves which, when excited, quicken the heart's beat, and may in a sense be called the motor nerves of the heart ; though, as is well known, the heart will continue to beat when all influences from outside nerves are cut off from it.

The vagus being the trophic nerve of the heart, it might be readily supposed *a priori* that it would be the nerve which contained the fibres for dilating the coronary arteries.   On the other hand we have the analogy of ordinary muscle where we know that the motor nerve branches which excite the organ to activity are those which contain the vaso-dilator nerves fibres.

At the beginning of this session I asked Mr. Lingle to study this problem with me, in the physiological laboratory of the Johns Hopkins University.   Our research is still far from complete, but we have, I think, reached some interesting results.   Our method has been to anæsthetize the animal, open the thorax, (of course starting artificial respiration) and then by opening the pericardium to expose the heart : we then selected some little artery on the surface of the ventricle for careful observation.   The best arteries are those that are in the etymological sense of the word capillaries, little arteries just as big as a hair, which one watches through a hand lens.   It is quite easy to observe them, but it is not easy always to observe their changes in diameter, but by selecting a little network on the surface of the myocardium and watching attentively, one can usually see any changes that occur in the diameter of its vessels.

We began by stimulating the pneumogastrics, and found that every time that the pneumogastrics were stimulated the arteries of the heart dilated; the heart became distinctly redder and the superficial arteries of the myocardium were very distinctly increased in diameter.   Then the query arose which led to the most interesting point in our work.

In order to watch accurately these changing blood vessels it was necessary to stop the artificial respiration, because the lungs moving up and down, kept heaving the heart up and down: It was hard enough to watch a given vessel during the beat of the heart itself; with the respiratory movements added it was practically impossible.   But the cessation of artificial respiration introduced a new factor ; and we therefore tried the effects of stopping the respiration without simultaneously stimulating any nerve.   Under these conditions we got *dilitation* of the conorary arteries, though dyopnœa causes constriction of the arteries in every other part of the body.

The diagram I exhibit is taken from a typical experiment. The top line is the chronograph line, each notch being a second.   The next is the respiration line.   Toward the far end of the diagram there are parts of two respiration curves. At the level of the first vertical line the respiration stopped, the stopcock having been turned which cut the lungs off from the pump, and towards the other end of the tracing respiration commenced again, as is indicated by the ñerves. The line C has one little notch in it.   That notch wàs worked by the observer with a little electric signal and indicated when he saw a change in the blood vessels of the heart.   The lowest line is a tracing of the blood pressure taken in the carotid artery, the beats being of course pulse beats.

The point I want to call attention to is this.   You see that for some time after the respiration is stopped there is no rise in the blood pressure and before there is any rise in the blood pressure the observer signals that he has seen a change in the diameter of the blood vessels.   That change was always an increase. Later on comes the dyspnœic rise of blood pressure and then, artificial respiration being used again, blood pressure returns to the normal.   .

In our first observations as to the diameter of the cardiac arteries during commencing asphyxia, we thought their dilatation might be due to the fact that there was a general rise of blood pressure, which rise mechanically distended the coronary arteries and their branches; but, as you see, the observer always signals before there is any rise of blood pressure in the carotid; therefore the phenomenon is a true vaso-dilator one.   The point of chief interest is that while in commencing suffocation the arteries of the body in general constrict, the arteries of the heart dilate.   The heart arteries dilate that the last remaining oxygen shall go to that fundamental vital organ. It is one of the most beautiful preservative mechanism that I know of in the whole physiological working of the body.

Report of the Section on Ophthalmology, Otology and Laryngology.

BLINDNESS IN THE UNITED STATES.

By Hiram Woods, M. D., *Chairman.*

Mr. President and Gentlemen of the Faculty:—The past year's work in ophthalmology has been, for the most part, along lines which so exclusively concern the specialist, and which touch at so few points the work of the general practitioner, that one finds some difficulty in choosing a subject which will be of both interest and profit to such an assembly as this. Moreover, the parts of this department of medicine which come under the notice of the general practitioner have been written upon so much that repetition is almost unavoidable. Research of late years pursued along one line, however, has revealed a condition of things which concerns not alone the eye specialist and the medical profession, but everyone who considers our national welfare. This is the alarming increase of blindness in the United States—an increase out of all proportion to the simultaneous growth of population. It is to a consideration of the causes of this increase and of the duty of the medical profession in the matter, that your attention is asked.

At the meeting of the American Ophthalmological Society at New London, Conn., in July, 1887, Dr. Lucien Howe,* of Buffalo, N. Y., presented a paper founded upon the following figures, taken from the U. S. census of 1870-80 :

Population of the United States in 1870, . 38,558,371.
Blind in the United States in 1870, . . . 20,320.
Population in 1880, ... 50,155,783.
Blind in 1880, ... 48,919.

*Transactions of the American Ophthalmological Society, 1887.

These figures show an increase for the decade 1870 to 1880 of 30.09 per cent. in the population, and 140.78 per cent. in the number of the blind. It was shown, also, from the same source, that the rate of blindness increased from North to South and decreased from East to West. Dr. Howe made careful inquiry into the methods of taking the census in 1870 and 1880. He found that substantially the same plan was pursued in both years. He obtained the returns for his own city, Buffalo, and found on investigation, that "that part of the report was quite as reliable as could be expected." He says that "there seems no escape from regarding them (*i. e.*, the census returns,) quite up to the average of relia- bility in showing that the blindness in this country has in- crèased more than four times as rapidly as the population." Among the significant facts brought out by Dr. Howe and by those taking part in the discussion of his paper, were the following : Blindness is greater, in proportion to the popu- lation, in the Eastern States ; that it is proportionately greater in these States, in the thickly populated, than in the rural districts ; that the crowding together of children in institu- tions seems to be a prolific cause ; that contagious eye dis- eases are often brought in by immigrants ; that the financial loss to the nation is immense, from the necessity of support- ing this great number of blind persons. To demonstrate this financial loss, Dr. Howe took the figures from the report of 1874 of the Perkins Institution and Massachusetts Asylum for the Blind, which give $2 per week, or $104 per year, for support, and $28 per year for clothing, as the minimum amounts required for each blind person. But, since these individuals are non-producers, there must be added to the cost of their maintenance what they would contribute to the national wealth were they able to work. Estimating the wages of the men at $1.20, and of the women at 40 cents for each working day, he finds that there was a loss in 1880 of $16,383,272, and at the same rate of increase from 1880 to 1887, as from 1870 to 1880, a loss of over $25,000,000 in 1887. If one estimates this loss on the basis of those reported in the census of 1880 as "totally blind" (22,717), and omits from this calculation the 56,202 "semi-blind," and "unknowns," the national loss even then was in 1880 nearly $8,000,000. It would be interesting to pursue the study of the economic side of this question still further, but the limits of this paper will not permit, and enough has been said to show its great and far-reaching importance. As the result of Dr. Howe's paper, the Ophthalmological Society appointed a committee to enquire into the correctness of these statistics, and to find the causes of this increase in the number of the blind. This committee, consisting of Drs. Howe, of Buffalo, Burnett, of Washington, and Andrews, of New York, reported to the Society at its meeting in July last.

The investigations were made in New York State. The census of 1880 had shown an increase in the blindness in this State between 1870 and 1880 of 125.7 per cent. with a simultaneous increase of population of 15.9 per cent. In other words, blindness had increased 8.2 times as rapidly as had the population. It will be remembered that in 1887 Dr. Howe expressed the opinion that blindness had increased certainly four times as much as had population from 1870 to 1880. The words of the committee's† report in regard to the census three years later are: "While the increase was decidedly exaggerated, still the proportion of these unfortunates is certainly greater than the increase of population warrants." The report, moreover, states that "a more recent examination of the statistics presented . . . . . three years ago confirms what was stated then." That is, I take it, that in the committee's opinion, blindness in New York State increased from '70 to '80, about four times as much as population. Before looking into the second part of the committee's report—the causes of blindness—it will be well to glance for a moment at the figures in our own State. The census of 1870 gives the population of Maryland as 780,894, and the number of blind as 427. In 1880 the population was 934,943, number of blind 946 ; an increase in the population of about 20 per cent., in the number of the blind of 121 per cent. What the figures of the last census will show cannot yet be told. I have, however, through the kindness of Mr. F. D. Morrison, Superintendent of the Maryland School for

†Transactions of the American Ophthalmological Society, 1890.

the Blind, obtained a list of the blind under the age of 21, in this State and the District of Columbia, according to the census of 1890. This list gives 357 blind under 21 in Maryland, 338 of them being in the "School Age," between 6 and 21. The census of 1880 gives 173 blind of the "School Age," in this State. So there is an apparent increase of 95 per cent. in the blind of ages from 4 to 21 for the decade of 1880 and 1890. A similar comparison of "School Age" blindness for the District of Columbia for 1880 and 1890 shows an increase from 13 to 75—177 per cent. The simultaneous increase in population has been in Maryland about 14 per cent., in the District of Columbia about 30 per cent. Mr. Morrison is not inclined to place a great deal of reliance upon these statistics. He says there are counted as blind some who have one good eye, others with sight, impaired indeed, but not enough so to force them to give up work requiring eyesight, while again some children are on the blind list who are going to the public schools—no doubt unwisely —and whose trouble is only excessive nearsightedness. There are good reasons for regarding such children as belonging to the class of physical delinquents, and many of them should be taken from the schools and taught in other ways than by eyesight; but this subject, though of great importance, can be only mentioned here.

Among the pupils at the blind school are several children with high degrees of myopia ahd choroidal atrophy. These children are being educated without doing close eye work and this will probably save what sight they have. The effort the authorities of the blind school are making to get hold of such children is worthy of the highest commendation.

Again, Mr. Morrison knows of several blind children who are not enumerated by the census, and I am personally aware of three or four others whose names do not appear on the list. The conclusion seems justifiable that if investigations were made in Maryland of the amount of blindness, from a medical standpoint, nearly the same results would be found as in New York: less than the census gives, but much greater than the increase of population justifies.

Returning now to the work of the committee of the Ophthalmological Society‡, we find that of the blind in the State of New York, the members of the committee were able to get at the exact condition of the eyes of 509 individuals of all ages. It is impossible to give in detail the various causes of blindness found by these investigators, and a few summary notes must suffice. 2.27 per cent. was congenital, 14.51 per cent. was caused by ophthalmia neonatorum, 7.78 per cent. was due to trachoma or granular lids, 12.51 per cent. come from primary or secondary corneal disease, and 8.21 per cent. from sympathetic ophthalmia. Omitting for our present purpose the 2.27 per cent. of congenital blindness, it is seen that 43.01 per cent. of the blindness in New York State came from four diseases, two of which, ophthalmia neonatorum, and sympathetic ophthalmia, are preventable by prophylaxis, and three, ophthalmia neonatorum, trachoma and corneal diseases, either altogether curable or capable of marked benefit if proper treatment be instituted soon after the diseases are established.

After reading the report from which I have so largely quoted, I asked Mr. Morrison to allow me to examine the pupils at the School for the Blind on North Avenue, and the School for Colored Blind, Deaf and Dumb on Saratoga Street. Mr. Morrison and his assistants gave me every possible facility for conducting the examinations, and I desire to express my thanks to him and them for their courtesy. At the white school I examined 74 pupils, and although many interesting things were noted, I shall confine myself to the four diseases mentioned in connection with the New York report. The ages of Mr. Morrison's pupils, (two, however, were teachers,) ranged from seven to twenty-eight. Only four were above twenty, and the large majority between eight and eighteen. Some gave the history of their cases clearly and could evidently be relied upon. The records of other cases were obtained from Mr. Morrison, while in others, sole reliance was put upon the objective appearance. The percentage of blindness caused by the diseases mentioned was: Ophthalmia

‡Transactions American Ophthalmological Society, 1890.

neonatorum 17.9, corneal diseases 4.5, sympathetic ophthalmia 6.7, trachoma 1.5. At the colored school no reliance whatever could be placed upon the histories obtained. Twenty cases were examined, two being men of 40 years of age, blind from nerve atrophy. The other eighteen were under twenty. One case of trachoma was found—a most unusual disease in the negro—two were blind from sympathetic ophthalmia, six from corneal diseases, and four from choroido-iritis. Syphilis and scrofula were evidently the potent agents in causing most of the blindness at this school. I found no case which, in the absence of a reliable history, I could attribute to ophthalmia neonatorum, although one child in all probability became blind in this way. If these cases be added to those from the white school, the percentages of the four diseases are very nearly the same as found in New York, except in the case of trachoma, which is much less, probably owing to the smaller number of foreign-born persons examined. If the white school alone be considered, we have more blind from ophthalmia neonatorum than in New York by four per cent., and considerably less sympathetic ophthalmia and corneal blindness.

It may be objected that the 509 cases in New York and the 94 in our own schools—603 in all—are not enough to justify any conclusions. They would not be if unsupported by outside evidence. This evidence is right at hand, however, in the statistics of Magnus,§ based upon the examination of 3,204 cases of blindness under twenty years of age, and of 2,528 cases of all ages observed by Schmidt-Rimpler, Hirschberg and others. One who feels sufficiently interested to go farther into the matter will find the tables in Noyes' Text Book valuable sources of information. Of the four diseases mentioned, these tables give the following percentages: Under 20 years, ophthalmia neonatorum 23.50, of all ages, 10.87 per cent.; corneal, under 20, .47 per cent., of all ages .35 per cent.; trachoma under 20, .47 per cent., all ages 9.49 per cent.; sympathetic ophthalmia 4.58 per cent., under 20, of all ages 4.5. The falling off in corneal diseases is most

‡Noyes' Text Book. Diseases of the Eye.

interesting and somewhat difficult to explain, but apart from this, the large numbers of these European investigators practically confirm what has been found in this country.

What, after all, is to be gained from a study of these tables, and why do they constitute an appropriate theme for a paper to be read before a body of physicians? In the remainder of this paper I hope to make this clear. In 1884, Dr. Samuel Theobald,| then chairman of the section to which I now have the honor to belong, presented to the Faculty an interesting paper upon "Preventable Blindness." Ophthalmia neonatorum, scrofulous ophthalmia, iritis, trachoma, sympathetic ophthalmia and glaucoma were carefully considered as causes of blindness, and the way pointed out to avoid this dire result. In this paper I wish to consider but one of these diseases, and to study it from a point of view different from Dr. Theobald's. This disease is ophthalmia neonatorum, or "babies' sore eyes:" the cause, according to Magnus, of 23.5 per cent. of blindness in Europe among persons under 20 years of age; of 10.87 per cent. of *all* the blindness; of 14.51 per cent. of the blindness in New York State, of the loss of sight in 817 out of 1,178 blind persons, (69 per cent.) according to Dumas' experience to 1879 (J. Lewis Smith, *Dis. of Children*, 7th edition,) and of 17.5 per cent. of the blindness in our Maryland schools; this, too, with the disease almost entirely preventable, and in certainly 98 cases out of 100 curable, if properly and promptly treated. Nor is it my purpose to go over the various methods of treating the disease or to urge promptness in beginning treatment. This has been done over and over again, and there is probably no one before me or who may hereafter read this paper, to whom the treatment of ophthalmia neonatorum would be more than a twice-told tale. The medical men who know nothing of the treatment of the disease are those who have never received instruction in ophthalmology, (or they have forgotten it,) and who do not read journals. It is pretty hard to reach them. The question before us is:

Why does ophthalmia neonatorum continue to cause so much blindness? The answer can be given in one word—ignor-

---

|Transactions Medical and Chirurgical Faculty of Maryland, 1884.

ance ; ignorance of its great dangers on the part of parents, ignorance on the part of midwives, and, too often, ignorance on the part of medical men. It is, I think, a proper work for our State Society—nay, its duty—to take some steps to enlighten parents, to compel midwives to give the babies under their care a chance, at least, for eye-sight, and to force, if possible, such medical men as will not voluntarily learn how to prevent and cure the disease, to do so anyway, or else to hand over the case to some one else. Oculists cannot prevent the greater part of the blindness from this disease, because they do not see the majority of cases soon enough. To an obstetrician, Credé, belongs the great credit of giving to us the means of prevention, and upon the obstetrician and general practitioner, with the aid of the health authorities, must rest the responsibility of stamping it out. I say "stamping out" advisedly, for I believe it can be done.

What Crede's method is, is generally known : The instillation into the conjunctival sac of the infant, immediately after washing, of one small drop of a two per cent. solution of nitrate of silver from a glass rod. There is usually slight reaction, such as reddening of lids and lachrymation. What the silver does is this : It (1) disinfects the conjunctival sac, and (2) destroys the outer layer of epithelium, thus getting at, so to speak, any micro-organisms which may have lodged in this structure. Objections have been made from time to time against the general use of a prophylactic measure on the grounds: 1. That its universal use is not justifiable, and, 2, that Credé's method is unnecessarily severe. The first objection is well presented by Dr. Rob't Tilley, of Chicago, in an interesting paper read before the Chicago Medical Society, and published in the *American Journal of Ophthalmology*, for February, 1891. He states that about one baby in every ten has ophthalmia, and he does not think that we are justified in "inflicting a punishment, however slight, on the infants of 90 or 95 women who are not affected with gonorrhœa in order to save the remaining ten or five, who may or may not have inflamed eyes." There is more or less force in this objection. I was told a few days ago by a friend who has a large experience in obstetrics, that he had never seen a case of *purulent* conjunctivitis in a new-baby in his private practice.   In such a class of patients as this gentleman has the good fortune to have, the disease is rarely seen, and prophylaxis may not be necessary unless there is a vaginal discharge.

The second objection is founded upon the pain which a two per cent. nitrate of silver solution (10 grs. to ʒi,) causes when used in the eye.   As Dr. Tilley says :   If one has ever used this solution in the eye, "he will not ask for its reapplication as a source of pleasure."   By some the strength of the solution has been reduced to 1, ½, ¼ per cent., while others have substituted corrosive solutions, boric acid in saturated solution, two per cent. carbolic acid solution, etc. Most of the authorities whom I have been able to consult, seem to think that, on the whole, Credé's method is the surest.   As Dr. Tilley says, Credé has arrived at the strength of his solution after a vast experience, and it is safest to stick to his directions.   The following table, taken from an article by Dr. Jacob M. Falk, of Buffalo, published in the *Buffalo Medical and Surgical Journal*, February, 1891, shows the superiority of carbolic acid over no prophylaxis, and of Crede's solution over carbolic acid.   The statistics are those of Königstein, of Vienna.

In 1,092 new-born, without treatment, there was 19.26 per cent. ophth. neonat.
" 1,541   "   use of 1 p. c. carb. ac.   "   7.42   "   "
" 1,250   "   "   2   "   nit. silver   "   5.44   "   "

The chief reason for making the solution as strong as 2 per cent. seems to be that a weaker solution will not always destroy the epithelium of the conjunctiva ; unless this is done, organisms may escape the antiseptic, and subsequently produce the disease.   The same objection holds against other agents than nitrate of silver.   Statistics might be easily lengthened out to show the good prophylaxis has accomplished.   It will suffice, however, to make two or three quotations from the tables of Dr. Falk's article, and to refer any one still skeptical to this article, Noyes' Text Book, or the chapter on ophthalmia neonati in the seventh edition of J. Lewis Smith's *Diseases of Children*.   From this table I quote :

Crede, before prophylaxis,	10.8 p. c. opthal. neonatorum in 2,897 children
" after using 5 p. c. nit.silver	0.2 " " " " 1,160 "
Felsenrich. before prophylaxis,	4.3 " " " " 1,887 "
" after using 2 p. c. nit. sil'r	1.9 " " " " 3,000 "
and a 2nd series of	1. " " " " 2,100 "
Bayer, before prophylaxis,	12.3 " " " " 1,106 "
" after using 2 p. c. silver,	00.0 " " " " 361 "

The foregoing can be claimed, I think, Mr. President, to prove that blindness is alarmingly on the increase, and that the cause of nearly one-fifth of it can be eradicated. The disease is rarely seen outside the circles of the poor. As far as our own city it concerned, the general use of Credé's method in our large lying-in hospitals has almost completely removed it from these institutions. The problem for our State Society to solve is how to protect the babies of the poor, outside of the hospitals—children born under the care of medical men who do not realize the dangers of infantile ophthalmia, or of midwives who may have never heard of it. The most important step in this direction will be instruction on the prophylaxis of ophthalmia neonatorum in the obstetrical lectures in our medical schools. In some of the medical colleges of the country instruction in eye diseases is only clinical; while even in those where didactic lectures are delivered, there is always a certain number of men who will tell you that they never expect to "practice on the eye," and will consequently pay little or no attention to lectures upon ophthalmology. During my own career I have met several such, and at the hospital I have seen blind babies who had been under the care of two or three of them when something could be done. Dr. Swan M. Burnett (*Medical Record*, February 22, 1890,) states that "in more than thirty standard works on obstetrics in English . . . . . . there were only four which considered the preventive measures of which we have spoken : Encyclopedia of Obstetrics and Gynæcology and the treatises of Barnes, Lusk and Cazeaux and Tarnier. In only six others, and they were mostly old works, was there any consideration given to the treatment of the disease when it had once been established." The works which Dr. Burnett mention are the most recent books on obstetrics and those which are, I believe, usually recommended to students. His statement, then, is rather encouraging than otherwise. I have looked through several standard English books upon diseases of children. In most of them nothing is said of the prophylaxis of ophthalmia neonatorum, and very little about its dangers or treatment. Three marked exceptions are Keating's Encyclopœdia, Edward's Therapeutics of Disease of Children, and the last (7th,) edition of Dr. J. Lewis Smith's book. In former editions of Smith there is nothing on prophylaxis, and, in my opinion, his treatment is not above criticism. Here again is evidence that our educators are working toward the prevention of the disease, and the fruits of their work will surely be seen during the next few years.

To teach the poor of the dangers of opthalmia is a task which presents many difficulties. Personal contact with medical men must be the main reliance, but other things can be done. The Eye Infirmary at Sheffield,¶ England, distributes among the poor by means of the poor physicians the following card :

IMPORTANT NOTICE : If a baby's eyes run with matter and look red a few days after birth, take it *at once* to a Doctor. *Delay is dangerous*, and one or both eyes may be destroyed if not treated *immediately*.

Dr. Burnett, in the paper from which I have already quoted, recommends the distribution of such cards by the health department of the District of Columbia. It seems to me that much good might be accomplished in this way. Such cards could be kept in a small rack in the waiting room of every dispensary, and their presence would soon attract attention. In addition, such a notice, framed, could hang on the wall of each dispensary waiting room and in the city police stations. A little effort in this direction might save many children from incurable blindness. Dr. Rohé, our health commissioner, tells me he thinks no difficulty would be experienced in bringing this about in Baltimore.

Finally, we have to deal with the midwives. This part of the subject is most difficult of all, in our own State at least. Our laws require nothing but self-confidence on the woman's

---

¶ Burnott, (loc. cit.)

part to entitle her to a license. These women attend many
more poor women in confinement than do physicians, and
are naturally interested in covering up their mistakes. In
various parts of Europe—Saxony, Austria, Prussia, etc.—
there are laws of more or less stringency regulating the
licensing of these women, compelling them to know Credé's
method before obtaining their licenses, and to use it in practice. A bill more strictly regulating the practice of midwives was introduced a year ago in the British Parliament.
It was temporarily laid aside, but will almost surely be made
a law. The Legislature of the State of New York, at its
last session, passed " An Act for the Prevention of Blindness." Nurses and midwives are required to report in
writing to the health officer or some legally qualified practitioner of medicine the mattering or reddening of babies'
eyes any time during the first two weeks of life, within twenty-
four hours after such conditions have been noticed. A
penalty of fine or imprisonment is attached for violation.

What would be *best* to do is hardly a matter of doubt : to
have a law requiring both doctors and midwives to show
that they know enough to practice before giving either
licenses. But we know from experience that there are certain obstacles in the way of this in Maryland. What is the
best possible, then, is what we want. To find this out and to
put it in practice will require work and careful thought.

It is, Mr. President, in my opinion, and I believe in yours
too, the legitimate work of the Faculty to attend to such
matters as this. I would, in conclusion, suggest the appointment of a committee of four—two obstetricians and two
oculists—to take charge of this matter, to have the power to
urge upon dispensaries, physicians and midwives in the State,
in the name of the Faculty, the importance of lessening the
number of blind from curable diseases, to go before our City
Council or Legislature, if the committee deems best, to ask
for necessary legislation—in a word to be clothed with power
to act for the Faculty in the great work of preventing blindness.
Reports from the committee should be presented to the Faculty at its semi-annual meetings. I believe there are men in
the State sufficiently interested in this matter to go ahead on

their own responsibility if necessary. If they can, however, have the Faculty's endorsement, the work will be easier and more effective.

DISCUSSION.

Dr. A. Friedenwald said this was the best paper he had ever read on the subject. The difficulty is not so much the want of knowledge but carelessness, as the cause of blindness.

Dr. Geo. H. Rohe said the strength of the nitrate of silver solution used at the Maryland Maternite was one per cent., that at one time during the year it was accidentally reduced to a one-half per cent. solution, when several slight cases occurred. In over two hundred births that had occurred there in the last two years, there had been but two of ophthalmia neonatorum. Before that time, the cases of ophthalmia neonatorum were not infrequent.

Dr. R. L. Randolph said, one point which I think should be especially emphasized is the quantity of the silver nitrate solution used. One might think that where one drop would ward off the disease, two drops would accomplish the result beyond a doubt. But this is not the case, for an excess of a two per cent. solution acts as a caustic. I certainly remember one case where the zeal of a physician resulted in a total and permanent cloudiness of the cornea from too much nitrate of silver. Again, it should be remembered that in a child a few hours old the secretion of serus is scant, and so there is less chance of an excess of the agent being neutralized. The agent, then, as presented by Credé is potent for good, but care should be taken to use no more than one drop, for it is also an agent potent for harm.

Dr. J. C. Harris thought that extreme cleanliness at the time of birth most important. Oculists do not usually have the opportunity to use those measures.

ENLARGED TONSILS, AND THEIR HARMFUL EFFECTS ON HEALTH AND DEVELOPMENT.

By William T. Cathell, M. D.

If it be true that the more important the disease, and the more frequently it is encountered by the physician, the more necessary it is for him to be awake to every theoretic probability and practical fact, regarding its cause, pathology, course and sequelæ, and familiar with every good plan in its treatment, then I am sure there exists valid reasons for asserting that the subject of Hypertrophy of the Tonsils in early life, is one of special importance in our ever-changing climate, and deserving of our most careful and thoughtful attention, both on account of its frequency and of its harmful and far-reaching effects on health, growth and general development.

Believing thus, and desiring to do some slight share of the work in the section of Opthalmology, Otology and Laryngology, I broach this subject to-day, with the hope that my flail may find some straw left unbeaten by former threshers.

I shall not at this time consider the inflammatory enlargement of the tonsils that temporarily follows attacks of acute and sub-acute tonsillitis, nor discuss hypertrophy of the tonsils in the mature adult, but shall limit myself to the genuine hyperplastic disease, or true hypertrophy, that begins in one or both tonsils at various periods of childhood, from teething to puberty, oftenest about the 7th, 8th or 9th year; consisting histologically of an increased nutritive activity and growth, affecting all the constituents of the tonsils: follicles, stroma, vessels, lymph-passages and cells ; which hypertrophy, although possessing a natural tendency to diminish between adolescence and full adult life, and to then allow the tonsils to return to somewhat their normal size; yet is pathological during the time it exists, and not only renders the tonsils unable to perform their physiological functions, but their presence as abnormal masses in this important portion of the upper air passages, by diminishing its lumen, makes a harmful and far-reaching impress on the mental and physical development of the individual.

Bear in mind that the nasal passages are not only the seat of smell, but their extensive surface also contains a number of hairs, cilia and follicular glands; also a very rich supply of blood in its membranes; which serve to warm and filter, cleanse, refine and moisten the air before its entrance into the throat and lungs; on the contrary air entering by the mouth is not thus prepared.

Among the commoner effects of this long continued interference with the functions of the tonsils, and with the lumen and physiological action of the pharynx and neighboring parts are:

1st. Interference with free and normal respiration through the nose, which necessitates a corresponding degree of mouth-breathing.

2nd. There being less than the normal amount of air passing through the nares, the circulation and constructive activity in all the tissues of that region are lessened; and neither the fleshy structures nor the bony framework of the nose and palatal arch, becomes normally developed, hence, the nose, the nasal passages and the naso-pharynx, all remain permanently narrower in breadth than normal breathing and free circulation would have caused. It also tends to allow the alveolar process of the upper jaw to remain abnormally small in size, crowding the teeth together and necessarily making the face unnaturally thin and pinched looking.

3rd. The partial stenosis of the faucial passages, besides limiting the volume and force of air passing through the nose, also interferes with natural drainage, and allows an accumulation of the products of its large number of follicular glands, and other secretions, which obtunds and injures the functions of smell, taste and hearing, and almost invariably excites nasal and faucial catarrh and chronic pharyngitis.

4th. The effete cheesy matter, and other debris that accumulates in the large and often ragged lacunæ of the tonsils;

consisting of epithelium, cholesterine, broken-down gland tissue, pus corpuscles, particles of food, and other caseated or decomposing matter, is prone to taint the breath with a disagreeable and characteristic odor, and may also be the unsuspected cause of an annoying spasmodic cough.

5th. The constant swallowing of these catarrhal and diseased tonsillar and pharyngeal secretions, and hurrying half-masticated food from the mouth to the stomach, because the mouth must be cleared for use in respiration, cannot fail to injuriously affect the sufferer's stomach and appetite.

6th. Chronic swelling and congestion about the mouths of the eustachian tubes, possibly involving the tubes themselves, and the partial plugging of them with mucus is apt to accompany the other disorders, and to cause labyrinthian deafness, varying in degree from a slight dulness to marked obtundity, contributing very much to the peculiar physiognomy, viz.: the vacant or silly expression, dull eyes, drooping eye lids, slow speech, nasal tone of voice, aural catarrh, otorrhœa, etc., so often seen in children with hypertrophy of the tonsils.

7th. The respiratory tract being thus interfered with, inspiration takes place to a minimum, instead of to a maximum degree, and there is not sufficient air supply to the lungs to resist the external atmospheric pressure, the natural result of which, to the child's yielding frame, is more or less thoracic deformity, occasionally even to the extent of the so-called "chicken-breast" or sunken sternum, since the entire chest, and especially its upper portion, remains smaller, narrower and flatter than it would, if there were a free and full admission of air to the lungs.

Among other characteristic results, we are apt to find the individual thin, pale, nervous, and inclined to persistent frontal headache; with a dry, tickling pharyngeal or uvular cough, worse at night; more or less dyphagia, and a peculiar throaty and thick, or nasal tone of voice, bad-smelling mouth, coated tongue, indigestion and palpitation. General indifference and inability to study. Sleep snoring, dreamful and disturbed, due in part to pressure of the tonsils diminishing the supply of arterial blood to the brain, and their pressure on the jugulars preventing the prompt venous return. Mouth open, especially during sleep; and both it and the throat unnaturally dry, especially on waking, and during the early hours of morning; also pharynx, larynx, trachea and bronchi all exposed to the free action of whatever irritating agents the air may contain.

A limited degree of mouth breathing may long escape detection since the person may be able to close the mouth while awake and attentive, and yet open it to breathe as soon as consciousness is lost in sleep, closing it again on waking, and thus remain ignorant of the fact that he ever resorts to mouth breathing.

Diphtheria has, in my opinion, a constant invitation to visit mouth-breathers with hypertrophied tonsils and finds in them excellent subjects.

When hypertrophy of the tonsils is once established it seldom wholly disappears spontaneously before about the thirtieth year of life, at which period, as a rule, liability to all tonsillar affections lessen, and natural absorption and atrophy of the tonsillar glands begins; but earlier; even during adolescence the natural broadening of the palatal arch, and the gradual increase of the intra-tonsillar space, brings some relief, but unfortunately, not before the affection has done the most harmful part of its work on the mental and physical development of the individual.

The symptoms of hypertrophy itself are more passive than active, and accompanied by but little or no pain, hence, hypertrophy of one or both tonsils may exist in various degrees unsuspected, or be discovered ɩ nly after having created concomitant affections of neighboring parts, yet, it is one of the most easily diagnosed of all internal abnormalities: the tonsils, instead of being rarely more than half an inch long, almond shaped and lying at each side of the fauces in the niche between the anterior and posterior pillars, and scarcely reaching up to the level of the half arches, as is normal, are visibly enlarged, globular, spongy or indurated, somewhat pale, and insensitive looking, ranging in size, from a slightly bulging prominence, up to almost complete occlusion of the isthmus faucium, sometimes presenting a rotated, globular, or even pediculated appearance, and arching far into the isthmus; their surface sometimes jagged but usually smooth, except at the depressions corresponding to the orifices of the small crypts, about which the mucous follicles are grouped, with their aperatures dilated and closed, instead of being rounded and open.

We may in exaggerated cases, even find the tonsillor masses encroaching boldly upon the naso-pharyngeal space, forcing up the velum palati, and touching or crowding the uvula on one or both sides, and almost hiding the posterior wall of the ph trynx from view; perhaps their lacunæ and crypts studded with cheesy accumulations, which can be expressed by slight pressure; their decomposition and fetid odor naturally tainting the breath as it passes in and out over them; all uniting to show both the nature aud extent of the affection.

The frequency of hypertrophy of the tonsils is attested on all sides, Chappell (Internat. Journal of Med. Sciences, Feb., 1889,) who examined 2,000 children found it present in 270. It may exist in early infancy and during teething, sometimes appearing to depend on this for its origin. I have seen well marked cases in children less than three years old, and on the contrary in persons who have reached full adult life, but it is most frequent and most harmful in this climate between the seventh and fifteenth year.

Causes:—I shall not detain you with theories, and opinions of interest chiefly to specialists in this department, but will merely state that among its common causes may be enumerated the catarrhal diathesis, chronic pharyngeal catarrh, exposure, unfavorable hygiene and debil.tating influences in general. It is a frequent expression of struma, and is occasionally the sequela of scarlatina, measles and small pox. It may aiso arise from frequent attacks of tonsillitis, and from any irritation of the lymphatic glandular system sufficient to excite an increase of the tonsillar connective tissue; so also, from frequent attacks of pharyngitis, and the prolonged atmospheric union of cold and dampness with insufficiency of sunlight as we often see during the winter months. We sometimes meet cases in otherwise healthy subjects for which no special cause can be assigned. It may, as I have already said, follow frequent attacks of tonsillitis, but some are subject to these without any such result. Rheumatism and the rheumatic diathesis have also been assigned as leading causes, but my experience does not support that conclusion.

Two varieties may be mentioned according to the existing degree of density or sponginess, with every intermediate grade: the soft hypertrophy or spongy variety in which the stroma attains the greater growth, and the true fibrous or hard variety in which the follicles are comparatively more enlarged. The soft variety is by far the most frequently seen and attains the greater size. Clinically we also meet with what is called a "ragged" variety, which condition is due to frequent abscesses and sloughing of portions of the hypertrophied tonsillar tissue.

Methods of Examination :—If we cause a mild effort to retch by slightly titillating the pharynx, the tonsils are at once protruded and rotated into full view. They may also be viewed in their normal location by having the patient to widely open his mouth and then cough or take a deep inspiration, but the most useful and complete information regarding their size, density and other qualities may be obtained by pressing the tonsillar region of the neck inwardly with all the fingers of one hand externally, while it is examined internally with the index finger of the other. Being poorly supplied with nerves of sensation, a properly conducted examination of the tonsils is rarely complained of.

The function or role of the tonsils which are nothing more or less than congeries of minute glands, or follicles, bound into almond shape masses by connective tissue, is yet not fully understood, but among the functions of their acinous glands is the secretion of a clear viscid fluid, which flows from their lacunæ, more abundantly while eating, and is intended to lubricate the bolus of food and assist its downward passage. They also exercise some ill-understood influence on the lymph and blood, but their services must be unimportant and easily spared, for their loss of function, and even their removal, when enlarged, is not only not followed by harm, but by a decided benefit.

Treatment :—Anyone who confines himself to any single method, or fixed mode of treatment, for hypertrophy of the tonsils, shuts his eyes to much else that is valuable. The great object in all plans of treatment is to bring about either resolution, or permanent fibrous or cicatricial contraction; and this requires good judgment and skill, and no difference how this reduction is effected, if it be done before the hypertrophy has continued long enough, to permanently prevent sufficient development of the nasal passages or to ever allow the proper quantity of air to pass through them to the lungs, we may expect the hearing to improve, the facial expression to brighten, the cervical adenitis, if present to disappear, the nutrition to increase, and the patient to be placed on a brighter, more pleasing, more intellectual and decidedly healthier road.

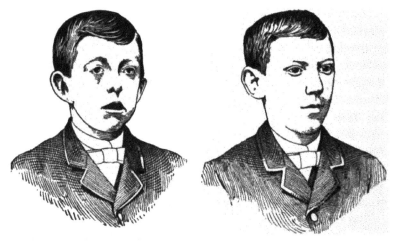

The first of the above kodacks is of W. J. K., a mouth-breathing boy 13 years and 5 months of age, on whom I performed double tonsillotomy October 3rd and 10th, 1889, followed by a systemic course of iron, cod liver oil and other restoratives. The other is of the same youth, now a nose breather taken a few days ago. It shows a great and gratifying improvement.

The age of the patient, the peculiarities of his case, and of his surronndings, all enter into the question of how to reduce his hypertrophy.

No difference what local or operative plans, short of surgical removal are pursued, constitutional and reconstructive treatment must be steadily used, else the return of the hypertrophy may be looked for.

Two of these auxillary agents I have found of special benefit and both were used in the above case, viz: the compound syrup of phosphates (chemical food) U. S. P., and syr. ferri iodidi. To a child 8 years of age, either one teaspoonful of the former before, and nine drops of the latter in sweet water after·every meal, or the two alternated day and day about, are highly beneficial. Iodide of iron seems to exert a decided and specific influence over glandular enlargement in children, but is apt to blacken the tongue and teeth, owing to the presence of the sulphide of iron. The blackening of the tongue is temporary, consequently of no moment, and the parents should be so informed, but that of the teeth is more permanent and should be prevented by giving the remedy sweetened until it is syrupy, or if they are already blackened they can be beautifully whitened by brushing them with equal parts of tannic acid and charcoal.

Pure cod liver oil, made pleasant by the addition of about one-fourth of its volume of syr. pruni Virginianæ and a tinge of creosote, is also very beneficial. Kalii iodidum also does good, and the older the patient the more likely it is to be useful.

Of topical or surface applications, astringents, absorbents, nitrate of silver, chromic acid and other caustics, I must confess that as far as permanent results are concerned, I can say but little in praise. I do not remember a single case in which they have fully and permanently removed the hypertrophy, and in many they have seemed practically useless, I have seen the persistent application of equal parts: tinc. iodini, glycerine, and syr. simplicis, lessen the size at a snail-like rate, and even then not to complete resolution or cure. I have also found good results, in a few cases, from the local use of a mixture composed of equal parts of muriated tincture of iron and glycerine.

It is very necessary in the use of these, and all other strong topical applications, to wipe the surplus from the brush or mop, before applying, lest it trickle down over the arytenoid cartilages into the larynx, and cause alarming spasm of the glottis.

The nearer to full adult age the patient, the more benefit have I seen from another good remedy, the iodide of zinc applied in the following manner: First thoroughly cleanse the tonsil with Dobell's solution, or better still, Gleason's excellent combination, the formula of which is as follows:

R.—Sodii bicarb,	.	.	.	.	.	a a.
Sodii biborat,	.	.	.	.	.	℥ i.
Sodii salicylat,	.	.	.	.	.	gr. iii,
Thymol,	.	.	.	.	.	gr. i.
Menthol,	.	.	.	.	.	grs. s.
Glycerinæ,	.	.	.	.	.	℥ i.
Aq. fervid, ad	.	.	.	.	.	℥ iv.

M.—Add to a quart of water.

Now make repeated applications of a 10 per cent. solution of antipyrin, for a period of 10 to 12 minutes, otherwise this treatment will fail, after which apply the zinc by any suitable means. I usually employ absorbent cotton twirled upon a pharyngeal applicator.

The treatment should be made at the office every third day until the object is accomplished; according to my experience the average time required is about two months. A keen smarting is the only inconvenience, and this remains but a few minutes. Neither of the two agents has any eschorotic power, therefore we have no formation of a slough but absorption and shriveling. A great advantage in this treatment is, that the zinc when thus applied will not invade the neighboring healthy structures, and therefore may be used with little fear of injury from being swallowed. Finally, one thing must not be lost sight of; that is this, in order to confirm a cure, the applications should be continued a few times after the tonsil is apparently shriveled to its normal size.

Experience gradually leads me to greater belief that while topical applications may occasionally be useful, yet, more potent methods are necessary for the fullest benefit to the vast majority of cases, but it may be stated as an axiom, that no operative procedure should be undertaken for reduction of the hypertrophied tonsils while they are in a state of inflammation or soreness.

I have found nothing better for removing soreness, erosions and foul breath than the following gargle:

℞.—

> Kalii chloratis—3 x.
> Acidi pheinci—gr xxiv.
> Olei gaultheriæ—gr xii.
> M. Fiat Pulv. No. 1.

Sig.   Add one quart of warm water.   Gargle 4 or 5 times a day.

One fact is worthy of remembrance: if pharyngeal catarrh is present with a tonsillar hypertrophy, whether as the presumable cause or as a result, it also, will require appropriate treatment for its removal.

In operative procedures, the choice with me is always between the tonsillotome, the Jarvis snare and the galvanocautery, with a decided leaning towards the former, since its whole work is done in a few seconds, and if skillfully done, is limited to exactly what the cure requires.   There are no large blood vessels in the tonsils of children, and the strong pharyngeal fascia lies between them and the internal carotids, and unless the whole tonsil is either lifted or pulled from its bed before being cut, or the small branch of the tonsillar artery that runs in the palato-glossal fold close to its edge is reached by accident, there can be no harmful hæmorrhage.   This is certainly the most thorough and effectual measure at our command, and if preceded by properly mopping with a 10 per cent. solution of cocaine, it is either painless or nearly so, and can then be done carefully and deliberately.

By gaining the patient's confidence during the preparatory examination, I rarely meet with unsurmountable opposition to the necessary operation; but when we have for the patient a puny, half sick or refractory child, whom it would be necessary to hold, pry open the jaws, force the instruments into the mouth, and operate amid his terror, struggles and shock, mild chloroform anæsthesia becomes an invaluable factor, both to him and to us, as it simply wraps him in a brief dream, while it gives us complete control over the patient and every feature of the operation.

Among the advantages that I have found in chloroform over ether, in nose and throat cases in young people is, that they take it more willingly, it induces its effects very much more rapidly, anæsthesia in children sometimes even following a few whiffs, and it does not, like ether, excite an abundant flow of viscid mucus into the mouth and pharynx.

My aim in all tonsillotomies is to carefully slice off the projecting growth down to its natural level with the half arches of the pillars of the fauces, and no more. The removal of more is unnecessary, and might wound the edge of the anterior pillar, in which runs a branch of the tonsillar artery, and expose it to hæmorrhage. Examination will show whether there exists any adhesion between the tonsils and pillars; if so, it should be broken up with a bent probe before proceeding to ablate. ·Bear in mind while ablating, that the cicatization and contraction which follows the removal will materially assist in further reducing the size.

I have performed a considerable number of tonsillotomies and never yet encountered serious hæmorrhage in these cases in young patients, in whom the tonsils are soft or only semi-indurated and never canaliculated. I have had but one case in the adult. Her's was controlled by using masses of ice in the mouth while I was preparing to use Levi's method of torsion of the base of the tonsil with an ordinary tenaculum.

Neither have I ever met with what might be truly called a calculus of the tonsil.

I am prepared to admit that each method has its advantages, and that no one plan of local treatment aiming at the removal or destruction of the hypertrophied tissue is all that could be desired. Some of the ablest of those who have given special thought to the subject prefer the galvano-cautery loop or snare for adults, and the galvano-cautery puncture for children, making six or eight punctures, about one-fourth of an inch deep, into the tissues, or the same number of plunges into the orifices of the follicles with the thermo-cautery point at each sitting, with intervals between the sittings of from two or three days to a week or two, according to the resulting soreness, until six or eight sittings are had, when the tonsil will be nearly restored to its normal condition ; provided the patient does not get disgusted with the odor of burning flesh, and absent himself before he becomes accustomed to it. If you can persuade these patients to continue the treatment until the number of sittings are more than half over, they will then usually continue to attend until all is accomplished.

After the hypertrophy is reduced or removed, no difference by which means, our next aim must be to prevent its recurrence and to efface the evil impress : the impaired nutrition, the arrested, diminished or irregular development, the general debility, etc., and to accomplish this, we must bring the patient's general health back into as perfect a condition as possible by good food, pure air, proper exercise, iron, cod liver oil, compound syrup phosphates, quinine, &c.

In conclusion, I have brought forward the subject of hypertrophy of the tonsils, for the following reasons : 1st. Because it is an affection so frequently encountered by the physician of this region that it must possess both value and interest to all. 2d. Because its presence is fraught with special danger during the period of development and growth. 3rd. Because it can be so quickly and surely diagnosed that no one has a reason for mistaking or overlooking it.

Finally, because its timely removal or reduction, is of such far-reaching benefit, that every physician should be wide awake to its importance and treatment.

FOUR CASES OF DIPHTHERITIC LARYNGITIS IN WHICH INTUBATION WAS PERFORMED WITH ONE RECOVERY, AND ONE CASE OF RECOVERY WITHOUT OPERATION.

By J. W. Humrichouse, M. D., of Hagerstown, Md.

CASE 1.—Kitty McC., aged six years, was taken sick December 26, 1890. When I made my first visit on above date, two small patches on left tonsil and one on right were seen. The voice was changed, being sometimes muffled, but becoming rather clear when an unusual effort to talk was made.

For the throat a twenty-five per cent. solution of Marchand's peroxide of hydrogen was ordered to be freely used as a wash and gargle, and for the larynx the frequent inhalation from a steam atomizer of a mixture of trypsin and bicarbonate of soda. Ten drops of tincture of chloride of iron in half an ounce of sherry wine were given every three hours. During the following six days the patches on tonsils became smaller, but the symptoms of laryngeal stenosis became gradually more and more pronounced.

Jan. 2nd. The child's breathing could be heard all over the room. On the morning of this day, the seventh of the sickness, to avert impending death from suffocation an O'Dwyer tube was put into the larynx and the operation was followed by immediate relief. After resting two hours the little patient managed to take two ounces of milk by slowly drawing it through a nipple from a nursing-bottle. She drank it lying down, with her head lower than her body. She slept well this night.

Jan. 3rd. There was a violent coughing spell attended with such dyspnœa that the nurse thought the child would be suffocated. Fortunately, however, three large and thick pieces of membrane were coughed through the tube.

Child begged to be allowed to drink water from a glass. She succeeded by sipping it slowly. After this attempt, beef juice, milk, and the iron and wine were taken in a sitting posture.

Jan. 4th. After spraying the throat there was a paroxysm of coughing which ended with the expulsion through the tube of a thick curled up piece of membrane. In this paroxysm the nurse suspended the child, head downwards, and slapped the chest, in order to force out the tube. It remained fast, however and its lumen became cleared of the obstruction before I arrived.

Jan. 6th. On the fourth day after its insertion the tube was removed. Immediately the breathing became distressed; so much so, that after waiting half an hour I was obliged to put it back in the larynx.

Jan. 8th. Another piece of membrane was coughed up. Urine at this date contained albumen and casts. Temperature throughout the sickness ranged from 99 to 102.

Jan. 10. Took tube out after being in larynx eight days. Child from this time had no further trouble.

CASE 11.—Nov. 15th, 1890, was called to see Clarence H., six years old. Two days previously Dr. Brotemarkle had diagnosed diphtheria and the child had been sick five days before his visit. At the time of my visit the respiration was so labored, the cyanosis and restlessness so marked, that it was apparent that relief could only be afforded by operative interference. Intubation accordingly was done on the eighth day of the sickness and caused the disappearance of the stridor, the cyanosis and the restlessness. The parents thought the boy would now certainly get well.

Nov. 16th. Breathing easy, with no symptoms of obstruction in larynx, and no rales in bronchi. Pharynx, however, covered with membrane.

Nov. 17th. The tenth day of his sickness the patient showed great weakness. He could not be induced to take enough nourishment. A part of the fluids given produced cough. He wanted me to extract the tube. Hoping that stimulants and food would be taken more freely after the removal of the tube, it was extracted after having been in the larynx two days. Unfortunately this did not prove to be the case and a few hours after the extraction the patient suddenly expired.   .

False membrane covered tonsils and pharynx was present in this case throughout its whole duration. Its persistence, the pallor of the boy's face, and his great weakness showed how profoundly he was affected. He escaped death by strangulation, to die on the eleventh day from exhaustion.

In addition to the above cases I will refer to two reported in the MARYLAND MEDICAL JOURNAL, March 10, 1888. One was a boy two years and ten months old, who on the sixth day showed all the distressing signs of obstruction to breathing; cyanosis, drawing in of the parts above clavicles and between ribs upon inspiration, and restlessness, which were immediately relieved upon the insertion of an O'Dwyer tube. After the operation he slept the whole night and the following morning took semi-solid food. Crushed ice he could swallow, but when he tried to drink water some of it would get into the tube and cause cough. He died about 36 hours after the operation from broncho-pneumonia.

The other case, a boy eighteen months old, died three days after relief of laryngeal symptoms by intubation. Death, we thought, was caused by extension downwards of the membrane on account of absence of bronchial rales, and the presence of cyanosis and hurried breathing. The tube was extracted twice in the three days in order to ascertain whether it was clogged and also for the purpose of giving food.

CASE V.—Julia McK., four years old, had sore throat and croup four days before I saw her, Oct. 7, 1886. Tonsils covered with membrane, voice reduced to a whisper, respiration very much embarrassed upon exertion, were observed at visit. Treatment consisted in the alternate use of antiseptic and solvent sprays from steam atomizers every fifteen minutes during the day, and as often as possible during the night, and the administration internally every two hours of $\frac{1}{14}$ grain bichloride of mercury with· five minims tincture of chloride of iron, and two teaspoonsful of whiskey with milk every three hours. Two or three doses of medicine were vomited bringing up pieces of membrane. The bichloride was discontinued after three days. On the morning of the seventh day I left the patient, with the intention to return in half an hour prepared to do intubation. To my relief, however, the symptoms of laryngeal stenosis had subsided, and although always thereafter present to an extent that made me uneasy, yet not sufficiently so to justify intubation. The child recovered after an illness of fifteen days. Its recovery I consider due to the constant, almost continuous inhalation of steam impregnated with solvents, as trypsin and bicarbonate of soda, which softened and loosened the membrane in larynx and trachea so that it was easily coughed up.

We have endeavored to show in the four cases that intubation was done to avert death from laryngeal stenosis, that death from this cause was averted, and that great relief followed the operation even in the cases ending fatally.

Having presented tubage of the larynx in its favorable aspect, we will consider two objectionable features pertaining to it; one, the passage of fluids into the tube in the act of swallowing, the other the want of expulsive power in coughing. In the first difficulty a part of the liquid food taken, such as water and milk, runs down through the tube into the lowest part of the trachea, where it excites violent coughing attended sometimes with vomiting, which if often repeated exhausts the child and finally makes it unable. or unwilling to take nourishment.

The second difficulty, the want of expulsive power in the cough, is caused by the glottis being occupied by an open tube, which offers no resistence to the action of the diaphragm, thereby preventing compression of the air in the chest and its sudden and forcible discharge. Schluck-pneumonie, catarrhal, lobular or broncho-pneumonia are thus sometimes mechanically caused by the failure to remove irritating and obstiucting matters from the bronchial tubes by means of coughing.

All cases are not seriously affected by these difficulties. Some children learn to overcome them. In our successful case the tube was in the larynx eight days and the child learned to swallow milk, water, sherry wine and semi-solid food; it also had coughing spells strong enough to expel through the tube several large pieces of tough membrane.

To do away with the trouble in deglution various procedures have been recommended. Dr. O'Dwyer and Dr. Dillion Brown approved the plan of feeding suggested by Dr. Casselberry, of Chicago, in which gravitation of fluids into the tube is overcome by placing the head of the patient lower than the body. Dr. J. Mount Bleyer advises the use of the stomach tube. By feeding without it he says you will stop up the canula in larynx and produce Schluck-pneumonie.

It has been his custom in many of his late cases to extract the tube from the larynx every day to cleanse it, and after extraction to offer food. The risk of pushing down membrane before the distal orifice of the tube does not deter him; he lessens it by using the laryngoscope. Dr. S. J. Meltzer, of New York, advises the introduction of a soft catheter into the stomach through the nose, to be left there permanently. By means of a small funnel rubber tubing, nourishment is administered.

Of course as in other diseases where there is difficulty in swallowing, rectal feeding is resorted to. Milk, expressed juice of beef, whiskey, as injections every three or four hours in the quantity of an ounce or two are generally tolerated for a long time.

Other embarrassments and dangers which I in my limited experience have not encountered, but which are often referred to, such as pushing down membrane before tube, apnœa from repeated and futile attempts at introduction, the making of a false passage, and the putting the tube into the œsophagus, it is not necessary more than to allude to.

THE REVIVAL IN PHYSICAL EDUCATION AND PERSONAL HYGIENE.

By Edward M. Schaeffer, M. D., of Baltimore.

Dr. Osler, of the Johns Hopkins University recently told a popular audience that a desire to take medicines is perhaps the great feature which distinguishes man from other animals. His plea was that our patients shall follow suit in the advance taken by the profession and accept the prescription of "a little more exercise, a little less food, and a little less tobacco and alcohol," and I may add, in brief, evince a greater reliance upon what still constitutes the fundamental strength of our art outside of surgery, viz., the precepts of hygiene and dietetic science. Voltaire wittily defined the physician to be an unfortunate gentleman expected every day to perform the miracle of reconciling health with intemperance. "A man may boast that he has learned how to evade nature's laws, but the brag is on his lips," says Emerson. The conditions are in his soul, *and body*. When I read in a modern magazine the charge that "physicians are too busy studying disease to pay any attention to health," and that "in learning the nature and effect of remedies, there results no time or inclination to learn the laws by which remedies would be rendered useless," it seems evident that the time is ripe for the doctor to resume his etymological role of *teacher*, and the physician that of student of *health in nature*. Galen declared him to be the best doctor who is the best teacher of gymnastics; and, as he became physician or medical director, we would now say to the gladiatorial school of his native town, after eleven years of study, may it not have been this experience which was the foundation of an influence dominant for thirteen hundred years after his death?

A certain Herodicus was so famous for his application of gymnastics to the improvement of health that Plato accused him of doing an ill service to the state by keeping alive people who ought to die, because, being valetudinarians, they cost more than they were worth to the community.

"Physical culture in theory is the obtaining and maintaining of a properly formed, healthy body; in practice *right conduct about food, (clothing,) activity and rest.*" On this broad platform, hereafter, the specialists in health will minister to the great masses, and especially to growing youth in homes, schools, and colleges, as a sort of medical extension corps, and so educate the public and themselves in the great basic facts of living—casualties aside—free from ordinary sickness and dying at the call of that honorable but infrequent messenger of death, Old Age. "This world is not yet prepared, so far as we know," says a writer, "for the activities of bodiless spirits." The first thing is to develop a firm healthy body, strong muscle, pure blood, a clean mucous membrane. Such conditions would base a soul, upright and free." Hope, sunshine and fresh air have never been supplanted as tonics, and along with diet and medication, regulated exercise, and its correlative, rest, calls for the same therapeutic respect in the prescriptions of the careful practitioner. Joining a gymnasium or an athletic association *per se* as remedial measures for the sedentary, weak or semi-invalid, is a species of polypharmacy; or the administration of a crude drug in place of the purified and isolated extract—active (athletic) principle, if you prefer. Of exercise, as of dieting, it may be said, *mutatis mutandis*, in the language of the famous Code of Salernum:

" Doctors should thus their patients' food revise.
    WHAT is it? WHEN the meal? and what its SIZE?
    How OFTEN? WHERE? Lest by some sad mistake
    Ill-sorted things should meet and trouble make."

Believing that in the Swedish educational gymnastics this physiological refinement of bodily exercises has received the most attention, I have ventured in the present paper to bring more especially to your notice some of the distinguishing features of the same.   In what follows it is not my purpose to speak of Swedish medical gymnastics, an altogether distinct branch, but to refer to educational exercises simply.

It has been well charged against the usual athletic work of schools and colleges that it does not reach the very class most in need of bodily development, viz., the more studious and sedate element, who have no desire to pursue sport as an end in itself, such as winning a prize, breaking a record or being known as an athlete.   The worship of muscle appertains rather to the prize ring, and exhibitions of strength or prowess introduce with quite a doubtful advantage the claims of physical training in a university course.   We want in America to-day a sensible enthusiasm or ambition for good health by rational living!   Sir James Paget says, "I should like to see a personal ambition for renown in health as keen as that for bravery or for beauty, or for success in athletic games and field sports.   I wish there were such an ambition for the most perfect national health as there is for national renown in war, or in art, or in commerce."

What, if physiological laws are as sacred as moral laws, in their own proper spheres, and mankind as truly bound to obey them?   "Holy and healthy are synonymous terms," admits that arch dyspeptic, Carlyle, who thus philosophizes: "The healthy know not of their health, but only the sick. The true peptician was that countryman who said 'for his part he had no system.'   A state of health is denoted by a term expressing unity, when we feel ourselves as we wish to be, we say we are WHOLE.   Had Adam remained in Paradise there had been no anatomy and no metaphysics."   So much for wilful infraction of known laws in the physical decalogue.

Let me call the attention of those interested in the Swedish idea of physical education to a treatise entitled "The Gymnastic Progression," by Claes J. Enebuske, Ph. D., of the Boston Normal School of Gymnastics, to whom the writer is indebted for practical instruction in the system.   I cannot serve my theme better than to quote the following analysis as he gives it. "The functions of the heart and lungs are the fundamental functions of the body. It is the aim of Swedish educational gymnastics to develop these fundamental functions, and it endeavors to attain this end by a series of movements of the voluntary system which shall be so arranged and executed as to bring about a healthy response between the muscles and the will. It does not strive to develop physical specialists, but only to train the different organs of the body in a manner that may serve the great double purpose of promoting the efficiency of the circulatory and respiratory functions, and of increasing the volitional control of the whole body. Throughout its entire course the Swedish system of gymnastics proceeds upon the well-grounded theory that muscular strength must follow as the necessary consequence of a training so carried on as to promote the health and strength of these fundamental functions. Theory and experience show that a system of training may be followed which, while it develops muscular strength to a considerable degree, at the same time causes dilatation of the heart and lung cells, making their walls thinner and weaker. Upon such a training common sense stamps the seal of disapproval. Get the heart and the lungs right and the muscles will meet every reasonable demand. This is the teaching of experience.

'The gymnastic day's order' is composed of a certain number of movements succeeding each other in a well defined order, calculated to produce certain effects in a certain succession, all these movements together being designed to bring about a distinct hygienic and educational result.

Students and brain workers generally, from the conditions of their life, present a more or less temporary congestion or tendency to such congestion of the brain and abdominal organs, decreased respiration, and the mind tired from prolonged concentration. The first object of the gymnastic drill must be to counteract these evils, to relieve the brain and oppressed organs, to reinstate a healthy respiration and circulation; to tone up the body generally. First, '*Order movements*' call attention to that fundamental position and carriage best suited to the physiological interests of the body, from which all correct gymnastics start and to which they return before a relaxed position of rest is resumed.   Then a class called '*leg movements*,' intended to draw the blood in larger quantities down towards the lower extremities, thereby relieving the brain and the oppressed organs.   These also stimulate the general circulation.   Next follow movements called '*strain-bending movements*' and '*heave movements*,' which expand the chest and induce deeper and more energetic respiration.   The combined result of these four typical gymnastic movements in the order mentioned is this : More and better oxygenated blood is carried to the muscles and the venous drainage correspondingly facilitated ; the mind is relieved from its previous strain and the will is concentrated upon the muscular response.   These results unite to form a most favorable general foundation upon which to ground the following more specific movements : '*Balance movements*,' which bring about a co-ordination of muscular contraction in all parts of the body, and by demanding equilibrium in difficult positions, train the sense of correct and graceful posture.

'*Movements for the back*,' which correct the shoulder-blades and back, and by equalizing the strength of the muscles on both sides of the vertebral column counteract faulty growth of the spine.   '*Movements for abdomen and fore-part of the body*,' which stimulate the abdominal organs by an alternating increase and decrease of the abdominal pressure.   The movements strengthen the muscles of the abdominal walls, as do also the next following, called the '*alternate side movements*.'

These last train the legitimate mobility of the ribs and vertebræ and mechanically stimulate the spinal nerves. These movements are performed with gradually increasing force, compelling stronger and stronger action from the circulatory and respiratory organs, but never exceeding a certain point, the *optimum*, the test of which is a deep, free, undisturbed respiration during the movement.   Whenever the extreme limit is approached, as shown by breathlessness and uncomfortable heart action, the effects are immediately moderated by administering movements that quiet and nor-

malize respiration and heart action. By these movements
the system is prepared for the next following. These are
the more vigorous exercises of running and jumping, which
culminate the day's order; after which the accelerated action
of the heart must be normalized and the body prepared for
rest. This is accomplished by slow, measured '*leg movements*,' accompanied by deep rhythmic breathing movements." The above lengthy quotation must suffice by way
of description to indicate that the Swedes have wrought out
a truly scientific system, simplified and classified all possible
beneficial movements of the body through its different members, and presented a rational, practical and economical plan
of bodily education, a basis on which our American method
will yet be founded. "The exercises, not the apparatus, constitute the system, and the movements can be taken anywhere
where there is sufficient floor space to stand on, and sufficient
oxygen in the air"—with the adaptation at times of ordinary
chairs and desks or other furniture. It is known to many that
the Swedish system is now being introduced into the public
schools of Boston, under the supervision of Dr. Hartwell, assisted by Mr. Nissen ; and a demand for teachers has come to
one training school from fifteen New England towns. There
are also applications from Kentucky, a college and private
school, and some from California, Virginia and the Middle
West. Atlanta has promptly entered the field in her public
school course. Baltimore is peculiarly fortunate in the excellent opportunities offered for scientific bodily training at
the Woman's College and the Bryn Mawr School for Girls.
The Normal School has also its drill of part Swedish and
part Delsarte exercises, and all these institutions are doing
commendable work of great promise to the young women
of our community. Thus gradually is the conspiracy against
girlhood being broken. To the dress reform movement of
the day a meed of tribute is also justly due, for at the basis
of all the physical possibilities of the sex lies a rational un-
fettered costume. "In spite of the abuse in the use of clothing to which most women have subjected themselves for
centuries," says Dr. Sargent, "I am glad to be able to state
that the typical woman, as shown by several thousand

measurements in my possession, is not quite so ugly in her lines and contour as the dress she often wears would lead one to infer." If, among other fallacies which are constantly being exploded as to what women can and cannot do, in both the physical and mental realm, should be added the belief that her attractiveness is in any way legitimately enhanced, or her comfort and elegance maintained, by wearing the inane, inartistic and often indelicate corset, then the gymnasium will readily have accomplished a feat hitherto denied to the most vigorous phillippics of the medical profession. Thinking it would be of interest to some to know how women have taken up this new occupation, and with what success they are meeting as teachers, I have obtained the following data relative to the Normal School previously mentioned, for there are now five leading schools for physical education in the country :

Whole number of pupils (men, women and children) for
    1890 and 1891, ... 465
    of whom 401 were women and children.
Whole number of normal pupils, ... 39

The standard requiring the rejection of 27, chiefly on account of insufficient mental training, though several were physically incompetent.

The personnel of this class includes three full graduates of Smith and Wellesley Colleges and the Boston university respectively; also 14 normal school graduates, while no one is received who has not the equivalent of a full high school training, and is free from any organic disease or serious functional disorder.

The course, lasting generally two years, includes the instruction given during the first year of a graded medical school in anatomy, physiology, hygiene, etc., and will be broadened by the subsequent addition of anthropometry, pædagogy and special studies in applied physics and chemistry. About one-third of the class are taking medical gymnastics, not to become practitioners but safer teachers of educational gymnastics. Graduates are now receiving from $60 to $100 a month for their services, and the demand is greater than the supply.

Vassar, Smith, Wellesley, and Mt. Holyoke Colleges have now well organized physical departments, working on scientific principles with an educational and hygienic aim.   None are, however, better equipped than the two of which our city may justly be proud.

At the last meeting of the American Association for the advancement of physical education, held in Boston in April, Rev. Dr. Hyde, President of Bowdoin College, made the following good points in explaining the proper status of physical training in our American colleges :

1. That exercise is best which reaches the largest number and does most for the weakest men.

2. That exercise is best which makes the hardest work attractive.

3. That exercise is best which most co-ordinates body, will and mind.

Ninety per cent. of students are not reached by athletics.

The question is not what can be done with the apparatus, but what can the apparatus do for the young man? He realizes, practically, that mind and body stand together in the closest correlation and gives this branch of education its just ACADEMIC RECOGNITION.   It is made one full study and is obligatory upon every man.   To it is given one-thirteenth of the whole time devoted to the college course and regular and faithful attendance is necessary for graduation.   A carefully prepared 'athletic and scholarship' table giving the standing of 153 students, showed that excellent physical development is compatible with the highest mental development.   Professional and mercantile classes, especially need the physical education, systematic scientific training will give them.   It trains the student to find pleasure in the right things.   They become less noisy, better able to fix attention, and less boisterous in play, and fortified against animalism and sensualism.   Amherst and Havaford are conducted on the same principle.   The instructor in these institutions should be a medical man and a college graduate, by preference, so he may the better command respect; and he should rank as a full professor and be paid accordingly."   Dr. Scaver, of Yale, in examining the academic freshman class of this year, found out of the 260 men "about 30 whom he termed in bad physical condition, about 75 in fair condition, fully 100 in good condition, and the remainder, about 55, are ranked as first-rate in health. The latter class are men who have had athletic training before—mostly in the preparatory schools." Inasmuch as the critical periods of growth are passed during school life, how necessary does it seem that trained and qualified, physical supervision should be added to the public school regime. Jean Paul, in his quaint way says, "each generation of children begins the history of the world anew. The school-house of the young soul does not merely consist of lecture and lesson rooms, but also of the school ground, the sleeping-room, the eating-room, the play-ground, the staircase and of every place. What intermixture of other influences always either to the advantage or prejudice of education ! In revising a scheme of education, G—— had chosen that more attention should be paid to bodily health than to mental superfoetation; he thought the tree of knowledge should be grafted with the tree of life. Ah ! whoever sacrifices health to wisdom has generally sacrificed wisdom, too, and only *in-born* not *acquired* sickliness is profitable to head and heart."

Dr. Seaver urges that the child should come under the care of an experienced physical director from the day of entrance to regular school life. A physical examination should be made that would determine the condition of heart, lungs, spine, muscles, skin, eyes and ears. Many a case of incipient disease that eventuates in disaster would be discovered and put in the care of a physician, if necessary, or a correct regimen of diet, sleep, exercise, etc., inaugurated, with the aid of the parents, that would counteract the tendency to disease or deformity, and save the child as a useful member of society. Countries abroad with far less financial resources than our own, such as Switzerland, Germany, Sweden, Denmark, France and Italy have long since taken such a step; and there is a public school for girls in Massachusetts where a similar examination prevails.

The *Sun* in a recent editorial called attention to the unsatisfactory results attending military instruction in colleges; and it is a very significant fact that Dr. Charles R. Greenleaf, Lieutenant-Colonel and Surgeon U. S. A., was specially detailed by Secretary Proctor to attend the meeting in Boston, and read a paper on "Physical Training in the Regular Army," in which he spoke of the necessity of supplementing the drills and manual of arms by more complete and systematized gymnastic exercise. The outgrowth of his visit was the appointment of a committee of medical men to urge upon Congress the authorization of a professorship of physiology, hygiene and physical training, at the United States Military Academy of West Point. Gymnasia have been erected at many outposts and it is intended to use the revenue from the canteen fund for their support.

Dr. Wey's successful labors in effecting mental and moral progress through physical training of youthful criminals at the Elmira Reformatory is another most interesting phase of this movement. He believes that the primary education of many criminals and defects should be the education of the body and the building up and strengthening of the brain. To force or develop a brain whose habitation is attenuated and architecturally inharmonious, whose nervous system is vitiated, is to produce a mental dyspeptic—to cram the mind with scholastic lore and moral platitudes in excess of its physical strength. First, let the scheme of training or reformation embrace the bringing to the highest attainable degree of perfection the physical man, and coincidently the brain will participate in the work of physical improvement. The work of physical education to be successful should be carried on in a three-fold line ; muscular amplification and structural enlargement, not mere increase in size but increase in structure, to arrest defects transmitted or acquired through environment or defective modes of living; the bath (Turkish) as a stimulus and means of bringing the various members of the body into greater harmony; and a dietary suitable to supply energy of the kind best adapted to the adjustment of mind to body." I cherish the hope that physical training which has thus risen to the dignity of preventive medicine, will prove a helpful resource in the development of the FEEBLE MINDED brain. Plato said to train the mind and neglect the body was to *produce* a cripple. More and more is it being appreciated that mental development begins with and depends upon purely physiological processes. Dr. Seguin wanted a way into a dormant mind and found it through the "Training of an Idiotic Hand." The occupations of the Kindergarten represent a successful approach to this lethargic and unquickened realm. Permanency of result necessitates structural improvement. It is easier to act upon the centres from the periphery than upon the periphery from the centres (Seguin).

Physical training has proved itself in the case of youthful criminals and dullards "an end to cerebral activity and mental increase"—mental development and culture ignoring the fact of a physical basis soon resolves itself into a study of pathology and morbid anatomy (Wey).

The test of the "good and faithful servant" specifies the comforts and help accorded the *physical* man ; moralizing seems a better application afterwards.

There is abundant evidence that our disdainful brains are largely indebted to the muscles for their start in life and that there is a distinct order in which the various motor centres develop through outside stimulus; and presumptive proof that these transmitted stimuli not only lead to increased central growth, but may effect contiguous motor areas. The researches of Dr. Wilmarth, of Elwyn, Pa., on the pathology of feeble minded brains (a report of 100 cases) temper one's enthusiasm somewhat, but what else can you better invoke in behalf of these defective ones than aids to improved nutrition and circulation ? To such as have faith in physical methods, commends itself, in my judgment a trial of the Swedish educational gymnastics, and I am glad to have the encouragement of Dr. Fort's Institution near Ellicott City, Md., where this system is now being introduced. In conclusion, what of the influence of this awakening in bodily culture on the profession ? Is it not an opportunity to insist more and more in practice that "there is only one rational method of treating the sick and that it consists in so relating the individual affected to the cause of his disease, as to make him not only intelligent on the subject but at the same time conscientious regarding it?"

The Sanitaria of this country are doing effective work in thus stimulating an enlightened public conscience. These were the first temples of Aesculapius, and are to-day renewing their youth under the best medical auspices.

The great question of the future is more and more tending to the prevention of disaase. Hygiene and sanitation are opening the way. Brilliant as is the most recent discovery in bacteriology, its illustrious author would probably be the first to admit, in the words of another, that "exactly the kind of cases most likely to be benefited through its means, have long since been known to be greatly improved and often cured by hygiene and dietetic treatment." Let us invoke first the *natural* germicidal and antiseptic powers of healthy tissues and normal functions. A hopeful writer classes the tuberculoses among the preventable diseases and says, "fresh air and an abundance of it, the increased capacity of the chest, the disinfection of the products of disease thrown off by its victims, the inspection of animals and meat, the application of sufficient heat to all foods, these are the agencies which will eventually lessen the ravages of the 'bacillus tuberculosis.'"

Foods, habits and other incidents of life being daily and continuous must exert a far greater influence on constitutional tendencies than medicine or treatment which are occasional and varying. The man who improves on food products, ventilation, exercise, etc., will thus confer the greatest benefit on the community.

The combination of science and popular experiment represented by the work in Boston of Mr. Edward Atkinson's food laboratory and the New England Kitchen, is of the highest importance to every physician and practical philanthropist; for it does not seem likely that either will ever be independent of the problem of nutrition in their labors for the maintenance of health, the cure of disease or the social and moral amelioration of the poor and afflicted. "For the first time it is believed that standard dishes—one of which is beef broth for invalids—have been prepared on scientific principles with such exactness that they may be duplicated in every particular like an apothecary's prescription." If with renewed investigations into sanitary chemistry the future shall bring us those data on which an exact science can be based; and emphasis be laid on the sacredness of physiological laws and the duty of bodily training, then the importance of the physician to the State will be better realized, and the era of preventive medicine more generally and acceptably inaugurated.

N. B.—The Swedish System has given most encouraging results with the feeble-minded in the institution where I introduced it last winter.   (Dec. 15.)

THE PHYSICAL TRAINING OF THE FEEBLE MINDED.

By Sam'l J. Fort, M. D.

The need of Exercise is Physiological, the Desire for Exercise Inherent.

Every living being that has long been motionless experiences a need for action, and it is this need for exercise which cause human beings, and even those animals in a lower scale of development, to perform actions necessary to the preservation of health ; prolonged repose then, excites a desire for muscular exercise, just as sustained work produces a need for repose. Insufficient exercise causes the intricate machinery of the body to become clogged by the accumulation of reserve materials which should be consumed as fast as produced, and this accumulation of organic debris excites a desire for exercise, which shall, as it were open the draughts and start the fire into activity. The need for exercise may also arise from a general sluggishness of the bodily functions, and a consequent desire for a stimulus sufficient to whip up the torpid vital forces, Says Lagrange,* "the need for burning too abundant reserves, the need for drawing more oxygen into the system, these are the two causes which join in producing the manifestation of the instinct which leads every living being to perform muscular work."

"Bodily work" says the same author, "is work done with the object of perfecting the human organism from the point of view of strength, skill or health," and as may be readily seen the scientific analogy between actual work, such as is done by the laborer, is identical with the physical exercise taken by the gentleman of leisure or the man of sedentary pursuits. Now work is one or a series of movements, and

*Physiology of Bodily Exercise,

these movements are made by the muscles, the fleshy masses which surround the different parts of the skeleton. These muscles possess the power of contracting i. e., shortening and approaching of one end to the other. When a muscle or series of muscles contract, there is a tension made upon bones to which they are attached, and through the systems of levers made by the bones and joints, traction is converted into flexion, extension, supination and pronation. This ability to contract is latent, until excited by some stimulus outside of the muscle. The most common stimulus is the *will*, though mechanical, physical, electrical or chemical action will bring about decided contractions and movements. From the extreme quickness with which *willing* and *doing* takes place, it would seem that the will acts directly upon the muscle, but there are intermediate organs to transmit its orders, the intricate meshwork of nerves ramifying throughout the entire body, connecting the most distant parts of the body with the great nervous centres, the brain and spinal cord.

To study the esoteric effects of muscular work upon the organism is not within the limits of this writing; it is only necessary to lay down as a proposition that the results of such work vary, according to the quantity done and the method by which it is done.

Such work or exercise performed without rule and without moderation induces fatigue and subsequently actual injuries. Systematically pursued the same exercises satisfy a physiological need, and bring about a certain adaptability of the entire organism to more active and violent exercises. The machinery of the body improves in its working ability, its parts are all strengthened, and friction is reduced to the minimum. It must also be considered that, as all the bodily organs are not the same and do not perform the same work in exercising, the exercises must be adapted to such differences, and further, the *quantity* of work needed, the nature or *quality* of work, and the *mechanism* by which the work is to be performed, must be carefully planned.

In adapting a system of exercise to a body disordered by disease, it is readily seen why that body must be studied, its various members separately and together, the muscular groups mapped out and their mechanism thoroughly understood, and for such cases we have the well known Swedish Movement Cure, and the more recent, perhaps more thoroughly scientific, "Medical Gymnastics," an outgrowth of the system of gymnastics originated by the great Ling, which is destined to become an exceedingly interesting branch of medical science, an invaluable aid to the orthopedic surgeon; and the gynecologist and especially valuable to the neurologist. The feeble minded child may enjoy the best of physical health, and it is of such I desire to speak, referring those with actual deformities to the above named system which is better adapted to their physical needs. In making choice of a system which is intended to train the bodies of mentally defective children, very much the same movements would be given as would serve the same purpose with the normal child, except, that with the former we would find the necessity of great simplicity until the child might be made capable of utilizing more complicated movements. This brings us to the consideration of a question demanding the attention of scholars through all the ages of which we have records, and to which question each successive age has given its reply. To fill the requirements of the present age, such a system must* "develop the whole body and its parts symmetrically and harmoniously; must preserve, increase or produce bodily health, strength and proportion, and maintain and promote physical activity, dexterity and efficiency." As has been said, the child with feeble mind must have a simple series of movements at the beginning of its physical training, for if the normal child's brain may be considered similar to a seven-octave piano, that of the weaker would be equivalent to an instrument with but five or six, and moreover we shall find physical conditions in defective children not far removed from deformities which our system should correct; these are,—

Round shoulders.

Contracted chests.

*Enebuske.

Peculiar gaits.

Habitually walking and standing with feet and legs apart.

Lower jaw dropped.

Automatic movements.

Superflexion of extremities, with lack of perfect extension.

Insufficient peristaltic action.

Weak circulation.

Lack of voluntary and superabundance of involuntary co-ordination.

I had the honor to present to this Faculty the adaptability of the Kindergarten to the education of feeble minded children, and I desire to call your attention to-day to a system of gymnastics which seems theoretically satisfactory to the physical needs of that class of dependents, and which has been introduced with most gratifying results in my own home school.

It is known as the Ling system of educational gymnastics, first introduced into Sweden by P. H. Ling, in 1813. The fundamental proposition of this system is, "to make the body subservient to the will," at the same time increasing and maintaining health, strength, activity, dexterity and muscular efficiency. It begins by thoroughly developing the fundamental functions of the body, *i. e.*, the circulation and respiration, and following out this line of reasoning believes that muscular *strength* follows hard upon the heels of a training which promotes the physical well-being of the heart and lungs. We have seen that muscle has an innate tendency to contract, and that muscular work is nothing but resistance to this contraction; such a resistance is then a proper training for the muscles concerned and increases the supply of oxygenated blood to them, as well as increasing drainage of waste products from the system. Children pursuing the routine duties of the class-room, even those who are engaged in the more carefully planned exercises of the Kindergarten, are more or less in a condition in which the slightest physical distortions are exaggerated. The thorax is compressed, the shoulders thrown forward or perhaps sagged to one side, the head sinks forward, the back is arched, the limbs are twisted or flexed, and the circulation and respiration embarrassed. Now, to obviate these distortions, which readily become habits, it is necessary to first overcome them by proper training, and then carry on this training until the physique becomes impressed or habituated to a proper self control; in other words to substitute a bad habit by a good habit. This is the sum and substance of all training, to so saturate mind and body with ideas that willing and doing become automatic. To properly comprehend the educational gymnastics a general idea of which is called a "day's order," is necessary. There would be first, "order movements," which serve to attract the child's attention and bring him into the so-called "fundamental position," which is nothing more than a position best adapted to the proper exercise of physiological function, from which correct movements start, and to which they return before a relaxed position of rest is assumed. Second, "leg movements," which increase the circulation of the extremities, relieving any passive congestions of the trunk and brain. Third, movements called "strain-bending and heave movements," which expand the chest and induce more complete inspiration and expiration. These may be termed typical movements, and their combined results are : more richly oxygenated blood is sent to the muscles, the mind is relieved from one line of thought and placed upon another, the will is centred upon muscular response, and the body prepared for the more specific movements. These are first, the "balance movements," which bring, about a co-ordination of muscular contraction in all parts of the body, and by demanding equilibrium in difficult positions, train the sense of graceful and correct posture.

Second, "movements of the back," which correct the carriage of the back and the shoulder blades, and by equalizing the strength of the muscles on both sides of the vertebral column, counteract the faulty growth of the spine.

Third, "movements for the abdomen and forepart of the body," which stimulate the abdominal organs by an alternating increase and decrease of abdominal pressure.

These movements strengthen the muscles of the abdominal walls, as do the next following, the "alternate side movements;" these latter also training the mobility of the ribs and vertebra, and stimulating the spinal nerves.* All these movements are graduated in force, culminating in what is termed the "optimum," which is the point where a full, free and undisturbed respiration may be taken during the movement. This is an absolute requirement, and if by inadvertence, breathlessness or over-action of the heart is brought about, resort is made at once to movements which quiet and bring the respiration and circulation to the normal.

Having now prepared the system for more vigorous movements, the running and jumping exercises are brought in, and for a short space of time involve a high degree of exertion, approaching, but never exceeding, the proper demands upon heart and lungs, and attaining the acme of complication in training the co-ordination of willing and doing. These are now followed by the slow measured "leg movements," accompanied by deep rhythmic breathing, which tranquilize the action of the heart and prepare the body for rest. Connected most intimately with the hygenic basis of the system is a natural progression in the intricacy of the movements, expressed by the term "gymnastic progression," each "day's order" bearing a distinct relation to the next following, but increasing the demand for volitional control, and efficiency of circulation and respiration, and each "order" may be modified or amplified by the teacher as occasion demands, the system being limited alone by the movements the body is capable of making. As a class attains a certain degree of precision of movement, marches and gymnastic games and dances are introduced. In these the pupils are trained to cooperate in movements gradually increasing in complexity, demanding a maximum of self-control, that each individual shall be able to maintain his place in line, a correct pose, and the closest possible attention to the movements of others, that the rhythm of the evolutions shall not be marred. While many of the marches and movements are

*Gymnastic Progression, by Claes Enebuske, Ph. D.

too complicated for use in classes of feeble-minded children, demanding an exactness of muscular co-ordination, puzzling to those with full complement of senses, the *natural progression*, the constant observation of physiological needs seem to mark this system as an ideal physical training. We find in it an easy method of overcoming the intense inertiæ of the child with arrested mental development, and having stimulated him to move and enjoy movement, there is still something ahead, something to look forward to, and practically an unlimited series of movements within reach of the teacher from which may be selected those best adapted to develop the awakening will.

If the brain is imperfectly developed or weakened by overwork, or we have in hand the brain of a normal, but as yet undeveloped child, elementary exercises must be chosen and lead up from them to the more complicated. This is a point sadly neglected heretofore by physical instructors who have not appreciated the advantages of *easy exercises*, which may be summed up as follows!—production of *muscular* fatigue without a corresponding *nervous* fatigue, quickening of the blood current, more complete respiratory effort, and stimulation of the digestive functions, without excessive stimulation of the cerebral functions, that accompanies difficult exercises. Besides these points, the simple exercises we have mentioned are within the power of the spinal cord to reproduce at slight excitation ; in other words to become automatic.

If we have a normal child to train, until its reasoning powers are developed, we insist upon implicit obedience without explaining why the command is given, and presently when the child finds that effect follows cause, that punishment invariably follows disobedience, even as the fire burns whenever his finger is placed in contact with it, then right behavior becomes a second nature, a habit.

In the individual whose mind is below the normal, the reasoning power is weak, in proportion, perhaps, to the brain defect, whatever its classification, and in training such persons it is necessary to furnish a programme of existence which shall embody the conditions demanded by polite society.   By persistent repetition the exercises of politeness and good behavior become fixed and need little, if any, exertion of the brain to produce.   Is it not clear, then, that given vicious physical habits, such as we find in feeble minded children, these must be eradicated by a system of training based upon what we know of anatomy and physiology, and by such training substitute habits we know to be correct?

The gymnasium of to-day is all very well in its place, but its province is surely not with children whose muscular and nervous systems are in a state of development or permanently weakened or defective.   Neither is it proper that the human body should be taught to ape the capers and contortions of the circus; its education should surely be placed upon a higher plane.   But, if considered a necessity to carry the youth on into a system of gymnastics, where other apparatus than his own body or ordinary furniture is necessary, let a plea be entered for this educational physical training, that at least, the growing, rapidly developing child may have some preliminary training which shall give him a certain control of his powers.

In adopting anything out of the ordinary routine it is well not to be too sanguine of results.   In my own school, I have already seen a marked improvement in carriage and ordinary movements of those children found capable of comprehending such movements as the teacher, trained by Dr. E. M. Schaeffer of our body and a pioneer worker in this line, has deemed properly adapted to the individual cases, and I hope later on to present you with certain statistics relative to the system as applied to our training.   I am of the opinion that every institution devoted to the care of feeble minded persons or epileptics, should have as a member of its official staff a physician, who should be thoroughly trained in medical and pedagogic gymnastics; whose duties should be to classify and train every child capable of receiving such training.   A set of assistants might be trained from among the corps of teachers, who could be trusted to give the "day's orders" under proper oversight.   He would also establish a clinic in which would be applied medical gymnastics, a treatment already foreshadowed by orthopedic surgeons.   I am

further of the opinion that the feeble-minded child has had
too little attention given to its physical training. If we have
these deformities of habit combined with a defective brain, is
it not logical to reason that one hampers the improvement of
the other? There are many children in this class whom I
would take at as early an age as possible and let the physical training begin with the mental training and be carried on
coincident with it, or as Enebuske says, "as soon as the child
is put to intellectual exercises which demand a volitional
concentration of mental force, there should begin, to counter-
balance it, a drill demanding the volitional concentration of
physical powers."

ONE HUNDRED CONSECUTIVE CASES OF LABOR AT THE MARYLAND MATERNITÉ.
WITH NOTES.

By George H. Rohé, M. D., Director,

AND

Samuel H. Allen, M. D., Resident Physician.

[Being the second series of one hundred cases and a continuation of the report read before the Medical and Chirurgical Faculty of Maryland at its annual session in 1890.]

The antiseptic methods practised in the Maternité Hospital, together with the care and treatment of the patients before, during and after labor, were described fully in a report read before the Faculty one year ago, and will therefore not be repeated in this paper. The results of the methods in use at this institution demonstrate beyond the shadow of a doubt that the advances of modern midwifery have placed this once sadly neglected science on the exalted plane now occupied by its sister sciences—modern surgery and gynæcology. Though this paper is chiefly statistical in its nature, yet we trust it will prove an addition of some value to the recent literature on obstetrics. Many unwarranted speculations and ancient errors must be relegated to the regions of eternal oblivion in the face of the carefully observed and properly interpreted phenomena and accurately recorded facts in hundreds of cases. These and these alone can form the foundation of any branch of medicine deserving the name of a science. The cases reported below are taken from the records of the Maternité in a consecutive series beginning with January 22, 1890, when the report presented last year ended.

Color.—Of the 100 cases included in this report there were 62 white and 38 black; total 100 patients.

Age.—The oldest was 40 years; the youngest was 14 years; average age 23.

Nativity.—Maryland 53, Virginia 21, Pennsylvania 8, North Carolina 3, West Virginia 1, Rhode Island 1, Massachusetts 1, Louisiana 1, Florida 1, District of Columbia 1, Germany 5, Ireland 2, Australia 1, Russia 1. Americans 91, foreigners 9 ; total 100.

Paræ.—There were 61 primiparæ and 39 multiparæ ; total 100.

Height.—Average height of patients 5 feet, 2½ inches.

Pelvic measurements.—Average, of the hundred cases, between the anterior superior spinous processes, 9⅔ inches, between the iliac crests 10 1-3 inches, from the symphysis pubis to the posterior part of last lumbar vertebra 7⅛ inches.

Beginning of menstruation: earliest at the 8th year, latest at the 19th year ; average time of beginning of menstruation between the 13th and 14th year.

Time when labor began : in 34 cases, between 9 P. M. and 3 A. M.; in 22 cases, between 1 and 7 P. M. It is a very common occurrence for labor to begin just after dinner or after supper.

Average length of the stages of labor.—First stage: primiparæ 17 hours, multiparæ 11 hours, combined average for both, 15 hours, 30 minutes. Second stage : primiparæ 1 hour and 40 minutes, multiparæ 1 hour, combined average 1 hour and 25 minutes. Third stage: primiparæ 19 minutes, multiparæ 16 minutes; combined average 17 minutes.

Rupture of the membranes.—Spontaneously in 88 cases, punctured in 12. Only when the non-rupture of the membranes delays the progress of labor are they interferred with. In two cases the child was born in a caul.

Hydramnion.—Case: registered No. 1657: M. M., white, æt, 28, multipara. Labor progressed very slowly, os dilated only sufficiently to admit two fingers. Excess of liquor amnii was diagnosticated by Dr. Samuel H. Allen, who punctured the membranes. Some water escaped, the pains became very strong, the os dilated rapidly and the child was soon born, followed by about 3 quarts of amniotic fluid.

Umbilical cord.—Longest 35½ inches, shortest 10 inches; average 22¼ inches. Spirals in cord, from right to left 60 cases, left to right 23, straight 13, irregular 4; total 100. The cord usually contained from 4 to 6 varicosities, rarely any knots, and was in the majority of cases inserted into the placenta 2½ inches from its edge.

About 20 per cent. of the cases were in labor when admitted to the hospital. In one case delivery took place while we were assisting the patient up the stairway, the child being born while the woman was in the erect posture. The umbilical cord broke about 6 inches from the child's abdomen and was not ligated for some time, as there was no hæmorrhage. The child was uninjured.

Placenta.—Method of delivery: Crede method 87, spontaneous delivery 10, manual extraction 3; total 100.

Weight.—Heaviest, 1 pound and 14 ounces; lightest, 11 ounces; average 1 pound and 4 ounces.

Position when delivered.—Maternal side out 21 cases; fœtal side out, 79 cases; total 100.

For about one hour after the birth of the child, the uterus is kept firmly contracted by the hand of the nurse or physician, applied to the fundus. Out of the last 200 confinements at the Ma'ernite, there has not been a severe case of postpartum hæmorrhage. Bleeding from cervical, vaginal and perineal tears has occasionally been quite free, but has never been such as to cause any apprehension or give rise to any trouble. With the proper management of the third stage of labor, we maintain that severe post-partum hæmorrhage should rarely occur. In one case the placenta was of the normal size; 8 inches long; 7½ broad, ½ inch thick and had attached to it by a narrow band composed of blood vessels, a small placenta, 3½ inches long, 2 inches broad and ¼ inch thick. There was only one child in this case. Since January 24, 1890, the date of the first case included in this report to the time of writing, there have been 4 pairs of twins born in the hospital. In the first of these there were two placentæ with separate sets of membranes. In the second case there was one large sac the cavity of which was occupied partly by the first fœtus and its liquor amnii and partly by another bag of membranes containing the second fœtus and liquor amnii.

A partition composed of four layers of membrane (amnion and chorion of each sac), separated the amniotic cavities in the last two cases. In the last three cases there was but one placenta in each case.

Perineum.—Ruptured to the 3rd degree 1 case, 2nd degree 20 cases; 1st degree 17 cases; intact 62; total 100.

Drugs used.—Ergot in 20, chloroform in 11, quinine in 5, no drugs used in 64 cases; total 100.

We never give ergot until the placenta has been expelled, and then only when there is hæmorrhage, or the uterus remains large and flabby, as after anæsthesia or very protracted labors.

In two cases the pains seemed to be increased by 15 gr. doses of quinine, though we have not used it in enough cases to claim for it any oxytocic properties.

Operations performed.—Forceps applied in 9, version in 2 cases.

Case: registered No. 1595, J. F., white, aged 23, primipara. Began to have convulsions January 25, 1890, at 12.30 A. M. Labor began at 10 A. M., same day. Simpson's forceps were applied to the head by Dr. W. J. Todd, at 9 P. M., after the patient had had 15 convulsions. Child still-born. Mother continued to have convulsions and died January 25, at 12.55 P. M.

Case: registered No. 1619, E. M., white, aged 33, multipara. Child delivered by Dr. Rohé with Simpson's forceps, March 1, 1890.

Case: registered No. 1612: twins, L. J., black, aged 19, multipara. Labor began March 7th, 1890, 12 M., and ended the same at 7.12 P. M. First child presented left sacro anterior and was born without any delay. Second child presented transversely. The patient was partially anæsthetised with chloroform and podalic version performed by Dr. Rohé, by introducing his hand into the uterus and securing the feet. The child was delivered alive without any difficulty.

Case: registered No. 1615: M. E. S., colored, aged 19, primipara. Fœtus presented right sacro anterior. Labor progressed very slowly. As there was evidence of uterine inertia and the patient was becoming exhausted, she was chloroformed and Dr. Rohe introduced his hand into the uterus bringing down the feet.   The after coming head was stopped by the rigid perineum.   Simpson's forceps were applied and the child delivered without lacerating the perineum. The child was apparently asphyxiated.   The funis was ligated at once and the infant dipped in cold then in hot water, rapidly alternating.   A towel was placed over its mouth and air blown into the lungs several times by the mouth-to-mouth method.   Then the Schultze method was tried and in 30 minutes after the child was born it began to breathe.   Mother and child discharged in good condition.

Case: registered No. 1624: M. B., white, æt., 17, primipara. Convulsions, death ; child lived.   Labor began April 25, 1890, at 9 A. M., and the first stage ended next morning at 7 A. M.   At 9.25, April 26, patient had a convulsion, also had another very severe one at 10 A. M.   Simpson's forceps were applied by Dr. Wm. S. Gardner, and the child delivered alive at 10.05 A. M.   Patient had eighteen convulsions after child was born, and died next morning at 2 A. M.

Case: registered No. 1650: F. R., black, æt., 40, primipara, admitted May 22, at 9 P. M., having been in labor five days. Her history was as follows: She had been married 24 years and had never been pregnant.   Twelve months before we saw her a physician dilated her cervix for dysmenorrhœa and soon after this she became pregnant.   Labor began May 18. The child presented left sacro anterior.   The labor dragged slowly on for five days, during which time three physicians had seen the case, but failed to deliver the woman.   At the end of the 5th day she was brought into the hospital and at once chloroformed.   The feet were brought down by Dr. Rohé inserting his hand into the uterus; while traction was made on the feet, pressure was made on the fundus uteri until the body was delivered.   The head was so firmly engaged that traction on the feet failed to move it at all.   Simpson's, Hodge's and Tarnier's forceps were applied in turn to the after-coming head by Drs. Rohé and W. S. Gardner, but all slipped.   The hook ends of the Hodge forceps were now inserted, one into the right orbital cavity, the other into the posterior fontanelle. Steady traction was made several times, when the head and placenta came away at the same time. The child was dead when the woman came into the hospital. The third day after delivery the patient's pulse and temperature rose, the lochia had a very offensive odor, the uterus was large, tender on pressure and hard to outline. For three days M.xv of ergot was given every two hours. Vaginal douches of a warm solution of corrosive sublimate, 1-4000, were given three times a day and once a day the uterus was washed out with the same kind of solution, 1-5000, by means of Dr. W. S. Gardner's intra-uterine catheter. The pulse and temperature came down, the abdominal tenderness disappeared and the patient made an excellent and speedy recovery.

Case : registered 1647: L. M., white æt. 36, primipara. Labor began June 27, 11.30 A. M.; in 24 hours the patient showed signs of exhaustion. The pains were weak from the first, though the first stage of labor was ended in 22 hours. The natural powers were plainly unable to expel the fœtus, and, after chloroforming the patient, the child, which presented right occiput anterior, was safely delivered with Simpson's forceps by Dr. W. S. Gardner.

Case: registered No. 1682: C. B., black, æt. 18, primipara. Labor began August 19, at 8.50 P. M.; at 11.40 P. M. patient began to have convulsions. After the second convulsion Simpson's forceps were applied by Dr. Samuel H. Allen, and the child delivered alive at 1 A. M., August 20th. The mother had seven convulsions after the child was born, but made a good recovery.

Case: registered No. 1694: placenta previa hæmorrhage; A. B., white, æt. 20, primipara. Hæmorrhage was noticed by the patient as soon as her pains began, which was on September 7th, at 1 P. M. It was quite profuse and coming from the os, which was dilated sufficiently to admit two fingers. The patient was put to bed, given bromide of potash and chloral, and the vagina tamponed by direction of Dr. Rohé. The hæmorrhage ceased. The child was lying transversely in the uterus. Next day the patient was chloroformed and cephalic version by external manipulation performed by Dr. Gardner.   The tampon was removed, but the hæmorrhage did not recur, though the placenta was attached near the margin of the internal os.   After version, the labor was allowed to go on naturally, but as it was lingering, and the mother becoming quite weak, Dr. Gardner applied Simpson's forceps and delivered the child alive at 6.30 A. M., September 9th.   Mother and child left the hospital September 25th in good condition.

Case: registered No. 1684: A. S., white, æt. 22, primipara. Pains began September 12th, at noon.   They were quite severe, though the labor was slow and exhausting the patient's strength.   The position of the child was left occipito anterior.   On the morning of September 14th the child was delivered safely by Dr. Gardner with Simpson's forceps, which were on the head 20 minutes.   On the second day after labor the patient's pulse beat 140 to the minute and the temperature rose to 101°.   Patient complained of tenderness over the bladder and was unable to pass her water.   The urine was offensive to the smell, of a whitish color, and was so thick it would hardly run through a catheter.   The bladder was washed out twice through a soft rubber catheter, with a weak boracic acid solution, and immediately the pulse and temperature came down to normal.

There were four other cases of cystitis which were treated successfully in the same way.

Presentation and position of children.—Left occipito anterior 56 cases, right occipito anterior 34, right occipito posterior 3, left sacro anterior 3, right sacro anterior 2, right scapula anterior 1, left mento anterior 1; total 100.   Born alive 97, still-born 4; total 101.   One child died from umbilical hæmorrhage.   The cord was tied by the nurse and the child wrapped in a blanket and placed near the stove, as it was a premature child and we had some difficulty in getting respiration started.   In two hours after it was born the nurse took it out of the blanket and noticed the hæmorrhage.   It had lost about an ounce of blood and died in half an hour.

Sex of the children.—Males 54, females 47 ; total 101.   Of the four cases of twins alluded to above, only one pair falls within the 100 cases included in this report.

Sex of the twins.—First and second pairs, all males; third pair 1 male and 1 female; fourth pair, both females. All were born alive.

Length.—Average length 19½ inches.

Weight of children at birth.—Heaviest, 10 pounds, 4 ounces; lightest, 3 pounds, 5 ounces ; average, 6 pounds, 12 ounces.

At the end of the third day the child loses about 6 ounces, while at the end of the sixth day it weighs about the same as at birth.

Diameters of the fœtal head.—Occipito frontal 4½ inches, occipito mental 5⅓, sub-occipito bregmatic 3¾, biparietal 3½.

Circumferences.—Occipito frontal 13, sub-occipito bregmatic 12, shoulders 12½; chest: expiration 11, inspiration 12½; hips 9½ inches.

It is not uncommon to find milk in the breasts of children soon after birth. It was present in seven cases: girls 4, boys 3. If the breasts become hard and the children restless, the breasts are rubbed with sweet oil and kept covered with warm wet cloths for a day or two. Two cases of infantile convulsions due to elongated and inflamed prepuce were cured by slitting the foreskin. Congenital hydrocele was noted twice.

Ichthyosis was present in one case. The child's skin was dry, shining and divided up into regular patches of scales, each scale being about ⅛ of an inch square. These scales would flake off freely, but there were large patches of them when the mother, a negress, brought the child back to the hospital for observation two weeks after it was discharged. Otherwise the child was all right. Wherever the scales had disappeared the skin was as dry and shining as at birth.

Icterus neonatorum was well marked in one case. It improved under minute doses of calomel.

Caput succedaneum in one case made a tumor on the occiput 3½ inches long ; it disappeared in six days.

One child had six fingers on the right hand and another had six on its left hand. One woman had six toes on her right foot.   There was an extra lobe attached by a thin pedicle to the left ear of one child.

Four children were tongue tied.   The parents of one child were mutes; but it cried vigorously as soon as it was born.

Ophthalmia neonatorum.—There were three cases, two of which developed on the first day.   The third was a case of ophthalmia simplex and under the use of simple astringent eye washes soon got well.   Vaginal douches of 1-4000 bichloride of mercury were given to each of the mothers of the first two cases before the child was born and a 1 pr. ct. solution of silver nitrate dropped into the children's eyes as soon as they were born.   In one of these cases the mother had several venereal warts on the labia and a decided case of specific vaginitis.   There was one slight opacity left in the right eye of the first child and a small one in each eye of the child of the patient with the venereal warts.   No eyes were lost. A one per cent. solution of silver nitrate is dropped into the eyes of every child as soon as it is born, and the vagina of the mother is thoroughly washed out with solution of mercuric chloride during the first and second stages of labor, partly as a prophylatic measure against ophthalmia.   Nitrate of silver, sulphate of zinc, boracic acid and iodoform are the drugs we use in the treatment of this disease.   During the inflammatory stage, most excellent results are obtained from applying to the eyelids every three minutes small strips of muslin taken from a piece of ice.   These applications are kept up for two hours at a time and made two or three times a day.

Syphilis in the mother.—A. J., colored aged 28, delivered of the seventh child, April 8th, 1890.   The child was stillborn.   Six of her children were still born, the seventh one lived two weeks.   Patient gave a clear history of syphilis and presented the characteristic lesions on different parts of her body.

Episiotomy.—Case: registered No. 1656, L. G., white, aged 21, primipara.   Confined June 6th.   In this case there was a very uncommon arrangement of the labia minora. They were continuous posteriorly forming a tough unyielding band which would not stretch sufficiently to allow the exit of the child's head from the vulvar fissure. After waiting half an hour episiotomy was resorted to by Dr. Allen and the child was born at once.

Fibroids.—Fibroid tumors were found on the uteri of two patients, one white and one black. In the former only one could be found while in the latter three were felt very plainly through the abdominal walls. All of them were small and did not interfere with labor. A small polypus was found growing from the cervix of a woman who had been a sufferer from menorrhagia and dysmenorrhœa some time before she became pregnant. It was torn off by the child during the second stage of labor.

Extreme after pains.—A. H., Black, aged 22, multipara, confined Sept. 7th, 3 53 P. M. The after pains were very severe. The patient suffered much; she became violent, tossed herself wildly about in bed and screamed with each pain. She was chloroformed and a piece of membrane and blood clot were removed from the uterus by the hand. The pains became less severe and the patient slept that night without any hypnotic.

Albuminuria.—Eclampsia.—The urine of each patient is analysed the first day after she is admitted, again on the first day after labor and also on the eighth day after labor. More analyses are made if the patient comes in two or three months before she expects to be confined or if any abnormal conditions point to renal disturbances. Albumin was found in the urine of 22 of the 100 cases. In six cases before and 19 cases after labor. In a few cases it was found before and after labor. In most of these cases the presence of albumin did not give rise to any disturbances of health, though in . some the feet and legs were much swollen. There were four cases of convulsions—two of the women died and two recovered. A glance at the following summary will give the salient points in each case.

CASE I.—Registered No. 1595; age 23, white, primipara; forceps used; delivered January 25, 1890; 17 convulsions before and 15 after delivery; no albumin present, treated with chloroform, jaborandi, morphine. Mother died, child was still-born.

CASE II.—Registered No. 1624; age 19, white, primipara; forceps used, delivered April 26, 1890; 2 convulsions before and 18 after delivery; albumin present before labor; treated with chloroform, jaborandi, morphine, venesection. Mother died, child lived.

CASE III.—Registered No. 1658; age 28, white, primipara; no forceps; delivered June 14, 1890; 4 convulsions after delivery; albumin after convulsions began; treated with chloroform, bromide, chloral; mother and child lived.

CASE IV.—Registered No. 1682; age 18, black, primipara; forceps used; delivered August 19th, 1890; 2 convulsions before and 7 after delivery; albumin present before and after labor; treated with bromide, chloral, chloroform. Mother and child lived.

Results in the 100 cases: discharged well, 98, died of convulsions 2.

DISCUSSION.

Dr. J. E. Michael wanted to know about the average elevation of temperature. He also noticed a large number of R. O. A. This is one of the rare positions. This must be due to some peculiar circumstances. There may have been cases where the occiput had gone around and rotated. In regard to the use of quinine to stimulate the uterus, he had no facts to hand, but he had used it in preference to ergot. The subject of ophthalmia neonatorum is an interesting one. He does not use the nitrate of silver solution as prescribed. When he first took charge of the Lying-in Hospital he found many eyes lost and going. He adopted Crede's method and used a two per cent. solution, which did little good. This was due to laxness in nursing. Since he took charge he has used this treatment regularly and had had few cases.

Dr. Geo. H. Rohé said in closing, that there was a large proportion of R. O. A. In the large majority of cases the diagnosis is made in the first stage of labor, but as many come into the hospital in labor, the diagnosis might not always be reliable. This position may be the result of partial rotation. His attention had, of course, been called to this by the known statements in the text-books.

ACUTE MILIARY TUBERCULOSIS TREATED WITH KOCH'S TUBERCULIN.

By John C. Hemmeter, M. D., Phil. D., of Baltimore.

On January 30th, 1891, the writer was called to attend a case of very sudden high fever in a young lady aged sixteen years. The thermometer indicated a temperature of 105.5 on the first visit. Among other symptoms there were loss of appetite, dullness, severe headache. Notwithstanding the high fever the complexion was markedly pale, the lips and tips of the ears cyanotic. The patient had for over a year been afflicted with aphonia. At the time she was first seen her voice was scarcely above a whisper. The bowels had been regular up to the attack ; there was no tympanites, no abdominal tenderness or gurgling, no rose spots ; the spleen and liver were enlarged to percussion. There were no evidences of physical changes in the lung except those of an intense bronchial catarrh. The pulse was 128, respiration 48. Since there were no other local affections to be discovered to explain the symptoms, the writer suspected typhoid fever and concluded to await further development. The therapy consisted of antipyretic agents, a supporting stimulating diet and baths. During the first week, notwithstanding systematic nursing and bathing, (whenever the mercury rose above 103°,) the temperature rose to 105, within one hour after the bath. The bowels became constipated. The tongue remained remarkably clear and healthy looking. There were numerous round and small and medium sized rales all over the right lung.

During the second week the fever remained high and even rose to 106° and cerebral symptoms appeared, there was loss of consciousness preceded by disturbances of sight, diplopia and disturbances in the inervation of the ocular muscles. On the 12th day after the beginning of the fever there were still no abdominal symptoms and physical examination of the lungs gave no definite results except evidence of bronchitis. On the 15th day a soft pleuritic friction sound was detected at the base of the right lung. The temperature on this day varied between 104-106, at times going down to 100, which was, as a rule, the result of bathing.

The tongue was surprisingly clear up to this date, the complexion intensely pale with a definite cyanotic hue. By this time the doctors' attention was called to a sister of the patient who began ailing with a lung trouble, which, on examination, revealed a consolidation of the left apex. The expectoration of this girl contained bacilli. It was also determined that the father of these patients had died with pulmonary tuberculosis, and a brother with tubercular meningitis. It was desirable to obtain some sputum of the patient with the high continued fever, but in the comatose condition she swallowed all of the expectoration. Another very careful examination of the lung gave a negative result as regards consolidation. Almost every positive evidence was wanting except that of pleurisy at the base of the right lung. The contrast between the labored breathing and dysponœa and the insignificance of the physical signs was inexplicable. As there were still no signs of enteric fever and no possibility of examining for bacilli, I confessed myself unwilling to make a definite diagnosis and expressed the necessity of consultation.

Dr. I. E. Atkinson examined the patient very thoroughly on the 23d day of the disease, inquired from the family into the history of the case, with the condition of the evacuations and urine, and concluded from the result of his study that we had before us undoubtedly a case of acute general tuberculosis. As the relation had insisted on knowing the prospects of the patient, an absolutely fatal prognosis was given:

Two days after Dr. Atkinson had made his examination, some of the thick, yellow, glue-like expectoration was obtained by wiping it out of the patient's mouth; it contained an abundance of bacilli, and some little elastic tissue, with red blood corpuscles. The bowels were still costive, the urine contained traces of albumen. The patient had now been comatose for seven days.

On the 26th day it was impossible for me to see the patient. Dr. C. W. Mitchell paid the visit for me, making an examination. It might be said right here that Dr. Mitchell made a careful microscopic examination of the sputum later on and also found tubercle bacilli in it.

On the 3rd day after Dr. I. E. Atkinson and myself had arrived at the diagnosis, the treatment with parataloid was begun, the patient being as a rule comatose, answering questions, however, when aroused, was fed on liquid peptones and milk punch occasionally per rectum, when capable of being aroused by warmth. During the first reactions from the tuberculin, the temperature, notwithstanding cold baths, hyperdermics of the quinia, etc., continued to stand at 106 for two hours. The first injection consisted of .5 milligram of 1 per cent. solution of parataloid. At the 3d injection there followed in the period of reaction an epistaxis. The blood being treated like sputum with Ziehl's carbol fuchsin and subsequent methyline blue and sulphuric acid stain showed bacilli, 9 to one field of the Zeiss $\frac{1}{12}$ homogeneous immersion. At the 4th injection the reaction went to 104. In the reaction from the 5th injection the patient passed about two pints of urine, which was thick with blood.

A second consultation with Dr. I. E. Atkinson was held two weeks after the first. The patient had in meanwhile received 12 injections. The last contained 2 ctg. of parataloid. Consciousness had returned. Dr. Atkinson, on making another careful study of the case, discovered what had escaped me, a tumor about the size of a goose egg to the left of the umbilicus, and about one inch below. The possibilities of impacted fæces, malignant growth, floating kidney, uterus or enlarged ovaries were excluded, and it was made probable that what Prof. Atkinson had found was an enlarged tuberculous mass of mesenteric glands. Dr. Mitchell, on being requested to see the case for a second time, agreed with us on this point.

Injections into the tumor of parataloid have so reduced its size that to-day it is felt as a nodule about ¾ in. broad and 1 in. long. Below the tumor the abdomen was somewhat puffy in an area about 3 inches square, tough fibrous bands could be felt, as if they were in the peritoneum, running from the linea alba to the ant. sup. spin. process. As there seemed to be some fluctuation, the region was punctured with a sterilized hypodermic syringe; the fluid showed blood corpuscles, no bacilli. About this time Dr. Ed. F. Milholland was invited to examine the patient; he did so and inquired about the history from the family and believed that the patient was suffering from acute miliary tuberculosis.

The only positive criterion enabling one to draw a line between typhoid fever and acute general tuberculosis is the demonstration of the Eberth bacillus. There is no more difficult thing to establish than this, as the bacillus of tuberculosis and that of typhoid fever cannot be differentiated by staining; the only positive proofs of the presence of the typhoid bacillus are its peculiar growth on sterilized potato and the negative result on subjecting suspected cultures to the so-called indol reaction. The recognition of a characteristic growth upon sterilized potatoes is a matter requiring much experience, however, and in addition to this, the fæces of this patient were, as a rule, hard, and not in the least resembling typhoid evacuations. To make the indol test, a pure culture was necessary from the fæces. This again was next to impossible from the nature and consistency of the fæces, the amount of work involved and the certain presence of tubercle bacilli in the fæces derived from swallowed expectorations. Concerning this test we might insert in parenthesis, that all pure cultures of bacteria occurring in fæces, spring, river and canal water give a rose-red coloration to the following treatment, viz.: 10 cub. cent. of peptonized alkaline bouillon are inoculated with the suspected culture and allowed to remain 24 hours in a temperature best suited for the culture of the bacteria. Then 1 cub. cent. of a potassium nitrate solution (0.02 pot. nitrite to 100 water), and after this, 2 to 3 drops of concentrated sulphuric acid were added. If indol is present a red color appears. This color does not appear in case of pure cultures of typhoid bacilli. Strumphel holds that miliary tubercles are demonstrable in the choroid by means of the ophthalmoscope in acute general tuberculosis. The consultation of an experienced ophthalmoscopist was refused by the family of the patient, on the ground that four physicians had already observed the case and there seemed to be perfect agreement regarding its nature. As the injections of tuberculin were continued, a stronger injection being given every second day, the patient's general condition improved more and more. After this treatment had been kept up for six weeks, Dr. A. C. Abbott examined the sputum of the patient. He was supplied with two kinds of sputum—one kind from the expectoration on days when an injection of tuberculin had been given, another kind from expectoration on days when no injection had been given. Dr. Abbott found tubercle bacilli in the sputum from days on which the patient had been injected, none in the other sputum.

The amount of the injection was increased until the patient received 150. milligrams per diem without reaction of any kind. The disease began January 30th, 1891. The patient was discharged on May 20th, 1891, to sojourn to the mountains. She had gained very much in weight, had not coughed or expectorated in four weeks. There were no evidences of pulmonary disease to auscultation and percussion, except an area of dullness over the lower lobe of the right lung, posteriorly; the breathing over this region was vesicular. The dullness was supposed to be due to a thickened pleura. The tumor to the left and below the umbilicus was still discernible on using moderate pressure. It can hardly be called a tumor ; it feels like a small hard nodule or an enlarged lymph gland, about ½ inch broad and ¾ inch long. The voice is very husky, but at times clear. Owing to these latter signs the patient was not pronounced cured, but will be kept under observation.

Whatever view we take of the etiology of tuberculosis, we will not be much aided in diagnosis—anatomically the disease is an extremely abundant development of miliary tubercles in a comparatively short time in many organs of the body. It has been compared to an overfilling of the body with tubercle bacilli, which in some way reach the different organs at the same time and there give rise to the eruption of tubercles. A long time ago* Buhl advanced the hypothesis that a cheesy focus could be found somewhere in the body in every case of acute miliary tuberculosis, and that the general infection of the body resulted from the absorption of these caseous masses by the blood. Ponfick first found in some of these cases an extensive tuberculosis of the thoracic duct, with destruction of the tubercular new growth. It is easy to see how in this way a large amount of tubercular material could be brought directly into the circulation from the free communication of the lymph duct with the subclavian vein. Still more frequently, however, the tuberculosis of the large venous trunks, discovered by Weigert, especially of the pulmonary veins, seems to be the starting point. Usually there are tubercular lymph glands, or sometimes other foci of tubercular disease, which unite with a wall of a neighbor- ing vein, gradually break through it and project into its lumen. If caseation or ulceration result in this spot the infectious material is of course constantly washed off by the blood current and carried to other organs. Since such a tubercular focus, like a tubercular bronchial gland, may remain for a long time entirely without symptoms, we can understand how miliary tuberculosis may break out in an acute form in persons who previously seemed perfectly well. In other cases the patient has already suffered from some tubercular affection until suddenly the conditions occur somewhere in the body which lead to development of miliary tuberculosis. Thus we see it break out in a patient who has had ordinary phthisis, though it is one of the rarities in advanced phthisis. Miliary tuberculosis is a rather frequent sequel to pleural effusion in tubercular patients; miliary tuberculosis is seen in people with old tubercular affection of bones and joints, like coxitis and vertebral caries, and with tuberculosis of the genito-urinary organs and lymph glands. In all such cases of source the tubercular affection which is discovered during life need not always be the source of the general miliary tuberculosis, but the discovery of the existence of such an affection is of greatest significance in the diagnosis, as in this way our attention is directed to the possibility of a general tubercular affection.

*We quote from Strumphel.

ADDENDUM, SEPTEMBER 16, 1891.

Patient having returned from the mountains, on physical examination evinces no evidences of pulmonary disease. There is still an area of dullness over the lower lobe of the right lung posteriorly. Breathing everywhere vesicular. A view of the case that was first suggested by Dr. Mitchell deserves mention because of its plausibility. This is, the possibility that we have been dealing not with a case of acute miliary tuberculosis, but with a case of typhoid fever, occurring in a subject with tuberculous consolidation of the lung. All the symptoms of enteric fever but the high temperature, were absent , there are, however, no positive methods to distinguish between enteric fever in a case of chronic tuberculosis, and a case of pure miliary tuberculosis, excepting the one to which we have previously referred.

EYE DISEASES OF THE UNBORN.

By Julian J. Chisolm, M. D.

Professor of Eye and Ear Diseases in the University of Maryland, and Surgeon-in-Chief of the Presbyterian Eye, Ear and Throat Charity Hospital of Baltimore city.

That man is born to trouble has been verified with the centuries. That he is exposed to diseases during his entire life, from the moment of birth until death ensues, and that no age is exempt from the resistless grip of the destroyer, is a matter of every day observation. The very act of being born brings with it its many troubles, some of which are serious enough to destroy a life which has had as yet no out-door existence.

The eyes of the human race are equally exposed with other parts of the human body to these destructive agencies. The most virulent of eye affections is waiting at the very door to lay hold upon the innocent victim, before the eyes even see the light for which they were made. In the initial effort of offspring to become independent beings, as they leave the warm abode to take the first whiff of the living ether in which they are hereafter to move, germs of disease squeeze themselves between the lids. In their new home these start an active colony of pathogenic bacteria, which after a short period of incubation, causes a violent and destructive inflammation. Of the blind children of the world—and they number millions,—one fourth it is said, have lost their sight during their first days of existence from organic poisons which have come in contact with the eyes as the head was traversing the vaginal passage. These cases of *ophthalmia neonatorum* are very familiar to us. Since the cause producing them has been so satisfactorily established, and its germ origin known, prophylaxis and antiseptic applications, when properly carried out, promise to reduce the source of permanent blindness in infants to a minimum.

The object of this paper; however, is not to discuss diseases of the outer world with which our every day experience as physicians make us so familiar. There are
numerous eye troubles which precede the birth of the child.
They exhibit all morbific phases from the simple to the most
serious, even to the destruction of the eye-ball. All these
detrimental acts are going on while the infant is supposed to
be safe in its mother's womb. An intra-uterine fœtus can
have inflammation of any of the eye tissues. Also a defective
nutrition might exhibit an arrest of development in one or
more parts of the eye-ball, which after birth remain as permanent deformities. In the enumeration of diseases which
follow, it is not my purpose to give an exhaustive treatise,
with facts sought from a voluminous literature; but I mean
to restrict myself to personal observation among the applicants for treatment at the Presbyterian Eye, Ear and Throat
Charity Hospital of Baltimore City.

To begin with faults of nutrition. I have seen a child
born with a defective upper lid, a fissure, or as it is called, a
coloboma, extending through the thickness of the lid from
the center of the lash border upward. The lid was split
into two portions, simulating the more familiar fissure in the
upper lip called hare-lip, and occasioned by a similar arrest
in development.

I have seen *erectile tumors* more or less extensive on the
lids of newly born children. They usually grow more rapidly
than the average growth of the child, look ugly from their
swollen discoloration, and need surgical interference for their
removal.

Thirty-three infants exhibited round, hard, elastic swellings l cated at the outer edge of the brow. These were
tumors of a cystic nature, over which the skin of the temple
would glide readily. When the swellings are seized, and an
attempt made to move them, they are found firmly and deeply
fixed to the periosteum. These are *congenital dermoid cysts*,
and can only be cured by extirpation. When they are cut
open, a quantity of grumous matter escapes, composed
chiefly of epithelium and fat, with strands of exfoliated hairs,
indicating the skin origin of the tumor.

In thirty children there existed a shelf of skin overlapping the inner angle of the lids. In some this shelf was so broad that the pupil was concealed by it during the forced convergence of the eye-ball. These are ugly deformities, destroying all agreeable and intelligent expressions of the face. The condition is known as *epicanthus*. It is occasioned by want of development in the nose bridge. The ample skin designed by nature to cover a properly formed nose, not being wanted, spreads out sideways over the eyes. In after years when the nose has grown to its adult size, the deformity usually disappears. Should the excess of skin remain, it can be taken away by the removal of an ellipse of skin vertically from over the root of the nose.

Infants are born with an inability to raise the upper eye lid —*Congenital Ptosis*. It may exist in one or both upper lids. Nature has either omitted the muscle necessary to pull the lid upward, the levator palpebrae superioris, or the nerve supply needful for its innervation is wanting. This latter contingency may arise from a defective nerve centre in the brain, or it may be the effect of a neuritis which has left the muscle permanently paralyzed. A very common popular expression is "laughing eyes," which, when properly interpreted means laughing eye lids. In Ptosis the eye not only looks sleepy and heavy, but the dropping lid covers more or less of the pupil; causing an ugly gait in walking, with the head bent far back to enable the person to see horizontally. This deformity is only partially removed by operation. By taking an oval piece of skin lengthwise from the lid, the breadth of the lid is shortened, tucking it up as it were, so that the pupil can be exposed without the backward bending of the neck.

Children have been born with eyes crossed—a *congenital squint*, detected by anxious parents with the first opening of the infants eyes. These are cases of true strabismus, all eye muscles acting. Still more rarely cases have been brought to the Hospital with paralyzed muscles, the cause of the eye deviation—*Congenital paralytic squint*. One case of unusual interest presented a paralysis of both sixth nerves, both eyes turning in towards the nose.

Nystagmus, an irregular and perpetual movement of the eye muscles, is also seen at birth, and is recognized as a congenital condition. The movement of the eyes may be a vertical or lateral oscillation, or a rotatory movement, depending upon the group of muscles which exhibit these choreic contractions. It is always associated with defective visions, either from imperfect retinal development or from congenital optic nerve defects. It is an incurable deformity, the incessant movement of the eye balls only stopping when life ends.

Tear drop is another congenital affection which attracts the early attention of an observing mother. The excessive moisture in one eye when the other remains dry is readily recognizable even in the early days of life. Infants have been brought to the Hospital with *lachrymal fistula*, the frequent oozing of a little dew drop from a point of skin overlying the lachrymal sac having attracted attention. No redness, swelling or mattering had ever existed since the birth of the child. During life, cases of fistula resulting from lachrymal abscesses opening upon the cheek are not very uncommon. In these we can trace the course of the inflammation from its beginning in the lachrymal sac with redness, swelling, pointing of the abscess, and final rupture with discharge of purulent contents. Then the slow subsidence of the inflammatory swelling to the disappearance of all purulent secretion: and lastly, the continual escape of drops of lachrymal secretion from the lachrymal sac through the contracted orifice, which refuses to close. This sequence is invariably as described. From analogy we must believe that a similar course is pursued in the formation of this congenital fistula during intra-uterine life, all inflammatory phenomena having disappeared before the birth of the child.

Sometimes we find curious lumps on the eye ball of the child at birth. They are more or less elevated from the surface of the eye, and are of a dull white color in the Caucasian infant, and of a brown or black color in the negro. Their location is on the temporal side of the eye ball, extending from the periphery of the cornea outward, even to the canthus with the larger lumps. Upon closer inspection they exhibit a striking similarity to ordinary skin, and fine hairs are seen growing upon them. The surface is covered with a coarse epithelium, and is dry in contrast with the lubricated conjunctiva. These tumors are islands of true skin, engrafted by a freak of nature upon the ocular conjunctiva. They are known to ophthalmologists as *dermie tumors*. They grow pari passu with the growth of the body and the normal development of the eye ball. Among the 49,000 eye patients on the Hospital books, thirteen patients had these curious congenital masses on the eye ball. They are ugly blemishes, and are removed by excision.

Corneal spots, or scars, apparently the sequel of intra-uterine corneal ulcerations, are at times brought to the attention of the Hospital staff. They are such spots as are seen by the hundreds in all large Eye Dispensaries as the remains of corneal ulcers which have been treated from the beginning of their pathological condition. When the congenital corneal spot is central, there is frequently seen a corresponding white hillock in the centre of the pupil and attached to the surface of the crystaline lens. Most frequently this elevated white spot on the lens capsule is found without any trace of corneal spot. It is called a *congenital pyramidal cataract.* Forty-nine such conditions are entered upon the Hospital books. The explanation for the formation of pyramidal cataracts in the unborn is, that at some stage of intra uterine life a central ulcer of the cornea has, in its extension, perforated the eye coat, allowing the anterior chamber to empty itself of its aqueous contents. The elasticity of the eye ball, shrinking on itself when the distending influence of the aqueous fluid is removed, obliterates the anterior chamber. This forces the iris, and through the pupil the lens in contact with the ulcerated cornea. Embryonic tissues with their excessive vitality cause a quantity of lymph to be exuded to fill up the corneal excavation. Some of it comes in contact with the capsule of the lens in its juxtaposition with the cornea. As soon as the leak through the corneal perforation has been stopped, a reaccumulation in the anterior chamber takes place. This collection of fluid pushes the iris and lens back again to their normal positions, rup-

turing the soft adhesive bands which had temporarily formed
between the capsule of the lens and the cornea. As there
are no vessels in the lens capsule, absorption of the white
exudate cannot take place. The white hillock remains as an
historic landmark of the event. The corneal exudate is often
absorbed, leaving no recognizable trace at birth. The iris
at this early stage of development is an imperforated septum.
The pupil opens towards the last months of uterine gestation by the absorption of the pupillary membrane. As the
pupil is open before this complication takes place, the period
of intra-uterine life at which the corneal ulcer occurred can
be approximated.

Keratitis is another disease which occurs in the unborn
child, as exhibited by more or less clouding of the cornea at
birth. These white corneal spots are as undoubtedly the
evidence of previous inflammatory processes as charred
wood would indicate the effects of a previously existing combustion. That a general breaking down of the cornea can
occur in the intra-uterine fœtus, just such destructive processes as are seen in children after birth, is recognized in
each instance by the similarity in appearance of the atrophic
eye balls.

Young infants have been brought to the Hospital for examination where only the *stump of a shrunken eye ball* could
be seen in one socket, the other eye ball being perfect.
There had been no inflammatory disease occurring in the eye
of the child since birth. The condition of the atrophic ball
could not have been brought about since the birth of the
child without accompanying and conspicuous evidences of
inflammation. In these stumps the sclerotic is perfect, the
cornea alone being absent. The shrunken and sightless eye
ball moves about in company with the good eye, indicating
that the eye muscles are all intact. All the manifestations
of disease must have existed in utero and would have been
detected had the child been prematurely born.

The iris does not escape the inroads of disease in the unborn. There are faults of omission and commission in this
interesting membrane. A very important preparation for
the usefulness of the iris is the presence of a blank pigment

which covers its posterior surface. Vision consists in presenting sharply defined pictures to the retina. This can only be done in a dark chamber, by letting in a stroug ray of light through a small orifice. The pupilary orifice which nature adjusts should be the only inlet for light. The heavy black pigmentation of the iris and choroid is designed to exclude the admission of light in any other direction. In the development of the eye, nature sometimes omits this pigment, as in *Albinos or pink-eyed persons*, in whom the entire iris is translucent and vision necessarily and permanently defective.

A patient has been among the Hospital applicants with faulty visions in one eye. Under ophthalmoscopic inspection the cause of defective vision was found to depend upon *remnants of the pupilary membrane* which nature had not altogether absorbed. Their presence in the pupil was a permanent, mechanical obstacle to good vision. In the formation of this important septum there is a growing together of two lateral folds to perfect the whole partition. Sometimes a hitch occurs in this fusion. The lower portion does not close up. A fissure is left extending downwards from the pupil to the corneal border, duplicating the condition so commonly seen in iredectomy. This appearance of the eye is known as *congenital coloboma of the iris*. It was observed at the Hospital in thirty-four patients. I have sometimes suspected other agencies in its formation. A marginal corneal perforating ulcer with prolapse of iris gives in the outer world similar results, and I have seen congenital artificial pupils which I fancied were caused in this manner.

Iritis with its sequelæ of closed puckered pupils takes place in intra-uterine life. With these evidences of a previous inflammation, infants are born. These congenital conditions are in every way similar to eyes lost by iritis in more mature years, and should be attributed to the same pathological condition.

The crystaline lens comes in for its full share of troubles in the unborn. Of the 4,047 cataract patients entered upcn the hospital books in the last thirteen years, 244 were classified as congenital. In two patients the crystaline lens had been entirely omitted in the making of the eye. Besides, the lymph stained capsule, the sequel of perforating ulcer of the cornea, and already referred to as pyramidal cataract, the pupil under illumination reveals opaque spots more or less extensive and in strong contrast with the red reflex of the choroid, as seen through the transparent margins of the lens. These spots are central and are black in appearance when viewed by the ophthalmoscope. The crystaline lens forms around a central germ upon which innumerable layers are deposited in the growing of the lens. Some of the early layers are defective and lose their transparency. In time healthy nutrition is restored and transparent lens substance is deposited over the unhealthy portions. The incarcerated zone retains its opaque character in the centre of the otherwise transparent lens, and as a *zonal cataract*, becomes a permanent obstruction to good vision.

Defects in nutrition may involve the whole lens substance, making it milky, destroying its transparency and establishing the whitish pupil detected at birth as *congenital cataract*. These cataracts are the most common congenital defects, and form one-fourth of the congenital eye troubles. Vision can be restored to such eyes by surgical operation.

The choroid lining of the eye comes in for its share in congenital eye troubles. In some infants its important normal black pigment is omitted, a serious detriment to good vision. Again, like the iris, it may be fissured, either partially or extensively, from the ciliary border to the very optic nerve entrance. This cause for impaired vision is known as *coloboma of the choroid*. Choroidal inflammations occur in the unborn, resulting in partial or complete atrophy of this very important backing of the retina, necessarily disturbing or even destroying sight. The retina is always implicated in these inflammatory disorganizations. Scotomato, or blind spots, always ensue when choroidal atrophies occur. Should the spot of atrophy be at the fovea or central axis of vision, all useful sight is permanently destroyed.

The retina has its peculiar intra-uterine troubles, in which inflammation plays a part more or less destructive. There is a slow progressive blindness accompanying the condition known as *retinitis*, (*pigmentosa*,) in which sclerosis of the retinal vessels occur, with obliteration of the same through invasion and proliferation of pigment cells. This is of congenital origin, although the complete destruction of vision may not occur until late in life.

That horrible disease known as cancer may invade the retina while the child is still in its mother's womb. *Glioma, or retinal cancer*, so fatal to both the eye and the life of the child, usually begins its ugly work before the child is born. As a small yellow nodule, possibly not larger than a pin's head when first observed in the depth of the eye ball, it grows more or less rapidly until it fills the eye chamber, infiltrates the eye tissues, develops in the orbit as well as externally between the lids, and usually destroys life after the fashion of cancer generally.

Neuritis and *optic nerve atrophy* are congenital causes of blindness, and are revealed by the ophthalmoscope in the early days of life.

Some children are born with defective sight, the causes for which the most rigid investigation of the eye itself cannot reveal, and we must seek for defects in the brain centres in explanation, as for instance, in *color-blindness* and in *amaurosis*.

In the eye ball as a whole we find at birth various lesions. In some the arrest of growth seems to have taken place after the eye had perfected its development, so that it retains a diminutive or dwarfed condition throughout the life of the individual—*micropthalmus*. A child may be born with a dropsical eye twice its normal size, a condition known in ophthalmic surgery under the name of *Buphthalmus*, of which 63 cases have been seen at the Presbyterian Hospital. In some cases the eye ball seems to have been blighted in its very conception, and is hardly rudimentary. The contracted socket seems empty at birth, and the case is called *anopthalmus*.

Deviations from the typical shape of an eye ball are as common as the absence of beauty in the faces of the masses, when the Apollo of Belvidere, or the Venus of Canova is accepted as typical of what the human race should look like. The eye may at birth be longer in its antero-posterior diameter than it ought to be. This condition,—a very common deformity,—includes all cases of *congenital myopia*. The reverse of this condition also holds good in which the eye is flatter from behind forwards than it ought to be. This condition is called *hyperopia*, and was illustrated in the hospital work by 3,156 persons. *Astigmatism*, another congenital fault in which the cornea deviates from its true curvature, was seen last year in 874 of the 6,464 patients who applied for treatment at the hospital.

The socket can also be invaded by disease during the intra-uterine residence of the fœtus. *Congenital cysts* may exist, causing prominence of the eye ball at birth. Also vascular growths of the socket tissues, involving the conjunctiva to a more or less extent have been present at birth under the name of *angioma*.

It is seen clearly from this long list of eye faults and diseases that the unborn babe is not at all safe from eye troubles in its incarceration. In fact there are very few of the eye diseases seen after birth that it is not liable to. If to the list of intra-uterine diseases is added those of the conjunctiva acquired in the passage of the head through the vagina in the act of being born, then, with few exceptions, the list of eye diseases of the unborn absorb nearly the entire catagory of ophthalmic affections found in the adult human race. This is a condition that would stagger belief, were it not substantiated by positive evidence, as seen daily in hospital practice.

TWO OBSTETRICAL CASES.

By Wilmer Brinton, M. D.

In reporting two cases of obstetrics I do so simply to bring to the notice of this Faculty the subject of hæmorrhage, either "ante" or "post-partum," which is a subject which must always be of great importance to the practical obstetrician, for it is only the working practitioner of midwifery in contra-distinction to the compiling or library obstetrician who recognizes the truth of the statement of one of our best authorities in speaking of the importance of obstetrical knowledge, "that very frequently the emergencies which occur in the practice of the art of obstetrics are sudden, and must be met promptly if met successfully. They may give no time for consulting books, or a fellow practitioner, but immediate as is the peril must be the means to avert it."

Hæmorrhages occurring in the pregnant woman have been designated "accidental," when due to the separation of a normally implanted placenta, and "unavoidable," when due to placenta prævia. Obstetrical literature and personal experience teach us the great danger of both forms. Goodell, in 106 tabulated cases of hæmorrhage occurring from detachment of a normally implanted placenta, reports 54 maternal deaths, and only six children out of the 107 survived. I have placed on record elsewhere a death occurring from this cause, the patient being in a dying condition by the time the family physician reached her house. The mortality in unavoidal hæmorrhage due to placenta prævia varies from 20 to 40 per cent., if we except the statistics of Hofmeier, Lomer and Behm, of Berlin, who claim a mortality of 4.5 per cent., or even much less in a selected class of cases. But it must be remembered that these are men of special attainments in obstetrical practice, with exceptional facilities. We know some of the causes of detachment of a normally implanted placenta, with subsequent hæmorrhage, such as external violence, nephritis, variola, acute atrophy of the liver, etc., but the etiology of placenta prævia is unknown unless multiparity be a factor. Admitting, then, the gravity of the antepartum hæmorrhages, I desire to impress upon all the necessity of a careful examination and watchful attention to all hæmorrhages occurring in a woman known or suspected to be pregnant. Not only is it important to make a diagnosis, but it is *absolutely imperative* that the physician should understand the state of affairs in *all* hæmorrhages occurring after the seventh month of pregnancy. Whenever hæmorrhage occurs, it must be due to a detached placenta or placenta prævia. This at once brings up the question of the differential diagnosis, which can only be decided by a thorough digital examination, the patient being under an anæsthetic, if necessary.

In placenta prævia the examining finger comes into contact with the peculiar firm fibrous mass constituting the placenta, which is situated in the lower segment of the uterus, and which may or may not overlap the internal os; whilst in hæmorrhage from a detached placenta normally implanted, no placental tissue can be felt by the examining finger, yet the lower uterine segment may contain more or less blood-clot, which can be distinguished from placental tissue by being softer, it breaks easily and is not attached. Again, if uterine contractions have set in, there is another point which will aid us in forming an opinion; namely, in placenta prævia the hæmorrhage is greater during a pain, whilst in hæmorrhage from detached placenta it is lessened by uterine contractions. Having thus very briefly mentioned causation and some diagnostic points, the question of treatment of these alarming hæmorrhages must be briefly considered.

I believe in the vast majority of cases of both accidental and unavoidable hæmorrhage occurring in the pregnant woman, there is no safety for the mother until the uterus is emptied of its contents and is thoroughly contracted and retracted upon itself. Dr. Barnes has long since written in his classical book on Obstetrics, "that in the treatment of placenta prævia, if the pregnancy has advanced beyond the seventh month it will, as a general rule, I think, be wise to proceed to delivery, for the next hæmorrhage may be fatal. We cannot tell the time or extent of its occurrence, and when it occurs, perhaps all that we shall have the opportunity of doing will be to regret that we did not act when we had the chance." The view thus expressed by Dr. Barnes in the treatment of placent prævia is, in my judgment, the correct opinion, and, judging from my personal experience with accidental hæmorrhage, will hold good in the vast majority of cases in the treatment of this unfortunate complication of pregnancy. I believe that when the obstetrician is conscious that he has to do with a case either of detached placenta or placenta prævia, with hæmorrhage, that his actions should be decided; no temporizing or vacillating should be indulged in. With these views, I submit the report of two cases of obstetrics coming under my care recently.

Case 1.—*Ante-partum hæmorrhage.* I was called at midnight of March 14th, to see, with Dr. D. S., Mrs. J., aged 40, who was pregnant for the fourteenth time, with the history of having had eleven full-term living children and two abortions. Supposed herself to be about eight and one-half months advanced in her present pregnancy, and, although a considerable amount of blood had been lost twenty-five days previous to this date, her present medical adviser, Dr. S., had not been sent for until a few hours before I saw her with him. An examination of the urine made at this time showed albumen and casts. The patient had complained of headache, had had vomiting, etc.

On the evening of March 13th she had considerable flowing with some slight pain ; as night advanced the hæmorrhage become more decided, and shortly before midnight, while urinating, a gush of blood came which filled the chamber over half full of blood. The patient becoming very weak and faint was assisted to bed by her attendant and her physician summoned. Upon examining the case with him shortly afterwards, we found the woman lying in bed, pale, faint and depressed ; pulse 108. Upon a thorough examination made by placing my hand in the vagina and finger in the cervix, we decided that we had to do with a case of decided accidental hæmorrhage from a partially detached

placenta. The same examination showed the child presenting vertex, and the occiput to the mother's left and front,
with the cervix rigid and not dilated to any extent. We
also found a considerable amount of blood oozing through
the cervix, although not coming with the gush which had
made her so faint and weak.

By auscultation the fœtal heart sounds, rapid and indistinct,
could be heard to the mother's left, and palpation confirmed
the digital diagnosis of the presentation of the child. After
waiting for about one hour, with more or less oozing of blood
and no special pain indicative of labor, we determined to bring
on labor. I ruptured the membrane with my finger, which
was immediately followed by the escape of a considerable
amount of amniotic fluid, and within a short time, uterine
contractions began, which were no doubt increased by ʒi of
fluid extract of ergot, which was given every hour. From
this time on, there were no special indications for any other interference. The labor pains became more severe, the bleeding ceased, and at 6.30 A. M. the woman was delivered of a
still-born child, of 6½ pounds. An examination of the placenta, which was expressed a few minutes after the birth of
the child, gave evidence of a recent hæmorrhage, and also
we were led to believe from this examination that a small
portion of the placenta had been detached when the first hæmorrhage occurred, some twenty-five days before. The patient
had an uneventful lying-in period, her pulse and temperature
remaining normal during this time. A note received within
the past two days from her attending physician informs me
that she has resumed her usual domestic duties, but that she
still continues under his treatment for nephritis, her water
containing large amount of albumen with casts.

Case 2.—*Placenta prævia lateralis, treated by internal podalic
version; mother and child saved.* Was requested at four
o'clock on the morning of April 23d, 1891, by two fellow
practitioners, to see with them Mrs. H., who was having exhausting hæmorrhages from placenta prævia. The patient,
Mrs. H., 36 years of age, was supposed to be ending the
eighth month of her sixth pregnancy. Her former labors
were normal, with the exception of her fourth, a twin

pregnancy. As on other occasions, a midwife was to officiate at this labor, and had been sent for in the early part of the night. The patient was then losing blood, but after midnight, the hæmorrhage becoming more decided, and the patient's symptoms becoming more alarming, the physicians were summoned, to whom the patient stated that besides the great hæmorrhages going on then, she had been losing blood continuously for four or five days previous. When I first saw the patient with her physicians, I found the bed saturated with blood. She was rolling from one side of the bed to the other, pulse rapid and weak, lips pallid, extremities cold, and exhibiting all of the characteristic symptoms of the so-called "air-hunger," indicating great loss of blood. A digital examination rapidly made indicated that we had to do with a case of placenta prævia lateralis, the placenta being attached to the left side of the lower segment of the uterus, extending and filling up about one-third of the dilating internal os. The child presented vertex, and the occiput was to the mother's left and front. The bag of water was unruptured, the cervix dilated and dilatable. As the woman at this time was seemingly in a dying condition, no time was lost for a more thorough examination, and I decided at once that version was the operative measure to be instituted in the interest of both mother and child. I ruptured the bag of water, performed internal podalic version and delivered the child in a very rapid manner. Some little delay in delivering the head caused the child to be born asphyxiated, but by the intelligent efforts of one of the physicians present, we soon had the pleasure of hearing the child cry. Immediately after the delivery of the child, I introduced my hand into the uterus and thoroughly removed the placenta and membranes. The uterus contracted well, and all hæmorrhage ceased. During and immediately after the operative measures, the patient received stimulants, by the mouth and hypodermically. For a time her pulse grew much better, but within an hour after the birth of the child, and without the loss of much blood, she had two attacks of syncope, and for a short time her pulse could not be felt at the wrist; however, by the continuation of stimulants, and other methods for combatting cerebral anæmia, she grew better, and under strict antiseptic care, which has been carried out in an intelligent manner by her attending physician, she has done well, and now, one week after delivery, her physician informs me that both mother and child are doing well, and indications are most favorable for speedy convalescence on the part of the mother.

A REPORT OF THREE SUPRA-VAGINAL HYSTE-RECTOMIES AND SIMILAR CASES TREATED BY ELECTROLYSIS.

By Thomas Opie, M. D.,

Professor of Gynecology, College of Physicians and Surgeons of Baltimore.

Mrs. L., age 48, was married at 28. Menstruation began at 16. This function continued regularly, painlessly, normally, throughout her unmarried life and during her married life until six months ago, when she began to menstruate on alternate months. She never conceived during her 22 years of married life, though her husband was a healthy man and both enjoyed to the fullest extent, the conditions of sexual union.

Five years ago, she first nóticed an enlargement of the abdomen; she observed that she was "short-waisted." Pressure symptoms manifested themselves in disturbances of the digestive system two years ago and were her only annoyance, save the mortification growing out of her abdominal development.

There has been no vesical nor renal disturbance, at least so far as the patient remembers, because like the uterus of advanced pregnancy, the tumor has for five or six years, been an occupant of the abdominal cavity.

The lady on her first visit to my office stated that she had been examired and an opinion obtained that she had an ovarian cystoma, but her friends were unalterably opposed to operative procedure.

The conditions of fluid contents were satisfactorily made out but my indecision as to its exact character was manifested, by my double equipment for the operation either as an ovariotomy or a hysterectomy.

After thorough aseptic, indeed absolute antiseptic preparation of the patient, operator and assistants, an incision was made from the ensiform cartilege to the symphysis pubis, a distance of 14 inches. The tumor was brought forward through the incision and Baker Brown's clamp supplemented by two Koeberle scissors clamps, were made to constrict the pedicle, which was the uterine neck. Despite this precaution hæmorrhage ensued but was promptly arrested by seizing the vessels with artery forceps, ligaturing them and tying the pedicle in three sections, the middle one, by the sadler's stitch.

The tumor weighed over 20 pounds, its antero-posterior circumference measured 23½ inches and its transverse circumference 22¾ inches. Its shape lying upon the table, might be similated by a bladder in the same position, three-fourths distended by water. The diameter from the pedicle to the fundus was 13 inches, the transverse diameter 12 inches and the vertical diameter 9½ inches. The intra-vaginal portion of the cervix was not enlarged; the body and fundus apparently monopolized all the pathological elements.

The general outline of the tumor was the smooth hypertrophied and symmetrical appearance of the uterus of advanced pregnancy, in strong contrast with the irregular and nodular characteristics of the typical fibroid. The ovaries are both intact in the specimen and are located near the section of the stump equidistant from it and exactly opposite each other. There were absolutely no adhesive bands or other evidences of there having been at any time inflammatory trouble.

The microscope showed a large preponderance of fibrous tissue and that the numerous dilated lymph spaces were filled with fibrin. The fluid contents of the tumor coagulated immediately after its removal.

In pregnancy the development of the uterus out of the pelvis into the abdominal cavity, so as to make the woman "short-waisted," would take at least four and a half months. In a measure there is a parallelism between the normal and this so-called abnormal growth, since both are nutritive in their character, the one in the main muscular, and rapid, the other fibrous and slow. It is set forth in the history of this case that since it began its abdominal development, five years have elapsed and it had now attained the size of the uterus at full term. In view of the law of uterine development, we might assume that this fibroma had an intra-pelvic existence of at least five years, and therefore the whole period of growth was at least ten years.

The early stage of the tumor was even more mysterious and inscrutable, than the early phases of pregnancy. The patient informs us that her first and only intimation of her condition was, that she was getting "short-waisted."

A pertinent and practical question is, when did this cystic degeneration begin and what is its significance as bearing upon the health and longevity of the patient?

The temperature has never risen since the day of operation above 99° nor the pulse over 78. The Koeberle clamps, were removed on the 2nd day, the Baker Brown clamp on the 10th day. The silk-worm-gut sutures with which the abdomen was closed, were removed on the 12th day. The whole extent of the wound has been sealed by primary union, except the lower end of the incision corresponding with the stump, of the pedicle which granulated healthily, the abdominal peritoneum being securely united to the peritoneum of the pedicle. I may say, at the time of this writing, the 12th day, that with a sensible and manageable patient like the one in question, there is but one possible danger ahead and of that we stand forewarned, viz : ventral hernia.

Two years ago I met with a similar case of fibro-cystic myoma and operated at a private house with the same fortunate results as in the case just described. The lady recovered without a single untoward symptom and is now plying an active and successful mercantile business.

My third case of Hysterectomy for a fibro-cystic myoma was performed 18 months since at a private residence. This patient died on the 6th day. While I cannot state positively the cause of death since a post mortem was refused, my belief is, she died from sepsis.

The length of the incisions in the two last cases referred to was about 12 inches and weight of each over 15 pounds.

The mode of operating in these cases is in dispute, though Keith, the most successful of all hysterectomists, advocates the extra-peritoneal plan, as do Pean, Hegar and Bantock, while Schroeder, Billroth and Koeberle, the author of the "serre noeud," practice the intra-peritoneal method.

It is not likely that any one will contend that Ergot administered by mouth or hypodermically would in any wise curtail growths like the specimen I have described. The removal of the appendices would, if it was practicable in such huge growths have but little if any influence. I have for two years past used electricity hopefully and for some time enthusiastically in fibroids of all kinds.

The intra-uterine electrode as well as the method of stabbing the tumor with the sharp platinum electrode has been tried frequently, and while the applications seemed to improve the general health of some cases, stopped hæmorrhages and greatly relieved dysmenorrhœal pain, I cannot claim to have dissolved any single fibroid or made even an arrest of growth of a cystic fibro-myoma. I caused an abdominal peritonitis by a puncture of a large fibroid through the abdominal wall and have seen one case where sepsis was caused by a physician, in the use of an intra-uterine electrode.

I have at this time under treatment two large fibro-myomata, both of which have developed above the umbilicus, one has had about 80 the other 50 intra-uterine applications, one case has ceased to have hæmorrhages, both have improved in general health.

I recall the case of a fibroid, which I detected when as small as a pea, located on the anterior lip of the cervix. It was not only favorably located for ready application of the current, but for the easy recognition of changes in its size. In the last 18 months I have made 25 electrolytic applications to it. It has trebled its size despite my currents.

I may not be as expert with my batteries as others who are claiming so much for electricity in the solution of fibroids, but I must insist that I have, after over two years of persistent effort with a considerable amount of material; some justification for having lost my enthusiasm and even in being discouraged as to this so-called conservative plan of dealing with fibroid tumors, pyosalpinx, cystic ovaries and the like disorders, which in many cases march straight on to death or what is worse, to chronic, hopeless invalidism.

The treatment of fibro-cystic myomata by electricity, is well nigh obsolete. Cases have been recorded, where abscesses have resulted and ended fatally. Whether aspiration and drainage of such tumors in conjunction with electro puncture will remove the dangers, is not yet proven.

As soon as fluctuation is determined in a fibroid, extirpation should be resorted to.

The rules of differentiation, the attendant dangers and the treatment of fibro-cystic myomata are the same as ovarian cystoma. Indeed the operation of gastrotomy for tumors involving the uterus has been evolved out of the work of the ovariotomist, in the last quarter of a century.

Whenever an ovariotomy is performed the equipment of the operator should embrace the additional instruments required in a Hysterectomy.

Rules for the Government of the Library.

Adopted May 9th and 12th, 1882.

I. The Librarian or Assistant Librarian shall attend at the Library Rooms daily except Sunday and legal holidays, from 12 o'clock until 6 o'clock P. M., during which hours only, books and journals may be taken from the Library.

II. Each member of the Faculty, paying the annual dues, shall be entitled to take out at one time, four volumes duodecimo, two volumes octavo, one volume quarto, or one volume folio. This rule may be suspended by the written order of three members of the Library Committee.

III. City members retaining books longer than two *weeks* and county members longer than four weeks, shall be subject to the following *fines* per week, viz: 10 cents for the first week, 20 cents for the second week, 30 cents for the third week, and 20 cents per week for every week thereafter. Such fines shall be appropriated exclusively for the benefit of the Library.

IV. No book shall be delivered to a member unless in person or to his written order. A member receiving a book shall be held responsible for it from the time of its delivery until its return to the Library.

V. A member not returning a book or books, belonging to the Library, within four weeks after the date of receiving them, shall be notified *by the Librarian* that he is incurring a fine ; and if they be not returned within three months, in the absence of satisfactory reasons therefor, the Librarian shall recover them, or if they be lost, their value, in behalf of the Faculty; otherwise, the defaulting member shall forfeit the privileges of the Library, and shall be reported at the next annual convention of the Faculty, by the Library Committee. Should any book be injured or defaced while in the possession of a member, he shall be fined, at the discretion of the Library Committee, or, at his option; may furnish such a copy of the same work as shall be acceptable to the Committee.

VI. If any member, upon returning a book, shall find that there has been no application for it while in his possession, he may take it again for the time allowed in Rule III, but

may not take it out a third time until after the expiration of one week succeeding its return to the Library. New books may not be taken by members for more than one term of two weeks, until after the expiration of one additional week after their return.

VII. Members are not entitled to receive books from the Library until all arrearages for fines are paid. Fines may be remitted or reduced, for just and sufficient reasons, by the Library Committee.

VIII. The Librarian shall appropriately number and stamp the books, pamphlets and periodicals, and place them in proper order on the shelves. He shall obtain and keep a correct list of the members p n the annual dues. He shall record, in a book kept foaything purpose, the names of members who receive books from the Library, the titles and sizes of the books, the time of their delivery and of their return. He shall continue the catalogue of the books, pamphlets, periodicals, etc.; keep an account of all moneys received by him for fines, contributions, sales, etc., which moneys he shall pay into the hands of the Chairman of the Library Committee on the last week-day of each month. He shall report during the last week in March of each year to the Library Committee, a statement of such donations of money or of books as may have been made to the Library, with the names of the donors, as well as of such books, pamphlets, periodicals, or other valuable matter as may have come into the possession of the Library by purchase, exchange, or otherwise. He shall keep a record of all books, periodicals, etc., upon the subscription list of the Library Committee, shall keep due record of their receipt at the proper time, and shall report to the Library Committee the non-receipt of any when over-due. He shall keep on file applications for such books as may have been let out of the Library; and may make any suggestions to the Committee he may deem necessary.

IX. Under no circumstances will members be permitted to remove new books, new journals, or other recently received matter, before such time as the Library Committee shall determine.

X. Scarce and valuable books, the loss of which it would be difficult to replace, shall not be removed from the Library rooms without the approbation of two members of the Library Committee.

XI. The Librarian is empowered to sell or exchange duplicate books, journals, etc., upon such terms as may appear advantageous, upon the approval of the Library Committee.

Resolutions, Amendments, &c., affecting the Constitution, from 1885 to 1891, inclusive.

May 16th, 1885, By Dr. J. Edwin Michael. Changing the word *gentlemen* to the word person in Article IV, Sec. 1, of the Constitution and changing phraseology throughout to correspond.

May 16th, 1885, By Dr. E. Cordell. Changing Article IX of the Constitution to read " The Annual Meetings of the Faculty shall be held in the City of Baltimore on the fourth Tuesday in April, or at such date as the Executive Committee, with the concurrence of the President, shall appoint. A Semi-Annual Meeting may be held at such time and place as the Executive Committee may designate."

May 16th, 1885, By the Library Committee, " That the Treasurer is hereby directed to deliver to the Library Committee, at the end of each calendar month, one half of the fees and dues received by him from members during the month, as provided for in Art. X, of the Constitution."

May 1st, 1886, By Dr. G. Lane Taneyhill. Article VIII, of the Constitution to read, "All resignations must be sent to the Corresponding Secretary, and can be accepted only by the Faculty, at any meeting except a memorial meeting."

May 1st, 1886, By Dr. G. Lane Taneyhill. "That the Corresponding Secretary, in giving notice of an Annual Meeting, shall do so at least two weeks before the date of such meeting."

April 29th, 1887, By Dr. John R. Quinan. Article III, Sec. 5 of the Constitution to read as follows between the words "referred to them" and "shall present:" He shall notify all members, by circular or otherwise, of the time and place of each meeting, and, if it be an annnal one, he shall issue such notice at least two weeks before said Annual Meeting.

April 27th, 1888, By the Secretary. *Resolved*, That the Treasurer is hereby instructed, annually, until otherwise ordered, to mail on April 1st, a printed statement of indebtedness to all members who are delinquent, stating the year of delinquency, and informing such members that by the Constitution, unless payment be made before the fourth Tuesday of April, they are temporarily deprived of the privileges of the Faculty, among which are voting, eligibility to office, and appointment on Standing Committees, sections, or as delegates to any Convention.

Resolved, That the Treasurer is hereby instructed, annually, until otherwise ordered, to hand up to the presiding officer at the adjournment of the third day's session a revised list of delinquents, resignations, deaths, and dropped for non-payment of dues of members, in order that the President may be enabled to complete a proper list of appointees for the ensuing year.

April 27th, 1889, By Dr. R. Winslow. Article VI, Sec. 2 of the Constitution so modified as to allow the publication of papers in any medical journal after being read before the Faculty and before the appearance of the "Transactions."

April 27th, 1889, By Dr. Chas. H. Jones, on motion to adopt the report of the Committee on Increasing Membership. "Change Art. X. of the Constitution, making dues from city members after the fourth Tuesday in April, 1890, $5.00, and those of county members $2.00. Also change the phraseology of Sec. 1, Art. IV, to read five instead of eight.

April 27th, 1889, By Dr. Randolph Winslow. Change Sec. 2, Art. VI, to allow the publication of papers read before the Faculty elsewhere than in the transactions, provided they have not been read previously before any medical society, and that such publication take place after they have been read before the Faculty.

April 25th, 1890, The following "Rules" offered by Dr. B. B. Browne, Chairman of the Library Committee were adopted. "City members retaining books longer than two weeks, and county members longer than four weeks, shall be subject to the following fines, per week, viz : 10 cents for the first week, 20 cents for the second week ; 30 cents for the third week, and 20 cents per week for each week thereafter. Such fines shall be appropriated exclusively for the benefit of the Library."

April 24th, 1890, On motion of Dr. B. B. Browne. *Resolved*, That at the Annual Convention, *an executive session* be held on Wednesday the second day of the Convention, at 8 P. M., that at this meeting the reports of all the Committees shall be read, miscellaneous business shall be considered, and the election of officers take place.

April 29th, 1891, By Dr. J. C. Hemmeter. The *titles* of all reports and papers must be sent to the Recording Secretary *at least one week before* the opening of the meeting at which it is desired to read the paper.

April 29th, 1891, By the Library Committee. *Resolved*, That the sum appropriated by the Faculty for the use of the Library, be disbursed to the Chairman of the Library Committee in equal payments, the first to be made on or before May 15th, the second on or before August 15th; the third on or before January 15th and the fourth on or before April 15th, of each year.

LIST OF PRESIDENTS—1799-1892.

Upton Scott—1799-1801.
Philip Thomas—1801-15.
Ennals Martin—1815-20.
Robert Moore—1820-26.
Robert Goldsborough—1826-36.
Maxwell McDowell—1836-41.
Joel Hopkins—1841-48.
Richard S. Steuert—1848-51.
William W. Handy—1851-52.
Michael S. Baer—1852-53.
John L. Yates—1853-54.
John Fonerden—1854-55.
Jacob Baer—1855-56.
Christopher C. Cox—1856-57.
Joshua I. Cohen—1857-58.
Joel Hopkins—1858-59.
Geo. C. M. Roberts—1859-70.
John R. W. Dunbar—1870-70.
Nathan R. Smith—1870-72.
P. C. Williams—1872-73.
Charles H. Ohr—1873-74.
Henry M. Wilson—1874-75.
John F. Monmonier—1875-76.
Christopher Johnston—1876-77.
Abram B. Arnold—1877-78.
Samuel P. Smith—1878-79.
Samuel C. Chew—1879-80.
H. P. C. Wilson—1880-81.
Frank Donaldson—1881-82.
William M. Kemp—1882-83.
Richard McSherry—1883-84.
Thomas S. Latimer—1884-85.
John R. Quinan—1885-86.
Geo. W. Miltenberger—1886-87.
I. Edmondson Atkinson—1887-88.
John Morris—1888-89.
Aaron Friedenwald—1889-90.
Thomas A: Ashby—1890-91.
Wm. H. Welch—1891-92.

ACTIVE MEMBERS.
1891.

Andre, J. Ridgeway, 1132 E. Baltimore Street, Baltimore.
Ankrim, L. F., 4 S. Broadway, Baltimore.
Aronsohn, Abram, 712 N. Eutaw Street, Baltimore.
Ashby, Thos. A., 1125 Madison Avenue, Baltimore.
Atkinson, Archibald, 2101 Maryland Avenue, Baltimore.
Atkinson, G. T., Crisfield, Somerset County.
Atkinson, I. E., 605 Cathedral Street, Baltimore.
Baldwin, Ed. C., 304 N. Exeter Street, Baltimore.
Barnes, Wm. M., 905 N. Stricker Street, Baltimore.
*Baxley, J. B., Jr., 1531 Madison Avenue, Baltimore.
Bayly, Alex. H., Cambridge, Dorchester County.
Belt, Alfred M., 1010 Cathedral Street, Baltimore.
Belt, S. J., 314 N. Exeter Street, Baltimore..
Benson, B. R. Cockeysville, Baltimore County.
Berkley, Harry J., 1303 Park Avenue, Baltimore.
Bevan, Chas. F., 807 Cathedral Street, Baltimore.
Biedler, H. H., 119 W, Saratoga Street, Baltimore.
Billingslea, M. B., 1206 E. Preston Street, Baltimore.
Birnie, C., Taneytown, Carroll County.
Blaisdell, W. S., 285 N. Exeter Street, Baltimore.
Blake, John D., 602 S. Paca, Street, Baltimore.
Blum, Joseph, 641 Columbia Avenue, Baltimore.
Bond, A. K., 311 W. Biddle Street, Baltimore.
Bond, Robert, Brooklyn, Anne Arundel County.
Bond, S. B., 1830 Madison Avenue, Baltimore.
Booker, Wm. D., 851 Park Avenue, Baltimore.
Bonnett, J. A., 1025 N. Caroline Street, Baltimore.
Bosley, James, 1701 Hollins Street, Baltimore.
Bowie, Howard S., 811 N. Eutaw Street, Baltimore.
Branham, J. H., 538 N. Arlington Avenue, Baltimore.
Branham, J. W., 538 N. Arlington Avenue, Baltimore.
Brawner, J. B., Emmittsburg, Frederick County.
Bressler, F. C., 1713 Bank Street, Baltimore.
Brinton, Wilmer, S. W. Cor. Preston and Calvert Streets, Baltimore.
Bromwell, J. E., Mt. Airy, Carroll County.
Browne, B. B., 1218 MadisonAvenue, Baltimore.
Brown, James, 131 W. Lanvale Street, Baltimore.

*Brune, T. Barton, 1815 N. Charles Street, Baltimore.
†Bubert, Charles Hy., 1926 Pennsylvania Avenue, Baltimore.
Buckler, Thos. H., 6 E. Centre Street, Baltimore.
Buddenbohn, C. L., 602 S. Paca Street, Baltimore.
Campbell, Wm. H. H., Owings Mills, Baltimore County.
Canfield, Wm. B., 1010 N. Charles Street, Baltimore.
Carr, M. A. R. F., Cumberland, Allegany County.
Cathell, D. Webster, 1308 N. Charles Street, Baltimore.
Cathell, W. T., 1308 N. Charles Street, Baltimore.
Chabbot, G. H., 1111 E. Preston Street, Baltimore.
Chamberlaine, J. E. M., Easton, Talbot County.
Chambers, John W., 18 W. Franklin Street, Baltimore.
Chancellor, C. W., 103 W. First Street, Baltimore.
Chatard, Ferd. E., Jr., 516 Park Avenue, Baltimore.
Chew, Sam'l C., 215 W. Lanvale Street, Baltimore.
Chisolm, J. J., 112 W. Franklin Street, Baltimore.
Chisolm, F. M., 114 W. Franklin Street, Baltimore.
Christian, J. H., 1801 Madison Avenue, Baltimore.
Chunn, W. P., 1023 Madison Avenue, Baltimore.
Clagett, Joseph E., 108 S. Eutaw Street, Baltimore.
Coffroth, H. J., 924 Madison Avenue, Baltimore.
Conrad, John S., St. Denis P. O., Baltimore County.
Cooke, Theodore, 910 N. Charles Street, Baltimore.
Cooke, Theodore, Jr., 910 N. Charles Street, Baltimore.
Cordell, Eugene F., 2111 Maryland Avenue, Baltimore.
Corse, Geo. F., Gardenville, Baltimore County.
Corse, Wm. D., Gardenville, Baltimore County.
Councilman, W. T., Johns Hopkins Hospital, Baltimore.
Crouch, J. Frank, 725 Greenmount Avenue, Baltimore.
Craighill, J. M., 1720 N. Charles Street, Baltimore.
Dalrymple, A. J., 2006 E. Pratt Street, Baltimore.
Dashiell, N. L., Jr., 700 S. Broadway, Baltimore.
Dausch, Pierre G., 1727 E. Baltimore Street, Baltimore.
Davis, R. G., 1307 N. Caroline Street, Baltimore.
Dickinson, G. E., Upper Fairmount, Charles County.
Dickson, I. N., Reisterstown, Baltimore County.
Dickson, John, 1018 Madison Avenue, Baltimore.
*Donaldson, Frank, 510 Park Avenue, Baltimore.
†Downey, Jesse W., New Market, Frederick County.
*Dulin, Alex'r F., 107 W. Monument Street, Baltimore.
Dwinelle, J. E., 1701 E. Baltimore Street, Baltimore.
Eareckson, R. W., Elkridge Landing, Howard County.
Earle, Sam'l T., 1431 Linden Avenue, Baltimore.
Eastman, Lewis M., 772 W. Lexington Street, Baltimore.
Ellis, E. Dorsey, 915 Light Street, Baltimore.
Ellis, R. H. P., 733 W. Fayette Street, Baltimore.

*Evans, Thomas B., 121 Jackson Place, Baltimore.
Fiske, John D., 11 S. Gay Street, Baltimore.
Flemming, Geo. A., 928 Madison Avenue, Baltimore.
Fort, Sam'l J., Font Hill, Ellicott City, Howard County.
*Forwood, W. Stump, Darlington, Harford County.
Finney, John T. M., 923 N. Charles Street, Baltimore.
Friedenwald, Aaron, 310 N. Eutaw Street, Baltimore.
Friedenwald, Harry, 922 Madison Avenue, Baltimore.
Friedenwald, Julius, City Hospital, Baltimore.
Fulton, John S., Salisbury, Wicomico County.
Funck, J. W., 1710 W. Fayette Street, Baltimore.
Gardner, Frank B., 424 N. Greene Street, Baltimore.
Gardner, W. S., 410 N. Howard Street, Baltimore.
Gibbons, Jas. E., 835 Edmondson Avenue, Baltimore.
Gibbs, E. C., 440 E. North Avenue, Baltimore.
Giles, A. B., 1340 Aisquith Street, Baltimore.
Gleitsman, J. W., 117 Second Avenue, New York.
Goldsborough, Brice W., Cambridge, Dorchester County.
Goldsmith, Robert H., 647 N. Calhoun Street, Baltimore.
Goodman, H. H., 410 Hanover Street, Baltimore.
Gorter, N. R., 1 W. Biddle Street, Baltimore.
Graham, Geo. R., 725 Columbia Avenue, Baltimore.
Griffith, L. A., Upper Marlboro, Prince George's County.
Grimes, J. H., 2100 Maryland Avenue, Baltimore.
Grove, B. Frank, 1321 E. Biddle Street, Baltimore.
*Gundry, Richard, Catonsville, Baltimore County.
Gwynn, H. B., 724 N. Gilmor Street, Baltimore.
Hall, Alice T., 708 N. Howard Street, Baltimore.
Hall, Reverdy M., 1019 Druid Hill Avenue, Baltimore.
Harlan, Herbert, 317 N. Charles Street, Baltimore.
Harris, John C., 773 W. Lexington Street, Baltimore.
Harryman, Harry G., 1512 E Preston Street, Baltimore.
Hartman, George A., 1121 N. Caroline Street, Baltimore.
Hartman, Jacob H., 5 W. Franklin Street, Baltimore.
Hartwell, E. M., Johns Hopkins Hospital, Baltimore.
Heldman, Joel A., 254 Pearl Street, Baltimore.
Hemmeter, John C., 633 W. Lombard Street, Baltimore.
Herman, H. S., State Line, Pa.
Hilgartner, H. L., E. Baltimore Street, Baltimore.
Hill, Chas. G., Arlington, Baltimore County.
Hill, Henry F., 1001 Edmonson Avenue, Baltimore.
Hill, Wm. N., 1438 E. Baltimore Street, Baltimore.
Hines, W. F., Chestertown.
Hocking, Geo. H , Mt. Savage, Allegany County.
Hoen, Adolph G., 713 York Road, Baltimore.
Hogden, Alexander Lewis, 1235 Lafayette Avenue, Baltimore.
Hopkins, Howard H., New Market, Frederick County.

Hopkinson, B. Merrill, 1524 Park Avenue, Baltimore.
Howard, Wm. T., 804 Madison Avenue, Baltimore.
Humrickhouse, J. W., Hagerstown, Washington County.
Hundley, J. M., 1002 Edmondson Avenue, Baltimore.
Hurd, Henry M., Johns Hopkins Hospital, Baltimore.
Iglebart, J. D., 1214 Linden Avenue, Baltimore.
Ingle, J. L., 1007 W. Lanvale Street, Baltimore.
Irons, Ed. P., 1835 E. Baltimore Street, Baltimore.
Jacobs, C. C., Frostburg, Garrett County.
Jacobs, J. K. H., Kennedyville, Kent County.
Jay, John G., 212 W. Franklin Street, Baltimore.
Jenkins, Felix, 400 Cathedral Street, Baltimore.
Johnson, Robt. W., 101 W. Franklin Street, Baltimore.
*Johnston, Christopher, 201 W. Franklin Street, Baltimore.
†Johnston, Christopher, Jr., 201 W. Franklin Street, Baltimore.
Johnston, Samuel, 204 W. Monument Street, Baltimore.
Jones, A. C., Crapo, Talbot County.
Jones, C. Hampson, 25 W. Saratoga Street, Baltimore.
Jones, Charles H., 1083 W. Fayette Street, Baltimore.
Jones, Edwin E., Pennsylvania and Wylie Aves., Baltimore.
Jones, Wm. J., E. Preston Street, Baltimore.
Keane, S. A.,—Druid Hill Avenue, Baltimore.
Kierle, N. G., 1419 W. Lexington Street, Baltimore.
Keller, Josiah G., 222 W. Monument Street, Baltimore.
Kelly, Howard A., 905 N. Charles Street, Baltimore.
Kemp, Wm. F. A., 305 N. Greene Street, Baltimore.
King, J. T., 640 N. Carrollton Avenue, Baltimore.
Knight, Louis W., 414 N. Greene Street, Baltimore.
Kremein, John D., 667 W. Lexington Street, Baltimore.
Krozer, J. J. R., 662 W. Lexington Street, Baltimore.
Kuhn, Anna L., 1435 Light Street, Baltimore.
Latimer, Thos. S., 103 W. Monument Street, Baltimore.
Lee, Wm., 323 W. Hoffman Street, Baltimore.
Lockwood, W. F., 201 W. Madison Street, Baltimore.
Lumpkin, Thos. M., 640 W. Barre Street, Baltimore.
MacGill, Chas. G. W., Catonsville, Baltimore County.
Mackenzie, Ed. E., 324 W. Biddle Street, Baltimore.
Mackenzie, John N., 205 N. Charles Street, Baltimore.
Magruder, W. E., Olney, Montgomery County.
Mann, A. H., Jr., 934 Madison Avenue, Baltimore.
Mansfield, Arthur, 129 S. Broadway, Baltimore.
Mansfield, R. W., 129 S. Broadway, Baltimore.
Marsh, Wm. H., Solomon's Island, Calvert County.
Mason, A. S., Hagerstown, Washington County.
Martin, H. Newell, 925 St. Paul Street, Baltimore.
Martin, James S., Brookville, Montgomery County.
Maxwell, Wm. S., Still Pond, Kent County.

McComas, J. Lee, Oakland, Garrett County.
McCormick, Thos. P., 1529 Eutaw Place, Baltimore.
McCormick, Jas. L., Trappe, Talbot County.
McKnew, Wm. R., 1401 Linden Avenue, Baltimore.
McSherry, H. Clinton, 642 N. Howard Street, Baltimore.
Merrick, S. K., N. Eutaw Street, Baltimore.
Michael, J. Edwin, 201 W. Franklin Street, Baltimore.
Miller, C. O., 836 N. Eutaw Street, Baltimore.
Miltenberger, Geo. W., 319 W. Monument Street, Baltimore.
Mittnicht, Jacob H., 307 N. Exeter Street, Baltimore.
Monmonier, John F., 824 N. Calvert Street, Baltimore.
Monroe, Wm. R., 1734 Bolton Street, Baltimore.
Moran, Pedro De S., 244 W. Hoffman Street, Baltimore.
Morgan, Wilbur P., 315 W. Monument Street, Baltimore.
Morison, Rob't B., 827 St. Paul Street, Baltimore.
Morris, John, 118 E. Franklin Street, Baltimore.
Mosley, W. E., 614 N. Howard Street, Baltimore.
Moyer, F. G., 4 S. Exeter Street, Baltimore.
Murdoch Thos. F., 8 W. Read Street, Baltimore.
Murdock, Russell, 410 Cathedral Street, Baltimore.
Neale, L. Ernest, 319 W. Monument Street, Baltimore.
Neff, John, 701 N. Carrollton Avenue, Baltimore.
Nihiser, Winton M., Keedysville. •
Norris, Amanda Taylor, 871 Harlem Avenue, Baltimore.
Norris, Wm. H., 1300 E. Baltimore Street, Baltimore.
O'Donavan, Chás., Jr., 311 E. Read Street, Baltimore.
Ohle, H. C., 1203 W. Fayette Street, Baltimore.
Ohr, Chas. H., Cumberland, Allegany County.
Opie, Thomas, 600 N. Howard Street, Baltimore.
Osler, Wm., 209 W. Monument Street, Baltimore.
Page, I. Randolph, 1206 Linden Avenue, Baltimore.
Piper, Jackson, Towson, Baltimore County.
Platt, Walter B., 802 Cathedral Street, Baltimore.
Pole, A. C., 2102 Madison Avenue, Baltimore.
Porter, Alex. Shaw, Lonaconing, Alleghany County.
Powell, Alfred H., 212 W. Madison Street, Baltimore.
Preston, Geo. J., 9 E. Townsend Street, Baltimore.
Prichard, J. E , 1010 S. Chesapeake Street, Baltimore.
Ragan, O. H. W., Hagerstown, Washington County.
Randolph, R. L., 211 W. Madison Street, Baltimore.
Rasin, Robt. C., 809 N. Eutaw Street, Baltimore.
Reid, E. Miller, 904 N. Fremont Street, Baltimore.
Redding, M. Laura Ewing, 930 Madison Avenue, Baltimore.
Rehberger, John H., 1709 Aliceanna Street, Baltimore.
Reiche, P. H., 906 Gorsuch Avenue, Baltimore.
Reinhard, G. A. Ferd., 220 W. Madison Street, Baltimore.
Rennolds, Hy. T., 2004 St. Paul Street, Baltimore.
Reynolds, Geo. B., 711 N. Calvert Street, Baltimore.

†Rickert, Wm., 1841 Pennsylvania Avenue, Baltimore.
Riley, Charles H., 1113 Madison Avenue, Baltimore.
Robb, Hunter, Johns Hopkins Hospital, Baltimore.
Robinson, J. H., 726 E. Preston Street, Baltimore.
Rohe, George H., Catonsville, Baltimore County.
Rowe, M., Deals Island, Somerset County.
Rusk, G. Glanville, 2000 E. Baltimore Street, Baltimore.
Salzer, Henry, 613 Park Avenue, Baltimore.
Sandrock, W. Christian, Broadway and Chase Street, Baltimore.
Sanger, Frank D., 712 N. Howard Street, Baltimore.
Saunders, J. B., 819 E. Chase Street, Baltimore.
Sappington, Purnell F., Arlington Avenue, Baltimore County.
Sappington, Thomas, 919 N. Calvert Street, Baltimore.
Schaeffer, E. Mortin, Lexington, Virginia.
Scott, John McP., Hagerstown, Washington County.
Scott, Norman B., Hagerstown, Washington County.
Seldner, Samuel W., 947 N. Caroline Street, Baltimore.
Sellman, W. A. B., 5 E. Biddle Street, Baltimore.
Shaw, W. Rutherford, 10 E. Read Street, Baltimore.
Shippen, Chas. C., 603 N. Charles Street, Baltimore.
Skilling, W. Quail, Lonaconing, Allegany County.
Smith, Alan P., 24 W. Franklin Street, Baltimore.
Smith, Nathan R., Mt. Royal Avenue, Baltimore.
Smith, Jos. T., 1010 Madison Avenue, Baltimore.
Spear, J. M., Cumberland, Allegany County.
Spicknall, Jno. T., N. Patterson Park Avenue, Baltimore.
Steiner, L. H., 1038 N. Eutaw Street, Baltimore.
Steuart, Jas. A., New York.
Stevens, Jas. A., Oxford, Talbot County.
Street, David, 403 N. Exeter Street, Baltimore.
Schwatka, J. B., 1003 N. Broadway, Baltimore.
Taneyhill, G. Lane, 1103 Madison Avenue, Baltimore.
Teakle, St. Geo. W., 702 Park Avenue, Baltimore.
Theobald, Samuel, 304 W. Monument Street, Baltimore.
Thomas, George, 550 Presstman Street, Baltimore.
Thomas, Jas. Carey, 1228 Madison Avenue, Baltimore.
Thomas, Hy B., 1710 Guilford Avenue, Baltimore.
Thomas, Richard H., 236 W. Lanvale Street, Baltimore.
Thompson, W. H., 526 St. Paul Street, Baltimore.
Tiffany, L. McLane, 831 Park Avenue, Baltimore.
Trimble, I. R., 214 W. Franklin Street, Baltimore.
Todd, W. J., Mt. Washington, Baltimore County.
Townsend, W. Guy, Samaritan Hospital, Baltimore.
Van Bibber, Claude, 26 W. Franklin Street, Baltimore.
Van Bibber, John, 1014 N. Charles Street, Baltimore.
Van Bibber, W. Chew, 26 W. Franklin Street, Baltimore.
Van Marter, J. G., Jr., Rome, Italy.
Vees, Chas. H., 1210 E. Eager Street, Baltimore.

Virdin, W. W., Lapidum, Harford County.
*Walker, E. R., 1703 N. Charles Street, Baltimore.
Warfield, Mactier, 719 N. Howard Street, Baltimore.
Warfield, R. B., 214 W. Franklin Street, Baltimore.
Waters, Edmund G., 1429 McCulloh Street, Baltimore.
Wattenscheidt, Chas., 2027 Druid Hill Avenue, Baltimore.
Welch, E. Giddings, Park Avenue and Mulberry Street, Baltimore.
Welch, W. H., 506 Cathedral Street, Baltimore.
White, W. W., 1101 N. Broadway, Baltimore.
Whitridge, Wm., 829 N. Charles Street, Baltimore.
Wiegand, Wm. E., 2023 Druid Hill Avenue, Baltimore.
Williams, Arthur, Elkridge Landing, Howard County.
Williams, E. J,. 1114 Chesapeake Street, Baltimore.
Williams, John M., Lonaconing, Allegany County.
Williams, J. Whitridge, 900 Madison Avenue, Baltimore.
Williams, Philip C., 900 Madison Avenue, Baltimore.
Wilson, Henry M., 1008 Madison Avenue, Baltimore.
Wilson, H. P. C., 814 Park Avenue, Baltimore.
Wilson, J. Jones, Cumberland, Allegany County.
Wilson, Robert T., 820 Park Avenue, Baltimore.
Wiltshire, Jas. G., 714 N. Howard Street, Baltimore.
Winsey, Whitfield, 1220 E. Fayette Street, Baltimore.
Winslow, Caleb, 924 McCulloh Street, Baltimore.
Winslow, John R., 924 McCulloh Street, Baltimore.
Winslow, Randolph, 1 Mt. Royal Terrace, Baltimore.
Winternitz, L. C., 25 S. Eden Street, Baltimore.
Woods, Hiram, Jr., 525 N. Howard Street, Baltimore.
Ziegler, Charles B., 920 N. Broadway, Baltimore.

HONORARY MEMBERS.

Bartholow, Roberts, M. D., Philadelphia, Pa.
Billings, John S., M. D., U. S. A., Washington, D. C.
Chaille, Stanford E., M. D., New Orleans, La.
Dunott, Thomas J., M. D., Harrisburg, Pa.
Goodell, Wm., M. D., Philadelphia, Pa.
Mallet, John W., M. D., University of Virginia.
Mitchell, S. Weir, M. D., Philadelphia, Pa.
Moorman, John J., M. D., Salem, Va.
Pepper, William, M. D., Philadelphia, Pa.
Toner, Joseph M., M. D., Washington, D. C.

DELEGATE MEMBER.

Shertzer, A. Trego.

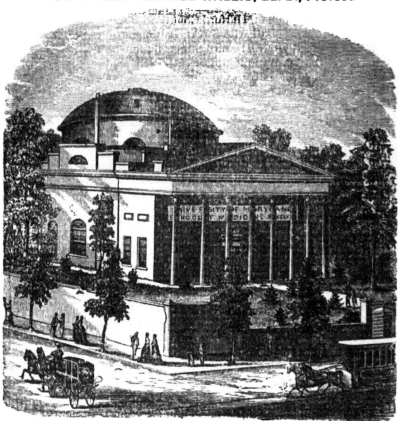

SCHOOL OF MEDICINE
N. E. COR. LOMBARD AND GREENE STS., BALTIMORE, MD.

The Eighty-sixth Annual Course of Lectures in this institution will commence on OCTOBER 1st, 1892.

FACULTY OF PHYSIC.

GEO. W. MILTENBERGER, M. D., Emeritus Professor of Obstetrics and Honorary President of the Faculty.

SAMUEL C. CHEW. M. D , Prof. of Principles and Practice of Medicine and Hygiene.

WM. T. HOWARD, M. D., Prof. of Diseases of Women & Children,& Clinical Medicine.

JULIAN J. CHISOLM, M. D., Professor of Eye and Ear Diseases.

FRANCIS T. MILES, M. D., Professor of Physiology and Clinical Professor of Diseases of Nervous System.

LOUIS McLANE TIFFANY, M. D , Professor of Surgery.

J. EDWIN MICHAEL, M. D , Professor of Obstetrics.

ISAAC EDMONDSON ATKINSON, M. D., Professor of Materia Medica and Therapeutics, Clinical Medicine and Dermatology.

FERD. J. S GORGAS, M. D , D D. S , Professor of Principles of Dental Science, Dental Surgery and Dental Mechanism.

JAMES H. HARRIS. M. D , D D. S , Professor of Operative and Clinical Dentistry.

R. DORSEY COALE, Ph. D , Professor of Chemistry and Toxicology.

RANDOLPH WINSLOW. M. D , Professor of Anatomy and Clinical Surgery.

JOHN NOLAND MACKENZIE, M. D , Clinical Prof. of Diseases of the Throat and Nose.

J. HOLMES SMITH, M. D. }
R. B. WARFIELD, M. D., } Demonstrators of Anatomy.

CHARLES W. MITCHELL. M. D., Lecturer on Pathological Anatomy.

CASPER O. MILLER, Demonstrator of Normal and Pathological Histology.

For further information apply to

I. EDMONDSON ATKINSON, M. D., Dean, 605 Cathedral St., Balto., Md.

PROFESSORS AND SPECIAL INSTRUCTORS.

FACULTY.

ABRAM B. ARNOLD, M. D.,
 Emeritus Professor of Clinical Medicine
THOMAS OPIE, M. D.,
 Professor of Gynæcology and Dean of
 the Faculty.
THOMAS S. LATIMER, M. D.,
 Professor of Principles and Practice of
 Medicine and Clinical Medicine.
AARON FRIEDENWALD, M. D.,
 Professor of Diseases of the Eye and
 Ear.
CHARLES F. BEVAN, M. D.,
 Professor of Principles and Practice of
 Surgery and Clinical Surgery.
WM. SIMON, Ph. D., M. D.,
 Professor of Chemistry.

GEORGE H. ROHE, M. D.,
 Professor of Materia Medica, Thera-
 peutics ,Hygiene and Mental Diseases.
J. W. CHAMBERS, M. D.,
 Professor of Anatomy and Clinical Sur-
 gery.
GEORGE J. PRESTON, M. D.,
 Professor of Physiology, and Clinical
 Diseases of the Nervous System.
N. G. KEIRLE, A. M. M. D.,
 Professor of Pathology and Medical
 Jurisprudence.
JOSEPH H. BRANHAM, M. D.,
 Lecturer on Obstetrics.
R. B WINDER, M. D., D. D. S.,
 Professor of Principles and Practice of
 Dental Surgery as Applied to Medicine.

ADJUNCT FACULTY.

WM. F. SMITH, A. B., M. D.,
 Demonstrator of Anatomy.
GEORGE THOMAS, A. M., M. D.,
 Lecturer on Diseases of the Throat and
 Chest.
WILLIAM S. GARDNER, M. D.,
 Lecturer on Obstetrics and Demon-
 strator of Chemistry.
G. A. LIEBIG, Jr., Ph. D.,
 Lecturer on Medical Electricity.
C. HAMPSON JONES, M. D. [M.B.Edin.]
 Demonstrator of Physiology.
HENRY P. HYNSON, Ph. G.,
 Demonstrator of Pharmacy.

HARRY FRIEDENWALD, A. B., M. D.,
 Lecturer on Diseases of the Eye and Ear
J. W. LORD A. B., M. D.,
 Lecturer on Dermatology.
FRANK C. BRESSLER, M. D.,
 Lecturer on the Diseases of Children.
LOUIS F. ANKRIM M. D.
FRANK C. BRESSLER, M. D.
R. G. DAVIS, M. D.,
 Assistant Demonstrators of Anatomy.
F. D. SANGER, M. D.,
 Prosector.

The Regular Winter Session will begin October 1st, 1892, and end April 1st, 1893, and for all students who enter after July 1st, 1892, is one of three annual sessions required for graduation.

The student of medicine is given unsurpassed clinical advantages at this school.

THE NEW COLLEGE BUILDING. The Faculty takes pride in announcing that the New College Building is complete in all its appointments. In it are provided the Physiological, Chemical, Pathological and Bacteriological Laboratories as well as the Lecture Halls which are equipped with handsome theatre seats.

The New City Hospital is a magnificent structure, with a capacity of 300 beds. situated in the centre of the city. Its position enables it to command most of the accident cases occurring in Baltimore. The Faculty have the exclusive medical control of it. A systematic course of bedside instruction is given in the wards.

The Maryland Lying-in Asylum, established by this school in 1874, was the pioneer institution of its kind in this State. It is full of obstetric cases throughout the year and furnishes each student with bedside instruction and experience.

The Maryland Woman's Hospital has been merged into and forms an important part of the New Baltimore City Hospital. New and handsome private rooms are set apart in the front of the main building for private Gynæcological patients and thoroughly equipped Operating Rooms have been provided for such cases.

The New Colored Hospital. The builing formerly known as the Woman's Hospital has been torn down and a handsome new structure is now in process of construction, which will be open for the reception of patients this Spring. This recent acquisition will be occupied as male and female wards for colored people. It is the first hospital which was ever established in the State of Maryland exclusively for the colored race.

Bay View, the Almshouse of Baltimore, which contains 1200 beds, has been thrown open for the clinical instruction of students of this school. Two Resident Physicians for the Medical and Surgical Departments are annually appointed at this institution, each with a salary of $500 and board. One from the University of Maryland and one from the College of Physicians and Surgeons. Two Assistant Resident Physicians are similarly appointed.

The City Hospital Dispensary, organized over twenty years ago, has become widespread in its influence and adds largely to the clinical attractions of the school.

Frequent post mortem examinations are made before the whole class, and the medico-legal bearings of cases are fully discussed

Attendance upon the demonstrations in the Physiological, Chemical and Pathological Laboratories is required of every student.

The Anatomical rooms are spacious and airy, and dissecting material abundant.

A Resident Physician and three Assistant Resident Physicians for the CityHospital, a Resident Physician for the Maternity Hospital and one for the Colored Hospital are appointed annually from the graduating class as awards of merit. A limited number of students will be admitted as residents in the hospital.

All students who enter this school of medicine after July 1st, 1892, will be subject to a preliminary examination.

The Medical Profession and Students of Medicine, are invited to call and inspect our equi ment.

The Maryland Lying-In Asylum,

115 WEST LOMBARD STREET,

BALTIMORE, MD.

Under the Exclusive Control of the College of Physicians & Surgeons.

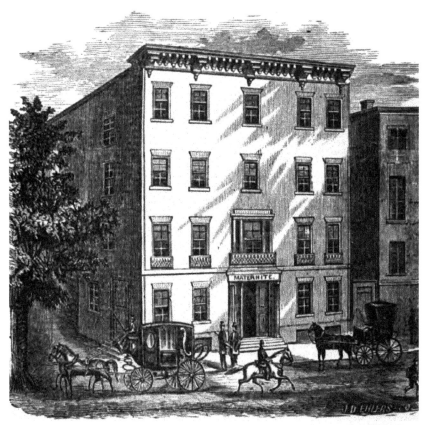

This Institution is open for the reception of patients. Indigent women of this City and State are admitted for their confinement, and carefully attended by scientific physicians and skilled nurses. Having been liberally aided by the Legislature, no cost or pains have been spared to render it as perfect as possible in all its departments. The Public Wards are spacious, well warmed and ventilated, and are supplied with all the appliances and conveniences which can conduce to the comfort and safety of the parturient woman.

Board, attention by a member of the Faculty nursing and medicines, are given free of charge to all patients in the Public Wards.

Every precaution is taken to prevent the recognition of inmates.

Private patients are furnished rooms at from $6.00 to $12 per week, according to the size and location of the chambers.

For additional information, apply to the Dean, or Charles E. Greene, M. D., House Physician.

THOS. OPIE, M. D., Dean of the Faculty.

OUR POLICY:

1ST.   Is to do, exclusively, a Prescription and Drug Business.

2ND.   To supply everything peculiar to the sick-room.

3RD.   To furnish all kinds of Surgical Dressings, Antiseptics, &c.

4TH.   To carry the most comprehensive Prescription Stock possible.

5TH.   To dispense always the very best products obtainable.

6TH.   To maintain an orderly and perfectly equipped Prescription Department.

7TH.   To employ only competent, courteous and experienced assistants.

8TH.   To abstain strictly from giving medical advice.

9TH.   To exclude all " Quack " Medicines, Nostrums, &c.

10TH.   To charge reasonable prices.

Hynson & Westcott,

Pharmaceutical Chemists,

421 N. CHARLES STREET, BALTIMORE.

CHARLES C. COOK'S

Beef Extract, With Iron, Wine and Coca-Pepsin. . . . . . .

The attention of the medical profession is respectfully called to this nutritive, digestive and invigorating tonic composed of the choicest Beef (free from fat or gelatin) Ammonia, Citrate of Iron, Imported Sherry Wine and Coca-Pepsin.

The Coca-Pepsin which makes this tonic an invaluable remedy for all stomach disorders and forms of indigestion caused by deficient secretion of gastric juice, contains in permanent solution the digestive ferments Pepsin, Ptyalin Pancreatin, Lactic and Hydrochloric acids, in combination with Coca, Celery; Caffeine and Chartreuse Cordial.

By the tonic action of the alkaloid Caffeine the digestive proper-ties of Coca-Pepsin are rendered more thorough and permanent, in-creasing the appetite, and digestive powers while tissue waste is diminished.

Celery and Coca are also good additions to this digestive compound, the former acts as an appetizer and nervous stimulant, while Coca pro-duces a general excitation or natural stimulus of the circulatory and nervous systems, and imparts increased vigor to the muscles and intel-lect, stimulating the stomach by imparting new tone to this organ when weakened or broken down. In combination with Beef and Iron, the effects of Coca are greatly prolonged.

The pleasant flavor and soothing properties of this tonic render it acceptable to the most fastidious palate, and agreeable to the most delicate stomach, and is adapted for delicate women, children and convalescents.

It will be found a prompt, safe and efficient remedy in nervous debility, headache, fullness of blood, loss of appetite, and depression of spirits. It overcomes that tired feeling and cures constipation by causing thorough digestion and proper assimilation of food.

It relieves nausea, fullness and oppression about the stomach, acidity and flatulency.

DOSE.– For adult, a tablespoonful after each meal.

For sale by all Wholesale and Retail Druggists.

PRICE $1.00 PER BOTTLE.

MANUFACTURED ONLY BY

CHARLES C. COOK,

COR. DRUID HILL AVE. AND LANVALE STREET,

BALTIMORE, MD.

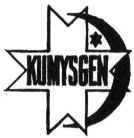 or **Carnrick's Kumyss Tablets,**

A PRODUCT OF PURE SWEET MILK,
PALATABLE, NUTRITIOUS,
EASILY DIGESTED,
AND WHEN DISSOLVED IN WATER
FORMS A DELICIOUS EFFER-
VESCENT KUMYSS.

(Put up in air-tight bottles, in two sizes; the larger holding sufficient Tablets for seven twelve-ounce bottles, and the smaller sufficient for three twelve-once bottles of Kumyss.)

THIS PREPARATION is presented to the Medical Profession in the convenient form of Tablets, and will be found superior in every respect to the ordinary *Kumyss, Wine of Milk, Fermented Milk,* or any similar preparation.

Kumysgen when prepared for use contains every constituent of a perfect Kumyss.

Kumysgen is made from fresh, sweet milk, and contains fully thirty per cent. of soluble casein, which is double the amount found in ordinary Kumyss preparations.

Kumysgen being in Tablet form, will keep indefinitely, is easily and readily prepared, less expensive than the ordinary variable and perishable Kumyss, and its *fermentative action* may be regulated at will, thus rendering it available at all times and under all circumstances.

Clinical tests gathered from every quarter of the globe attest its special value in all cases of *Gastric* and *Intestinal Indigestion* or *Dyspepsia, Pulmonary Consumption, Constipation, Gastric and Intestinal Catarrh, Fevers, Anæmia, Chlorosis, Rickets, Scrofula, Vomiting in Pregnancy, Bright's Disease, Intestinal Ailments of Infants, Cholera Infantum ;* for young children and for convalescents from all diseases.

The casein being finely subdivided, it is especially valuable for all who require an easily digested or a partially digested Food.

Kumysgen is a delicious effervescent Food-Beverage, relished alike by the sick or well.

Kumysgen is tonic, stimulant, diuretic, highly nutritious, easily digested, perfectly palatable, and always *permanent* and *uniform* in strength.

SAMPLE SENT ON REQUEST.

MANUFACTURED BY

REED & CARNRICK, New York.

✦HORLICK'S✦
MALTED MILK,

THE NEW MILK FOOD

For Infants, Invalids, Dyspeptics and Aged People.

**MALTED MILK IS EASILY SOLUBLE,
REQUIRES NO COOKING, CONTAINS NO STARCH.**

Samples of Horlick's Malted Milk sent free on application to

MALTED MILK CO.,

RACINE, WIS.

For the Speedy Relief of Nervous Headache and Brain Fatigue.

WARNER & CO.'S EFFERVESCING

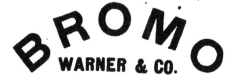

BROMO
WARNER & CO.
SODA

**Useful in Nervous Headache, Sleeplessness, Excessive Study,
Over Brainwork, Nervous Debility, Mania, etc., etc.**

DOSE.—A heaping teaspoonful in half a glass of water, to be repeated once after an interval of thirty minutes, if necessary. Each teaspoonful contains 30 grs. Bromide Sodium and 1 gr. caffein.

It is claimed by some prominent specialists in nervous diseases that the sodium Salt is more acceptable to the stomach than the Bromide Potassium. An almost certain relief is given by the administration of this Effervescing Salt. It is also used with advantage in Indigestion, Depression following alcoholic and other excesses, as well as Nervous Headache. It affords speedy relief for Mental and Physical Exhaustion.

PREPARED ONLY BY WM. R. WARNER & CO.

THOMAS & THOMPSON, Agts.,

BALTIMORE AND LIGHT STS.   BALTIMORE, MD.

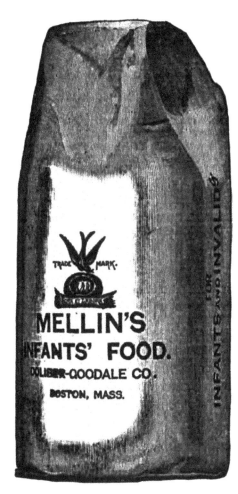

TRANSACTIONS

—OF THE—

edical and Chirurgical Faculty

—OF THE—

STATE OF MARYLAND,

Ninety-Fourth Annual Session

—HELD AT—

BALTIMORE, MARYLAND, APRIL, 1892.

—ALSO—

emi-Annual Session, Held at Rockville, Md., Nov., 1891.

BALTIMORE:
GRIFFIN, CURLEY & CO., PRINTERS,
202 E. Baltimore Street,
1892.

Officers, Committees, Sections and Delegates.

FOR THE YEAR 1892-93.

President.
L. McLANE TIFFANY.

Vice-Presidents.
J. W. DOWNEY,   J. W. CHAMBERS.

Recording Secretary.
G. LANE TANEYHILL.

Assistant Secretary.
ROBT. T. WILSON.

Corresponding Secretary.
JOSEPH T. SMITH.

Reporting Secretary.
W. B. CANFIELD.

Treasurer,
W. F. A. KEMP.

Executive Committee.
WM. H. WELCH,	T. A. ASHBY,	P. C. WILLIAMS,
DAVID STREETT,	GEO. H. ROHE,	L. McL. TIFFANY.

Examining Board, Western Shore.
WILMER BRINTON,	J. E. MICHAEL,	J. D. BLAKE,
S. K. MERRICK,	D. W. CATHELL,	AARON FRIEDENWALD,
	B. B. BROWNE.	

Examining Board, Eastern Shore.
W. F. HINES,	B. W. GOLDSBOROUGH,	MONMONIER ROWE,
G. E. DICKINSON,	J. M. BORDLEY.	

Library Committee.
B. B. BROWNE,	I. E. ATKINSON,	G. J. PRESTON,
G. LANE TANEYHILL,	R. W. JOHNSON.	

Publication Committee.
G. LANE TANEYHILL,	W. F. A. KEMP,	H. M. WILSON,
W. OSLER,	J. WHITRIDGE WILLIAMS.	

Memoir Committee.
E. F. CORDELL,	A. K. BOND,	ROBERT C. RASIN,
J. W. HUMRICHOUSE,	G. E. DICKINSON.	

Committee on Ethics.
G. W. MILTENBERGER,	JOHN F. MONMONIER,	T. S. LATIMER,
A. FRIEDENWALD,	J. E. M. CHAMBERLAINE.	

Curator.
W. T. HOWARD, JR.

Section on Surgery.

RANDOLPH WINSLOW,   J. T. M. FINNEY,   C. F. BEVAN,
JAMES BROWN,   R. B. WARFIELD.

Section on Practice.

CHARLES O'DONOVAN, Jr.,   W. F. LOCKWOOD,   J. D. IGLEHART,
CHARLES M. ELLIS,   A. S. PORTER.

Section on Obstetrics and Gynaecology.

J. WHITRIDGE WILLIAMS,   WILMER BRINTON,   HOWARD KELLY,
W. A. B. SELLMAN,   B. W. GOLDSBOROUGH.

Section on Materia Medica and Chemistry.

A. K. BOND,   R. H. P. ELLIS,   A. C. POLE,
R. B. MORRISON,   EDWARD ANDERSON.

Section on Sanitary Science.

JAS. T. McSHANE,   JOHN D. BLAKE,   ALICE H. CHAPMAN,
WM. B. CANFIELD,   C. BIRNIE.

Section on Anatomy, Physiology and Pathology.

J. M. CRAIGHILL,   JAS. G. WILTSHIRE,   L. R. TRIMBLE,
CHARLES W. MITCHELL,   O. H. W. RAGAN.

Section on Psychology and Medical Jurisprudence.

HARRY J. BERKLEY,   G. J. PRESTON,   H. M. THOMAS,
ALEX. L. HODGDON,   B. D. EVANS.

Section on Microscopy, Micro-Chemistry and Spectral Analysis.

C. O. MILLER,   A. G. HOEN,   DAVID STREETT,
SIMON FLEXNER,   W. T. HOWARD, Jr

Section on Ophthalmology, Otology and Laryngology.

HARRY FRIEDENWALD,   F. M. CHISOLM,   JOHN R. WINSLOW.
SAMUEL JOHNSTON,

Delegates to American Medical Association.

A. FRIEDENWALD,   JOS. H. STONESTREET,   W. A. B. SELLMAN,
T. S. LATIMER,   M. B. BILLINGSLEA,   I. F. MARTINET,
J. M. SCOTT,   A. H. MANN,   A. S. MASON,
J. E. DWINELLE,   WM. M. BARNES,   J. H. BRANHAM,
J. J. CHISOLM,   G. LANE TANEYHILL,   WM. LEE HOWARD,
H. H. BIEDLER,   J. W. HUMRICHOUSE,   THOMAS OPIE,
J. W. CHAMBERS,   THEODORE COOKE,   GEO. B. REYNOLDS,
DAVID STREETT,   JAS. G. WILTSHIRE,   ROBERT C. RASIN.
JOHN C. HARRIS,

Delegates to West Virginia State Medical Society.

H. H. BIEDLER,   A. S. PORTER,   I. M. SPEAR,
J. LEE McCOMAS,   A. C. POLE,   A. B. PRICE.

Delegates to North Carolina State Medical Society.

J. E. MICHAEL,   RANDOLPH WINSLOW,   W. E. MOSLEY,
J. M. CHAMBERS,   EDWIN GEER,   W. T. HOWARD, Jr.
GEO. H. ROHE,   K. B. BATCHELOR,

Delegates to Virginia State Medical Society.

T. A. ASHBY,   ROBERT T. WILSON,   B. D. EVANS,
H. P. C. WILSON,   S. K. MERRICK,   THOMAS OPIE.
S. T. EARLE.

DISCLAIMER. The Medical and Chirurgical Faculty of the State of Maryland, while formally accepting and publishing the reports of the various Sections and Volunteer Papers read at its sessions, *does not hold itself responsible* for the opinions, theories or criticisms therein contained.

TO AUTHORS. Contributors to any volume of the TRANSACTIONS are requested to observe the following : 1st, Write on one side of the paper only. 2nd, Write without breaks, *i. e.*, do not begin a new sentence on a new line ; when you want to begin a new paragraph, begin in the middle of the line. 3rd, Draw a line along the margin of such paragraphs as should be printed in smaller type—for instance, all that is clinical history in reports of cases, or that which is quoted, &c. 4th, Words to be printed in *italics* should be underscored once ; in SMALL CAPITALS twice ; in LARGE CAPITALS three times. 5th, Proofs sent for revision should be returned without delay ; authors who contemplate a temporary absence from their regular residence any time during the summer, should notify the Recording Secretary, thus avoiding vexatious delays in the delivery of proof. 6th, Authors whose papers have been "accepted" by the Faculty and referred to the Publication Committee—such papers thus becoming the property of the Faculty—are expected to place the original or a verbatim printable copy on desk of the Recording Secretary immediately after the reading of the same. 7th, The Publication Committee is instructed by the Faculty to publish no paper that has been read before a local medical society prior to the publication of the TRANSACTIONS of the Faculty. 8th, Alterations in manuscript should be limited to what is of essential importance, they are equivalent to resetting, and cause additional expense, such changes, if they exceed half a page of printed matter, as also all wood cuts, photographs and electrotypes, are invariably to be paid for by authors.

MEMBERSHIP. Applications for membership in the Medical and Chirurgical Faculty should be addressed to the Recording Secretary, Corresponding Secretary, Treasurer, or Chairman of the Examining Board, and should state name in full, post office address, where graduated in medicine, date of graduation, and by whom recommended. They must be accompanied by the *initiation fee* of five dollars : no membership dues are required for the first current year : a copy of the annual TRANSACTIONS is mailed gratuitously to each member. *Blank applications* for membership will be mailed to any address on application to the Recording Secretary or Treasurer.

CONTENTS.

EXPLANATORY.

On account of the scarcity of funds the Faculty directed the Publication Committee, this year, to omit the publication of all papers read before the Society except the address of the President and the Annual Oration. As the subjects that would be referred to in the "special meetings" have been fully set forth in the report of the Memoir Committee, they have judged it unnecessary to publish those minutes. After a half dozen ineffectual efforts to obtain the manuscript of the Annual Orator they despaired of their efforts, but have the pleasure of presenting the exhaustive and instructive address of the President on "*Acute Lobar Pneumonia, in the light of Bacteriological Investigation.*"

MINUTES.

Semi-Annual Meeting.

ROCKVILLE, MD., Nov. 17–18, 1891.

The Semi-Annual Meeting of the Medical and Chirurgical Faculty of Maryland was held at Rockville, Montgomery County, Maryland, November 17th and 18th, 1891, there being twenty-seven members of the medical profession present.

The meeting was called to order at 11.30 A. M., by the President, Dr. Wm. H. Welch, Dr. Robert T. Wilson, Assistant Secretary, and Dr. Wm. B. Canfield, Reporting Secretary were at their desks.

The address of welcome was delivered by Dr. E. E. Stonestreet, of Rockville, for the Montgomery County Medical Society.

The President thanked in a most fitting manner on behalf of the Faculty, Dr. Stonestreet for his cordial address of welcome.

The President then delivered his address—"*The Bacillus Coli Communis*"—the conditions of its invasion in the human body, and its pathogenic properties. The address was a masterly one on the subject. It was discussed by Dr. Black, of Australia.

On motion it was ordered that all doctors present who were not members of the Faculty be invited to take part in the deliberations of the Faculty. Dr. Ernest Black, of Australia, formerly of London,

England, was introduced to the Faculty and invited to take part in the discussions.

Dr. George J. Preston read his paper on "*Rest Cure, and Cases in which it is applicable.*"

Remarks were made on this paper by Drs. Ashby, Robert T. Wilson, Roger Brooks, Black and Welch.

Dr. Edward Anderson read his paper on "*Typhoid Fever.*" It was discussed by Drs. Ashby, Preston, Onderdonk, J. McP. Scott, Welch, Stonestreet, Hines and Anderson.

Dr. Anderson showed to the Convention several rare works, printed before the American Revolution.

Dr. Ashby brought up the subject of burial places in towns and cities and the danger of the same to the community.

There being no further business, Convention adjourned to meet next day.

ROBERT T. WILSON,
Assistant Secretary.

Second Day.

The Convention was called to order, Dr. W. H. Welch in the Chair.

The minutes of the previous meeting were read and approved.

Dr. Ashby read his paper on "*Appendicitis in the Female*," with report of two cases.

Remarks were made by Drs. Welch and Robert T. Wilson.

Dr. Robert T. Wilson read his paper on "*Laparotomy for Removal of a Purulent Tumor of the Right Ovary*."

Remarks were made by Drs. Ashby, Welch, Wilson.

Dr. Canfield read his paper on "*Occupation and Disease*," with special reference to the connection between the inhalation of dust and pulmonary disease.

Remarks were made by Drs. Welch, Preston, Canfield.

At this juncture arrived from Baltimore Drs. Bond, Chambers, Harlan, Hilgartner, Michael, Winslow, Randolph; also J. S. Stone and S. B. Muncaster, from Washington.

Dr. Michael read his paper on "*A Case Illustrating the Diagnosis of late Extra Uterine Pregnancy, and the Difficulty of Producing Abortion*."

Remarks were made by Drs. Stone, Winslow, Welch and Michael.

Dr. Bond read his paper on "*Notes on the use of Codeine.*"

Remarks were made by Drs. Stone, Canfield, Anderson, Wilson and Bond.

Dr. Winslow read his paper on "*A Case of Elephantiasis of the Scrotum.*"

Remarks were made by Drs. Welch and Winslow.

The paper by Dr. Charles E. Stone, on "*Early Diagnosis and Operation in Osteo-Sarcoma of the Lower Bones*," was read for Dr. Stone by Dr. E. E. Stonestreet, Dr. Stone being prevented by sickness from being present.

Remarks were made by Drs. Chambers, Winslow, Stonestreet and Welch.

Dr. Stonestreet reported an interesting case of this kind now under his care.

Dr. Randolph read his paper on "*Report of Fifty Consecutive Operations for Cataract.*"

Remarks were made by Drs. S. B. Muncaster, Harlan, Belt and Randolph.

On motion of Dr. Ashby, a vote of thanks to the "Montgomery County Medical Society" for their kind hospitality was unanimously adopted.

On motion of Dr. Wilson, a vote of thanks to the President, Dr. Welch, for the able manner in which he presided at this successful meeting was ordered.

Among the Physicians present were: Drs. T. A. Ashby, Ernest Black, Canfield, Preston, Robert T. Wilson, William H. Welch, J. McP. Scott, E. E. Stonestreet, Etchison, J. L. Lewis, Edw. Anderson, Hines, O. M. Linthicum, Elgin, S. B. Muncaster, Winslow, Michael, Chambers, Stone, Randolph, Onderdonk, Albert, Deets, Bond, Harlan, Farquhar, C. L. G. Anderson and Roger Brooks.

There being no further business, the Convention adjourned, *sine die*.

ROBERT T. WILSON, M. D.,

Assistant Secretary.

MINUTES.

Annual Meeting.

HALL OF THE FACULTY,
St. Paul and Saratoga Sts.

TUESDAY, April 26th, 1892.

The 94th Annual Convention was called to order this day, by the President, Dr. Wm. H. Welch, about 200 physicians being present. All the Secretaries and the Treasurer were at their desks.

On motion, the calling of the roll and reading of minutes were dispensed with. The Recording Secretary made the preliminary announcements as recorded on page 2 of the official programme, and on his motion the memoranda as there printed were adopted by the Faculty.

Dr. Joseph T. Smith, the Corresponding Secretary, made his report, which was accepted.

Dr. G. Lane Taneyhill, the Recording Secretary, read his report, which was accepted.

Dr. Wm. Fred'k Kemp, the Treasurer, read his report, which was received and referred to the Executive Committee to be audited and report on the same. It showed the total expenses for the year to have been - · - - $1,712 82
Total receipts - - - 1,671 36

Over paid during the year	-	$ 41 46
Unpaid rent - -	-	400 00
Deficiency of 1891 -	-	518 06
Total indebtedness - -	-	$959 52

The President, Dr. Wm. H. Welch, read his address. On motion of Dr. Philip C. Williams, the thanks of the Faculty were voted the President and a copy of the address requested for publication.

The Section on Surgery reported through its Chairman, Dr. R. W. Johnson.

Under this heading the following gentlemen read papers, all of which were referred for publication: Drs. R. W. Johnson, S. T. Earle and Walter B. Platt.

The Examining Board of Western Shore reported through their Chairman, Dr. J. W. Chambers. They recommended seventy-two candidates for election to membership in the Faculty. The list was posted on the Bulletin Board, the names to be voted on the following day.

At the appointed hour the Faculty adjourned, to meet at 8 p. m. this day.

G. LANE TANEYHILL,
Recording Secretary.

HALL OF THE FACULTY,

APRIL 26TH, 1892.

The Faculty was called to order by the President, Dr. Wm. H. Welch. The other officers were at their tables. The minutes of the day session were read and approved.

Under the head of *"Section on Practice,"* Dr. C. O'Donavan read a volunteer paper, which was received and referred for publication.

Under the head of *"Section on Obstetrics and Gynæcology,"* papers were read by Drs. L. E. Neale, Philip C. Williams, Hunter A. Robb and J. H. Kennedy. The papers were discussed by the readers, and also by Drs. Opie, A. B. Price, Mosley, Brinton, Ellis, Bond, Michael and Downey.

The paper of Dr. Mosley was, at his own suggestion, on motion, read by title on account of the lateness of the hour. That of Dr. Branham was postponed to a future time. The Examining Board submitted another list of candidates.

On motion of Dr. Michael, the President was authorized to announce to-morrow a committee of nine, who should submit nominations to be voted for as composing the Licensing Board of seven regular practitioners of Maryland, this list not preventing other nominations.

On motion adjourned.

G. LANE TANEYHILL,
Recording Secretary.

HALL OF THE FACULTY,
WEDNESDAY, April 27th, 1892, 12 M.

The Faculty was called to order promptly by the President, Dr. Wm. H. Welch. The minutes were read by the Secretary and approved by the Faculty.

The Corresponding Secretary read a letter from Dr. C. Johnston, Jr., donating the busts of Drs. N. R. Smith and John Buckler. On motion the thanks of the Faculty were ordered to be transmitted to Dr. Johnston, Jr.

The Corresponding Secretary read an invitation from the Maryland Historical Society inviting the members to visit the art gallery of the Society. On motion the thanks of the Faculty were ordered to be returned to the Historical Society.

The Recording Secretary read an invitation from the Secretary General of the Pan-American Congress inviting the Society to lend its influence to the furtherance of the objects of the same. On motion it was ordered that the present President appoint a committee of five, of which the present President shall be chairman, to act for this Faculty in all matters pertaining to the Pan-American Congress.

At this juncture, the President announced the committee on *nominating* a Licensing Examining Board of Regular Physicians of the State of Maryland as contemplated in an Act passed by the late Legislature of this State. The following are the names of the members of the *committee:* J. E. Michael, T. A. Ashby, Chas. H. Jones, Geo. J. Preston, Herbert

Harlan, John Neff, Hiram Woods, Jno. W. Humrichouse, Walter B. Platt.

The election of candidates to membership in the Faculty having now been entered into, with Drs. Iglehart, Cordell and Mann as tellers, resulted in the following members of the medical profession being admitted into the Society:

Edw. Anderson, Wm. S. Archer, Edw. Carey Applegarth, John H. Bolton, Thos. H. Brayshaw, Wm. B. Burch, K. B. Batchelor, Jas. Bordley, Edw. N. Brush, Jas. Cooper, A. A. Clewell, W. B. Clarke, Pinckney L. Davis, Jas. E. Deets, Rufus W. Dashiell, Emanuel W. Eilan, Wm. F. Elgin, B. D. Evans, W. R. Eareckson, Chas. E. Ellis, Robert Fawcett, Fred. H. F. Fincke, Jas. H. Fore, Louis F. Frey, Hugh Forsythe, Simon Flexner, W. W. Frames, Wm. B. Gambrill, A. L. Gage, Joseph Gichner, Edwin Geer, Wm. S. Halstead, Chas. B. Henkel, Wm. Travis Howard, Jr., Wm. Lee Howard, Albert K. Hadel, Eugene W. Heyde, Louis C. Horn, August Horn, M. L. Hooper, David C. Ireland, John J. Jones, Eugene H. Judkins, T. D. Kennedy, Marshall E. Leatherman, John Latane Lewis, Wm. Milton Lewis, Thos. W. Linthicum, Jas. T. McShane, Ellis Micheau, Stuart B. Muncaster, Thos. A. Milliman, Edw. P. McDeritt, Chas. W. Mitchell, Frank Martin, H. A. McComas, A. D. McConachie, John Henry O'Donovan, M. G. Porter, A. B. Price, Thos. Carnes Price, Abraham Shank, Edw. A. Smith, Cacilino C. Steuart, Jos. H. Stonestreet, A. Trego Shertzer, Edwin M. Schindel, Hiram L. Spicer, Solomon J. Ulman, A. G. Watson, J. E. Willing, A. S. Wagner, E. M. Wise, Chas. R. Winterson, Chas. Wattenscheidt, Geo. L. Wilkins, Lot Ridgeley Wilson, Thos. Chew Worthington, Wm. F. Wootten, Alfred Whitehead.

Under the head of "*Materia Medica and Chemistry*" the following gentlemen read papers: Drs. Joseph T. Smith, E. F. Cordell and Walter B. Platt. Drs. Bernie and Hines discussed the papers.

In the absence, temporarily, of the next reader, Dr. J. H. Branham read a paper from the *Obstetric Section*; it was discussed by Dr. Brinton and others.

The regular order being resumed, Dr. Jno. C. Hemmeter read a paper from the *Section on Anatomy, Physiology and Pathology*.

Dr. Chambers, the chairman of the Examining Board for Western Shore, in behalf of the Board, offered an additional list of candidates, whom the Board recommended for membership.

Dr. Walter B. Platt read an interesting paper on the necessity of an "*Inspection of Dairies and Milk.*"

After several announcements the Faculty adjourned to meet, in *Executive Session*, to-night at eight o'clock.

G. LANE TANEYHILL,
Recording Secretary.

HALL OF THE FACULTY,
BALTIMORE, MD., Wednesday, April 27th, 1892.
NIGHT MEETING.

The Faculty was called to order by the President, Dr. Welch; the Secretaries and Treasurer were at their desks. There were 213 physicians present. The minutes of the morning session were read and approved. The President informed the Faculty that this is the "*Executive Session,*" as ordered by the Constitution, and that no papers would be read to-night.

Dr. T. A. Ashby, Chairman of the Executive Committee, read his report, it was accepted, and the suggestions contemplating changes in the Constitution and By-Laws, etc., were ordered to be presented, subsequently, under New Business, as notices of amendments.

Dr. G. Lane Taneyhill, Chairman of the *Library Committee,* read the report; it was accepted and the suggestions contained therein were ordered to be presented under New Business.

Dr. G. Lane Taneyhill, Chairman of the *Publication Committee*, read his report; it was accepted and the resolutions appended were ordered to be presented under New Business.

Dr. E. F. Cordell, Chairman of the *Memoir Committee*, on his own motion had his report read "by title."

Dr. L. McLane Tiffany, the chairman of the *Ethics Committee*, reported verbally that no business had been presented and therefore the committee had nothing to hand in.

Dr. L. F. Ankrim, the *Curator*, had nothing, "pathologically," to report.

Dr. T. A. Ashby, Chairman of the special committee "*on Increasing the Membership*," reported verbally that not only the committee, but many members, and especially the Recording Secretary through his circular, had done some effective recruiting, and the committee had reason to believe that over 100 candidates would apply for membership, as already 86 names had been handed in. The report was accepted and the committee continued.

Dr. Hiram Woods, chairman of the special committee on "*Preventable Causes of Blindness in the United States*," read his report, which was accepted.

Under *Unfinished Business*, Dr. G. Lane Taneyhill, the chairman of the Library Committee, brought forward the following amendment to the Constitution, which had been offered by that committee in its report of 1891, and recorded on page 162 of the Transactions of 1891:

That one-half of all initiation fees and annual dues be paid to the Library, instead of five-eighths of dues from city and two-thirds of dues from county members, as at present.

After a short debate and some explanations the amendment received more than a constitutional majority.

Under the same head the amendment offered by Dr. Hiram Woods, proposed at the convention of 1891 and recorded in the Transactions of 1891, page 146, was called up by that gentleman; it is as follows:

Art. V, Sec. 2. The chairman of each Section shall select some member of the Faculty to open the discussion upon one of the papers to be read by his Section : he shall send to the Recording Secretary the name of the one selected when he sends the titles of papers to be presented by his Section.

After some explanatory remarks and after the withdrawal of certain proposed modifications, the amendment, in its original form, received a constitutional majority.

Dr. Michael, the chairman of a committee to nominate "seven regular physicians as a *Board of*

Medical Examiners for the State of Maryland, representing the Medical and Chirurgical Faculty of the
State of Maryland, said appointees to be physicians
actually engaged in the practice of medicine and of
recognized ability and honor," reported that the committee had decided to recommend to the Faculty the
names of the following gentlemen, but that this action did not prevent other nominations from the members of the Faculty :

Drs. Samuel T. Earle and *Wm. F. Lockwood,* of
Baltimore; *Dr. F. B. Smith,* of Frederick; *Dr. Wm.
F. Hines,* of Chestertown; *Dr. James Bordley,* of
Centreville; *Dr. J. McPherson Scott,* of Hagerstown,
and *Dr. W. W. Wiley,* of Cumberland.

There being no other nominations made, the
Faculty, by ballot, elected the above named gentlemen as the seven regular physicians, to serve for
four years from June 1, 1892, on the *Board of Medical Examiners* for the State of Maryland.

The Executive Committee reported that they had
audited the accounts of the Treasurer and found
them correct, thereupon the Report of that officer
was accepted.

Under *New Business,* Dr. T. A. Ashby, chairman
of the *Executive Committee,* gave notice of numerous *amendments* which they would offer at a future
meeting; the manuscript was filed with the Recording Secretary.

*Amendments offered by Executive Committee to
Constitution and By-Laws :*

In Article V, Section 1, omit the words "and Sections"—
and all that follows after the words "Committee on Ethics,"

insert "Committee on Programme" after "Committee on Ethics."

Omit the word Section or Sections (when used to designate Section on Surgery, Section on Practice of Medicine, etc., as enumerated in Article V, Section 1,) from Article III, Sections 1, 3, 5, 7, Article V, Section 2, and change the phraseology to correspond to these omissions. Omit the last paragraph beginning "each Section," etc., in Article V, Section 2. Change Article III, Section 1, paragraph 2, to read thus: He shall call a special meeting at such times as the interests of the Faculty may require.

In Article VI, after Section 5, introduce the following: "Section 6." *The Committee on Programme* shall procure papers to be read at the Annual and Semi-Annual Meetings of the Faculty.

Make membership of Executive Committee 7 instead of 6, including Recording Secretary and Treasurer *ex-officio* members of this Committee.

Under *By-Laws*, Section 1, omit "13, Report of Sections, in order of appointment," in the following line omit the word "Volunteer," and in order "18, announcement of Committees, Sections, etc.," omit the word "Sections."

In amendments of April 27, 1888, by the Secretary, omit the word "Sections.

Introduce motion limiting time for reading papers (with exception of the general addresses) to 20 minutes.

Dr. G. Lane Taneyhill, chairman of the *Publication Committee*, offered the following resolutions from said Committee, which, after some explanations and a slight amendment, were adopted by the Faculty:

Resolved, That, until otherwise ordered, every member reading an original paper or report before the Faculty shall, on the same day, deliver to the Recording Secretary, at his desk, after reading the same, the original manuscript or a perfect copy of said paper or report; and, if he fail in this, or fail to mail a copy to that officer *within ten days* after adjournment of the Convention at which said paper was read, the Publishing Committee is hereby authorized to proceed to publish the Transactions without such paper.

Resolved, That in future, the Publication Committee be and is hereby authorized to employ, at a reasonable salary, a competent person, a member of the medical profession, as *proof reader* for the Committee ; and, that, all manuscripts and proofs shall be edited and corrected by said proof reader, instead of, as at present, by the authors.

On motion of Dr. Samuel T. Earle, the following action was ordered :

Whereas, In the opinion of the Medical and Chirurgical Faculty of Maryland the means of public disinfection, in use, at this time, by the Health Department of Baltimore City have been found by actual experience, to be insufficient, therefore,

Resolved, That this Faculty does hereby urgently recommend to the Health Department, and, if it be unable to move in the matter—to the Mayor and City Council of Baltimore City, the advisability of at once adopting some approved system of Steam Disinfection under pressure ; a note of this action to be transmitted at once to the Health Department by the Secretary of the Faculty.

On motion of Dr. T. A. Ashby the following resolution was passed :

Resolved, That the Publication Committee, if they discover, this year, after consultation with the Treasurer, that they may not be able to publish the full volume of the *Transactions* on account of the scarcity of funds, that they, at least, publish the minutes, reports of officers and committees and the President's Address and Annual Oration.

The Recording Secretary, who had previously, alone, prepared the programmes, with a view of dividing up the work and securing early pledges of papers by members, offered the following resolution, which was adopted:

Resolved, That the outgoing President appoint a special "*Committee on Programme,*" to consist of three members, whose duty it shall be to collect from the Recording, the Corresponding and the Assistant Secretary, and, when necessary, from the members of the various Sections and Volunteer writers the *Titles of all papers* to be read at the meetings of the Faculty. This Committee shall be empowered to solicit papers from members and to make other arrangements calculated to enhance the success of the programme.

The resignation of Dr. J. A. Bonnett was on motion accepted.

The election of officers for the ensuing year resulted as follows:

President—Dr. L. McLane Tiffany.
Vice-Presidents—Drs. J. W. Downey and J. W. Chambers.
Recording Secretary—Dr. G. Lane Taneyhill.
Assistant Secretary—Dr. Robt. T. Wilson.
Corresponding Secretary—Dr. Joseph T. Smith.
Reporting Secretary—Dr. W. B. Canfield.
Treasurer—Dr. W. F. A. Kemp.
Executive Committee—Drs. Wm. H. Welch, T. A. Ashby, P. C. Williams, David Streett, Geo. H. Rohe, and *ex-officio*, L. McL. Tiffany.
Examining Board, Western Shore—Drs. Wilmer Brinton, J. E. Michael, J. D. Blake, S. K. Merrick, D. W. Cathell, Aaron Friedenwald and B. B. Browne.
Examining Board, Eastern Shore—Drs. W. F. Hines, B. W. Goldsborough, Monmonier Rowe, G. E. Dickinson and J. M. Bordley.

On motion the Faculty adjourned to meet at 12 M., Thursday.

G. LANE TANEYHILL,
Recording Secretary.

HALL OF THE FACULTY,
THURSDAY, April 28th, 1892.
DAY SESSION.

The meeting was called to order by the President, Dr. Wm. H. Welch. The minutes of the previous meeting were read and adopted.

The Faculty went into the election of new members. The chair appointed Dr. Randolph Winslow and Dr. Wilmer Brinton, tellers.

The resignation of Dr. Archibald Atkinson was read and accepted, also that of Dr. Caleb Winslow.

The chair announced the following committees:

On *Pan-American Congress—*

Drs. Wm. H. Welch, Geo. H. Rohe, Henry M. Hurd, I. E. Atkinson, T. A. Ashby.

Committee appointed under Dr. Rohe's resolution (amendment to Dr. Earle's resolution) to adopt proper measures to carry out more effectively Dr. Earle's resolution urging the adoption of heat under pressure as the method of disinfection for Baltimore, and to present the same to the Mayor and City Council of this city:

Drs. S. T. Earle, E. F. Cordell, A. K. Bond, P. C. Williams and J. D. Blake.

The tellers announced the following gentlemen elected to membership:

Henry M. Baxley, Jas. Edw. Benson, E. Tracy Bishop, Jas. B. Bennett, Merville H. Carter, Pearson Chapman, Wm. J. Craigen, Stephen Crowe, Wm. Green, A. E. F. Grempler, H. H. Hayden, S. V. Mace, J. Chas. Macgill, C. H. A. Meyer, F. P. Murphy, Chas. F. Nolen, John U. Pickel, Chas. W. Pfeffer, A. H. Price, C. R. Shoemaker, Thos. W.

Simmons, Wm. F. Smith, Reuben J. H. Tall, Geo. F. Taylor, A. S. Warner, Arthur Wegeforth, Thos. H. Williams, C. H. Wissler, T. A. Wright.

Dr. H. M. Hurd, chairman of the *Section on Psychology and Medical Jurisprudence*, read an interesting paper on "*Post-fibrile Insanity.*"

The paper was discussed by Drs. Harry Friedenwald, Chas. G. Hill, John C. Harris, Geo. H. Rohe.

The chairman of Examining Board of Western Shore announced an additional list of *candidates* for membership in the Faculty.

Dr. Samuel J. Fort read his paper on "*Diet and Exercise in the Treatment of Epilepsy.*"

The paper was discussed by Dr. Henry M. Hurd.

Dr. Charles G. Hill read his paper on "*Some Hints on the Relation of Sexual Organs to Nervous Diseases.*"

The paper was discussed by Dr. H. M. Hurd.

The volunteer paper on "*Paranoia*," by Dr. B. D. Evans, was read "by *title.*"

No report was made from the *Section on Micro scopy, Micro-Chemistry*, chairman, Dr. C. Hampson Jones.

Section on Ophthalmology, Otology and Laryngology, being called, its chairman, Dr. S. K. Merrick, read a paper on "*A Review of the Literature of Laryngology during the past year.*"

The Recording Secretary read, by request of the President, an invitation from the Sheppard Asylum Trustees to the Faculty to visit that institution on Saturday, the 30th. It was accepted.

The hour for adjournment having arrived, the reading of other papers on the *Section of Ophthalmology, &c.*, was, on motion, postponed until Friday's session.

On motion, adjourned.

G. LANE TANEYHILL,
Recording Secretary.

HALL OF THE FACULTY,

THURSDAY, April 28th, 1892, 12 M.

NIGHT SESSION.

The meeting was called to order by the President, Dr. Wm. H. Welch. The reading of the minutes of the previous meeting were, upon motion, postponed.

The president introduced the orator of the evening, Dr. Frederick E. Lange, of New York City, who delivered his able address upon "*The Pathology and Treatment of Acute Spontaneous Osteo-Myelitis.*"

On motion of Dr. Robert W. Johnson and Dr. L. McLane Tiffany, the thanks of the Faculty were extended Dr. Lange, and a copy of his address requested for publication in the Transactions.

On motion, the Society adjourned to meet at 12 o'clock, Friday.

G. LANE TANEYHILL,
Recording Secretary.

HALL OF THE FACULTY,

FRIDAY, April 29th, 1892.

DAY SESSION.

The Faculty was called to order by the President, Dr. Wm. H. Welch. The Secretaries and Treasurer were at their desks. The minutes of the day session of the 28th were read by the Assistant Secretary, Dr. Robert Wilson, and approved by the Faculty.

The minutes then of the night session of the 28th were read and were approved by the Faculty.

The election of other candidates to membership was temporarily postponed.

Dr. James M. Craighill was called to assist at the Secretary's desk.

The Faculty resumed the work on the unfinished reports from the *Section on Ophthalmology, Laryngology and Otology.* From this Section Dr. George Thomas read his paper on "*The Relation of Surgery to the treatment of Nasal Diseases.*"

The paper was discussed by Drs. Merrick and Woods.

Dr. H. Friedenwald, by unanimous consent, substituted a paper with the title, "*On Opening of the Mastoid Process,*" for the paper listed on the programme, which latter paper was ordered to be "read by title."

The next paper was by Dr. Hiram Woods, on "*Diphtheritic Conjunctivitis.*"

The paper was discussed by Dr. Wm. H. Welch and Dr. Chisolm.

The next paper was read by Dr. J. J. Chisolm, on the "*Dislocation of an Opaque Lens. Nature's Rare Method of Restoring Sight to a Cataractous Patient.*"

It was discussed by Drs. H. Woods and H. Fried-enwald.

At this juncture, the Faculty, on motion, went into an election of candidates to membership, Drs. Baker and Cordell being tellers. These gentlemen announced the following as having been elected to active membership:

C. L. G. Anderson, R. M. Dorsey, C. E. Downs, Elishe C. Etchison, P. S. Field, W. E. Gaver, Wm. Gombel, A. Van Hoff Gosweiler, H. A. Hyland, Henry M. Kemp, Geo. Lotz, J. H. McGaun, M. Sherwood, C. E. Sadtler, F. B. Smith, Henry M. Thomas, John R. Uhler, S. J. Windsor, C. Wattenscheidt.

Dr. P. C. Williams related an interesting case of a woman, who under the action of large doses of chloral, expelled an immense gallstone, measuring $1\frac{5}{8}$ inches long, $1\frac{1}{4}$ inches in diameter, and $3\frac{5}{8}$ inches in circumference at largest part. He produced the specimen.

On motion, it was ordered that the Treasurer pay the Janitor $10.00 extra for services during the convention.

On motion of Dr. Taneyhill, the President was authorized to complete his list of appointments of Delegates to the American Medical Association, and send transcript to the Secretary.

The President then ordered the Secretary to read the following as his appointments as Committees, Sections and Delegates for the ensuing year:

STANDING COMMITTEES.

Library.—B. B. Browne, I. E. Atkinson, G. J. Preston, G. Lane Taneyhill, R. W. Johnson.

Publication.—G. Lane Taneyhill, W. F. A. Kemp, H. M. Wilson, W. Osler, J. Whitridge Williams.

Memoir.—E. F. Cordell, A. K. Bond, Robert C. Rasin, J. W. Humrichouse, G. E. Dickinson.

Ethics.—G. W. Miltenberger, John F. Monmonier, T. S. Latimer, A. Friedenwald, J. E. M. Chamberlaine.

Curator.—W. T. Howard, Jr.

SECTIONS.

Surgery.—Randolph Winslow, J. T. M. Finney, C. F. Bevan, James Brown, R. B. Warfield.

Practice.—Charles O'Donovan, Jr., W. F. Lockwood, J. D. Iglehart, Charles M. Ellis, A. S. Porter.

Obstetrics and Gynæcology.—J. Whitridge Williams, Wilmer Brinton, Howard Kelly, W. A. B. Sellman, B. W. Goldsborough.

Materia Medica and Chemistry.—A. K. Bond, R. H. P. Ellis, A. C. Pole, R. B. Morison, Edward Anderson.

Sanitary Science.—Jas. T. McShane, John D. Blake, Alice Hall Chapman, Wm. B. Canfield, C. Birnie.

Anatomy, Physiology and Pathology.—J. M. Craighill, Jas. G. Wiltshire, I. R. Trimble, Charles W. Mitchell, O. H. W. Ragan.

Psychology and Medical Jurisprudence.—Harry J. Berkley, G. J. Preston, H. M. Thomas, Alex. L. Hodgdon, B. D. Evans.

Microscopy, Micro-Chemistry and Spectral Analysis.—C. O. Miller, A. G. Hoen, David Streett, Simon Flexner, W. T. Howard, Jr.

Ophthalmology, Otology and Laryngology.—Harry Friedenwald, Samuel Johnston, F. M. Chisolm, John R. Winslow.

DELEGATES.

American Medical Association.—A. Friedenwald, T. S. Latimer, J. M. Scott, J. E. Dwinelle, J. J. Chisolm, H. H. Biedler, J. W. Chambers, David Streett, John C. Harris, Jos. H. Stonestreet, M. B. Billingslea, A. H. Mann, Wm. M. Barnes, G. Lane Taneyhill, J. W. Humrichouse, Theodore Cooke. Jas. G. Wiltshire, W. A. B. Sellman, J. F. Martinet, A. S. Mason, J. H. Branham, Wm. Lee Howard, Thomas Opie, Geo. B. Reynolds, Robert C. Rasin.

West Virginia State Medical Society.—H. H. Biedler, A. S. Porter, I. M. Spear, J. Lee McComas, A. C. Pole, A. B. Price.

North Carolina State Medical Society.—J. E. Michael, J. W. Chambers, Geo. H. Rohe, Randolph Winslow, Edwin Geer, K. B. Batchelor, W. E. Mosely, W. T. Howard, Jr.

Virginia State Medical Society.—T. A. Ashby, H. P. C. Wilson, Samuel T. Earle, Robert T. Wilson, S. K. Merrick, B. D. Evans, Thomas Opie.

On motion of Dr. P. C. Williams, the thanks of the Faculty were voted to Prof. Wm. H. Welch for the able manner in which he had presided. This action was supplemented by a general vote of thanks to all the other officers, and the President declared the 94th Annual Convention adjourned *sine die*.

G. LANE TANEYHILL, M. D.,

Recording Secretary.

REPORTS.

REPORT OF RECORDING SECRETARY.

BALTIMORE, MD., April 26, 1892.

MR. PRESIDENT AND MEMBERS :—Your Recording Secretary begs leave to report that after taking counsel with the President and some of the members of the Executive Committee, he issued a *preleminary circular* to the 1383 regular practitioners of the State of Maryland, in which the subject of organization (which subject was written up by our honored President) was fully set forth, as also other inspiring topics. This, by the aid of some good friends of the Faculty, has been the means of bringing in over forty applicants for membership, and there are more to follow.

The expenses of printing, directing and mailing the circulars, was paid for by *the first day's mail*, in applications for membership, by initiation fees.

Your Secretary has, by circulars to drug dealers, &c., secured the whole floor of the Exhibition Hall by applicants for space, and after paying expenses will be able to add to our treasury at least $130 this year.

The programme which he presents this morning he modestly opines, will speak for itself—it is replete with interesting topics—he hopes it will be of service to the membership. The titles of *other* papers would have been listed had the authors transmitted them to this office. The proof was held back until yesterday, and the programmes are fresh and damp from the press of to-day. Provision is made for papers not listed, they can be read Friday morning. The edition is limited, and, as he desires to mail a copy to each member in the *counties* who is not fortunate enough to be in attendance, it is suggested that members bring their copies back with them if they take them to their residences.

All of which is respectfully submitted,

G. LANE TANEYHILL,
Recording Secretary.

REPORT OF EXECUTIVE COMMITTEE.

BALTIMORE, MD., April 26, 1892.

MR. PRESIDENT AND MEMBERS:—The Executive Committee begs leave to report that it has met at irregular intervals during the year, and given attention to such matters of business relating to the affairs of the Faculty as properly came under its authority.

At a meeting held in October last, arrangements were made for the semi-annual meeting, which was successfully held at Rockville, on the third Tuesday and Wednesday in November.

In consequence of loss by death of a large number of members, who were members of different committees and sections, the Executive Committee has been called upon to fill a number of vacancies. This duty has been discharged as follows: On the *Library Board* Dr. G. Lane Taneyhill was advanced to the chairmanship to fill the place of Dr. T. Barton Brune, deceased, and Dr. J. Whitridge Williams was added to the *Board*. Dr. R. W. Johnson was elected a member of the *Board*, to fill the vacancy occasioned by the resignation of Dr. B. B. Browne.

Dr. R. B. Warfield was added to the *Section on Surgery*, to fill the vacancy made by the death of Dr. E. R. Walker.

Dr. J. W. Humrichouse was advanced to the chairmanship and Dr. R. H. P. Ellis elected to fill the vacancy in the *Section on Materia Medica*, occasioned by the death of Dr. T. Barton Brune, chairman of the section.

Dr. W. Frank Hines was elected to fill the vacancy in the *Section on Sanitary Science*, made by the death of Dr. A. H. Bayley, and Dr. J. E. M. Chamberlaine was elected to fill the vacant position on the *Board of Examiners for the Eastern Shore*, occasioned by the same death.

The President of the Faculty, Dr. Welch, called the attention of the Executive Committee to the anticipated reduction of the Congressional appropriation to the Library of the Surgeon General's Office, and asked that action be taken in the way of a protest at a special meeting of the Faculty.

In view of the importance of this matter, the Executive Committee called a special meeting of the Faculty, at which resolutions were adopted, and by the authority of the Faculty, were mailed to the members of the Senate and House of Representatives in Congress from this State.

Dr. W. F. A. Kemp, Treasurer, having called the attention of the Executive Committee to the financial condition of the Faculty, he was requested to furnish a statement of the assets and liabilities of the Faculty for the consideration of the Committee.

The Treasurer's report will be presented at this meeting, and the Executive Committee only feels called upon to make suggestions in view of the deficiency which now exists.

An examination of the Treasurer's accounts will show that deficiencies have been carried forward for some three or four years past, until they now assume a larger liability than the Faculty should carry. The increase of expenditure over receipts has been due to the large increase in the cost of the annual volume of Transactions, and to incidental expenses incident to the work of the Faculty. A large deficiency in the receipts is due to non-payment of annual dues by members, part of which is not available.

In view of these facts the Committee recognizes that the only course the Faculty can adopt at this time to recover from financial embarrassment is, to recommend the suspension for the present the publication of the annual volume of Transactions as far as papers are concerned, and that the minutes of its meetings, reports of officers and committees, oration and presidents' addresses, be published in such form and number as will meet the wants of the Faculty. It is, however, urged that each member who shall read a paper before the Faculty be requested to furnish the Recording Secretary and the Library Committee with one or more printed copies of the same for preservation in the Library. It is believed by the Executive Committee that this plan will save an annual expense to the Faculty of some $500.00, without materially injuring its usefulness and prosperity. Of the large number of papers now published in the volume of Transactions, all or nearly all have previously appeared in other publications.

After careful consideration by the Committee of Ways and Means of promoting the growth, influence and prosperity of the Faculty, the Committee ventures to suggest such changes in the Constitution and By-Laws as will do away with the present system of work by sections, and to substitute, therefor, a "*Committee on Programme*," which shall arrange all the work to be brought before the Faculty at annual and semi-annual meetings.

At a proper time these suggestions will be offered, under the head of Resolutions and Amendments, when they will be brought before the Faculty for discussion.

The Committee would recommend to the Faculty that the present plan of having a special memorial meeting after the decease of any one member be abolished, and that a general memorial meeting be held during the annual convention.

The Executive Committee decided that a banquet be held on Thursday night, after the delivery of the annual oration, and appointed Drs. Ashby, Rohe and Brinton as a committee to arrange the details.

Your Committee takes pleasure in announcing that Dr. Frank E. Lange, of New York, has accepted its invitation to deliver the annual oration on "The Pathology and Treatment of Acute Spontaneous Osteo-myelitis." His oration will be delivered on Thursday, the 28th inst., at 8 P. M.

All of which is respectfully submitted,

T. A. ASHBY, M. D., *Chairman*,
J. EDWIN MICHAEL, M. D.,
WILMER BRINTON, M. D.,
GEORGE H. ROHE, M. D.,
PHILIP C. WILLIAMS, M. D.

REPORT OF TREASURER.

MR. PRESIDENT AND GENTLEMEN :—The report of your Treasurer at this 94th session of the Medical and Chirurgical Faculty of Maryland should engage your most careful attention. We ought thoroughly to understand our condition and legislate wisely that our expenditures may not exceed that which we are able to do, in justice to all our creditors.

Our income for the coming year will still be far from reaching our obligations unless radical changes are made in our expenditures or an assessment levied upon our membership. This latter would, in your reporter's opinion, be very undesirable.

This past year has been our second year under reduced membership dues and lessened initiation fees. Our increase in members has made our income nearly that reported from dues before the reduction occurred, and what we lack in total is due to the smaller income from rent of hall to local societies and advertisements. In the past year we received $175 from rent of hall, and we cannot expect more in the year we are just entering.

For the telephone we received last year one-half of what it cost us, and we can expect no more for the next.

We have every prospect of acquiring at this session a large number of new members, the application of forty having already been handed to the Chairman of the Examining Board.

Of our expenditures we might say much, but a comparison of income and disbursements will be sufficient to show that we must retrench—must economize. Your Treasurer for the use of members here appends the total of a few years, that your membership may the better understand, for they will have the figures at hand :

1887, Income $1,767.26, Paid out $1,902.03,   A deficit $134.77.
1888,   "   1,944.50,   "   1,911.72, excess $32.78.
1889,   "   2,134.25,   "   1,985.67, excess 148.58.
1890,   "   1,752.91,   "   1,889.97,   a deficit 137.06.
1891,   "   1,740.89,   "   2,026.98,   a deficit 286.09.
1892,   "   1,671.36,   "   1,712.82,   a deficit   41.46.

To which we should add $400 still unpaid by us on rent of hall. Some of our expenses it is impossible to anticipate, especially our incidentals. This year we report $92.45, whilst last year it was $162.16.

Our published transactions have also been an uncertain quantity in our expenses, a brief comparison of the cost for printing, directing and postage is seen to be as follows : 1889, $355.51 , 1890, $435.31 ; 1891, $591.61. A moment's reflection will convince one that this item is a growing one and calls for yearly, a greater outlay of our income.

The Library Board will report concerning their expenses, and your attention is especially solicited to their showing. This Board has received from your treasury the sum of $503, which includes the sum of $47.10 as directed by a resolution adopted by the Faculty, April 29, 1891. See pages 139 and 140 of transactions for 1891. In this connection, allow your Treasurer to state that he is aware of the fact that the resolution appended to the Library report, and adopted last year, has not been complied with. He disavows any intention of going contrary to that which the Faculty has directed him to do, either by the constitution or by resolution ; the state of our finances and the treasury did not allow it. On this point the Library Board may speak with emphasis. It becomes us to consider our course step by step and prepare to meet the emergencies as they arise. I read in this connection from a letter received from the official head of the Library Board: "1103 Madison Ave., April 22, 1892, enclosed find the receipt for $250, a partial payment to the Library Board for a part of the money ordered to be paid to said Board by Treasurer at intervals of three months. I wish personally, Doctor, you could be *let off* as easy by *other* creditors, but remember, the Library Board next year, will-be prompt in their requisitions unless some more of them die or resign." Mr. President, we ought to stop and consider the lesson here presented. Look not every man on his own things, but also on the things of his brother. This report already sets forth that we still owe $400 on rent. The rent of the hall is a just debt, we are bound by action of a former Executive Committee, in which action this Faculty agreed when it came into these premises, and your reporter does hold the opinion that for this we are as justly liable as is the Treasurer to pay the Library Board as per a resolution adopted at ANY meeting.

Mr. President, may your Treasurer ask for his successor your kind protection, for if the Faculty be legally pressed for rent and the Library Board adhere to their intention as expressed above, the demise of the Treasurer can be but a matter of the near future. The end of all these things is a matter for your most serious consideration.

Could we reduce our rent, we would experience a relief to the extent of the reduction, but this seems at best problematical. The only items upon which we can legislate with a view to retrenchment, are in the publication of the *Transactions* and the subsidy allowed Library Board. Our income must be increased if possible, and our expenditures decreased *by all means.*

With this state of affairs, we are brought face to face with kind and considerate creditors, the Library Board have already, through their Chairman regretted that others have not been as considerate as they, had they claimed all the adopted resolution to last year's report entitled them, they would have received $123.55 more than they report.

The agent for the owners of this building, to whom we owe $400 has not made so considerate a claim, but has dealt

leniently with us, considering our present condition.   It does
appear that simple justice demands a wiser course than has
been possible to pursue, and that of the first available funds
this $400 ought to be paid—even though the present Library
Board carry out the intention as expressed in the letter to
which reference has before been made.   It is but just to the
Library Board that we appreciate their action in not demanding the utmost penny.   Your Treasurer takes pleasure in
reading the following letter from the Chairman of the Library
Board :

> "1103 MADISON AVENUE,
>
> "BALTIMORE, MD., April 15, 1892.

"*Dr. W. Fred. A. Kemp:*

"DEAR SIR:—As Chairman of the Library Board I have the honor to
make formal request this day—15th April—for the proportion allowed
the Library Committee of the Medical and Chirurgical Faculty of the
State of Maryland as per resolution, adopted at the session of April,
1891.   A conference is respectfully solicited at a very early day, with
you at which the committee, as represented by me, desires to express
its willingness to accept $253 instead of $376.55, the remaining proportion allowed it.

> "Respectfully,
>
> "G. LANE TANEYHILL, M. D.,
>
> "*Chairman.*"

In accordance with the spirit and import of this letter,
your Treasurer will place no amount as "due" the Library
Board, when he records our liabilities.

Your Treasurer reports that in accordance with a standing resolution, that on April 1st all delinquents received
notice of the amount due the Faculty from each of them.

We report accessions in membership of the following gen-
tlemen: Alex. Shaw Porter, E. Gittings Welch, Edward
Morton Schaeffer, Theodore Cooke, Jr., J. H. Robinson, J.
B. Schwatka, Julius Friedenwald, W. Guy Townsend, Pedro
J. S. Moran, J. Frank Crouch, Jacob H. Mittnick, J. A.
Bonnett, Frank D. Sanger, Harry G. Harryman, Robert C.
Rasin, Hy. B. Thomas, I. R. Trimble, J. T. M. Finney, Jas.
L. McCormack, Howard A. Kelly, Charles Wattenscheidt,
Philip Briscoe, A. C. Jones, Jas. A. Stevens, J. H. Kennedy.

We erase from our active membership the names of eleven members, who are numbered among our *honored dead*: J. Brown Baxley, Jr., T. B. Brune, Frank Donaldson, Alex. F. Dulin, Thos. B. Evans. W. Stump Forwood, C. Johnston, Sr., Wm. H. Norris, Lewis H. Steiner, Edmund R. Walker.

We *drop* from membership for non-payment of dues three, viz.: Charles Hy. Bubert, Christopher Johnston, Jr., Wm. Rechert.

Receipts for the year ending April 25, 1892 :

RECEIPTS.

From Initiation Fees at Annual Meeting, . . .	⌐ 125 00
" " " " Semi-Annual Meeting, . .	25 00
" Delegate Fees, ...	2 00
" Pharmaceutical Exhibit, ...	120 00
" Rent of Hall, ...	175 00
" Rent of Telephone, ...	36 00
" Dues of Members, ...	1,172 00
" Sales and Fines at Library, ...	16 36
	$ 1,671 36

DISBURSEMENTS.

Advertising 93d Annual Session, ...	⌐ 19 67
Janitor, ...	60 00
Chairs for Annual Meeting, ...	15 00
Gas, ...	10 75
To Library Board, ...	505 00
" " from Sales and Fines, . . .	16 36
For Rent of Hall (still owe $400), ...	200 00
" " Telephone, ...	72 00
Transactions—Printing, &c..	549 11
" Stamps, ...	32 50
" Directing, ...	10 00
Corresponding Secretary, ...	33 88
Reporting Secretary, ...	21 00
Semi-Annual Meeting, ...	25 00
Commissions Collecting Dues, ...	15 10
Treasurer's Expenses, ...	37 00
Carry forward,	$ 1,620 37

Amt. brought forward,	$ 1,620 37
Ice at Library, ...	15 70
Ribbons for Diplomas, ...	2 00
Circulars, ...	2 50
Griffin, Curley & Co., Election Tickets and Programs,.	21 25
Sumers Letter Heads, ...	1 00
Stamps for Recording Secretary, ...	2 00
Insurance, 3 years, ...	48 00
	$ 1,712 82
Total Receipts, ... , . . .	1,671 36
Deficiency of 1892, ...	$ 41 46

ASSETS.

Amount to Credit Building Fund, ...	$ 192 00
Library and Fixtures (estimated), ...	7,500 00
	$ 7,692 00

OBLIGATIONS DUE THE FACULTY.

From Delinquent Members, ...	$. 279 00
" Advertisers, ...	30 00
	$ 309 00

INDEBTEDNESS OF THE FACULTY, APRIL 25, 1892.

For Deficiency April, 1891, ...	$ 518 06
" " " 1892, ...	41 46
" Unpaid rent " 1892, ...	400 00
	$ 959 52

Gentlemen—you have heard the report. Your Treasurer regrets the length of it as much as any of you, the times demanded in his opinion as full a statement as you have received, he has tried to be concise and to the point. Let him remind you that our dues are payable in advance, and within thirty days from the adjournment of this session. Our necessities have been placed before you. Yours is to do your part promptly, that our present may be made less grievous and our future more glorious.

In conclusion, let your Treasurer indulge the hope, that who ever may make the statement of our finances at our next convention, may report liabilities, none. To do this we must act more wisely in our legislation, we must increase our income, so adjust our necessities as to live within our income ; we must pay all just debts and deny ourselves of some of the luxuries we have thus far enjoyed. Then, indeed, as we step from our completed century of existence we may lift a proud head—unincumbered by any debt—we may, unimpeded march confidently into a second century wiser for our mistakes, for they have taught us economy and prudence ; more influential for with wisdom comes power, and wisdom with power will make this Faculty a potential factor in the medical affairs of the State.

Respectfully submitted,

W. F. A. KEMP,
Treasurer.

REPORT OF THE LIBRARY COMMITTEE.

MR. PRESIDENT AND MEMBERS :—Before proceeding to the consideration of the usual subjects considered in a report of a Library Board, your Committee are compelled reluctantly and sadly to make reference to the painful fact that their honored Chairman, Dr. T. Barton Brune, who so assiduously guarded the interests of the Library, and who so bravely and successfully contended for its rights, fell a victim to typhoid fever last autumn, was removed from the activities of this mundane sphere, and commenced that new life of the soul in the great future that has received so many of our members during the last twelve months.

In consequence of the decease of Dr. Brune, under whom the work of the Library had been so auspiciously begun, Dr. B. B. Browne acted for a short time as Chairman, and subsequently resigned from the Committee. At the next meeting of the Executive Committee, Dr. G. Lane Taneyhill, was advanced to the Chairmanship of the Library Board.

In the early part of the fiscal year the previous Librarian and Assistant Librarian, namely, Drs. A. K. Bond and W. Guy Townsend, were re-elected. These gentlemen gave faithful service until the fall of 1891, when other duties in more inviting fields caused them to resign, and the offices were filled by the election of Dr. C. Hampson Jones and his father, Mr. Isaac Jones. These latter gentlemen have faithfully continued to give the same efficient service that was rendered by their predecessors, and are at present well versed in the duties pertaining to their offices.

At a late meeting of the Executive Committee Drs. Robt. W. Johnson and John Whitridge Williams were, on nomination of the Library Board to the Executive Committee, elected to the vacancies caused by the death of Dr. Brune and the resignation of Dr. Browne.

Your Committee on the Library regrets to continue the complaint of the usual confronting perplexity of an insufficiency of funds available to properly equip and manage this "most valued and noble inheritance," the *nucleus* of which was established in 1832, and which, to-day, in the opinion of those who appreciate it, is a "valuable and honored possession, a force and influence of wide-reaching importance and significance, an aid and stimulus to professional ambition and culture," alike of use and available to the astute professors, as to the youngest tyros as they emerge from the medical colleges of our rapidly increasing city.

Despite the hampered condition of the finances of the Faculty, caused in part apparently by inefficiency in collections, but more probably by remissness on the part of members in settling their accounts early in the fiscal year with the Treasurer, the Library has been kept open six hours daily, during the past fiscal year, (except Sundays,) and the patronage has increased.

There has been, though small, an actual gain in periodicals, pamphlets and a few new books. Some of the new books subscribed for, your Committee regret to say, will not be received until after the Convention adjourns. A moderate amount of binding has been ordered, especially of frequently used numbers of medical journals, some of which have already become defaced in consequence of not having been bound at an earlier date. In order to preserve other valuable journals considerable binding must be done this coming year.

The Committee is glad to report that a large space, during the last month has become available for the placing of books, by the removal of a number of books by the Historical Society from its shelves in this room. The Committee desire to receive more donations from the members. They will also have more journals bound, and thus made available, especially to country members.

The Library has received the regular issues of forty domestic publications and thirty-three foreign journals by subscription and exchange during the year.

Books and journals have been donated by Drs. James Stuart, F. T. Miles, A. K. Bond and Archibald Atkinson. Any donations received after April 1, '92, will be noticed in a future report.

The Transactions of forty-two Societies have been received by exchange, and twenty-three reports of the United States Consuls and Bureau of Education.

Finances.—If it would help this struggling Library your Committee would vote for free coinage in more than one sense.

They have received from fines and sales at the
Library . . . . $ 16 36
They have received from the Treasurer of the
Faculty 503 00

Making a total from the Faculty proper of . $ 519 36

This, as is well known by our Treasurer, is $123.00 *less* than the appropriation, but your Committee being *one of the family* will not, this year, demur, for, policy, if not justice, requires that we pay our outside debts first. However, no bureau or interest of the Faculty more deserves the fostering care of this Faculty than the *Library ;* and now, as its Committee has, during the past year, worked personally to increase the membership, and has the intense gratification of having influenced at least 47 out of the 94 candidates that have been elected, and who have paid into the treasury the good sum of $470.00 during the past two days, they not only pray for but *expect* that the appropriation for the *coming* year will be more liberal. All the money received from the Treasurer has been appropriated for journals—domestic and foreign—for a few new books, and for binding. A few unpaid bills for journals, inadvertantly overlooked by a previous chairman, have been personally guaranteed by members of the Board.

Nurses Directory.—This bureau of practical information of decided value to the profession and to the citizens of this and even other States, has become, under the prudent management of the present Registrar and his predecessors, a marked source of revenue to the Faculty. Its claim, as stated by a previous President, Dr. T. A. Ashby, upon the profession of Maryland is now established, and is worthy of every care and support, for it has *already* assumed a position of importance not to be disregarded by this august body.

Dr. C. Hampson Jones, our energetic and courteous Registrar, reports that 102 nurses have been supplied since the 1st of September, 1891, and 18 new nurses added to our list. He goes on to state that there are now in active service 61 nurses, 6 male and 55 female. 16 of these are regular graduates of training schools for nurses, 9 are graduates of a Maternite. That during the busy season, in December, January, February and March, it frequently occurred that the Directory could not supply the full demand for nurses. This has been, to a great extent, due to the difficulty of prevailing upon the nurses to promptly report when they are disengaged.

The fact that many nurses *consider themselves independent* of the Directory, leads them to neglect the obligation to report promptly to it. They *do* report, however, after being some time without work. An opportune hint, just here, let us drop, viz : That members of the Faculty procure their nurses *through this Directory* instead of *privately* making that arrangement. If fifty per cent. of the general practitioners of this Faculty would report the names of nurses on their private lists *to this Directory,* and those nurses offer their names for record, your Committee is confident that there would be in the next year an increase of $300.00 in the annual revenue. Without going into fine figures, from the Registrar's report to the Library Committee, we may say here in passing, that the revenue from the Directory, has, during the past few months, paid the salaries of the Librarian, the Assistant Librarian and Registrar, and the income bids fair to increase during the coming year, in consequence of an improvement already instituted in the manner of advertising the usefulness and availability of the Directory to the general profession.

In attempting to impress upon the members the *claims of the Library* your Committee finds its sentiments so well set forth in the address of a previous President, Dr. T. A. Ashby, that with slight modification they quote a half page of his address, delivered April, 1891. "Every intelligent and thoughtful physician must feel the need of literary assistance in his medical work, and yet how few there are of us who fully appreciate the value of such a repository of medical literature as this properly conducted Library can and does present. This single agency should entitle the Faculty not only to the respect, but the support and liberality of the entire profession of Maryland.

"It is a common centre around which we should unite as a means of the highest advantage to an educated class of men. Its value and usefulness has not been sufficiently appreciated because we have not fully made a personal application of its advantages. Its importance at once grows upon our attention if we consider the opportunities which it offers the profession as an entirety. No man at this time will question the assertion that *libraries,* whether technical or general in their scope and characteristics, are essential to the successful practitioner of the day. They create intellectual wants, stimulate ambition, promote culture and refinement to a degree

not within the reach of any other single educational influence."

With this appeal your Committee on Library closes its
report.

All of which is respectfully submitted,

G. Lane Taneyhill, M. D., *Chairman*,
S. T. Earle, M. D.,
Wm. Osler, M. D.,
R. W. Johnson, M. D.,
J. Whitridge Williams, M. D.

REPORT OF PUBLICATION COMMITTEE.

APRIL 26, 1892.

Mr. President and Members:—Your Publication Committee began their work early in the fiscal year, but were
very much annoyed by the carelessness and inexcusable delays on the part of authors in transmitting original manuscript to your Committee, and subsequently in neglecting to
promptly return proofs. Your Committee is painfully convinced of the necessity for a radical reform in the manner of
conducting its business, and will submit the following resolutions for adoption by this Faculty at the proper time, viz:

Resolved, That until otherwise ordered, all members reading any original paper or report before this Faculty shall, on
the same day, deliver to the Recording Secretary, at his
desk, after reading the same, the original manuscript or a
perfect copy of said paper or report; and, if he fail in this,
or fail to mail a copy to that officer within *ten days* after the
adjournment of the Convention at which said paper was
read, the Publishing Committee is hereby authorized to proceed to publish the Transactions without such papers.

Resolved, That in future the Publication Committee be,
and is hereby authorized to employ, at a reasonable salary,
a competent person, a member of the medical profession, as
proof reader for the Committee; and that all manuscripts and

proofs shall be edited and corrected by said *proof reader*, instead of, as at present, by the authors.

Your Committee has complied with the order of the Faculty at its last meeting, requesting it to publish in the Transactions all amendments and resolutions adopted by the Faculty from the last issue of the Constitution up to and including April, 1891. They have also had a transcript of same pasted in the copies of the Constitution. Copies are on the officers' desks for distribution.

The lowest competent bidders for the publication of the 700 volumes ordered by your Committee was the firm of Griffin, Curley & Co., and the clean cut typographical execution of the work demonstrates their ability to meet the exacting demands of your Committee. Including the semi-annual papers read at Cambridge the volume is over 400 pages, the largest issued for many years ; the only feature your Committee regrets is the *lateness* at which the volume appeared, this was in consequence, as indicated above, of the tardiness on the part of the authors to transmit manuscript and return proof promptly.

Of the 221 city members only 90 have, until the meeting of this convention, called at the Library for the copies. Your Committee on Publication urges the other 131 members to call at the room of the Nurse's Directory and procure their copies, even if they have not paid their dues. Mr. Jones, the Assistant Librarian, will wait on them at any hour of the day. It would cost the Committee over $15 to mail these remaining copies.

Many commendatory criticisms on this volume of Transactions have been received from appreciative editors of medical journals.

Copies have been mailed to all State Medical Associations and to the prominent libraries and medical journals throughout the world. In consequence of this liberal distribution the Faculty has received many valuable exchanges,

Your Committee recommends the adoption of this report without the resolutions.

All of which is respectfully submitted,

G. Lane Taneyhill, *Chairman,*
. W. F. A. Kemp,
J. Edwin Michael,
H. M. Wilson,
Chas. H. Riley.

REPORT OF MEMOIR COMMITTEE.

Baltimore, Md., April, 1892.

Mr. President and Fellow-Members: Death has been busy with his scythe amongst us, during the past year, and eleven of our colleagues have fallen before his stroke. In no previous year has our loss been so great, either in numbers or quality. Amongst those whom we are called upon to mourn are at least two who had reached the highest position in the profession of this State and may I not truthfully say of this country? one who had acquired eminence in politics and in superintending the founding and development of what is now our largest library; three others who were well known from their connection with medical schools and from the influence and activity of their lives, and two country members who were leading citizens and practitioners in their respective sections.

I have the honor in behalf of the Memoir Committee to present at this time brief memoirs of the following in the order of their decease :

J. Brown Baxley, Jr., M. D.; Edmund Rhett Walker, M. D.; Christopher Johnston, M. D.; Thomas B. Evans, M. D.; Thomas Barton Brune, A. M., M. D.; Francis Donaldson, M. D.; Alexander F. Dulin, M. D.; William Stump Forwood, M. D.; William H. Norris, M. D.; Lewis H. Steiner, A. M., M. D.; Alexander H. Bayly, M. D.

In preparing these memoirs every effort has been made to secure correct and trustworthy information, and in every instance material has been directly obtained from the families of the deceased and in some cases biographical notes left by the subjects of the memoirs themselves have been availed of.

J. BROWN BAXLEY, JR., M. D.

Dr. Baxley was the eldest son of the well known druggist of the same name and was born in Baltimore, September 5, 1856. He was educated partly in the public schools, partly by a private tutor. At the age of seventeen he entered the drug business, and in 1876 graduated from the Maryland College of Pharmacy. He then took charge of the drug store, corner Park Avenue and Dolphin Street. In 1877 he entered into partnership with his father, establishing the drug store corner Madison Avenue and McMechen Street. In 1880 he withdrew from this firm and was elected apothecary to the Baltimore General Dispensary. While serving in this capacity during two years, he was thrown in with the various attending physicians and was thus led to study medicine. With the aid of an occasional substitute he attended two courses at the University of Maryland and graduated there in 1884. He was then elected one of the attending physicians to the Dispensary and held the position up to the time of his death.

Dr. Baxley's health had not been good for some years previous to his death. About five years ago, when examining a specimen of urine at the Dispensary, he was led for comparison to examine his own, when to his surprise and alarm he found it loaded with albumen. In December, 1890, he began to fail rapidly, and was confined to the house off and on from that time up to the following June, when he seemed to recuperate a little and went to the country. While there he complained of pains in the chest, on account of which he returned to the city and consulted Dr. James Brown, his attending physician. A diagnosis of pneumonia was made and from this attack he never recovered. Four days before his death he had a uræmic convulsion, and he died in a second convulsion on July 12, 1892, after an illness of two weeks.

Dr. Baxley was never married.

EDMUND RHETT WALKER, M. D.

Dr. Walker was born in Beaufort, S. C., in 1836, being the son of Rev. Joseph R. Walker, D. D., and Mianna Rhett (Walker), both of that place.

In 1852, at the age of 16, he entered the University of Virginia where he graduated in Latin, Greek and other branches. Being too young to begin the study of medicine at that time he returned to South Carolina and attended the College at Columbia, where he obtained the degree of B. A. In 1856 he re-entered the University of Virginia, as a student in the Medical Department, and took the degree of M. D. therefrom in 1857. He then went to New York and graduated at Bellevue Hospital Medical College and became one of the assistant surgeons at the hospital. After two years thus spent in New York, he returned to Beaufort and was practicing his profession in that town when the late war began. Enlisting with the Beaufort artillery, he held the rank of full surgeon in the Confederate army, and had charge of hospitals at Charlottesville, Petersburg and Richmond, and also served in the field with General Longstreet. After the close of the war he practiced for a short time in Suffolk, Va., but the climate there not agreeing with his family, he removed to Baltimore, where he continued in active practice up to the time of his death.

Dr. Walker held several professional positions of honor in this city. For several years he was a coroner and subsequently post mortem examiner. He was professor of surgery in Washington University in 1876-7, the last year of the independent existence of that institution. For eighteen years he was chief examiner for the Equitable Life Assurance

Society and one of the attending physicians to the Church Home and Infirmary. He was a member of the University Club of Baltimore ; of the Clinical Society of Maryland, and of the Alumni Association of Bellevue Hospital Medical College, New York. For several years he had filled most acceptably the chair of principles and practice of surgery in the Baltimore Medical College.

For some years prior to his death his health had been failing. He suffered with symptoms of locomotor ataxia and he often spoke of his expectation that he would be taken away suddenly. But he had been feeling quite well for several weeks and was as bright and cheerful as he had ever been, when he left home on the evening of September 30, 1891, to attend the ceremonies connected with the opening of the session at his college. Shortly after the speaker of the evening, Dr. Ellis, had commenced the inaugural address, he suddenly sprang from his seat, placing his hand over his heart, as if in pain there. As he was being assisted out of the hall he exclaimed, "angina pectoris !" he then sank to the floor. At his own request he was removed to the adjoining hospital ward. He survived about two hours after the onset of the attack. His wife—nee Miss Perkins, of Charlottesville—a son and a daughter, the latter the wife of Rev. A. H. Miller, an Episcopal clergyman of Philadelphia, survive him.

Dr. Walker was a man of pure and elevated character, refined, modest, simple and an unaffected Christian. In his domestic life he was a model husband and parent. As a surgeon he was painstaking, thorough, conservative and conscientious. Averse to writing and public speaking, he left but little record of his labors, and his worth and virtues are fully appreciated only by a narrow circle of friends and colleagues, who keenly feel his loss.

CHRISTOPHER JOHNSTON, M. D.

The subject of this memoir was of Scotch descent. His grandfather emigrated to Baltimore in 1766, and pursued a mercantile career. His mother was Miss Elizabeth Gates, a daughter of Major Lemuel Gates, U. S. A. Inheriting the name of his father and grandfather, Dr. Johnston was born in Baltimore, September 27th, 1822. On the death of his father in 1835, in Cincinnati, where the family spent several years, he was adopted by his aunt, Miss Mariah S. Johnston, of Baltimore. He was educated at St. Mary's College, Cincinnati, and at the institution of the same name in Baltimore, and then began the study of medicine under Dr. John Buckler. He received his medical degree at the University of Maryland in 1844, and then entered the Baltimore Almshouse, which at that time was a popular resort for postgraduate clinical experience. About 1848 he joined with Drs. Frick, Theobold and Stewart to found the Maryland Medical Institute, a preparatory school of medicine, "organized to elevate the standard of office instruction in accordance with the design of the National Medical Convention." About 1851 he went abroad and studied for two years in the hospitals of Paris and Vienna; he also traveled extensively in Spain. In 1855 he became a "Lecturer on Experimental Physiology and Microscopy" at the University and Curator of the Museum. His course was highly popular with the students and the second year it was made obligatory. He next held the chair of Anatomy in the Baltimore Dental College. The battle of Gettysburg seems to have been the turning point in Dr. Johnston's medical career,—that period which Shakspeare says comes to all of us at some time, and which rightly used "leads on to fortune." He volunteered his services after this battle and was on the field for some time rendering surgical aid to the Southern wounded. After his return the friends of the South residing in Baltimore presented him with a valuable testimonial and his fame and practice were both greatly augmented. In 1864 he was elected Professor of Anatomy and Physiology in the University of Maryland, and in 1869 he succeeded Professor N. R. Smith in the chair of Surgery. In 1881 he resigned this chair and was appointed Emeritus Professor.

Dr. Johnston's ill-health was attributed by him to an attack of diptheria contracted in performing an operation in 1884. He never fully recovered, but manifested increasing infirmity from this time on, and an impediment in his speech gave his friends much concern. Notwithstanding the end came rather suddenly. On Friday evening, October 10th, he complained of feeling unwell, and on the following morning after getting up and coming down stairs, he was compelled to return to bed, where he suffered for some hours with indigestion and abdominal cramps. At two o'clock Sunday morning he became unconscious and died at 11.15 A. M. In the death certificate "indigestion and colic" are assigned as the cause of his death. His funeral took place from St. Paul's Church, of which he was an active member, and his remains were interred in Loudon Park Cemetery. Dr. Johnston married Miss Sallie L. C. Smith, the daughter of Benjamin Price Smith, of Washington, D. C.; she died a few years ago. He leaves four sons (the eldest, bearing his name, being a member of the Faculty of Johns Hopkins University,) and one daughter.

Dr. Johnston early manifested a strong taste for scientific studies and research, which continued up to the very last days of his life. He devoted himself with ardor to the study of histology and pathology and acquired great expertness in the use of the microscope at a time when such knowledge was possessed by very few. He had unusual skill as an artist and was thus enabled to illustrate his own articles and lectures. He was one of the founders of the Pathological (1853) and what may be considered its legitimate successor, the Clinical Society (1875), and held the highest office in both. He was also President of the Baltimore Medical Association, of the Medical and Chirurgical Faculty of Maryland (1876-7), and for several years of the Maryland Academy of Sciences. He was a member of the American

Medical and American Surgical Associations, of the International Medical Congress, Philadelphia, 1876, and a delegate from this Faculty to the International Medical Congresses held at London in 1881, and at Copenhagen in 1884.

He was a frequent contributor to scientific and medical literature, and a list of his writings was given in the Catalogue of Scientific Papers published by the Royal Society of London some years ago. In the summer of 1886 he visited Europe for the fifth time, and traveled extensively through Russia, Norway and Sweden, and on his return wrote a very interesting description of his journey and observations. He was Consulting Surgeon to the Church Home, the Baltimore Hebrew Hospital and the Johns Hopkins Hospital. He was a warm friend of Edwin Booth (with whom he first became acquainted when called to attend the actor for a wound accidentally received in a fencing scene on the stage of the Holliday Street Theatre); also of the distinguished lawyers, Reverdy Johnson, I. Nevitt Steele and S. Teackle Wallis.

Dr. Johnston's personal appearance was very striking and commanding. He was of medium height, and had a graceful and erect carriage. His hands and feet were small. He had red hair, which he parted in the middle, and a long red beard. He was neat, somewhat prim in his attire. His most striking feature, however, was his head, which was large and of classical shape and well poised upon his shoulders. His forehead was broad and massive and betokened a superior intellect. He was not a fluent speaker, but expressed himself in choice, precise and scientific terms.

Of the large number of contributions made to literature by Dr. Johnston, the most important perhaps are these:

"Auditory Apparatus of Culex Mosquito," *Jour. Mic. Sci.*, vol. 4, 1855; "Color of Blood Corpuscles," same, 1857; "Microscopy of the Blood," *Trans. Int. Med. Congress*, Philadelphia, 1876; "Experts, Registration and Microscopy," Presidential Address before Medical and Chirurgical Faculty of Maryland, 1877; Plastic Surgery and Skin Grafting," *Ashhurst's Encyclopædia of Surgery, 1881.*

In contemplating Dr. Johnston's life we are at once struck with his lofty character. In him we see combined the courteous gentleman, the erudite scholar, the cultivated man of taste, the dignified and skillful physician. He knew what was due to himself and to his profession and he had the courage to exact it. He was particularly noted for insisting upon adequate compensation for his professional services and for maintaining a due standard of rates for which the younger generation of physicians felt particularly grateful to him. Professional honor and ethics found their truest exponent in him. He was strict and conscientious in meeting and discharging his duties and engagements and he *never slighted* or hurried through his work. He was always ready to respond to the calls of his brethren or the appeals of the poor.

His religion was of that sort whose depth is scarcely suspected by the superficial observer, who judges by the commotion on the surface of the stream. In the death of such a man—father, citizen, scholar, scientist, investigator, physician, benefactor, christian, exemplar—words are incapable of expressing our loss, and we can only bow in silence to the divine behest, which has called him away.

Appended are the remarks made at the memorial meeting by Drs. Miltenberger, Howard and J. Carey Thomas.

REMARKS OF DR. GEO. W. MILTENBERGER.

I second the resolutions just read, and would pay my feeble tribute to one whose life is his own best eulogy.

It has been my sad privilege, Mr. President, during a prolonged professional life, to see one after another of my revered elders, my esteemed and respected cotemporaries, and my juniors, the characters of some of whom I had assisted to form, and whose career I had watched with interest and pride, fall by the wayside, in the ripe fullness of old age, in the maturity of manhood, or in the pride and vigor and earnestness of early professional life.

And then, as now, standing as I do almost alone, the old unsolved problem forces itself upon me, why one should be taken, often the brightest, and another left.

Of all this bright throng, who in the past half century have gone over to the majority, I feel deeply and sincerely thankful that in no single instance has there been one drop of bitterness at the side of the grave, and that with all, due to their kindness, their courtesy and consideration, I have enjoyed the ties of friendship, personal and professional.

Among the brightest and most esteemed has been our late departed brother, whose worth as man and as physician has been so justly, so truly and without exaggeration depicted.

I have known Dr. Johnston from his earliest student days, and I have known him well, and while our association has ever been a source of pride and profit to me, I owe him much for counsel and assistance in sickness and in trouble, ever rendered promptly, cheerfully and with his characteristic grace and geniality.

His presence in the sick room, with his kindness of heart, his polished courtesy of manner, his brightness of spirit, his ready wit, was as a sunbeam, and I always expected his visits with pleasure, and was comforted physically and mentally.

Dr. Johnston was a rare type of man.

We all recognized his full and ripe knowledge of his profession, his researches and attainments in the wider circle of general science, his varied, and in many instances, deep culture, the beauty and brightness of his mind, his marked and in some respects exceptional manipulative skill.

He was always courteous, personally and professionally, ever considerate, recognizing what was due to others, while realizing what was due to himself, fastidious and chivalrous in his honor, he never, in the minutest detail violated the strictest rules of professional ethics.

He was above all true, a true man, a true gentleman. He was true to himself, true to his convictions, true to his friends, true to his profession, true to the world at large.

"To thine ownself be true,
And it must follow as the night the day,
Thou can'st not then be false to any man."

May his life, his conduct, his character, be in the future a bright exemplar to the profession he so loved, so honored, so adorned.

DR. WM. T. HOWARD'S REMARKS.

There are times and occasions in the lives of most men of ardent natures and warm sympathies when the lips refuse to give adequate utterance to the feelings that oppress the heart. And such are my feelings on the present occasion. Our late lamented *confrere* was my room-mate in the old Baltimore City and County Alms House Hospital, where we were students of medicine, the friend of my early manhood, and of all succeeding years, and for many years my beloved colleague in the school of physic of the University of Maryland. Of the four young students of medicine who occupied the large elliptical blue room in the hospital, I alone in the Providence of God, am the sole survivor. Often in my professional rambles over this large city and in the solitude of a desolate home, do I recur to those days, the most profitable, if not the most pleasant of my life, and in no moments does memory mingle more of melancholy with such delightful sweetness. During that epoch was laid the foundation of whatever of success I may have attained in professional life.

Dr. Johnston displayed as a student the qualities of mind and heart that distinguished him in after life. It was difficult to determine what branch of the profession was most attractive to him, or in which his genius shone brightest, for he seemed to acquire all knowledge with equal facility. Of the eight young students in the hospital, he was incomparably the most gifted of all and socially the most charming. His genial good nature, his quick perception of the humorous, and his keen wit, often enlivened the tedium of student life and rendered his presence a perpetual joy. After serving a year or more in the hospital, Dr. Johnston prosecuted his studies for four years abroad. He spoke the French and German languages with almost equal facility, and so well that in the opinion of competent judges he might have been readily mistaken as a native of either country. He was an accomplished artist, and some of his drawings, especially those of the brain and spinal cord, are of unsurpassed excellence. As a microscopist he was for many years *facile princeps* in this city, and many of his microscopical specimens are of the highest order.

After perfecting his professional education abroad, Dr. Johnston returned to this city to battle for the honors and emoluments of his profession, and early learned the great lesson to quietly bide his time ; not in idleness and feverish impatience, but in constant endeavor, so that when occasion came, he was found ready and equal to it. In all his professional relations, alike to the public and the profession, he was a *model prototype* for the rising race of young medical men.

The unusually large number of physicians and of the best and brightest men and women of our beloved city, who attended his funeral, attested the high and honorable position he held in their confidence and esteem. And I do not hesitate to declare, as my sincere conviction, that *Dr. Christopher Johnston*, take him for all in all, was the most variously accomplished medical man I have ever known.

In conclusion, sir, let me express my belief that our efforts to do good and to be useful in our day and generation do not perish forever at death. I believe there is a superior intelligence, which concerns itself in human affairs and that there will be a recompense for those who make sacrifices to uprightness and the good of their fellow creatures. Whatever we accomplish in this brief life, though so imperfectly done, so far below our aspirations, will not be lost. "Human existence has a purpose, and human virtue an *unfailing friend.*"

REMARKS OF DR. JAS. CAREY THOMAS.

I wish to add a few words to that which has been so well said by the gentlemen who have already spoken. Dr. Christopher Johnston was an accomplished surgeon and physician, a cultivated man of varied interests and a good citizen. In all these aspects of his character he has been well presented by his other friends and colleagues. It must suffice for me to refer for a moment to the relations into which scientific pursuits, which were so prominent in his history brought him. As early as 1855 he wrote a dissertation on the auditory apparatus of the mosquito (illustrated) —which was reprinted. Copies of this reprint are now quite scarce.

I well remember forming one of his first class on the use of the microscope in medicine—then a comparatively new theme to the profession. He had studied microscopy in Paris and his lectures were illustrated by his own brilliant drawings. From this time onward in addition to his strictly professional pursuits—he employed his leisure moments in some scientific investigation. This naturally caused him to take an intelligent interest in the scientific work of the Johns Hopkins University.

He was one of the first to encourage this work—not only by his frequent enquiries and presence, but by constant contributions to the departments that interested him. As an example of this—when he was studying the intimate structure of the teeth—he gave to the biological museum of the University a set of fossil teeth of various animals—afterwards a number of casts of the skulls of apes.

He was a frequent visitor at the pathological laboratory, often bringing with him microscopic slides of his own preparation and discussing the newer questions of the day.

His love of crystals, drew him at once into sympathy and co-operation with Dr. Williams in that department of geological study, though his own studies were not in the line of microscopical mineralogy, but pertained to the optical study of crystals in polarized light. He had found out many facts of interest about many substances mostly artificial compounds which have never, as far as is known been published.

Dr. Johnston was an extensive and intelligent traveller, and often brought on his return from European trips some addition to the collections of the university—showing the best new work of the professors of optical crystals abroad.

The teachers of science in the University will miss his wise and generous appreciation of their work and his personal encouragement.

At the very time of his being taken ill, he had been investigating by crystal sections, the characters of some supposed apophyllite sent him by Dr. Day from California.

Dr. Johnston was an example of a physician whose broad sympathies and scientific spirit impelled him to recognize and foster what was best whether at home or abroad. He often entertained at his hospitable board and introduced to his friends in Ba'timore—distinguished men from at home and abroad. In all these ways Dr. Johnston fostered high aims, and scientific progress, leaving in these respects a commendable example to other members of the profession of which he was an ornament.

As a memorial of his lasting interest in the work of the Johns Hopkins University he has bequeathed to it, his medical and surgical instruments, his cabinet of microscopical preparations, his cabinet of crystals prepared for optical purposes and his medical library, which includes a large number of anatomical illustrations prepared by himself as illustrations for his lectures when professor of surgery at the University of Maryland.

Mr. President, I have only attempted to emphasize one side of Dr. Johnston's life, his own devotion to and earnest encouragement of others in purely scientific research and to commend his example to all. His loss will be greatly felt by a wide circle of clients and friends, by whom his personal kindness and professional service will always be remembered with gratitude and affection.

Thomas B. Evans, M. D.

Dr. Evans was the eldest son of the Rev. David Evans, a minister of the Methodist Episcopal Church, who died about two years ago. He was born in Baltimore, November 5, 1832. He obtained an elementary education at private schools and at the age of seventeen entered a drug store, where he acquired a knowledge of pharmacy and conceived the idea of pursuing a medical career. He began his medical studies under Dr. John Monkur, a prominent physician of the eastern section of the city, and obtained his degree at the (old) Washington University before he had attained his majority. He at once entered upon a lucrative practice. He was intensely fond of his profession and indefatigable in his pursuit of it, allowing himself but little recreation. Besides this society he was a member of the Maryland Academy of Sciences, the Baltimore Medical Association, the Baltimore Medical and Surgical Society and the American Medical Association ; he was vice-president of the latter in 1889, and was twice president of the Baltimore Medical and Surgical Society (1873 and 1880). He took an active interest in all these societies and held many positions in them. He contributed numerous papers, addresses and reports to medical journals. For many years (1855-60, 1866-67) he was vaccine physician of the city, and he was surgeon of the Baltimore City Guards under Governor Bradford, with the rank of major. The first vote which he ever cast was for Abraham Lincoln, as President, and he was one of the corps of physicians sent to the relief of the victims of the Bull Run disaster. He held the chair of ophthalmology, and later of pathology, in the Baltimore University and at the time of his death was dean of that school. In June, 1891, he was thrown from his carriage and sustained injuries from which he never recovered. But the immediate cause of his death was a carbuncle, due to a complication of diseases. He died at his residence on Jackson Place, on October 30, 1891, aged not quite 59. He married Miss Maggie J. Myers, of Frederick City, Md., in 1861, who with one daughter, survives him.

Dr. Evans was a man of genial disposition, of open, frank and hearty manners. He was gifted with ready speech and was a good debator, arguing his points with clearness and tenacity, yet with considerateness and politeness. His style was highly ornate and rhetorical and he had many of the elements of the natural orator. He was a member of the Unitarian Church.

Thomas Barton Brune, A. M., M. D.

Dr. Brune was the second son of the late Frederick W. Brune, a prominent lawyer, and Emily S. Brune, and was born at "Oak Lawn," Waverly, in the suburbs of Baltimore, June 4, 1856. His early education was received under the private tutorship of Rev. Mr. Johnston, the rector of St. John's P. E. Church, Waverly, and later at the "Penn Lucy School" of Colonel Richard Malcolm Johnson, where he remained until he entered college. He began his collegiate career at St. John's College, Annapolis, and graduated with special distinction (delivering the salutatory) in 1875. Three years later, he studied for and obtained the degree of A. M. He never failed to receive "first-grade certificates" and marks during any one of the college terms. He was also captain of the College base ball nine, between whom and the U. S. Naval Cadets there were continual contests. His devotion to athletics was a feature of his career. He was singularly successful in all field sports, and was an earnest advocate of such exercises. Law was first chosen as his profession, but almost at once he decided to change the study of it for that of medicine. He began his medical studies under Dr. Frank Donaldson and entered the School of Medicine of the University of Maryland, receiving his degree of M. D. in 1878. He then spent a year in Europe, chiefly in attendance at the hospitals in Berlin and Vienna. On his return he became resident physician at the University Hospital, 1879-80. In March, 1880, he began private practice, and for several years he was also attached to the U. S. Marine Hospital service. For some years he served as corresponding secretary of this society. Through his persistent efforts the

Nurses' Directory of this society was inaugurated, and he took the deepest interest in the success of the library. He was one of the physicians of St. Joseph's Hospital and was also at the time of his death physician to the "Maryland School for the Blind," on North Avenue. He likewise held for a short time the position of professor of practice of medicine in the Baltimore Polyclinic, and he was, a lecturer on clinical medicine in the University of Maryland. In urinary analysis, both qualitative and quantitative, he was unusually skillful and his translation of Hoffman and Ultzmann's work upon this subject (begun while he was in Vienna) has passed through three editions and is now a leading text book in our colleges. He did not write a great deal, as his private practice grew very rapidly and occupied his time very fully, and he had a great horror of writing unless he had something really important and interesting to claim attention for. The articles which he wrote appeared chiefly in the Boston Medical and Surgical Journal. It was a frequent source of regret to him that the exactions of his large practice prevented his attending more frequently the meetings of the various medical societies of which he was a valued member. He loved his profession dearly, particularly its scientific departments, and was always a hard student, studying and reading frequently until nearly daybreak after a hard day's practice. He took special interest in microscopic work and gave much time and study to it. He was one of the Board of Visitors and Governors of St. John's College, his alma mater, and to her service he devoted half of his last day of work, working untiringly over business connected with a trustees' meeting to be held that night, with a temperature of 103° after a severe chill. He then drove in a heavy rain, 18 miles, in and out, to a very ill country patient and returned still more ill and never left his room again.

Dr. Brune's death was due to typhoid fever and occurred after an illness of 38 days, November 9, 1891, when he had reached the age of 35 years and 5 months. Dr. Brune married Miss Agnes Randall, daughter of the late Alexander Randall, of Annapolis, who survives him with two daughters.

Dr. Brune was noted for the thoroughness of his work and for the earnestness with which he held and maintained his convictions. He was unquestionably a man of very superior abilities and this fact together with his grave and impressive manner, his industrious and studious habits, and his accurate and extensive professional knowledge gained for him early in his career a wealthy and cultured clientele rarely obtained by the young physician and pointed him out as one destined to attain the first rank in his profession had he lived.*

FRANCIS DONALDSON, M. D.

Dr. Donaldson was a native of Baltimore and was born July 23rd, 1823. He was the fifth and youngest son of John Johnston Donaldson, President of the Franklin Bank and of the Baltimore Insurance Company. He was educated at Dr. Prentiss' School, near Baltimore, but his father was unable to give him the advantages of a college education, a source of much regret to himself. He attended the University of Maryland and graduated in medicine in 1846. He continued his studies in the hospitals in Paris, which was then the great resort of medical students from America, for two years. In 1848 he returned to Baltimore and began his career as a physican. He held positions as attending physician to the Baltimore General Dispensary and the City Almshouse, and was also resident physician at the Marine or Pest Hospital ; serving for two years in each one of these. During his service at the last named institution there was an epidemic of typhus fever here, and he was the only one of the physicians connected with the hospital who did not contract the disease. From 1863 to 1866 he was Professor of Materia Medica in the Maryland College of Pharmacy, and in the latter year was elected Professor of Physiology and Hygiene, and Clinical Professor of Diseases of the Throat

------

*It is deserving of mention that Mrs. Brune has presented the entire medical library of her husband to the University Hospital.

and Chest in the University of Maryland. In 1880 he resigned his didactic chair, but retained the clinical professorship until 1888, when he withdrew from that also, and was
made emeritus professor.

Dr. Donaldson had not been well since an attack of the
grippe from which he suffered in the winter of 1890-91. It
was noticed that he was short of breath and he attended to
his professional duties with difficulty. He spent the summer
at the Isle of Shoals, but was not benefitted. Symptoms of
Bright's Disease also appeared. For some weeks prior to
his death he was confined to his house with this complication,
which terminated his life December 9th, 1891, at 1 A. M.
The immediate cause of his death was heart failure. The
cause of death assigned in the death certificate was "Fatty
Heart and Albuminuria." He was buried two days later
from St. Paul's Church, of which he was a member. Dr.
Donaldson married Miss Elizabeth Winchester, the daughter
of William Winchester, of Baltimore, who together with
three daughters and two sons (the elder of whom, bearing
his name and also a physician, resides in Germany) remain
to mourn his loss.

Hardly had we laid away our friend Dr. Johnston when
Dr. Donaldson claimed a like service from us. It was a
singular coincidence that these two, born in the same city
within a year of each other, commencing their careers about
the same time, moving along side by side and each achieving
the highest eminence in his department, should both pass
away within a period of less than two months. One of the
last appearances in public of Dr. Donaldson was at the
memorial meeting held to do honor to his life-long friend
and associate. It was a very impressive scene, witnessing
his faltering attempt to speak and seeing him overcome with
emotion. Looking back upon it, I cannot help thinking he
must have then had in his own mind his own early departure.

In personal appearance Dr. Donaldson was below the
average height, but compactly built. He was a man of active
and energetic habits of mind and body and gave one—as has

been said—the impression that he was always busy. His face was always cleanly shaven. Whilst his features were not handsome there was something striking about them, and one could not look upon him without recognizing his superiority. He had a peculiarly bright expression and winning smile and his manners were charming. He was of a sensitive disposition and very considerate of the feelings of others. He was devoted to his profession and an enthusiastic student and teacher and had the faculty of communicating his enthusiasm to others. The driest subjects acquired a fresh interest under the magic of his voice and earnest manner. A favorite expression of his when he wished to impress a fact or statement particularly on his audience (as his old students will remember) was, "Gentlemen, stick a pin there!" He was particularly happy and in his element in the clinics. Few men have had such a deep hold on the hearts of their patients and a visit from him was worth more than medicine.

Beginning his studies under the masterly guidance of Power, he paid great attention while abroad to physical diagnosis and came back thoroughly imbued with the teachings of the modern French school, which claimed physiology as the basis of all rational medicine. For many years he was *facile princeps* in diseases of the chest and throat in Baltimore. But although so eminent in this department he did not confine himself to it ; he had also a large general and consultation practice, and during his office hours his office was always thronged with patients. In all his relations, both professional and lay, he was courteous, courageous, conscientious, pure-minded and public-spirited, an ideal physician and an ornament to his profession and city. He took a deep interest in all measures and enterprises for the advancement of his fellow men, and he was a warm friend and a generous contributor to our library. He was deeply but not obtrusively pious. He was especially interested in medical education and at the beginning of his connection with the University of Maryland urged the adoption of the three-year course and other advanced methods, which his colleagues, however, at that time deemed impracticable.

As an author he enjoyed an extensive reputation, for he wrote with studious care and always upon subjects with which he had familiarized himself by long study or practical experience. Besides numerous papers and addresses he contributed several articles to Pepper's System of Medicine. Dr. Donaldson was a member of the Maryland Academy of Sciences, of the American Association of Physicians, of the American Medical Association, the American Laryngological and Climatological Associations and an Honorary Fellow of the College of Physicians of Philadelphia. He had held the office of President in the American Climatological Association and also of this Faculty in 1881-82. He was for many years an examining physician to the New York Mutual and other leading Life Insurance Companies, and he was one of the consulting physicians to the Johns Hopkins Hospital.

I append to this memoir the remarks which were made at the Memorial Meeting held in honor of Dr. Donaldson, by Dr. Louis H. Steiner, who, alas, himself, was summoned away within a few weeks after he penned them, and of Dr. S. C. Chew. Dr. Van Bibber's remarks were published in the Maryland Medical Journal, January 9th, 1892.

REMARKS OF LEWIS H. STEINER, M. D.

Notwithstanding my hearty concurrence in whatever has been said or shall be said in the way of deep regret for the loss and high commendation of the estimable qualities of our brother, I feel that the many years of friendly intercourse that I enjoyed with him require a few words on this occasion. Thirty-nine years ago I took up my residence in Baltimore, comparatively a stranger, although a native Marylander, and among those who then extended a cordial welcome to me, closely connected in my memory, were Drs. Donaldson and Johnston. It seems but a few days since we met in this room to utter our lamentations that the latter had been taken from us, and to listen to the loving words which friends uttered over the loss so deeply felt then and now. And now a like sorrowful purpose brings us together again, and the former, who then united so feelingly in the earnest tributes paid to Dr. Johnston, is no longer with us, and, alas, we are called upon to recount his beautiful traits of character as these occur to friend after friend in this venerable Faculty.

It was my privilege to be a colleague of Dr. Donaldson in the early days of the Maryland College of Pharmacy. When Dr. Frick was transferred from that institution to the medical department of the University of Maryland, the vacancy created was filled by the appointment of Dr. Donaldson. Through several winters we were brought very closely together, and then I learned to know the accuracy of his knowledge and his wonderful skill in imparting information to the students under his care. No pains were ever spared by him to acquire all attainable information that could be of practical utility, and this was so carefully and systematically arranged, so clearly brought to the apprehension of his hearers, who never tired of his teachings, that he speedily established his reputation as a successful teacher.

But this career was only a preparation for a more extended one, when called to follow his predecessor to the medical university, where he carried with him the zeal, care, earnest love of research, honest disposition to secure full knowledge of the subject under investigation, conjoined with such a hearty sympathy with his audience that he speedily confirmed the prophecies of his friends that he would soon take high rank as a medical teacher. With this part of his life some of you are more familiar than the speaker. All must agree that his success did not depend alone upon his knowledge of the subject, the earnest study he gave to it, so that he might bring his hearers up to the latest information known to the profession, or even to his kindly face and charming voice, but still more to the sympathetic relations which he established with his class, the earnest, loving desire he felt that they should possess all that he knew and the brotherly interest he took in their success. There never was a professional teacher within the range of my acquaintance who exhibited these delightful qualifications so strikingly as our departed brother. He always spoke as one who loved his subject, as one who loved his class. Pecuniary advantages were to such a lecturer of but little value as compared with his earnest desire to aceomplish the task he had undertaken, honestly, conscientiously. He had assumed obligations which were to be filled to the best of his ability, earnestly, laboriously,. if need required, but at all events to the best of the ability that his Master had given him.

These qualities entered into his relations with his patients. Few physicians have been more beloved by those who with such unhesitating confidence placed their own lives and those of their dear ones in his skillful hands. They were charmed with that happy sunshine that seemed to spring from his transparently honest face, that winning glance of the eye that seemed to know no guile, and were won by what for want of a better word we call that magnetic power that wins friends and disarms prejudice. While his professional knowledge was equal to the demands of the case, faith was aroused, which made its employment most successful against the attacks of disease, and the good physician brought with him all the necessary adjuncts that enabled the fight with disease to be carried on with the greatest hope for success. I know that these words but poorly express the wonderful influence he had over his patients and their friends. I have experienced in my own household this influence which he brought with him and exercised, but it is fitting that it should be emphasized on the present occasion.

And all the qualities named made him a true professional brother, dear to all his associates, and a citizen whose reputation as a man extended far beyond the city of his birth. Born to win friends, his loving soul had no enmity for anything but that which was vicious. He found himself surrounded by those who prized his friendship as inestimable, and who felt honored by the same as one of their dearly prized possessions.

That such a man, such a teacher, such a physician, was a christian need not surprise one. Indeed there was that in his character, his peculiarities, his very being, that could only thrive and attain its highest development in the christian life.

And so as a scholar, a physician, a citizen, a christian, our brother lived, went in and out among us, and was taken away just when we thought that we needed him most. He did not die—the good never die. They are taken away from the toils and cares of the world, leaving us their precious memories, and bidding us cherish their example. We shall no longer hear the bright, cheerful sound of his voice, no longer see the sunny smile that lighted up his kind countenance, but we still have his memory with us. May our own record be such that when the time of departure comes there may be those who have been made happier, if not better, by our lives, and who shall be able to say with deep affection, as we now say, farewell, brother beloved, farewell. *Auf wiedersehen* on the *other* side!

ALEXANDER F. DULIN, M. D.

Dr. Dulin was a native of Baltimore and was the son of Dr. Alexander F. Dulin. He was born October 5th, 1856. When a boy he attended school in Europe and later entered the University of Virginia, where he also took a preliminary medical course. He graduated in medicine at the University of Maryland in 1878, and immediately after went abroad. He spent eighteen months attending the hospitals of London, Paris and Dublin. Returning to Baltimore he entered upon practice, but gave it up after two or three years. His circumstances were such that he had not the stimulus of necessity to work. For a time he was one of the vaccine physicians of the city. He died December 19th, 1891, after an illness of two weeks.

WILLIAM STUMP FORWOOD, M. D.

Dr. Forwood, son of Samuel Forwood, was born on Deer Creek, near Darlington, Harford County, Maryland, where his ancestors had resided for several generations, January 27th, 1830. His father is still living in Alabama, and is nearly a centenarian, having been born in the same year in which this Society was organized. Dr. Forwood obtained his elementary training at the Darlington and Grove Hill (Clarke Co., Ala.) Academies. He entered upon the study of medicine in May, 1851, under the preceptorship of Dr. Robert H. Archer, Sr. In October, 1852, he matriculated at the University of Pennsylvania, from which he received his degree April 1st, 1854. He first began practice at Darlington, where he continued until 1869, when he removed to Philadelphia. In December, 1870, he removed to Gosport, Alabama, where he practiced until 1873, when he returned to Darlington. In 1876 he bought a property in the village of Darlington, where he continued to reside up to the period of his death.

Dr. Forwood was a leading and one of the most public-spirited citizens of Harford County, but on account of ill-health had been prevented from showing that active interest in public affairs during the past ten or twelve years, which he felt. He was possessed of the highest moral character, was firm as a rock when he knew he was in the right and was never afraid to express his views on any subject. He loved the truth. He was devoted to his home and family and was a most indulgent parent, entering into all the enjoyments and interests of his household. He loved his profession and never slighted its duties in the least degree, but often sacrificed his personal comforts and inclinations to its demands and interests. His death was due to an attack of the grippe, which in his delicate state of health he was unable to withstand, and occurred January 2nd, 1892. He was buried in Darlington Cemetery, a spot which he had always taken great pleasure in beautifying. He knew he could not survive the disease, and expressed himself as ready, willing and anxious to go. Death had no dread or fears for him. He said he had always lived a life such that at any time he felt prepared to die and he looked for his reward. Dr. Forwood was twice married, his last wife dying in 1888. The following enumeration of his services and writings will show that Dr. Forwood led an exceptionally busy and useful life:

He aided in organizing the Medical Society of Harford County, 1866, was its President and for many years its

Secretary and repeatedly its delegate to the American Medical Association. He joined the Medical and Chirurgical Faculty of Maryland in 1868, and in 1883 was its first Vice-President.

He aided in organizing the "Clarke County (Ala.) Medical Society" in 1872, and was its first President. In the same year he became a member of the Alabama State Medical Association.

He has been a member of the "Pennsylvania and Maryland Union Medical Association" since 1879—the second year of its organization, and was its President in 1882.

He aided in forming the Harford County Historical Society in 1885, and was President of it from its foundation up to his death. He contributed papers to it entitled, respectively, "Sketches in the Early History of Harford County," "The Passage of General Lafayette through Harford County in 1781," and "A Memoir of Junius Brutus Booth, the Elder."

In 1882 he took an active part in the establishment of the Darlington Cemetery.

He was one of the Trustees of the Darlington Academy for fifteen years, during the last eight of which (up to the period of his death) he was the President of the Board.

When typhoid fever prevailed in Harford County so extensively in 1881, as a member of a committee appointed by the County Society to investigate the subject, after consulting many physicians and others, he prepared a report pointing out the dangerous character of the offensive offal about the numerous canning houses and its proper distribution. This report, entitled "An Address to the Canners," was published in the county newspapers, and its effect in improving the health of the community and in ridding it of the horrible odor was most beneficial.

During the past thirty-five years Dr. Forwood published numerous medical papers, chiefly in the Medical and Surgical Reporter, of Philadelphia. His chief literary work was entitled "An Historical and Descriptive Narrative of the Mammoth Cave of Kentucky; Including Explanations of the Causes concerned in its Formation, its atmospheric conditions, Its Chemistry, Geology, Zoology, etc., with full Scientific Details of the Eyeless Fishes," with a map of the Cave. [J. B. Lippincott & Co., Phila.; 12 mo. pp. 241; 1st edition 1870; second edition 1875.] This work is referred to in the last edition of the Encyclopœdia Britannica as an authority upon the subject of which it treats.

WILLIAM H. NORRIS, M. D.

Dr. Norris was born in Carroll County, Md., in 1829. He received his preliminary education at Oxford College, Ohio, and his degree in medicine from the University of Maryland in 1854. He was health warden from 1855 to 1862, vaccine physician, 1855-61, and again in 1873; examiner of recruits, 1861-2; Surgeon United States Army, 1861-65; in charge hospital at Hampton and on staff of General Weber, 1862; on staff of Generals Kelly, Morris and Jeffries, 1862-3; chief medical officer in charge of 14,000 Confederate prisoners at Fort Delaware, 1863; at Petersburg, Va., during engagements of 1862; at McKimm's Mansion Hospital, Baltimore, in 1865; in the Custom House, Baltimore, 1872; resident eastern dispensary, from 1880 until time of death, and medical director of G. A. R., 1882. He had held the office of president in the Medical and Surgical Society and in the Clinical Society of Maryland. He was the author of several articles, a list of which is given in Quinan's Annals. During the war he married Miss Mollie E. Suter, daughter of James E. Suter, and his wife, and three sons and one daughter survive him. Dr. Norris died February 8, 1892, suddenly of heart disease.

Dr. Norris took much interest in medical organizations and frequently joined in the discussions. He was much esteemed for his upright character and for his faithful services to the poor.

LEWIS H. STEINER, A. M., M. D.

Dr. Steiner, the late librarian of the Enoch Pratt Library, of this city, was born in Frederick City, Md., in 1827. He was descended from German ancestors who settled in the western part of the State in the early part of the last century.

He attended Marshall College, at Mercersburg, Penn., an
graduated there as bachelor of arts in 1846. Three yea
later he obtained his medical degree of the University c
Pennsylvania. He removed from Frederick to Baltimore i
1852, and held chemical chairs in the Maryland Institute
the Maryland College of Pharmacy, Columbian College an
the National Medical College, Washington, D. C. In 186
he returned to Frederick. During the war he was chief in
spector of the United States Sanitary Commission in th
Army of the Potomac, and at its close he reorganized th
public schools of his native county and served for nearl
three years as president of the school board. Since 1868 his
time was mostly given to literary and scientific pursuits. In
1869 he received the honorary degree of A. M. from Yale
College. In 1871 he was elected to the State Senate and
was re-elected in 1875. In the Senate he wielded great influence and was respected by all for his manhood, his sterling
integrity and his devotion to the public interests. In 187
he was a member of the Republican National Conventior
which nominated Rutherford B. Hayes. When the Enoc
Pratt Library was established six years ago he was electe
librarian and in this position he found a wide and congenia
field for his talents. This library (including its fou
branches) now numbers 107,000 volumes. Dr. Steiner'
death occurred in his library at his home in this city, sud
denly of apoplexy, on the evening of February 18, 1892.

Dr. Steiner was a member of the Reformed Church an
took an active interest in its affairs. He leaves a widov
three daughters and two sons. His eldest son succeeds hi
as librarian.

Dr. Steiner was a close student, an eloquent speaker and
ready writer. At the age of twenty-four he published hi
first work, entitled "Physical Science." He subsequentl
published numerous volumes, addresses, etc., and was at on
time editor of the American Medical Monthly. He was
member of the American Medical Association, of the Mary
land Academy of Sciences, of the American Association fo
the Advancement of Science, of the Maryland and Ne
Haven Colony Historical Societies, and a correspondin

member of the Academy of National Sciences of Philadelphia; he was also a member of the American Public Health Association and its vice-president for one year, of the American Academy of Medicine and its senior vice-president for two years, and he was a trustee of several collegiate and literary institutions. "No brighter example," says Professor Raddatz, "of high and earnest ardor in his country's cause, of manhood, integrity and energy, shines in the galaxy of sterling citizens which the sturdy race from which he sprang has given to our State."

ALEXANDER H. BAYLY, M. D.

Dr. Bayly was the son of Josiah Bayly, once Attorney-General of Maryland and an eminent lawyer, and was born on the Eastern Shore of Maryland in 1814. Early in life he married Miss Delia Eccleston, daughter of the late Washington Eccleston, for many years register of wills in Dorchester County. He graduated at the University of Maryland in 1835. He died at Cambridge, Md., after a long illness, March 14, 1892, aged 78. He was one of the most prominent men in his section. For many years he enjoyed a very large practice, from which he gradually withdrew in the latter years of his life.

He was mayor of Cambridge for over thirty years, until age compelled him to resign. He is said to have managed the business and finances of the corporation very wisely and carefully and to him more than to any one else the citizens owe their beautiful shade trees and gardens. He was universally beloved in Dorchester and his charity was widespread and generous. He is said to have left a considerable fortune to his heirs, who consist of three sons and three daughters. Dr. Bayly was the president of the State Lunacy Commission.

All of which is respectfully submitted.

E. F. CORDELL, *Chairman*,
J. McP. SCOTT,
G. T. ATKINSON,
C. F. BEVAN,
ALICE T. HALL.

REPORT OF COMMITTEE TO DEVISE MEANS FOR LESSENING THE AMOUNT OF BLINDNESS FROM CURABLE DISEASES.

MR. PRESIDENT AND GENTLEMEN:

The committee appointed at the last annual meeting to devise ways and means for the prevention of blindness in the city and state begs to report as follows: The work of the committee has been confined to one disease: Ophthalmia Neonatorum.

After considering various plans which have been tried in other places, the committee concluded that the work assigned it must be accomplished by an educational process. Ignorance, and not indifference or carelessness, is the cause of so much preventable misfortune. It is hard to conceive of a parent, midwife or physician being careless or indifferent, if they really know the nature of the disease. There is no doubt that most of this ignorance prevails, just where one expects to find it, among parents and midwives; but no thoughtful man will deny that it is not confined to these persons. Of six blind babies, recently observed by the chairman of your committee, three had been attended by midwives, two by physicians, while to the last a physician had been called in when too late. In all the cases save the last the treatment reported was entirely inadequate.

A circular letter to the midwives of Baltimore was prepared by the committee, and mailed through the City Health Department to each midwife in the city. A copy of this letter, with an accompanying explanatory note, was mailed by the committee to each physician in the city and to many in the State. This letter to the midwives reads as follows:

"BALTIMORE, OCT. 16, 1891.

"TO THE MIDWIVES OF BALTIMORE:

"The undersigned practicing physicians of Baltimore were appointed by the Medical and Chirurgical Faculty of Maryland to take measures tending to diminish the blindness in our city and state. About *one-third of the blind* in our Blind

Asylums have lost their sight through a disease which is common among the newly-born. This *fearful disease* which causes so much suffering and unhappiness *can be prevented by proper care. It can nearly always be cured and sight saved if treatment is begun early and kept up.* The disease shows itself by redness and such swelling of the eyelids that the baby cannot open its eyes; the eyes discharge yellow matter. The disease usually begins during the first few days of life. This disease will often cause incurable blindness in forty-eight hours, unless properly treated.

"We ask you to impress upon the mothers you attend *the great danger of delaying treatment.* Do not let them waste valuable time in using breast-milk, chamomile tea, quince water and other home remedies, for *a day lost may rob the infant of its sight.* Insist upon sending the child, as soon as the disease begins, to a physician, or, if the parents are unable to procure one, to a dispensary.

"You can do much towards *preventing* the disease by thoroughly cleansing the child's eyes immediately after it is born. Wash the eyes carefully with fresh, warm water and a piece of perfectly clean soft linen. Do not use water or linen which has been used on other parts of the body, but wash the eyes first of all. You will assist greatly in the important work of diminishing blindness:

"1. By washing the eyes of the newly-born as described above, in order to prevent the disease from attacking them.

"2. By instructing the mothers whom you attend concerning the *importance of watching the eyes closely during the first and second week.*

"3. By calling attention to the *dangers of the disease,* and the *great urgency of prompt medical treatment.*

> "HIRAM WOODS, M. D., *Chairman,*
> "GEORGE H. ROHE, M. D.,
> "J. EDWIN MICHAEL, M. D.,
> "HARRY FRIEDENWALD, M. D.,
> "*Committee.*"

Placards, designed to call the attention of parents to the necessity of watching the eyes of new-born babies now hang in the waiting rooms 'of most of our dispensaries. In the distribution of these placards a few dispensaries were unintentionally overlooked, but they will be supplied. These placards read as follows: "Watch a baby's eyes carefully for a week after birth. If they look red or run matter, take it at once to a doctor. The child may become blind, if not treated properly."

Your Committee believes more than ever that such work as was assigned it a year ago is of great importance. That it belongs indeed to the most important work the Faculty has to do—educating the public in matters pertaining to health. We are just on the threshold of this work, and your Committee respectfully asks to be continued, with the same powers given it last year.

If any physician in the State can make use of these letters and placards in the city or town where he lives, the Committee will gladly supply him. Such co-operation as this is earnestly asked.

Finally, the Committee wishes to thank Dr. James F. McShane, Health Commissioner of Baltimore, for his kindness in mailing the circular letters to the midwives.

Respectfully submitted,

HIRAM WOODS, M. D., *Chairman*,
J. EDWIN MICHAEL, M. D.,
GEORGE H. ROHE, M. D.,
HARRY FRIEDENWALD, M. D.,
Committee.

PRESIDENT'S ADDRESS.

THE ETIOLOGY OF ACUTE LOBAR PNEUMONIA, CONSIDERED FROM A BACTERIOLOGICAL POINT OF VIEW.

By WILLIAM H. WELCH, M. D.

Professor of Pathology, Johns Hopkins University.

MEMBERS OF THE FACULTY:

I had the honor at the last Annual Meeting of this Faculty of addressing you upon the *Causation of Diphtheria*, and I endeavored then to present the results of the bacteriological study of this disease in a manner which might be helpful to the practitioner of medicine. It has seemed to me that it may be acceptable on this occasion to consider *Acute Lobar Pneumonia* from a similar point of view.

Various names have been given to the bacterium which we now believe to be the specific cause of acute lobar pneumonia, such as micrococcus Pasteuri (Sternberg), micrococcus of sputum septicæmia (A. Frænkel), diplococcus or diplobacillus or pneumococcus of Frænkel and Weichselbaum, diplococcus pneumoniæ (Weichselbaum), micrococcus or diplococcus lanceolatus capsulatus (Foà and Bordoni-Uffreduzzi), micrococcus pneumoniæ cruposæ (Sternberg). Of these names micrococcus or diplococcus lanceolatus, diplococcus pneumoniæ and pneumonia coccus or pneumococcus have gained the widest currency and will be used in this article. Perhaps the name micrococcus lanceolatus is the least objectionable. Such names as pneumococcus, micrococcus pneumoniæ cruposæ suggest an exclusive relationship of this organism to croupous pneumonia, whereas this same organism is concerned in the causation of epidemic cerebro-spinal meningitis and many other affections independent of pneumonia.

The micrococcus lanceolatus was discovered by Sternberg in September, 1880, by inoculation of rabbits with his own saliva. It was next found by Pasteur in December, 1880, by inoculating rabbits with the saliva of a child dead of hydrophobia. Pasteur's observations were the first to be made public in January, 1881. Sternberg's first publication on this subject appeared in April, 1881.

At this time there was no suspicion that this micrococcus of the saliva is concerned in the causation of lobar pneumonia.

No little sensation was made by Friedländer's publication in November, 1883, in which he described cultures of a bacterium to which he gave the name pneumococcus. We now know that the so-called pneumococcus of Friedländer is an organism entirely distinct from the micrococcus lanceolatus and is to be regarded as a bacillus. This pneumobacillus of Friedländer is probably in no way concerned in the causation of genuine acute lobar pneumonia in man. Friedländer's method of cultivation in nutrient gelatine at ordinary temperatures precluded his obtaining the genuine pneumonia coccus. The historical importance of this publication of Friedländer, is that he was the first to describe cultures obtained from croupous pneumonia by using Koch's solid nutritive media, that his pneumobacillus was widely accepted until the year 1886 as the specific cause of croupous pneumonia and especially that his results gave an impetus to the further bacteriological study of this disease by modern methods.

For a while there was much confusion of the genuine pneumonia coccus with Friedländer's bacillus. Thus the observations of Talamon in 1883, of Salvioli in 1884 and of Sternberg in 1885, unquestionably pertained to the micrococcus lanceolatus but these writers thought they were working with the pneumococcus which had been described by Friedländer.

This period of confusion was brought to an end by the exhaustive and fundamental researches of A. Frænkel, published in 1886. His articles furnished a full and accurate description of the leading characters of the micrococcus lanceolatus, rendered probable its causal relation to acute lobar pneumonia, separated this organism clearly from the pneumobacillus of Friedländer and recognized its identity with the micrococcus of sputum septicæmia.

Not less important were the independent investigations of Weichselbaum, published in October, 1886, and based upon the study of a much larger number of cases. Foà and Bordoni-Uffreduzzi also deserve mention among the pioneer investigators of this period. In the same year they reported their observation of lanceolate diplococci in the exudate of epidemic cerebro-spinal meningitis. They identified correctly this micro-organism, which they called meningococcus, with Frænkel's pneumonia coccus.

Since these fundamental researches, each year has been rich in contributions to the literature of our subject.

As the name lanceolate coccus implies, the typical form of the pneumonia coccus is oval, with one end somewhat more tapering than the other. It is often compared in shape to the flame of a candle or to a grain of barley. Regularly oval and spherical forms, however, are not uncommon and there may be actual rods or bacilli. The propriety of calling this organism a coccus is open to question. Its typical form is transitional between a coccus and a bacillus. Usage is in favor of calling it a coccus, but some good authorities prefer to regard it as a bacillus.

The arrangement in pairs is so characteristic that this has given origin to the name diplococcus pneumoniæ. Pneumococci not infrequently appear in short chains and, especially in old cultures and when devoid of virulence, they may grow in long and curved chains, regular streptococci.

In fact, there is good reason to believe that the micrococcus lanceolatus belongs to a species presenting varieties which are represented by every transition from single and double cocci to long streptococci and which are endowed with varying degrees of virulence and that some of these varieties are almost constantly present in the mouth. This relation of the pneumococcus, which ordinarily in croupous pneumonia appears as a diplococcus, to streptococci is of much interest in view of the increasing importance attached to primary and especially secondary streptococcus infections. I shall have occasion throughout this article repeatedly to refer to the extraordinarily variable characters of the pneumonia coccus, which render a concise and accurate description of the organism difficult.

The third morphological characteristic of the pneumonia coccus is the presence around it of a clear gelatinous capsule which can be stained with various aniline dyes. The combination of the three traits mentioned suggested the descriptive name diplococcus lanceolatus capsulatus. Capsules are as a rule readily demonstrable only around the cocci growing in the animal body, although they may be present also in cultures.

Degenerating and dead pneumococci, which are very common in old inflammatory exudates caused by this organism, often leave behind them empty or faintly staining capsules.

The micrococcus lanceolatus is not motile. It never forms spores. It stains well with Gram's and Weigert's fibrin stain.

It grows best at temperatures approaching that of the human body. Below 24° C. (75° F.) the growth may cease, but sometimes there is development at as low a temperature as 18° C. (64.4° F.), especially when the organism has been cultivated for some time outside of the body and has lost virulence. Nutrient gelatine, therefore, which melts at 22°-24° C., is not a medium adapted for obtaining first cultures of the pneumococcus, and as already mentioned it was doubtless in consequence of the use of this medium that Friedländer failed to isolate the genuine micrococcus of croupous pneumonia.

The pneumococcus is capable of growing on all of our ordinary culture media but there is no other known organism which will grow on so many media and at the same time is so particular as to the exact composition of the medium. Slight differences in the reaction of the medium, in the quality of the peptone or of the meat used to prepare the medium often determine whether or not growth takes place.

The most suitable and generally employed culture medium for this organism is feebly alkaline nutrient agar or a mixture of agar and gelatine. The growth is usually delicate and grayish in color, but it may be more abundant and opaque. Gelatine is not liquefied. Milk is usually soured and coagulated. No visible growth on potato usually appears. The culture in bouillon may be diffusely cloudy or in the form of a granular sediment. Growth occurs without as well as with the presence of free oxygen.

The variability in the properties of this coccus is manifested not less in its behavior in culture media than in other respects. Decided modifications in cultural characters, particularly as to luxuriance of growth and capacity of development at low temperatures can often be brought about by artificial cultivation. Abundant growth at low temperatures is generally associated with loss of virulence and is often observed in late generations of artificial cultures of primarily virulent pneumococci.

One of the most striking properties of the lanceolate coccus both in the animal body and especially in cultures is its short viability, a property, however, which like most of the others is not without exceptions. The maximum development in cultures at body temperature is attained in twenty-four hours or less. After this there is usually progressive and rapid death of the bacteria so that at the end of four to seven days the cultures are usually dead. Cultures capable of surviving two weeks or more are generally not virulent, but to this rule there are exceptions.

In order to be sure of keeping the cultures alive they should be planted over every day or two. But even this care will not as a rule preserve the virulence of the organism.

After the third or fourth generation it is not uncommon to find marked diminution of virulence and after ten generations, and often sooner, virulence has generally nearly or entirely disappeared. To keep up the virulence of the organism the plan is usually adopted of transmitting it frequently through rabbits, but even this will not always succeed.

This short viability and rapid loss of virulence give to the micrococcus lanceolatus a quite exceptional position among pathogenic bacteria and they constitute an annoying obstacle to systematic experiments with this organism.

The limited duration of life of the lanceolate coccus is a matter of great practical interest. It is capable of longer life in the virulent state in susceptible animals and in human beings than in artificial cultures but it is apt to die even in the living body sooner than most other pathogenic bacteria. Dead pneumococci are found often in large number in empyæmas and in the exudate of croupous pneumonia. This short vitality is doubtless one reason why empyæmas and other local inflammations caused by the lanceolate coccus usually afford a more favorable prognosis than those caused by the longer lived streptococcus pyogenes and why a single aspiration of a pneumococcus empyæma may be followed by a permanent cure. But here as well as with other properties of this peculiar micro-organism it is necessary to keep in mind the frequent exceptions to the rule, instances occurring in which virulent pneumococci are found in empyæmas and other inflammatory exudates at least six months old.

The pneumococcus may suffer a progressive loss of virulence during the course of croupous pneumonia so that at the end of the disease the cocci may be nearly devoid of virulence, but this behavior is not sufficiently constant to establish a rule.

Pneumonia cocci in blood and sputum are in general tolerably resistant to drying, living and retaining their virulence in the dried state sometimes for at least four months, although they may die much sooner. This resistance to desiccation as well as other reasons indicate the propriety of destroying or disinfecting pneumonic sputa.

According to Sternberg the pneumonia coccus is killed by exposure for ten minutes to a temperature of 52° C. (125.6°

F.). The action of sunlight is injurious to this as well as to other bacteria.

Experiments upon animals and observations on human beings prove that the micrococcus lanceolatus is an organism of the most manifold and varied pathogenic possibilities. It is the cause in human beings of a large number of affections formerly regarded as etiologically distinct. Before considering these it is desirable to say something concerning the results obtained by inoculation of animals.

We meet under natural conditions and we can readily obtain by artificial cultivation pneumococci totally devoid of any virulence to animals and at the other extreme we find pneumococci capable of killing rabbits by septicæmia in eighteen hours or less. Between these extremes occur pneumococci of all possible degrees of virulence and capable of causing manifold pathological lesions.

The experimental results vary with the animal, with the number and virulence of the bacteria inoculated and with the site of the inoculation. Rabbits and mice are the most susceptible animals. The principal symptoms which may be observed in rabbits inoculated with virulent pneumococci are fever, diarrhœa, albuminuria and shortly before death convulsive seizures. Pulmonary œdema sometimes accompanies the death agony.

Septicæmia with multiplication of the cocci in the blood is regarded as the leading type of experimental pneumococcus infection of rabbits. With this the rabbit usually dies in one to three or four days. The more common and important lesions are serous, fibrinous or fibrino-purulent exudation around the point of inoculation if this has been subcutaneous, swelling of the spleen, which may be either hard or soft, small, opaque foci of necrosis in the liver, fatty degeneration of the heart, ecchymoses, and sometimes hyaline thrombi in the renal capillaries. Sometimes there is fibrinous inflammation of the peritoneum or other serous membrane. Cocci are usually abundant in the blood but they may be scanty. They are always numerous in recent local exudates.

The attempt has been made to establish distinct biological varieties of the micrococcus lanceolatus on the basis of diverse pathological effects in these septicæmias, especially on the basis of the consistence of the spleen and the character of the exudate at the point of inoculation. But these alleged distinctive characters have not been found to be sufficiently constant to justify a sharp separation into distinct varieties.

A second type of pneumococcus infection in rabbits, not sharply separated from the septicæmic type, is that characterized by spreading, localized, usually multiple fibrino-purulent inflammation without many cocci in the blood. There is evidence that this exudative type depends upon weakened virulence of the cocci. Rabbits affected with this form of the disease live usually four to fifteen days and sometimes longer. Very virulent pneumococci may produce this exudative type in rabbits rendered partly immune from infection. In the majority of cases there are associated with extensive subcutaneous exudation spreading from the site of inoculation, similar fibrino-purulent inflammation of one or more serous membranes and sometimes hepatized pulmonary areas. The spleen is often little or not at all changed. Cocci are usually few in the blood but in enormous numbers in the exudates, in which in the course of time many degenerate and die. The animal becomes emaciated and anæmic, commonly with marked leucocytosis.

Croupous pneumonia in human beings belongs to the exudative rather than to the septicæmic type of pneumococcus infection. Inasmuch as the occurrence of such spreading inflammations with little invasion of the blood by pneumococci is experimentally shown to depend chiefly upon the relation existing between the virulence of the coccus and the resistance of the animal and as we cannot suppose that the pneumococci which cause croupous pneumonia are of weakened virulence, the inference seems warranted that man ranks among those relatively insusceptible to this organism.

A third type of disease caused by subcutaneous inoculation of the diplococcus pneumoniæ is the formation of an abscess at the point of inoculation. This occurrence indicates either still less virulence than in the preceding types or, with the same virulence, greater resistance on the part of the animal. Rabbits which have been rendered sufficiently immune to be protected from septicæmia often acquire a local abscess at the point of inoculation. Under these conditions the micrococcus lanceolatus is an exquisitely pyogenic micro-organism, as it may also be in man. Usually the animal recovers after evacuation of the abscess.

A rare form of experimental pneumococcus disease is pyæmia, with multiple suppurative foci in the joints and other parts of the body.

It is noteworthy that in animals as well as in man the micrococcus lanceolatus is capable of producing not only fibrinous but also genuinely purulent inflammations of the serous membranes.

The efforts to reproduce in animals a form of pneumonia in all respects identical with acute lobar pneumonia as it occurs in man have been only moderately successful. To accomplish this it is evident that the animal must not die of quick septicæmia. Hence these experiments have been made either with virulent cultures on relatively insusceptible animals such as the dog, or with attenuated cultures on rabbits. A few experimenters claim to have produced by intrapulmonary or tracheal inoculations typical lobar fibrinous pneumonias, but the usual result if the organism is sufficiently virulent, is the production of pleurisy and pericarditis with or without circumscribed areas of pulmonary hepatiza-
-tion.

So far as known the domestic animals are not subject to a form of pneumonia etiologically and anatomically identical with croupous pneumonia of man. We do not usually in our experimental tests with pathogenic micro-organisms on animals reproduce the exact counterparts of human diseases nor is it necessary or to be expected that we should do so in order to rest satisfied with our experimental evidence. We possess conclusive experimental proof that the pneumococcus is capable of producing spreading inflammatory exudates with all of the histological and bacteriological characters of the exudate in croupous pneumonia as it occurs in man.

As the micrococcus lanceolatus is the cause of many cases of cerebro-spinal meningitis, (hence the synonym, meningococcus) the attempt has been made by submeningeal inoculation to reproduce this lesion in animals and with occasional success.

Endocarditis which is a very rare result of simple subcutaneous or intravenous inoculation of the pneumococcus can be readily produced by the well known method adapted to cause infectious endocarditis, viz.: by first injuring the valves by means of a sterilized probe passed from the carotid artery into the left ventricle and then injecting the cultures. This is an illustration of the predisposing influence to localized infection of a locus minoris resistentiæ.

Various other special localizations such as arthritis and periarthritis, ostitis and otitis media have been produced by special methods of inoculation, in order to demonstrate the possibility of reproducing in animals similar affections caused by the same organism in human beings.

It is evident from the foregoing review, which is only partial, of the pathogenic effects which may be produced by the micrococcus lanceolatus in animals that we possess a rich mass of experimental data to aid us in explaining the multiform manifestations of infection by this micro-organism in human beings. The pathogenic effects produced are a function on the one hand of the number and virulence of the infecting cocci and on the other hand of the degree of susceptibility of the individual and according to these differences the result is now septicæmia, now single or multiple sero-fibrinous or fibrinous or fibrino-purulent or purulent or hemorrhagic exudations or now a localized abscess.

The transmission of pneumococci from mother to fœtus has been demonstrated both in human beings and in animals. It is interesting to note that in the few hitherto reported observations in human beings in which the pneumococci have been demonstrated in the embryos of mothers affected with croupous pneumonia, there has been no pneumonia in the fœtus although the organisms were present in the blood, whereas in infants congenitally infected who had lived some hours after birth, actual pneumonia has existed. Netter concludes that it is necessary that the child should have breathed in order to acquire localization of pneumococcus infection in the lung. This is an illustration, and there are others in the case of different diseases, of the difference in susceptibility between the embryo and the infant after birth.

To produce intra-uterine infection of the fœtus the pneumococci must of course have circulated in the blood of the mother and have broken through the placental barrier, which as is well known is a perfect physiological filter for inanimate particles. But living micro-organisms are capable of damaging in various ways the placental tissue and opening a passage into the fœtal vessels. Some micro-organisms do this often, others only exceptionally or not at all.

It is probable that the transmission of pneumococci from mother to fœtus is exceptional in the case of human beings. The toxic substances produced by micro-organisms, being soluble, can of course pass much more readily through the placental vessels to the fœtus than the micro-organisms themselves, and these poisons often cause the death of the fœtus. It is well known that pneumonia developing during pregnancy is likely to bring about miscarriage. The same is to be noticed in mice and rabbits inoculated with virulent pneumococci. Neither in human beings nor in animals does abortion necessarily attend pneumococcus infections.

Pneumococci have been found in the milk of rabbits inoculated with the virulent organism and suckling rabbits have been infected by the ingestion of this milk. Pneumococci have been detected also in the milk of women affected with croupous pneumonia. As to the frequency of this occurrence we have not sufficient information.

Evidence is constantly accumulating that pathogenic bacteria do injury chiefly by their toxic chemical products. It was thought at one time that the most important of these poisonous products are crystallizable alkaloidal substances called ptomaines, but it is now known that the toxic products

which produce the more characteristic and specific manifestations of an infectious disease are of an entirely different
nature. These more specific poisons are believed for the
most part to be proteids and are called toxalbumins or toxic
proteids. We know very little of their chemical constitution
and identify them chiefly by their biological effects.
They have not been separated in a state of purity but are
contained usually in albuminous precipitates. They are
formed both in the body of the infected animal and in cultures,
often more abundantly in the former. In fact with some
pathogenic bacteria which give evidence of the formation of
toxins in the infected body, there has been difficulty in
demonstrating poisonous substances in cultures.

The most powerful toxic bacterial proteids are produced
by the bacilli of diphtheria and of tetanus which multiply as
a rule only or chiefly locally near the point of entrance. In
the experimental septicæmic infections, such as may be
caused by the pneumococcus, where there are abundant invasion and multiplication of the bacteria in the circulating
blood, we do not find such concentrated and powerful
poisons as in the more distinctively toxic diseases like
tetanus and diphtheria.

Cultures of the pneumonia coccus as a rule do not contain
in a concentrated form toxic substances. As much as thirty
to forty cubic centimeters of beef broth cultures of virulent
pneumococci, sterilized or deprived by filtration of bacteria,
can sometimes be injected into the circulation of rabbits
without grave symptoms. Cultures concentrated by evap-
oration at low temperature cause death when injected in
smaller quantities. As might be expected with an organism so variable in all of its properties, some cultures are
more poisonous than others, so that much smaller quantities
than those mentioned may cause intoxication.

There is clinical evidence both for human beings and
animals that the pneumococcus may produce toxic substances in the living body. In fact we find in the blood
of rabbits dead of pneumococcus infection, more concentrated toxic substances than we are able to demonstrate in

cultures. The blood of human beings affected with croupous pneumonia is often highly poisonous for rabbits, three to six cubic centimeters of such blood injected into the circulation of rabbits sufficing to cause grave symptoms and even speedy death. This blood may retain its toxic properties for a time after the crisis.

With the exception of the unconfirmed observation of Bonardi no toxic ptomaines have been found in pneumococcus cultures. There have, however, been obtained from cultures and from the blood and tissue juices of animals dead of infection albuminous substances, possessing poisonous properties. It is believed therefore that the specific poison produced by the pneumococcus, as well as the poisons of most pathogenic bacteria, belong to the group of toxic albumins. It has received from the Klemperers the name pneumotoxin. The name is a convenient one but it must not be inferred that it refers to any substance which has hitherto been isolated in a state of chemical purity or which has been demonstrated to be of an albuminous nature.

Grave constitutional symptoms and some of the local lesions of pneumococcus infection are referable to the poisonous substance or substances called pneumotoxin. It is questionable, however, whether this substance is concerned in the production of local inflammatory exudates. These exudates must be caused by bacterial products possessed of powerful positive chemotactic properties, that is, of the power of attracting leucocytes. Experiments indicate that the specific toxalbumins repel rather than attract leucocytes. It is held by Buchner and others that substances called bacterio-proteins, set free from degenerating and dead bacteria, are the chief agents which manifest positive chemotactic properties. This view fits in with the fact that it is especially bacteria of weakened virulence in susceptible individuals or virulent bacteria in more resistant individuals which attract leucocytes and set up local inflammations. There is evidence however, that living and vigorous bacteria may also attract leucocytes so that we cannot accept Buchner's observations as excluding other explanations of the accumulation of inflammatory products, more particularly leucocytes, around bacteria.

Whether we suppose that the positively chemotactic substances are derived from pneumococci already damaged by the living cells and fluids of the body in accordance with Buchner's view, or from still active and thriving pneumococci, there is good reason to believe that these substances are not identical with the toxalbumins which, by their absorption into the circulation, cause the graver constitutional symptoms often observed in croupous pneumonia and other pneumococcus infections. The variability in these clinical manifestations may depend partly on the susceptibility of the patient and partly on the virulence of the pneumococcus. Varying degrees of virulence of a micro-organism are to be interpreted usually as varying capacity to produce toxic substances.

A class of bacterial products of great importance are those which are capable of producing immunity. Rabbits can readily be rendered insusceptible to fatal doses of virulent pneumococci. All of the known principles of producing artificial immunity have been successfully employed in protecting rabbits from the micrococcus lanceolatus. These principles of immunization are:

1. Inoculation of small, not fatal, quantities of virulent cultures of the specific micro-organism causing the disease.

2. Inoculation of the specific micro-organisms partly or wholly attenuated in virulence. The ways by which virulence can be weakened or annulled are various, and consist chiefly in exposure to agencies injurious to bacteria. In the case of the pneumococcus we often meet under natural conditions the organism so weakened in virulence as to serve as a vaccine against the virulent variety.

3. Injection of products of the bacteria causing the disease, either products contained in sterilized cultures or in the germ-free filtrate of cultures or products obtained from the body of an infected individual. These substances may be used when still toxic, or better, as a rule, after diminution or removal of their toxicity by heat, mixture with chemical

antiseptics or other means. This class constitutes the so-called chemical vaccines in distinction from the living vaccines just described.

4. Injection of the blood serum or other fluids from animals artificially rendered immune from the disease. This method is different in principle from the first three, and the resulting immunity presents important peculiarities. As this immune serum possesses also curative properties, it is called curative or healing serum.

Inasmuch as it is by their chemical products that bacteria confer immunity, as well as cause disease, the distinction which appears in the preceding classification between living vaccines and chemical vaccines is not so fundamental as at first glance it might appear.

The immunizing bacterial products are believed to be proteids, and especially of the class derived from the bacterial cells, but we recognize them by their physiological properties rather than by any known chemical tests. The relation in which they stand to the toxic proteids is not definitely known. Inasmuch as the vaccinating power of sterilized or filtered cultures deprived partly of toxicity by heat or by other means is greater than that of the unaltered toxic products, it is held that the immunity-conferring products are either distinct from the toxic products or are derived from them.

When we introduce vaccinating substances, belonging to the first three methods just described, immunity does not ensue at once, but there is a period of reaction, often severe, with fever, local inflammation and other symptoms, which precedes the establishment of immunity. In the case of the pneumococcus this period of reaction lasts three or four days after intravenous injection and about two or three weeks after subcutaneous injection. The resulting immunity may be augmented by repeated successive injections of vaccines of increasing strength and finally of increasing quantities of the virulent organism. In this way rabbits may be protected against subsequent inoculation with several times the fatal dose of virulent pneumococci. Such very high degrees of immunity as have been secured from tetanus by vaccination, have not, however, been obtained from pneumococcus infection.   The immunity may last at least two years, but usually disappears sooner.

The protection which is afforded by injecting the blood serum of an animal already rendered by vaccination or by recovery from the disease immune from the pneumococcus rests upon a different principle from that afforded by vaccination with the living micro-organism or its products.   By the former method we inject a fluid which is already endowed with properties upon which immunity depends, whereas by the latter methods these properties must be developed before immunity is established. . In using immune serum we simply transfer a part of the immunity possessed by one animal to another, or at least we introduce substances which quickly bring about that change in the body upon which immunity depends.   Hence this is called passive immunity, in distinction from the active immunity induced by vaccination. Passive immunity appears at once or within a few hours after the injection of immune serum, and is not preceded or attended by any noteworthy reaction.   To compensate for this speedy and safe development, passive immunity lasts a shorter time than active immunity, and is in direct proportion to the quantity of immune serum introduced and the degree of immunity possessed by the animal from which the serum is derived.   It is only a fraction of the immunity of the animal yielding the serum.

Acquired immunity is the result of a specific reaction of the living body, which in the case of the pneumococcus can be produced only by the direct or indirect products of this organism.*   Hence when we find that the blood and fluids of persons recently convalescent from pneumonia is capable of protecting rabbits from infection with the pneumococcus, and that this property is absent from the blood before an attack of pneumonia, we feel justified in inferring that the pneumococcus has been operative in the causation of the pneumonia.

---

*To this general statement an exception must be admitted if Bonome's assertion be confirmed that rabbits may be protected from the pneumococcus by the sterile filtrate of cultures of the bacterium of rabbit septicæmia.

Different explanations of artificial immunity from pneumococcus infection have been offered. One theory is that the blood and fluids of the immune individual have acquired the power of destroying the specific poison or pneumotoxin. A second theory is that the blood and fluids exert a direct germicidal action on the pneumococci. A third theory is that the leucocytes and other cells act as phagocytes and eat up the bacteria.

The first or antitoxic theory is advocated especially by the Klemperers. According to this view immunity from pneumococcus infection depends upon the same principle as has been proven for immunity from tetanus and diphtheria. The substance in the blood and fluids which acts as a direct antidote to the specific bacterial poison is called antitoxin, in the present case anti-pneumotoxin. The Klemperers explain the crisis of pneumonia by the sudden or critical production of the antitoxin. As soon as the poisonous weapons of bacteria are destroyed, these organisms, even if they survive for a time, are reduced to the level of ordinary saprophytes, and are as incapable of doing harm as a venomous snake is after extraction of its poison fangs.

The observations upon which the Klemperers base their fascinating theory, are opposed by those of several other investigators, and we cannot by any means consider the antitoxic theory of immunity from pneumococcus infection as proven.

Nor are the results of different experimenters regarding the second and third theories in accord. As might be predicted, Metchnikoff and his students find abundant evidence for the phagocytic theory of acquired immunity from the pneumococcus as from all other infections. As with immunity from many other infectious diseases, it cannot be said that we possess at present any thoroughly demonstrated explanation of the basis of immunity from this organism.

A most important characteristic of the blood serum and some other fluids from animals or human beings who have recently acquired immunity from pneumococcus infection is that they are capable not only of protecting a susceptible animal from subsequent inoculation with the organism, but also of protecting after such inoculation. This is the so-called healing property which, in some degree, belongs to the blood and fluids in most cases of solid acquired immunity from infectious bacteria. Protection after reception of the virus, however, is by no means so simple a matter as mere immunization before reception.

When the immune serum is introduced soon after the inoculation with the virulent organism, it must be given in larger quantity than is required a few hours before inoculation. With each succeeding hour the difficulty of conferring protection increases, and as soon as the symptoms have appeared only large doses of serum of high immunizing power offer chance of recovery. In rapidly fatal pneumococcus infections, soon after the onset of the symptoms it is no longer possible to rescue the animal. With slower infections cure has been effected when treatment has begun twentyfour hours after the appearance of the first symptoms.

It is well to have clearly in mind the factors which, according to our present knowledge, control the results of this so-called blood-serum therapy. These factors relate to the dose, the immunizing power of the serum used, and the stage and intensity of the disease when treatment is begun. The larger the animal the greater must be the dose, and in the case of tetanus, where the principles of serum therapy have been worked out more fully than for any other disease, the dose is in approximately direct ratio to the weight of the individual. With serum, therefore, of only moderate immunizing power, the quantity required to protect a large animal or man may be so great that its introduction would amount to a transfusion of blood, or might exceed any amount which could be injected. It is of the first importance, therefore, to secure the highest possible degree of immunity in the animal yielding the serum, or else to find some way of obtaining the healing substance in a concentrated form. So far as pneumonia is concerned, neither of these conditions has been fulfilled to an extent analogous to that for tetanus and diphtheria. In fact we do not possess any such satisfactory experimental basis for the adoption of serum therapy in the treatment of human pneumonia, as we do in the case of tetanus, and it is desirable that laboratory work should supply this basis in the case of an infectious disease, before the general introduction of this principle of treatment for that disease. It is entirely comprehensible from what we know as to the nature of passive immunity and the properties of immune serum, upon which blood-serum therapy depends, that there may be no difficulty in obtaining by this method powerful therapeutic effects in small animals, such as mice and rabbits, and yet we may not be able to attain with the same serum any curative effect in a large animal or man. A person may possess blood and fluids of sufficient immunizing power to protect himself and still not furnish serum of sufficient power to cure another person. It remains yet to be demonstrated by a process such as is successful for tetanus, or by any other process, that animals may be rendered so highly immune from pneumo-coccus infections as to furnish serum curative for human pneumonia.

Whether or not human beings who have recently recovered from an attack of pneumonia or in other ways have acquired immunity from the pneumococcus may yield serum of suffi-ciently high immunizing power to exert a curative influence in human pneumonia, cannot at present be positively stated. Some observations indicate that the injection of serum obtained under these circumstances may influence favorably the course of the disease, but it does not appear that any such constant and specific therapeutic effects have been attained as to justify sanguine hopes that by this procedure with its present possibilities the treatment of pneumonia is to be revolutionized.

The immunity in man following an attack of pneumonia appears to be variable both in degree and in duration. How long it may last we cannot say, but repeated attacks of this disease are common. In fact it has been held that one attack increases susceptibility to subsequent attacks. These facts would suggest that the protection temporarily afforded by a single attack of pneumonia is not due to the production of a very large amount of immunity substance, but we know too little of the real conditions on which immunity from this disease depends and as to the conditions determining duration of immunity to establish such an inference.

The practical difficulties in the way of obtaining, preserving and applying healing serum are sufficiently obvious to require no especial comment. Inasmuch as the blood of pneumonic patients at and soon after the crisis may, as I have found by experiments on rabbits, possess marked toxic properties, the use of such blood serum cannot be said to be free from possibilities of danger.

The future may succeed in surmounting difficulties which are now apparent. With a clearer understanding of the basis of immunity from the pneumococcus means may be found to heighten this immunity. Methods may be discovered by which curative substances may be separated in a more concentrated, permanent and easily handled form, than that in the original serum of immune individuals.

The present outlook for the successful employment of the direct chemical products of bacteria and more particularly of the active vaccinating products, in the treatment of acute infectious diseases is not promising. Inasmuch as it is by such actively immunizing products that immunity is under natural conditions acquired from an infectious disease, and as we have reason to believe that natural recovery consists essentially in the development of this immune condition, it did not seem unreasonable to hope that the injection of such vaccinating bacterial products might exert a curative influence. It was soon observed, however, that the immediate effect of such injection, corresponding to the period of reaction before establishment of immunity, is often distinctly unfavorable and is attended with increased susceptibility to the micro-organism yielding the products.

Whether this unfavorable influence may be checked by further purification of the vaccinating products and removal of toxic substances is not at present clear. Some experiments, especially with the pneumococcus, seem to indicate such a possibility, but it cannot be said that we have yet succeeded in wholly separating the protective from the toxic properties of bacterial products and it may be that retention of some toxic property is essential for the production of immunity.

A further obstacle to the successful application of these vaccinating substances to the treatment of infections, is that unlike the healing serum they require an interval of time, often of days, before insusceptibility to the disease is manifested and hence they cannot be expected to do any good in rapidly fatal infections. By concentration of the vaccinating fluids this interval may be shortened, and in this way Klemperer has succeeded in curing slow pneumococcus infection of moderate severity in rabbits. At the present moment however, hopes of finding specific curative agents rest in healing serum rather than in cultural bacterial products. We are in the midst of a period of active experimentation revealing new and unexpected facts and points of view concerning this whole subject, and it would be hazardous to pass any verdict at the present moment.

We have now passed in review the more important facts concerning the known morphological and biological properties of the diplococcus pneumoniæ. It now remains to consider the observations relating to the presence and effects of this interesting micro-organism in human beings.

That the diplococcus pneumoniæ is the specific cause of at least the great majority of cases of acute lobar pneumonia is no longer open to dispute. This organism is present regularly and in large number in the pulmonary exudate of this disease, and also in most of the complicating inflammations, such as pleurisy, pericarditis and meningitis. In the majority of cases it is the only bacterial species present. The pathogenic effects obtained by inoculation of its cultures in animals, form an important link in the chain of evidence. The proof is clinched by the demonstration in the bodies of those affected with or convalescent from croupous pneumonia of specific toxic and immunizing proteids, which, so far as known, can be produced only through the activities of the pneumococcus.

The only point in this connection which can be considered at all unsettled, is whether this organism is the specific cause of all cases of genuine acute lobar pneumonia. The pioneer investigators of this subject, A. Frænkel and Weichselbaum, expressed opposite opinions on this point, Frænkel believing that the pneumococcus is the sole cause of lobar pneumonia, and Weichselbaum contending that it is the most common and important cause, but that in some cases other organisms play the causal role.

The number of competent bacteriologists—and this question is purely a bacteriological one—who hold to Weichselbaum's eclectic view is much smaller now than formerly, and is decreasing w th advance in our knowledge of the peculiar properties of the micrococcus lanceolatus.

Failures to find this organism in the affected lung in cases of croupous pneumonia date for the most part from a period in which all of the requirements necessary to establish its absence were not completely understood. Ordinarily there is no particular difficulty in demonstrating the presence of the pneumococcus in croupous pneumonia by microscopical examination, by culture and by inoculation of mice and rabbits with a bit of the hepatized lung. But it may happen that one or two of these procedures give a negative result, when the other succeeds. Therefore when all three methods have not been employed, a negative result of the bacteriological examination is not conclusive. At the time of the examination it may be that most of the cocci are dead or incapable of development in our cultures. This is particularly common in old metapneumonic empyæmas.

From what has already been said regarding the assumption by pneumococci of the form of streptococci, it is probable that some investigators have described under the latter name in cases of croupous pneumonia forms of the pneumococcus.

It is not very uncommon to find associated with the pneumococcus in croupous pneumonia other bacteria, particularly the pyogenic staphylococci and streptococci, and less frequently Friedländer's pneumo-bacillus. The co-existence of these other bacteria, although it may influence the course and character of the disease, cannot of course detract from the etiological primacy of the pneumococcus.

It will be remembered that the micrococcus lanceolatus was first discovered by Sternberg and by Pasteur in the human saliva, and hence it received the name of micrococcus of sputum septicæmia, as the injection of saliva containing virulent lanceolate cocci causes septicæmia in rabbits and mice. The pneumococcus is a frequent inhabitant of the mouth in health, occurring in the virulent state in this situation in fifteen to twenty per cent. of healthy adults. It is even more common in the mouths of those who have recovered from pneumonia. According to Netter it is to be found in sixty-six per cent. of such persons. It is less common in the mouths of children, the estimates varying from five to fifteen per cent.

If we include pneumococci with little or no virulence, the percentage of cases in which it is present in the mouths of healthy persons is much greater. In fact Kruse and Pansini bring good evidence to show that the pneumococcus, or some of its varieties, with or without virulence, is a regular inhabitant of the mouth.

The diplococcus pneumoniæ is present regularly in the expectoration of acute lobar pneumonia, but its presence is deprived of diagnostic value by the facts just stated.

The presence of the pneumococcus in the mouth in health is not an argument against the pathogenic powers of this organism in man. We have several other examples of the frequent presence of undoubtedly infectious bacteria in the mouth, intestinal canal and other exposed situations in the human body in health. Indeed the existence of the pneumococcus in healthy persons is a help, rather than a hindrance, to our understanding of the etiology of pneumonia. It permits, even compels, us to give due weight to all of the so called predisposing, secondary or accessory causes of this disease, causes often so manifestly operative that they may seem to be, as they were once believed to be, the efficient causes.

Pneumonia is one of those infectious diseases in which predisposition is an important etiological factor. In what way such predisposing or secondary causes as exposure to cold, season, climate, pre-existing disease, alcoholism, old age, injuries to the chest, act in favoring the onset of pneumonia, we do not know. We can imagine that some may enhance the virulence of the pneumococcus, or facilitate its ingress to the deeper air passages, or render the pulmonary tissues less resistant to its invasion and multiplication, or weaken the general insusceptibility of the system. But with our present imperfect knowledge it is not profitable on this occasion to discuss these speculations. Certain diseases, notably measles and perhaps influenza, have been found to be associated with exaltation of virulence of the pneumococci contained in the mouth. We cannot say how often infection resulting in pneumonia is due to pneumococci received from without, as would seem to be the case in some instances of epidemic and contagious pneumonia, or to pneumococci already present in the body.

The distribution of the specific micrococci in cases of croupous pneumonia is subject to considerable variation. In most cases the number of diplococci in the affected part of the lung is large. Living pneumococci are particularly abundant at the margin of an advancing pneumonia, which is evidence that they are not merely secondary settlers in a soil already prepared for them by pre-existing disease. They are often contained within leucocytes.

Pneumococci are generally numerous in the fibrinous pseudo-membrane on the pleura, which accompanies all croupous pneumonias reaching the surface of the lung. They are usually present in the bronchial lymph glands.

In the majority of cases the cocci are not abundant in the circulating blood. The larger the quantity of blood used for inoculating culture media or animals, the greater the chances are of demonstrating the presence of pneumococci. It is probable that in most, if not all, cases a certain number of cocci get into the blood, but it may be in such small number or for such short sojourn that their presence will readily escape detection.

Sometimes the number of cocci found after death in the blood in the heart and vessels is large, exceptionally as large as in pneumococcus septicæmia of the rabbit. Often, although not invariably, this extensive invasion and reproduction of the cocci in the blood corresponds to the so-called asthenic or typhoid pneumonias.

Inasmuch as the pneumococci are not infrequently carried by the circulation in cases of croupous pneumonia, it is not surprising to find them in distant organs, as the spleen, kidneys, liver, joints, bone marrow, brain and meninges. In these situations they may be present without doing demonstrable injury, or they may multiply and cause lesions. It is not rare to find the specific cocci in the intestinal canal, and they may penetrate the bile.

It is a noteworthy fact that the complications of croupous pneumonia, in contradistinction to those of typhoid fever and many other diseases, are, in the majority of instances, referable to the same micro-organism which causes the primary disease. Our consideration of the manifold pathogenic possibilities of this variable organism has prepared us for this fact. Complicating pleurisy, pericarditis, meningitis, peritonitis, endocarditis, nephritis, enteritis, parotitis, arthritis may all be due to special secondary localizations of the pneumococcus. In fact each of these and many other local inflammations may be caused by the same organism, independently of the existence of croupous pneumonia as either a primary or secondary affection.

This general rule as to the etiology of complications of pneumonia is subject to many exceptions. As in typhoid fever, scarlatina, diphtheria, tuberculosis, pyogenic staphylococci and streptococci, may find the way open in pneumonia for their entrance and multiplication within the body, and these secondary invaders may cause various local inflammations and septicæmia.

The occurrence of abscess of the lung as a complication or sequel of pneumonia is usually the result of secondary infection with pyogenic cocci. In gangrene of course the putrefactive bacilli are present.

It is interesting to consider what lesions are attributable to the actual presence and multiplication of the pneumococci and what to the absorption of soluble chemical products into the general circulation. In all acute exudative inflammations the cocci are present in the exudate. The diffuse fatty and parenchymatous degenerations are due to the absorption of chemical products. There are probably few at the present day who any longer attribute these degenerations in pneumonia to high temperature. There is evidence that swelling of the spleen, which is common, although not constant, in pneumonia is also due rather to the action of absorbed chemical products than to the actual presence of the microorganism in this organ. Focal necrotic lesions of the liver, such as are extremely common in pneumococcus infections of the rabbit, I have occasionally met with in the human liver in pneumonia. I have experimental evidence that the toxic chemical products of the pneumococcus are capable of producing these focal necroses. To the action of the products of the pneumococcus we can attribute the increase of the fibrin factors in the blood, which characterizes many cases of pneumonia.

The decision as to the relative influence of the actual presence of the pneumococcus, or of the action of its absorbed products in causing the renal complications of pneumonia, is not at present altogether clear. Pneumococci are more frequently, in my experience, to be found in the kidneys in cases of croupous pneumonia than in any other extra-thoracic organ. Faulhaber, who has carefully studied this question, thinks that it is improbable that the purely parenchymatous changes, such as desquamation, cloudy swelling, fatty degeneration and necrosis of epithelium, the hyaline degeneration of vessels and the formation of casts are referable directly to the bacteria. These changes are more probably attributable to bacterial products. On the other hand he considers that the inflammatory alterations, particularly the exudation of white and red corpuscles and of fluids and the interstitial infiltration with small round cells are probably directly dependent upon the presence of bacteria in the kidney. Inasmuch, however, as it is possible to produce experimentally by the chemical products the enumerated inflammatory changes, there is no strict proof that these also may not be due to bacterial toxic products. In other words, I think it probable that all of the lesions of an acute diffuse nephritis may be caused by toxic substances, without the necessary presence of bacteria.

Pneumococci have been found only exceptionally in the urine of pneumonic patients.

It has been shown by experiments upon animals that the injection of bacteria or their products into the circulation causes primarily a diminution in the number of leucocytes in the circulating blood. In rapidly fatal infections this diminution is often extreme, and may continue until death. If recovery takes place there is an increase in leucocytes, often considerably beyond the normal. In infections of protracted course there is no general law, often a notable oscillation in the number of leucocytes being observed within short intervals. If the infection is characterized by local inflammatory exudation, there is leucocytosis, proportionate within limits to the extent and character of the inflammation. This leucocytosis is attributed to the absorption by the blood of positively chemotactic substances, such as we know to be frequently formed by bacteria, but it cannot be said that this explanation of leucocytosis is proven beyond question. In accordance with these experimental observations we find that leucocytosis, in greater or less degree, is commonly present in pneumonia. The absence or disappearance of leucocytosis in this disease is an unfavorable prognostic sign.

The pneumococcus has been demonstrated to be the specific cause of all the varying types of genuine acute lobar pneumonia, the sthenic, the asthenic, the bilious, the typhoid, the alcoholic, the epidemic, etc.

We owe to Jürgensen the distinction between primarily and secondarily asthenic pneumonias. So far as the secondarily asthenic pneumonias are concerned, that is, pneumonias which assume an asthenic type as the result of alcoholism, old age, pre-existing disease or other debilitating influences, it is not necessary to assume any increased virulence on the part of the infecting pneumococci. The greater gravity of the symptoms can be explained by the lessened resistance of the system to the pneumococcus and its poisons.

There is more reason to assume more than ordinary virulence on the part of the pneumococci in primarily asthenic pneumonias, especially in times and places where nearly all who are attacked, including the previously vigorous, acquire the asthenic type. The extraordinary variability in the degree of virulence manifested by the different varieties of the diplococcus pneumoniæ renders this view permissible. Nevertheless, even under these conditions, it is possible that the asthenic type is due to influences, which, acting perhaps upon many persons in a household or community, weaken resistance to the pneumococcus.

Although enlightened physicians have often recognized that the gravity of acute lobar pneumonia cannot be measured by the extent of the pulmonary inflammation, nevertheless it is not uncommon to find writers even at the present day who attribute the principal dangers of the disease to such elements as hyperæmia of the lungs, accumulation of inflammatory products, obstacles to the pulmonary circulation, removal of lung surface from the respiratory function. Indications for treatment are sometimes based chiefly upon this mechanical conception of the disease.

The degree and extent of the pulmonary inflammation afford an index of the severity of the disease much in the same way as high temperature does. They are not the real dangers in the majority of cases, although they are of course not to be ignored as sometimes the direct cause of grave symptoms, and as affording indications for treatment. Both clinical experience and the bacteriological study of this disease support the view that in the majority of cases the grave constitutional manifestations of lobar pneumonia are due to toxic substances circulating in the blood and acting injuriously on the respiratory centres and other parts of the nervous system, on the heart, the kidneys and other parts.

There are indeed reasons which lead us to think that local inflammatory exudations in infectious diseases may subserve a useful, conservative, protective purpose. We cannot regard the inflammatory exudate in pneumonia as *per se* a good thing, but it may be the most desirable occurrence possible under the circumstances of the invasion of virulent pneumococci into the lungs of susceptible persons. Experiments upon animals show that it is just those infections with the pneumococcus which are unattended by marked inflammation at the point of entrance which run a rapidly fatal course, and that there is often a direct relation between the development of local inflammation and the severity of the disease in the sense indicated.

Even if it were within our power to arrest the hyperæmia and exudation of leucocytes and other products of inflammation, we should confer a very doubtful benefit upon the patient, unless at the same time we injured the bacteria. It is very likely that in so doing we should rob nature of a weapon which she is using as efficaciously as possible against these invading micro-organisms. It is doubtless often a fortunate thing for the patient that it is not within the power of the physician to accomplish what he considers to be indicated in the way of treatment.

Rules for the Government of the Library.

Adopted May 9th and 12th, 1892.

I. The Librarian or Assistant Librarian shall attend at the Library Rooms daily except Sunday and legal holidays, from 12 o'clock until 6 o'clock P. M., during which hours only, books and journals may be taken from the Library.

II. Each member of the Faculty, paying the annual dues, shall be entitled to take out at one time, four volumes duodecimo, two volumes octavo, one volume quarto, or one volume folio. This rule may be suspended by the written order of three members of the Library Committee.

III. City members retaining books longer than two *weeks* and county members longer than four weeks, shall be subject to the following *fines* per week, viz: 10 cents for the first week, 20 cents for the second week, 30 cents for the third week, and 10 cents per week for every week thereafter. Such fines shall be appropriated exclusively for the benefit of the Library.

IV. No book shall be delivered to a member unless in person or to his written order. A member receiving a book shall be held responsible for it from the time of its delivery until its return to the Library.

V. A member not returning a book or books, belonging to the Library, within four weeks after the date of receiving them, shall be notified *by the Librarian* that he is incurring a fine ; and if they be not returned within three months, in the absence of satisfactory reasons therefor, the Librarian shall recover them or if they be lost, their value, in behalf of the Faculty ; otherwise, the defaulting member shall forfeit the privileges of the Library, and shall be reported at the next annual convention of the Faculty, by the Library Committee. Should any book be injured or defaced while in the possession of a member, he shall be fined, at the discretion of the Library Committee, or, at his option, may furnish such a copy of the same work as shall be acceptable to the Committee.

VI. If any member, upon returning a book, shall find that there has been no application for it while in his possession, he may take it again for the time allowed in Rule III, but

may not take it out a third time until after the expiration of one week succeeding its return to the Library.   New books may not be taken by members for more than one term of two weeks, until after the expiration of one additional week after their return.

VII.   Members are not entitled to receive books from the Library until all arrearages for fines are paid.   Fines may be remitted or reduced, for just and sufficient reasons, by the Library Committee.

VIII.   The Librarian shall appropriately number and stamp the books, pamphlets and periodicals, and place them in proper order on the shelves.   He shall obtain and keep a correct list of the members paying the annual dues.   He shall record, in a book kept for the purpose, the names of members who receive books from the Library, the titles and sizes of the books, the time of their delivery and of their return.   He shall continue the catalogue of the books, pamphlets, periodicals, etc.; keep an account of all moneys received by him for fines, contributions, sales, etc., which moneys he shall pay into the hands of the Chairman of the Library Committee on the last week day of each month.   He shall report during the last week in March of each year to the Library Committee, a statement of such donations of money or of books as may have been made to the Library, with the names of the donors, as well as of such books, pamphlets, periodicals, or other valuable matter as may have come into the possession of the Library by purchase, exchange, or otherwise.   He shall keep a record of all books, periodicals, etc., upon the subscription list of the Library Committee, shall keep due record of their receipt at the proper time, and shall report to the Library Committee the non-receipt of any when over-due.   He shall keep on file applications for such books as may have been let out of the Library; and may make any suggestions to the Committee he may deem necessary.

IX.   Under no circumstances will members be permitted to remove new books, new journals, or other recently received matter, before such time as the Library Committee shall determine.

X.   Scarce and valuable books, the loss of which it would be difficult to replace, shall not be removed from the Library rooms without the approbation of two members of the Library Committee.

XI.   The Librarian is empowered to sell or exchange duplicate books, journals, etc., upon such terms as may appear advantageous, upon the approval of the Library Committee.

Resolutions, Amendments, &c., affecting the Constitution, from 1885 to 1892, inclusive.

May 16th, 1885, By Dr. J. Edwin Michael. Changing the word *gentlemen* to the word person in Article IV, Sec. 1, of the Constitution and changing phraseology throughout to correspond.

May 16th, 1885, By Dr. E. Cordell. Changing Article IX of the Constitution to read "The Annual Meetings of the Faculty shall be held in the City of Baltimore on the fourth Tuesday in April, or at such date as the Executive Committee, with the concurrence of the President, shall appoint. A Semi-Annual Meeting may be held at such time and place as the Executive Committee may designate."

May 1st, 1886, By Dr. G. Lane Taneyhill. Article VIII, of the Constitution to read, "All resignations must be sent to the Corresponding Secretary, and can be accepted only by the Faculty, at any meeting except a memorial meeting."

May 1st, 1886, By Dr. G. Lane Taneyhill. "That the Corresponding Secretary, in giving notice of an Annual Meeting, shall do so at least two weeks before the date of such meeting."

April 29th, 1887, By Dr. John R. Quinan. Article III, Section 5 of the Constitution to read as follows between the words "referred to them" and "shall present:" He shall notify all members, by circular or otherwise, of the time and place of each meeting, and, if it be an annual one, he shall issue such notice at least two weeks before said Annual Meeting.

April 27th, 1888, By the Secretrry. *Resolved*, That the Treasurer is hereby instructed, annually, until otherwise ordered, to mail on April 1st, a printed statement of indebtedness to all members who are delinquent, stating the year of delinquency, and informing such members that by the Constitution, unless payment be made before the fourth Tuesday of April, they are temporarily deprived of the privileges of the Faculty, among which are voting, eligibility to office, and appointment on Standing Committees, sections, or as delegates to any Convention.

Resolved, That the Treasurer is hereby instructed, annually, until otherwise ordered, to hand up to the presiding officer at the adjournment of the third day's session, a revised list of delinquents, resignations, deaths, and dropped for non-payment of dues of members, in order that the President may be enabled to complete a proper list of appointees for the ensuing year.

April 27th, 1889, By Dr. R. Winslow. Article VI, section 2 of the Constitution so modified as to allow the publication of papers in any medical journal after being read before the Faculty and before the appearance of the "Transactions."

April 27th, 1889, By Dr. Chas. H. Jones, on motion to adopt the report of the Committee on Increasing Membership. "Change Art. X of the Constitution, making dues from city members after the fourth Tuesday in April, 1890, $5.00, and those of county members $2.00. Also change the phraseology of Sec. 1, Art. IV, to read five instead of eight."

April 27th, 1889, By Dr. Randolph Winslow. Change Sec. 2, Art.VI, to allow the publication of papers read before the Faculty elsewhere than in the transactions, provided they have not been read previously before any medical society, and that such publication take place after they have been read before the Faculty.

April 25th, 1890, The following "Rules" offered by Dr. B. B. Browne, Chairman of the Library Committee, were adopted. "City members retaining books longer than two weeks, and county members longer than four weeks, shall be subject to the following fines, per week, viz.: 10 cents for the first week, 20 cents for the second week, 30 cents for the third week, and 20 cents per week for each week thereafter. Such fines shall be appropriated exclusively for the benefit of the Library.

April 24th, 1890, On motion of Dr. B. B. Browne. *Resolved*, That at the Annual Convention, *an executive session* be held on Wednesday, the second day of the Convention, at 8 P. M. That at this meeting the reports of all the Committees shall be read, miscellaneous business shall be considered, and the election of officers take place.

April 29th, 1891, By Dr. J. C. Hemmeter. The *titles* of all reports and papers must be sent to the Recording Secretary *at least one week before* the opening of the meeting at which it is desired to read the paper.

April 29th, 1891, By the Library Committee. *Resolved*, That the sum appropriated by the Faculty for the use of the Library be disbursed to the Chairman of the Library Committee in equal payments, the first to be made on or before May 15th, the second on or before August 15th, the third on or before January 15th, and the fourth on or before April 15th, of each year.

April 27th, 1892, By the Library Committee. *Resolved*, That *one-half* of all the *initiation fees* and *annual dues* be paid to the Library instead of five-eighths of the dues from city and two-thirds of dues from county members, as at present.

April 27th, 1892, By Dr. Hiram Woods. The Chairman of each Section shall select some member of the Faculty to open the discussion upon one of the papers to be read by his Section. He shall send to the Recording Secretary the name of the one selected when he sends the titles of papers to be presented by his Section.

LIST OF PRESIDENTS—1799-1892.

Upton Scott—1799-1801.
Philip Thomas—1801-15.
Ennals Martin—1815-20.
Robert Moore—1820-26.
Robert Goldsborough—1826-36.
Maxwell McDowell—1836-41.
Joel Hopkins—1841-48.
Richard S. Steuert—1848-51.
William W. Handy—1851-52.
Michael S. Baer—1852-53.
John L. Yates—1853-54.
John Fonerden—1854-55.
Jacob Baer—1855-56.
Christopher C. Cox—1856-57.
Joshua I. Cohen—1857-58.
Joel Hopkins—1858-59.
Geo. C. M. Roberts—1859-70.
John R. W. Dunbar—1870-70.
Nathan R. Smith—1870-72.
P. C. Williams—1872-73.
Charles H. Ohr—1873-74.
Henry M. Wilson—1874-75.
John F. Monmonier—1875-76.
Christopher Johnston—1876-77.
Abram B. Arnold—1877-78.
Samuel P. Smith—1878-79.
Samuel C. Chew—1879-80.
H. P. C. Wilson—1880-81.
Frank Donaldson—1881-82.
William M. Kemp—1882-83.
Richard McSherry—1883-84.
Thomas S. Latimer—1884-85.
John R. Quinan—1885-86.
Geo. W. Miltenberger—1886-87.
I. Edmondson Atkinson—1887-88.
John Morris—1888-89.
Aaron Friedenwald—1889-90.
Thomas A. Ashby—1890-91.
Wm. H. Welch—1891-92.
L. McLane Tiffany—1892-93.

ACTIVE MEMBERS.

1892.

Andre, J. Ridgeway, 1132 E. Baltimore Street, Baltimore.
Ankrim, L. F., 4 S. Broadway, Baltimore.
Aronsohn, Abram, 712 N. Eutaw Street, Baltimore.
Ashby, Thos. A., 1125 Madison Avenue, Baltimore.
Atkinson, G. T., Crisfield, Somerset County.
Atkinson, I. E., 605 Cathedral Street, Baltimore.
Anderson, Edw., Rockville, Md.
Archer, Wm. S., Bel Air, Md.
Applegarth, Edw. Carey, 1511 W. Fayette Street, Baltimore.
Anderson, C. L. G., Hagerstown, Md.
Baldwin, Ed. C., 304 N. Exeter Street, Baltimore.
Barnes, Wm. M., 905 N. Stricker Street, Baltimore.
*Baxley, J. B., Jr., 1531 Madison Avenue, Baltimore.
*Bayly, Alex. H., Cambridge, Dorchester County.
Belt, S. J., 314 N. Exeter Street, Baltimore.
Belt, Alfred M., 1010 Cathedral Street, Baltimore.
Benson, B. R., Cockeysville, Baltimore County.
Berkley, Harry J., 1303 Park Avenue, Baltimore.
Bevan, Chas. F., 807 Cathedral Street, Baltimore.
Biedler, H. H., 119 W. Saratoga Street, Baltimore.
Billingslea, M. B., 1206 E. Preston Street, Baltimore.
Birnie, C., Taneytown, Carroll County.
Blaisdell, W. S., 285 N. Exeter Street, Baltimore.
Blake, John D., 602 S. Paca Street, Baltimore.
Blum, Joseph, 641 Columbia Avenue, Baltimore.
Bond, A. K., 311 W. Biddle Street, Baltimore.
Bond, Robert, Brooklyn, Anne Arundel County.
Bond, S. B., 1830 Madison Avenue, Baltimore.
Booker, Wm. D., 851 Park Avenue, Baltimore.
Bosley, James, 1701 Hollins Street, Baltimore.
Bowie, Howard S., 811 N. Eutaw Street, Baltimore.
Branham, J. H., 538 N. Arlington Avenue, Baltimore.
Branham, J. W., 538 N. Arlington Avenue, Baltimore.
Brawner, J. B., Emmittsburg, Frederick County.
Bressler, F. C., 1713 Bank Street, Baltimore.

Brinton, Wilmer, S. W. Cor. Preston and Calvert Streets, Baltimore.
Brisco, Philip, Island Creek, Calvert County.
Bromwell, J. E., Mt. Airy, Carroll County.
Browne, B. B., 1218 Madison Avenue, Baltimore.
Brown, James, 131 W. Lanvale Street, Baltimore.
*Brune, T. Barton, 1815 N. Charles Street, Baltimore.
Buckler, Thos. H., 6 E. Centre Street, Baltimore.
Buddenbohn, C. L., 602 S. Paca Street, Baltimore.
Bolton, John H. 1201 N. Broadway, Baltimore.
Brayshaw, Thos. H., Glen Burnie, Md.
Burch, Wm. B., 509 Hanover Street, Baltimore.
Batchelor, K. B., 708 Madison Avenue, Baltimore.
Bordley, James, Centreville, Md.
Brush, Edw. N., Sheppard Asylum.
Baxley, Henry M., 1531 Madison Avenue, Baltimore.
Benson, Jas. Edw., Cockeysville, Md.
Bishop, E. Tracy, Smithsburg, Md.
Bennett, Jas. B., Broadway & Gough St., Baltimore.
Campbell, Wm. H. H., Owings Mills, Baltimore County.
Canfield, Wm. B., 1010 N. Charles Street, Baltimore.
Carr, M. A. R. F., Cumberland, Allegany County.
Cathell, D. Webster, 1308 N. Charles Street, Baltimore.
Cathell, W. T., 1308 N. Charles Street, Baltimore.
Chabbot, G. H., 1111 E. Preston Street, Baltimore.
Chamberlaine, J. E. M., Easton, Talbot County.
Chambers, John W., 18 W. Franklin Street, Baltimore.
Chancellor, C. W., 103 W. First Street, Baltimore.
Chatard, Ferd. E., Jr., 516 Park Avenue, Baltimore.
Chew, Sam'l C., 215 W. Lanvale Street, Baltimore.
Chisolm, J. J., 112 W. Franklin Street, Baltimore.
Chisolm, F. E., 114 W. Franklin Street, Baltimore.
Christian, J. H., 1801 Madison Avenue, Baltimore.
Chunn, W. P., 1023 Madison Avenue, Baltimore.
Clagett, Jos. E., 108 S. Eutaw Street, Baltimore.
Coffroth, H. J., 924 Madison Avenue, Baltimore.
Conrad, John S., St. Denis P. O., Baltimore County.
Cooke, Theodore, 910 N. Charles Street, Baltimore.
Cooke, Theodore, Jr., 910 N. Charles Street, Baltimore.
Cordell, Eugene F., 2111 Maryland Avenue, Baltimore.
Corse, Geo. F., Gardenville, Baltimore County.
Corse, Wm. D., Gardenville, Baltimore County.
Crouch, J. Frank, 725 Greenmount Avenue, Baltimore.
Craighill, J. M., 1720 N. Charles Street, Baltimore.
Cooper, Jas., 1353 Hull Street, Towson, Md.
Clewell, A. A., 1741 Harford Avenue, Baltimore.
Clarke, W. B., Quarantine Hospital, Port of Baltimore.

Carter, Merville H., 1800 W. Baltimore Street, Baltimore.
Chapman, Pearson, Perryman's, Md.
Craigen, Wm. J., Cumberland, Md.
Crowe, Stephen, 1526 N. Caroline Street, Baltimore.
Dalrymple, A. J., 2006 E. Pratt Street, Baltimore.
Dashiell, N. L., Jr., 700 S. Broadway, Baltimore.
Dausch, Pierre G., 1727 E. Baltimore Street, Baltimore.
Davis, R. G., 1307 N. Caroline Street, Baltimore.
Dickinson, G. E., Upper Fairmount, Charles County.
Dickson, I. N., Reisterstown, Baltimore County.
Dickson, John, 1018 Madison Avenue, Baltimore.
*Donaldson, Frank, 510 Park Avenue, Baltimore.
*Dulin, Alex'r F., 107 W. Monument Street, Baltimore.
 Dwinelle, J. E., 1701 E. Baltimore Street, Baltimore.
DeKraft, S. Chase, Cambridge, Md.
Davis, Pinckney L., 746 Dolphin Street, Baltimore.
Deets, Jas. E., Clarksburg, Md.
Dashiell, Rufus W., Princess Anne, Md.
Downs, C. E. 400 Park Avenue, Baltimore.
Dorsey, Reuben N., St. Denis, Md.
*Eareckson, R. W., Elkridge Landing, Howard County.
Earle, Sam'l T., 1431 Linden Avenue, Baltimore.
Eastman, Lewis M., 772 W. Lexington Street, Baltimore.
Ellis, E. Dorsey, 915 Light Street, Baltimore.
Ellis, R. H. P., 733 W. Fayette Street, Baltimore.
*Evans, Thomas B., 121 Jackson Place, Baltimore.
Eilan, Emanuel W., 1523 E. Baltimore Street, Baltimore.
Elgin, Wm. F., Bethesda, Montgomery County.
Evans, B. D., Morris Plains, N. J.
Eareckson, W. R., Elk Ridge, Md.
Ellis, Chas. E., Elkton, Md.
Etchison, Elishe C., Gaithersburg, Md.
Fiske, John D., 11 S. Gay Street, Baltimore.
Flemming, Geo. A., 928 Madison Avenue, Baltimore.
Fort, Sam'l J., Font Hill, Ellicott City, Howard County.
*Forwood, W. Stump, Darlington, Harford County.
Finney, John T. M., 923 N. Charles Street, Baltimore.
Friedenwald, Aaron, 310 N. Eutaw Street, Baltimore.
Friedenwald, Harry, 922 Madison Avenue, Baltimore.
Friedenwald, Julius, City Hospital, Baltimore.
Fulton, John S., Salisbury, Wicomico County.
Funck, J. W., 1710 W. Fayette Street, Baltimore.
Fawcett, Robert, 550 Mosher Street, Baltimore.
Fincke, F. H., 113 W. Preston Street, Baltimore.
Fore, Jas. H., Bay View.
Frey, Louis F., 2414 Druid Hill Avenue, Baltimore.

Forsythe, Hugn, 1931 Pennsylvania Avenue, Baltimore.
Flexner, Simon, Johns Hopkins Hospital.
Frames, W. W., 115 W. Lombard Street, Baltimore.
Field, P. S., 642 N. Fulton Avenue, Baltimore.
Gardner, Frank B., 424 N. Greene Street, Baltimore.
Gardner, W. S., 410 N. Howard Street, Baltimore.
Gibbons, Jas. E., 835 Edmondson Avenue, Baltimore.
Gibbs, E. C., 440 E. North Avenue, Baltimore.
Giles, A. B., 1340 Aisquith Street, Baltimore.
Gleitsman, J. W., 117 Second Avenue, New York.
Goldsborough, Brice W., Cambridge, Dorchester County.
Goldsmith, Robert H., 647 N. Calhoun Street, Baltimore.
Goodman, H. H.. 410 Hanover Street, Baltimore.
Gorter, N. R., 1 W. Biddle Street, Baltimore.
Graham, Geo. R., 725 Columbia Avenue, Baltimore
Griffith, L. A., Upper Marlboro, Prince George's County.
Grimes, J. H., 2100 Maryland Avenue, Baltimore.
Grove, B. Frank, 1321 E. Biddle Street, Baltimore.
*Gundry, Richard, Catonsville, Baltimore County.
Gwynn, H. B., 724 N. Gilmor Street, Baltimore.
Gambrill, Wm. B., Alberton, Md.
Gage, A. L., 522 N. Broadway, Baltimore.
Gichner, Joseph E., ——, Baltimore.
Geer, Edwin, Park Avenue and McMechin Street, Baltimore.
Green, Wm., 1124 N. Charles Street, Baltimore.
Grempler, A. E. F., 517 Scott Street, Baltimore.
Gaver, W. E., Mt. Airy, Md.
Gombel, Wm., 837 W. Fayette Street, Baltimore.
Gosweiler, A. Von Hoff, 1300 E. Baltimore Street, Baltimore.
Hall, Alice T., 708 N. Howard Street, Baltimore.
Hall, Reverdy M., 1019 Druid Hill Avenue, Baltimore.
Harlan, Herbert, 317 N. Charles Street, Baltimore.
Harris, John C., 773 W. Lexington Street, Baltimore.
Harryman, Harry G., 1512 E. Preston Street, Baltimore.
Hartman, George A., 1121 N. Caroline Street, Baltimore.
Hartman, Jacob H., 5 West Franklin Street, Baltimore.
Hartwell, E. M., Johns Hopkins Hospital, Baltimore.
Heidman, Joel A., 254 Pearl Street, Baltimore.
Hemmeter, John C., 633 W. Lombard Street, Baltimore.
Herman, H. S., State Line, Pa.
Hilgartner, H. L., E. Baltimore Street, Baltimore.
Hill, Chas. G., Arlington, Baltimore County.
Hill, Henry F., 1001 Edmondson Avenue, Baltimore.
Hill, Wm. N., 1438 E. Baltimore Street, Baltimore.
Hines, W. F., Chestertown.
Hocking, Geo. H., Mt. Savage, Allegany County.

Hoen, Adolph G., 713 York Road, Baltimore.
Hogden, Alexander Lewis, 1235 Lafayette Avenue, Baltimore.
Hemmett, S. B., Bowens, Calvert County.
Hopkins, Howard H., New Market, Frederick County.
Hopkinson, B. Merrill, 1524 Park Avenue, Baltimore.
Howard, Wm. T., 804 Madison Avenue, Baltimore.
Humrickhouse, J. W., Hagerstown, Washington County.
Hundley, J. M., 1002 Edmondson Avenue, Baltimore.
Hurd, Henry M., Johns Hopkins Hospital, Baltimore.
Halstead, Wm. S., Madison Avenue and Lanvale Street, Baltimore.
Henkel, Chas. B., Annapolis, Md.
Howard, Wm. Travis, Jr., 804 Madison Avenue, Baltimore.
Howard, Wm. Lee, Calvert Street near Biddle, Baltimore.
Hadel, Albert K., 1143 Park Avenue, Baltimore.
Heyde, Eugene W., Parkton, Md.
Horn, Louis C., 697 Mulberry Street, Baltimore.
Horn, August, 697 Mulberry Street, Baltimore.
Hooper, M. L., 1327 Hanover Street, Baltimore.
Hayden, H. H., City Hospital.
Hyland, H. A., 953 N. Gay Street, Baltimore.
Iglehart, J. D., 1215 Linden Avenue, Baltimore.
Ingle, J. L., 1067 W. Lanvale Street, Baltimore.
Irons, Ed. P , 1835 E. Baltimore Street, Baltimore.
Ireland, David C., 1420 Chase Street, Baltimore.
Jacobs, C. C., Frostburg, Garrett County.
Jacobs, J. K. H., Kennedyville, Kent County.
Jay, John G., 212 W. Franklin Street, Baltimore.
Jenkins, Felix, 400 Cathedral Street, Baltimore.
Johnson, Robt. W., 101 W. Franklin Street, Baltimore.   •
*Johnston, Christopher, 201 W. Franklin Street, Baltimore.
†Johnston, Christopher, Jr., 201 W. Franklin Street, Baltimore.
†Johnston, Sam'l, 204 W. Monument Street, Baltimore.
Jones, C. Hampson, 25 W. Saratoga Street, Baltimore.
Jones, Chas. H., 1083 W. Fayette Street, Baltimore.
Jones, Edwin E., Pennsylvania and Wylie Avenues, Baltimore.
Jones, Wm. J., E. Preston Street, Baltimore.
Jones, A. C., Carpo, Talbot County.
Jones, John J., Frostburg, Md.
Judkins, Eugene H., 314 N. Charles Street, Baltimore.
Keane, S. A. 1520 Druid Hill Avenue, Baltimore.
Kierle, N. G., 1419 W. Lexington Street, Baltimore.
Keller, Josiah G., 222 W. Monument Street, Baltimore.
Kelly, Howard A., 905 N. Charles Street, Baltimore.
Kemp, Wm. F. A., 305 N. Greene Street, Baltimore.
King, J. T., 640 N. Carrollton Avenue, Baltimore.
Knight, Louis W., 414 N. Greene Street, Baltimore.

Kremein, John D., 667 W. Lexington Street, Baltimore.
Kennedy, J. K., Aberdeen, Md.
Krozer, J. J. R., 662 W. Lexington Street, Baltimore.
Kuhn, Anna L., 1435 Light Street, Baltimore.
Kemp, Henry M., 1709 E. Eager Street, Baltimore.
Kennedy, T. D., Annapolis, Md.
Latimer, Thos. S., 103 W. Monument Street, Baltimore.
Lee, Wm., 323 W. Hoffman Street, Baltimore.
Lockwood, W. F., 201 W. Madison Street, Baltimore.
Lumpkin, Thos. M., 640 W. Barre Street, Baltimore.
Leatherman, Marshall E., Mechanicstown, Md.
Lewis, John Latane, Kensington, Montgomery County.
Lewis, Wm. Milton, 1209 Presstman Street, Baltimore.
Lintbicum, Thos. W., Savage, Md.
MacGill, Chas. G. W., Catonsville, Baltimore County.
Mackenzie, Ed. E., 324 W. Biddle Street, Baltimore.
Mackenzie, John N., 205 N. Charles Street, Baltimore.
Magruder, W. E., Olney, Montgomery County.
Mann, A. H., Jr., 934 Madison Avenue, Baltimore.
Mansfield, Arthur, 129 S. Broadway, Baltimore.
Mansfield, R. W., 129 S. Broadway, Baltimore.
Marsh, Wm. H., Solomon's Island, Calvert County.
Mason, A. S., Hagerstown, Washington County.
Martin, H. Newell, 925 St. Paul Street, Baltimore.
Martin, James S., Brookville, Montgomery County.
Maxwell, Wm. S., Still Pond, Kent County.
Martinett, J. F., 1441 N. Gay Street, Baltimore.
McCormic, J. L., 1421 Eutaw Place, Baltimore.
McComas, J. Lee, Oakland, Garrett Co.
McCormick, Thos. P., 1529 Eutaw Place, Baltimore.
McKnew, Wm. R., 1401 Linden Avenue, Baltimore.
McSherry, H. Clinton, 612 N. Howard Street, Baltimore.
Merrick, S. K., 420 W. Biddle Street, Baltimore.
Michael, J. Edwin, 201 W. Franklin Street, Baltimore.
Miller, C. O., 836 N. Eutaw Street, Baltimore.
Miltenberger, Geo. W., 319 W. Monument Street, Baltimore.
Mittnicht, 307 N. Exeter Street, Baltimore.
Monmonier, John F., 824 N. Calvert Street, Baltimore.
Monroe, Wm. R., 1734 Bolton Street, Baltimore.
Moran, Pedro De S., 244 W. Hoffman Street, Baltimore.
Morgan, Wilbur P., 315 W. Monument Street, Baltimore.
Morison, Rob't B., 827 St. Paul Street, Baltimore.
Morris, John, 118 E. Franklin Street, Baltimore.
Mosley, W. E., 614 N. Howard Street, Baltimore.
Moyer, F. G., 4 S. Exeter Street, Baltimore.
Murdoch, Thos. F., 8 W. Read Street, Baltimore.

Murdock, Russell, 410 Cathedral Street, Baltimore.
McShane, Jas. T., 2 S. Patterson Park Avenue, Baltimore.
Micheau, Ellis, 526 S. Sharp Street, Baltimore.
Muncaster, Stuart B., Washington, D. C.
Milliman, Thos. A., 1048 Hopkins Avenue, Baltimore.
McDeritt, Edw. P., 208 Aisquith Street, Baltimore.
Mitchell, Chas. W., 937 Madison Avenue, Baltimore.
Martin, Frank, 859 Park Avenue, Baltimore.
McComas, H. A., Oakland, Garrett Co., Md.
McConachie, A. D., 311 N. Charles Street, Baltimore.
Mace, S. V., Rossville, Baltimore Co., Md.
Macgill, J. Chas., Catonsville, Md.
Meyer, C. H. A., 1019 N. Caroline Street, Baltimore.
Murphy, F. P., 2307 York Road, Baltimore.
Neale, L. Ernest, 319 W. Monument Street, Baltimore.
Nihiser, Wintou M., Keedysville.
Norris, Amanda Taylor, 871 Harlem Avenue, Baltimore.
*Norris, Wm. H., 1300 E. Baltimore Street, Baltimore.
Nolen, Chas. F., 606 N. Charles Street, Baltimore.
O'Donavan, Chas., Jr., 311 E. Read Street, Baltimore.
Ohle, H. C., 1203 W. Fayette Street, Baltimore.
Ohr, Chas. H., Cumberland, Allegany County.
Opie, Thomas, 600 N. Howard Street, Baltimore.
Osler, Wm., 209 W. Monument Street, Baltimore.
O'Donovan, John Henry, 3 E. Read Street, Baltimore.
Page, I. Randolph, 1206 Linden Avenue, Baltimore.
Piper, Jackson, Towson, Baltimore County.
Platt, Walter B., 802 Cathedral Street, Baltimore.
Pole, A. C., 2102 Madison Avenue, Baltimore.
Porter, Alex. Shaw, Lonaconing, Allegany County.
Powell, Alfred H., 212 W. Madison Street, Baltimore.
Preston, Geo. J., 819 N. Charles Street, Baltimore.
Prichard, J. E., 1010 S. Chesapeake Street, Baltimore.
Porter, M. G., Lonaconing, Md.
Price, A. B., Frostburg, Md.
Price, Thos. Carnes, Frostburg, Md.
Pickel, John U., 1312 Ashland Avenue, Baltimore.
Pfeffer, Chas. W., 48 E. Montgomery Street, Baltimore.
Price, A. H., Monkton, Md.
Ragan, O. H. W., Hagerstown, Washington County.
Randolph, R. L., 211 W. Madison Street, Baltimore.
Rasin, Robt. C., 809 N. Eutaw Street, Baltimore.
Reid, E. Miller, 904 N. Fremont Street, Baltimore.
Redding, M. Laura Ewing, 930 Madison Avenue, Baltimore.
Rehberger, John H., 1709 Aliceanna Street, Baltimore.
Reiche, P. H., 906 Gorsuch Avenue, Baltimore.

Reinhard, G. A. Ferd., 220 W. Madison Street, Baltimore.
Rennolds, Hy. T., 2004 St. Paul Street, Baltimore.
Reynolds, Geo. B., 711 N. Calvert Street, Baltimore.
†Rickert, Wm., 1841 Pennsylvania Avenue, Baltimore.
Riley, Charles H., 1113 Madison Avenue, Baltimore.
Robb, Hunter, Johns Hopkins Hospital, Baltimore.
Robinson, J. H., 726 E. Preston Street, Baltimore.
Rohe, George H., Catonsville, Baltimore County.
Rowe, M., Deals Island, Somerset County.
Rusk, G. Glanville, 2000 E. Baltimore Street, Baltimore.
Salzer, Henry, 613 Park Avenue, Baltimore.
Sandrock, W. Christian, Broadway and Chase Streets, Baltimore.
Sanger, Frank D., 712 N. Howard Street, Baltimore.
Saunders, J. B., 819 E. Chase Street, Baltimore.
Sappington, Purnell F., Arlington Avenue, Baltimore County.
Sappington, Thomas, 919 N. Calvert Street, Baltimore.
Schaeffer, E. Mortin, Lexington, Virginia.
Scott, John McP., Hagerstown, Washington County.
Scott, Norman B., Hagerstown, Washington County.
Seldner, Samuel W., 947 N. Caroline Street, Baltimore.
Sellman, W. A. B., 5 E. Biddle Street, Baltimore.
Shaw, W. Rutherford, 10 E. Read Street, Baltimore.
Shippen, Chas. C., 603 N. Charles St., Baltimore.
Skilling, W. Quail, Lonaconing, Allegany County.
Smith, Alan P., 24 W. Franklin Street, Baltimore.
Smith, Nathan R., Mt. Royal Avenue, Baltimore.
Smith, Jos. T., 1010 Madison Avenue, Baltimore.
Spear, J. M., Cumberland, Allegany County.
Spicknall, Jos. T., N. Patterson Park Avenue, Baltimore.
*Steiner, L. H., 1038 N. Eutaw Street, Baltimore.
Steuart, Jas. A., 1611 John Street, Baltimore.
Streett, David, 403 N. Exeter Street, Baltimore.
Swatka, J. B., 1003 N. Broadway, Baltimore.
Stevens, J. A., Oxford, Md.
Shank, Abraham, Clear Spring, Md.
Smith, Edw. A., Francis Street, Baltimore.
Steuart, Cacilino C., 120 W. 23rd Street, Baltimore.
Stonestreet, Jos. H., Barnesville, Md.
Shertzer, A. Trego, 101 W. Preston Street, Baltimore
Schindel, Edwin M., Hagerstown, Md.
Spicer, Hiram L., 855 W. Lombard Street, Baltimore.
Shoemaker, C. R., 403 St. Paul Street, Baltimore.
Simmons, Thos. W., Hagerstown, Md.
Smith, Wm. F., 926 Madison Avenue, Baltimore.
Sherwood, Mary, The Arundel, Baltimore.
Sadtler, C. E., 2100 Druid Hill Avenue, Baltimore.

Smith, F B., Frederick, Md.

Taneyhill, G. Lane, 1103 Madison Avenue, Baltimore.

Teakle, St. Geo. W., 702 Park Avenue, Baltimore.

Theobald, Samuel, 304 W. Monument Street, Baltimore.

Thomas, George, 921 N. Charles Street, Baltimore.

Thomas, Jas. Carey, 1228 Madison Avenue, Baltimore.

Thomas, Hy. B., 1710 Guilford Avenue, Baltimore.

Thomas, Richard H., 236 W. Lanvale Street, Baltimore.

Thompson, W. H., 526 St. Paul Street, Baltimore.

Tiffany, L. McLane, 831 Park Avenue, Baltimore.

Trimble, I. R., 214 W. Franklin Street, Baltimore.

Todd, W. J., Mt. Washington, Baltimore County.

Townsend, W. Guy, 1918 N. Charles Street, Baltimore.

Tall, Reuben J. H., 524 S. Sharp Street, Baltimore.

Thomas, Henry M., 1228 Madison Avenue, Baltimore.

Ulman, Solomon J., 1325 Linden Avenue, Baltimore.

Uhler, John R., 661 W. Fayette Street, Baltimore.

Van Bibber, Claude, 26 W. Franklin Street, Baltimore.

Van Bibber, John, 1014 N. Charles Street, Baltimore.

Van Bibber, W. Chew, 26 W. Franklin Street, Baltimore.

Van Marter, J. G., Jr., Rome, Italy.

Vees, Chas. H., 1210 E. Eager Street, Baltimore.

Virdin, W. W., Lapidum, Harford County.

*Walker, E. R., 1703 N. Charles Street, Baltimore.

Warfield, Mactier, 412 Cathedral Street, Baltimore.

Warfield, R. B., 214 W. Franklin Street, Baltimore.

Waters, Edmund G., 1429 McCulloh Street, Baltimore.

Wattenscheidt, Chas., 2027 Druid Hill Avenue, Baltimore.

Welch, E. Giddings, Park Avenue and Mulberry Street, Baltimore.

Welch, W. H., 506 Cathedral Street, Baltimore.

White, W. W., 1101 N. Broadway, Baltimore.

Whitridge, Wm., 829 N. Charles Street, Baltimore.

Wiegand, Wm. E., 2023 Druid Hill Avenue, Baltimore.

Williams, Arthur, Elkridge Landing, Howard County.

Williams, E. J., 1114 Chesapeake Street, Baltimore.

Williams, John M., Lonaconing, Allegany County.

Williams, J. Whitridge, 900 Madison Avenue, Baltimore.

Williams, Philip C., 900 Madison Avenue, Baltimore.

Wilson, Henry M., 1008 Madison Avenue, Baltimore.

Wilson, H. P. C., 814 Park Avenue, Baltimore.

Wilson, J. Jones, Cumberland, Allegany County.

Wilson, Robert T., 820 Park Avenue, Baltimore.

Wiltshire, Jas. G., 714 N. Howard Street, Baltimore.

Winsey, Whitfield, 1220 E. Fayette Street, Baltimore.

Winslow, John R., 924 McCulloh Street, Baltimore.

Winslow, Randolph, 1 Mt. Royal Terrace, Baltimore.

Winternitz, L. C., 25 S. Eden Street, Baltimore.
Woods, Hiram, Jr., 525 N. Howard Street, Baltimore.
Watson, A. G., 1301 N. Central Avenue, Baltimore.
Willing, J. E., 508 N. Fremont Avenue.
Wagner, A. S., Hebrew Hospital, Baltimore.
Wise, E. M., 706 N. Howard Street, Baltimore.
Winterson, Chas. R., Elk Ridge, Md.
Wilkins, Geo. L., 226 S. Broadway, Baltimore.
Wilson, Lot Ridgeley, 1729 W. Lombard Street, Baltimore.
Worthington, Thos. Chew, 840 W. Fayette Street, Baltimore.
Wootten, Wm. F., Frederick, Md.
Whitehead, Alfred, 330 N. Charles Street, Baltimore.
Warner, A. S., 1120 Highland Avenue, Baltimore.
Wegeforth, Arthur, 805 Aisquith Street, Baltimore.
Williams, Thos. H., Cambridge, Md.
Wissler, C. H., Baltimore and Eden Streets, Baltimore.
Windsor, S. J., Dames Quarter, Somerset Co., Md.
Ziegler, Charles B., 920 N. Broadway, Baltimore.

HONORARY MEMBERS.

Bartholow, Roberts, M. D., Philadelphia, Pa.
Billings, John S., M. D., U. S. A., Washington, D. C.
Chaille, Stanford E., M. D., New Orleans, La.
Dunott, Thomas J., M. D., Harrisburg, Pa.
Goodell, Wm., M. D., Philadelphia, Pa.
Mallet, John W., M. D., University of Virginia.
Mitchell, S. Weir, M. D., Philadelphia, Pa.
Moorman, John J., M. D., Salem, Va.
Pepper, William, M. D , Philadelphia, Pa.
Toner, Joseph M., M. D., Washington, D. C.

DELEGATE MEMBERS.

Gilchrist, T. C., 317 N. Charles Street, Baltimore.
Mittrick, J. H., 406 N. Exeter Street, Baltimore.